Medical Radiology

Diagnostic Imaging

For further volumes:
http://www.springer.com/series/4354

A. Mark Davies • Andrew J. Grainger
Steven J. James
Editors

Imaging of the Hand and Wrist

Techniques and Applications

Springer

Editors
A. Mark Davies
Royal Orthopaedic Hospital
MRI Centre
NHS Foundation Trust
Birmingham
UK

Steven J. James
Royal Orthopaedic Hospital
Birmingham
UK

Andrew J. Grainger
Department of Radiology
Chapel Allerton Hospital
Leeds Teaching Hospitals
Leeds
UK

ISSN 0942-5373
ISBN 978-3-642-42849-4 ISBN 978-3-642-11146-4 (eBook)
DOI 10.1007/978-3-642-11146-4
Springer Heidelberg New York Dordrecht London

Printed on acid-free paper

Springer is part of Springer Science+Business Media (www.springer.com)

Contents

Contributors

Waqar A. Bhatti Consultant in Musculoskeletal and Sports Radiology, University Hospital South Manchester, Manchester, UK, e-mail: Waqar.bhatti@uhsm.nhs.uk

Stefano Bianchi Clinique des Grangettes, Chemin de Grangettes 7, 1224 Geneva, Switzerland; CIM SA Cabinet Imagerie Medicale, Route de Malagnou 40, 1208 Geneva, Switzerland, e-mail: stefanobianchi@bluewin.ch

D. A. Campbell Consultant Hand and Wrist Surgeon, Leeds General Infirmary, Leeds LS1 3EX, UK

R. S. D. Campbell Department of Radiology, Consultant Musculoskeletal Radiologist, Royal Liverpool University Hospital, Liverpool L7 8XP, UK, e-mail: Rob.Campbell@rlbuht.nhs.uk

Jim Carmichael Department of Paediatric Radiology, Guys and Thomas'/Evelina Childrens Hospital, London, UK

Georgios Christopoulos Institut für Diagnostische und Interventionelle Radiologie, Herz- und Gefäss-Klinik GmbH, Salzburger Leite 1, 97616 Bad Neustadt an der Saale, Germany

S. G. Davies Consultant Radiologist, Radiology Department, Royal Glamorgan Hospital, Rhondda Cynon Taf, Llantrisant CF72 8XR, UK, e-mail: Stephen.Davies1@wales.nhs.uk

A. Mark Davies Department of Radiology, Royal Orthopaedic Hospital, Birmingham B31 2AP, UK, e-mail: wendy.turner1@nhs.net

René de Gautard CIM SA Cabinet Imagerie Medicale, Route de Malagnou 40, 1208 Geneva, Switzerland

Milko C. de Jonge Department of Radiology, Academic Medical Center, Amsterdam, The Netherlands; Department of Radiology, Zuwe Hofpoort Ziekenhuis, Woerden, The Netherlands

A. M. De Schepper Department of Radiology, University Hospital Antwerp, Wilrijkstraat, 10, 2650 Edegem, Belgium

Andrew Dunn Department of Radiology, Royal Liverpool University Hospitals NHS trust, Prescot Street, Liverpool L7 8XP, UK

Ignac Fogelman Consultant Physician in Nuclear Medicine, Department of Nuclear Medicine, St Thomas' Hospital Guy's and St Thomas' Hospital NHS Foundation Trust, Lambeth Palace Road, London SE1 7EH, UK

J. L. Gielen Department of Radiology, University Hospital Antwerp, Wilrijkstraat, 10, 2650 Edegem, Belgium

Thierry Glauser CH8, Cabinet de Chirurgie de la Main, Rue Charles Humbert 8, Geneva, Switzerland

Gopinath Gnanasegaran Consultant Physician in Nuclear Medicine, Department of Nuclear Medicine, St Thomas' Hospital Guy's and St Thomas' Hospital NHS Foundation Trust, Lambeth Palace Road, London SE1 7EH, UK, e-mail: gopinath.gnanasegaran@gstt.nhs.uk

Andrew J. Grainger Department of Musculoskeletal Radiology, Chapel Allerton Orthopaedic Centre, Leeds LS7 4SA, UK, e-mail: Andrew.grainger@leedsth.nhs.uk

Giuseppe Guglielmi Department of Radiology, University of Foggia, Viale L. Pinto 1, 71100 Foggia, Italy; Department of Radiology, Hospital "Casa Sollievo della Sofferenza", Viale Cappuccini 1, 71013 San Giovanni Rotondo, Italy, e-mail: g.guglielmi@unifg.it

Greg J. Irwin Consultant Paediatric Radiologist, Diagnostic Imaging, Royal Hospital for Sick Children, Dalnair Street, Glasgow G3 8SJ, Scotland, UK, e-mail: Greg.irwin@ggc.scot.nhs.uk

Steven L. James Department of Radiology, Royal Orthopaedic Hospital, Birmingham B31 2AP, UK

R. Jonges Department of Biomedical Engineering and Physics, Academic Medical Center, Amsterdam, The Netherlands

James J. R. Kirkpatrick Consultant Plastic and Hand Surgeon, Canniesburn Plastic Surgery Unit, Glasgow Royal Infirmary and Royal Hospital for Sick Children, Dalnair Street, Glasgow G3 8SJ, UK

Anand Kirwadi Department of Radiology, Northern General Hospital, Sheffield Teaching Hospitals NHS Foundation Trust, Herries Road, Sheffield S5 7AU, UK, e-mail: anandkirwadi@doctors.org.uk

Nikhil A. Kotnis 77 Elm Street, Toronto, ON M5G 1H4, Canada; Department of Radiology, Royal Orthopaedic Hospital, Birmingham B31 2AP, UK, e-mail: nkotnis@hotmail.com

M. Maas Radiology Room C1-120, Meibergdreef 9, 1105A2 Amsterdam, The Netherlands; Department of Radiology, Academic Medical Center, Amsterdam, The Netherlands, e-mail: m.maas@amc.uva.nl

Stefan Mariacher Chefarzt und stv. Vorsitzender der Klinikleitung, aarReha Schinznach Badstrasse 55P, 5116 Schinznach-Bad, Switzerland

Lucio Molini Struttura Complessa di Radiodiagnostica, Ospedale Galliera, Via Volta, 16128 Genoa, Italy

Nicola J. R. Mulholland Department of Nuclear Medicine and Radiology, Kings College Hospital, London, UK

Silvana Muscarella Department of Radiology, University of Foggia, Viale L. Pinto 1, 71100 Foggia, Italy; Department of Radiology, Hospital "Casa Sollievo della Sofferenza", Viale Cappuccini 1, 71013 San Giovanni Rotondo, Italy

Tishi Ninan Imaging Directorate, Department of Radiology, Plymouth Hospitals NHS Trust, Derriford Road, Crownhill, Devon, PL, PL6 8DH, UK

Lil-Sofie Ording Müller Section for Paediatric Radiology, Oslo University Hospital, HF, Ullevål, Oslo, Norway

Bo Povlsen Department of Orthopedics, Guy's and St Thomas Hospital NHS Foundation Trust, London, UK

Nigel Raby Department of Radiology, Westen Infirmary, Glasgow G11 6NT, UK, e-mail: nigel.raby@ggc.scot.nhs.uk; N.Raby@clinmed.gla.ac.uk

Karen Rosendahl Department of Paediatric Radiology, Haukeland University Hospital and University of Bergen, Bergen, Norway, e-mail: rosenk@gosh.nhs.uk; karen.rosendahl@helse-bergen.no

Emma L. Rowbotham Royal United Hospital, Bath, UK, e-mail: emmarowbotham@doctors.org.uk

Vikram S. Sandhu Imaging Department, Royal Orthopaedic Hospital, Bristol Road South, Birmingham B31 2AP, UK, e-mail: viksandhu@doctors.org.uk

Rainer R. Schmitt Institut für Diagnostische und Interventionelle Radiologie, Herz- und Gefäss-Klinik GmbH, Salzburger Leite 1, 97616 Bad Neustadt an der Saale, Germany, e-mail: schmitt.radiologie@herzchirurgie.de

Marie Claude Schenkel Cabinet de Rhumatologie, Rue de la Faïencerie 6, 1227 Carouge-Geneva, Switzerland

Emily J. Stenhouse Consultant Paediatric Radiologist, Royal Hospital for Sick Children, Dalnair Street, Glasgow G3 8SJ, UK, e-mail: Emily.Stenhouse@ggc.scot.nhs.uk

S. D. Strackee Department of Plastic, Reconstructive and Hand Surgery, Academic Medical Center, Amsterdam, The Netherlands

G. J. Streekstra Department of Biomedical Engineering and Physics, Academic Medical Center, Amsterdam, The Netherlands

Sri Priya Suresh Imaging Directorate, Department of Radiology, Plymouth Hospitals NHS Trust, Derriford Road, Crownhill, Devon, PL6 8DH, UK, e-mail: sureshpriya2000@yahoo.com

Giorgio Tamborrini Rheumaklinik, Universitäts-Spital Zürich, Rämi-Strasse 100, 8091 Zürich, Switzerland

P. Van Dyck Department of Radiology, University Hospital Antwerp, Wilrijkstraat, 10, 2650 Edegem, Belgium

F. M. Vanhoenacker Department of Radiology, University Hospital Antwerp, Wilrijkstraat, 10, 2650 Edegem, Belgium; General Hospital Sint-Maarten Duffel-Mechelen, Rooienberg 25, 2570 Duffel, Belgium, e-mail: filip.vanhoenacker@telenet.be

Radiography and Arthrography

S. G. Davies

Contents

S. G. Davies (✉)
Consultant Radiologist, Radiology Department,
Royal Glamorgan Hospital, Rhondda Cynon Taf,
Llantrisant, CF72 8XR, UK
e-mail: Stephen.Davies1@wales.nhs.uk

Abstract

The main emphasis of this chapter is a description of basic radiography of the wrist and hand with detailed description of radiographic technique and evaluation of the different projections. Static and dynamic carpal instability evaluation is vital for the assessment of ligamentous disruption. These techniques are covered in this chapter. There are a whole variety of measurement techniques which can be used in the assessment of wrist pathology. Following distal radial fracture, radial inclination, radial length and palmar tilt are important. Ulna variance is also assessed following distal radial fracture and in the context of ulnar-sided wrist pain. The scapholunate angle and capitate lunate angle are assessed when intercalated instability is suspected. Finally, the carpal height is a measurement which is applied when there is evidence of carpal collapse or loss of joint space. Arthrography still has a place in the modern assessment of the wrist. Radiocarpal and to a lesser extent midcarpal injection techniques may be employed.

1 Introduction

Plain film radiography has a fundamental role in the evaluation of the hand and wrist following trauma, in cases of suspected arthropathy, as part of an evaluation for certain systemic disorders with hand manifestations and in other miscellaneous situations such as tumour masses and pain.

A. M. Davis et al. (eds.), *Imaging of the Hand and Wrist*, Medical Radiology. Diagnostic Imaging,
DOI: 10.1007/174_2010_136,

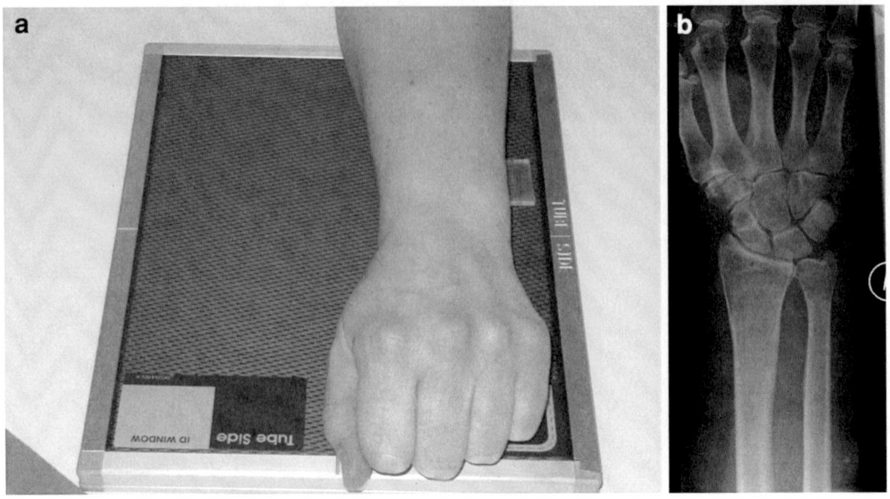

Fig. 1 **a** Patient positioning for posteroanterior (PA) wrist radiograph. **b** PA radiograph of wrist

2 Radiographic Projections

2.1 Radiographic Projections of the Wrist

The standard wrist projections are postero-anterior (PA) and lateral (Whitley 2005). Occasionally an oblique projection is added.

2.1.1 PA and Lateral Projections of the Wrist

Technique

The PA projection is performed with the patient seated. The shoulder is 90° abducted and the elbow is 90° flexed. The forearm is held in a neutral position with the hand flat on the table top. The tabletop should be at the same height as the forearm. The centering point is midway between the radial and ulnar styloid. The field of projection should include the distal half of the radius and ulna extending distantly to include the proximal two-thirds of the metacarpals (Fig. 1).

There are two different methods for obtaining the lateral projection of the wrist. The simplest method is to rotate the hand 90° maintaining the elbow in a flexed position. With this method, the ulna stays in a fixed position and the radius rotates through 90° along with the carpus. The second method involves rotation of both ulna and radius through 90°. This is achieved by extending the elbow and rotating the humerus through 90°. This latter method has the benefit of enabling a second projection at 90° to the first of the ulna. The centering point for both methods is the radial styloid (Fig. 2).

Evaluation

The PA projection of the wrist is useful in the evaluation of injuries to the distal radius and ulna, carpus and proximal metacarpals. It is also helpful in the evaluation of pathology such as erosions to the distal radius and ulna and carpus. The PA wrist should profile the extensor carpi ulnaris tendon groove which should be at the level of, or radial to the base of the ulnar styloid (Fig. 1) (Goldfarb and Yin 2001).

The positioning of the lateral projection of the wrist is evaluated with reference to the palmar cortex of the pisiform (Yang and Mann 1997). A well-positioned and centered lateral projection results in the palmar cortex of the pisiform lying between the palmar cortices of the distal scaphoid and capitate (Fig. 2).

The PA view of the wrist displays the carpal anatomy (Fig. 3). The carpal bones are arranged in proximal and distal rows. The proximal row comprises the scaphoid, lunate and triquetral, whilst the distal row is made up of the trapezium, trapezoid, capitate and hamate. The normal anatomic relationships of the wrist should demonstrate parallel opposing articular surfaces with symmetrical width of all intercarpal joints (Resnik 2000). The articular surfaces of the carpal bones should be normally aligned in three arcs (Fig. 4) (Gilula 1979). Arc I describes the outer proximal convexities of

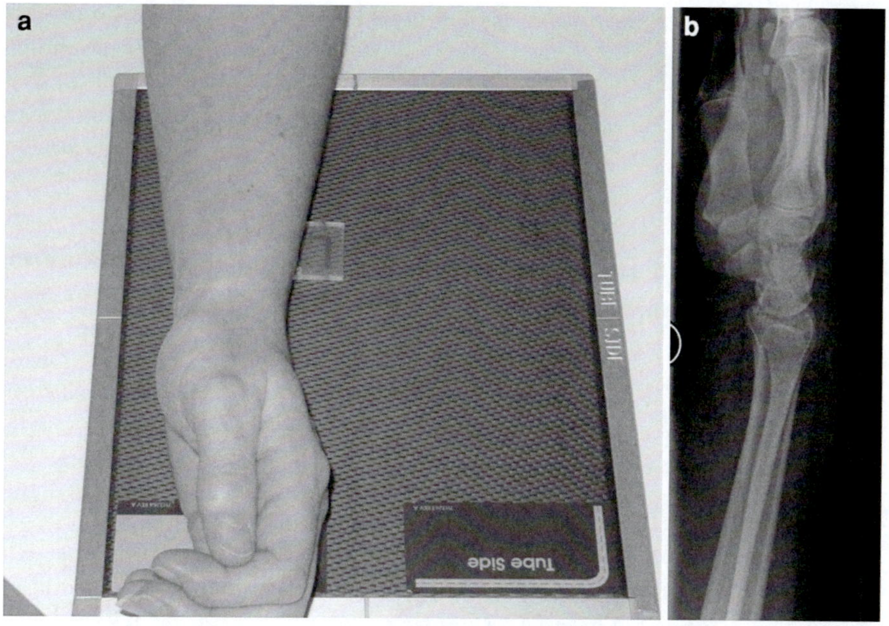

Fig. 2 **a** Patient positioning for lateral wrist radiograph. **b** Lateral radiograph of wrist

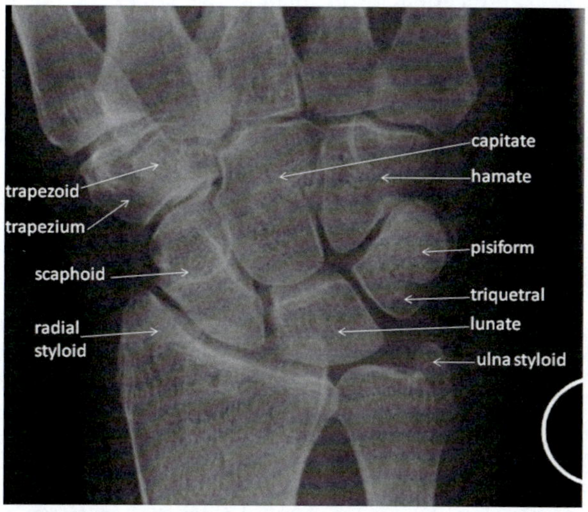

Fig. 3 Carpal anatomy

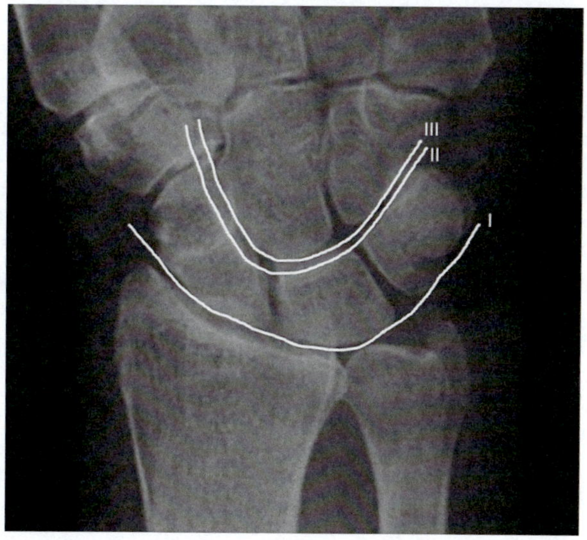

Fig. 4 Carpal arcs

scaphoid, lunate and triquetrum. Arc II describes the distal concavities of the scaphoid lunate and triquetrum. Arc III describes the proximal convexities of the capitate and lunate. For optimal demonstration, the wrist must be imaged PA in the neutral position. Two normal anatomical variants of the arcs are recognized (Loredo and Sorge 2005). The first variant is that the triquetrum may be shorter in its proximal–distal dimension than the adjacent lunate. This gives rise to discontinuity of arc I. The second variant is that the proximal hamate may be unusually prominent and rounded thereby creating discontinuity of arc III. Evaluation of the integrity of the arcs is important when assessing for fractures, dislocations and instability.

An important feature of the lateral wrist is the alignment of the radius, lunate and capitate (Fig. 5). These structures should be within 10° of coaxial alignment (Gilula 1979). It is noted that they are truly co-axial in only 11% of cases.

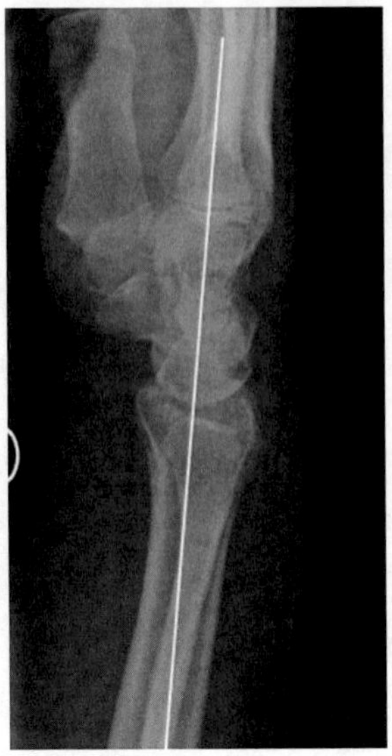

Fig. 5 Lateral wrist demonstrating axis for lateral alignment (not co-axial in this case)

2.2 Radiographic Projections of the Scaphoid Carpus

There are four standard projections for radiography of the scaphoid. They are the AP with ulnar deviation (plus or minus tube angulation), anterior oblique (pronated oblique), posterior oblique (supinated oblique) and lateral. This series is designed to provide tangential projections of the carpal bones with particular emphasis on evaluation of the scaphoid. The prime indication for these projections is the presence of trauma to the carpus particularly if there is associated tenderness in the region of the scaphoid.

2.2.1 AP with Ulnar Deviation

Technique

The patient sits to the side of the table with a flexed elbow and pronated forearm. The elbow and wrist are at the level of the tabletop. The hand is deviated in the ulnar direction (Fig. 6). The purpose of the deviation is to reduce the foreshortening of the scaphoid seen on the standard PA projection. When the wrist is in the normal neutral position the scaphoid is tilted (Gilula 1979). Additionally, the X-ray tube may be angled towards the elbow by 20° (Fig. 7) which further compensates for the normal scaphoid tilt.

The centering point is midway between the ulna and radial styloid processes. The film should include the distal radius and ulna and proximal metacarpals.

Evaluation

The PA projection should produce a good projection of the length of the scaphoid aiming at visualisation of clear joint space around the whole of the scaphoid (Fig. 6). Occasionally, there is some distal overlap. The radial styloid and ulnar styloid should be clearly seen.

2.2.2 Anterior Oblique (Pronated Oblique)

Technique

The wrist is externally rotated from the PA neutral position by 45° (Fig. 8). The radial styloid is, therefore, elevated from the tabletop. The centering point is midway between the ulnar and radial styloid. The fingers may be slightly flexed with the thumb held in front.

Evaluation

This projection (Fig. 8) gives a good demonstration of the distal scaphoid and trapezium. It is also a useful projection for evaluating the trapezoid and bases of the first and second metacarpals. The radial styloid and dorsal surface of the triquetrum is visible. Consideration may be given to applying a degree of ulnar deviation to this projection for better visualisation of the scaphoid.

2.2.3 Posterior Oblique (Supinated Oblique)

Technique

From the anterior oblique the wrist is externally rotated a further 90° (Fig. 9). The fingers are held together. The centering point is the ulnar styloid.

Evaluation

This projection demonstrates the pisiform and the piso-triquetral joint (Fig. 9). It is also useful for evaluating the hook of the hamate and bases of the fourth and fifth metacarpals. The long axis of the scaphoid lies perpendicular to the cassette.

2.2.4 Lateral

Technique

The technique is as described for the standard lateral view of the wrist (Sect. 2.1). However, a narrower field of view is generally used including only the

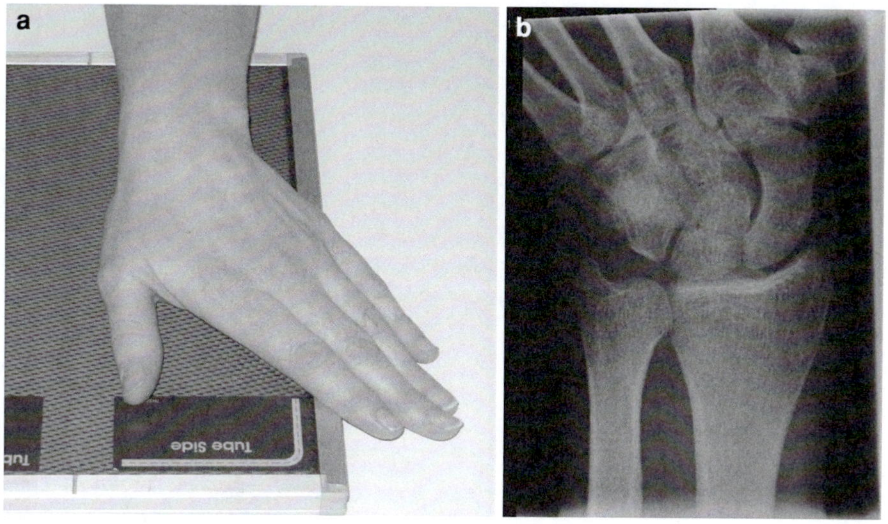

Fig. 6 **a** Patient positioning for AP carpus with ulna deviation. **b** AP radiograph with ulna deviation of carpus

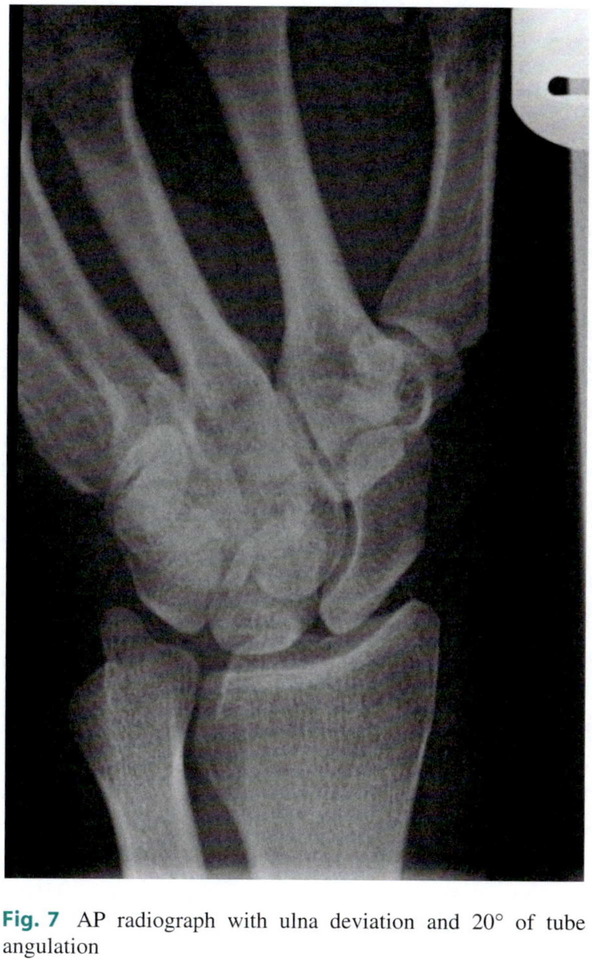

Fig. 7 AP radiograph with ulna deviation and 20° of tube angulation

distal aspect of the radius and ulna and proximal metacarpal bases (Fig. 10).

Evaluation

The lateral projection is particularly valuable in assessing the dorsal surface of distal radius for fracture. This projection enables an evaluation of the alignment of the distal radius, lunate and capitate (Fig. 10). This projection is useful when assessing for dislocation and carpal instability.

2.3 Radiographic Projections of the Hand

There are two standard projections for the hand which are the PA and anterior oblique projections. Supplementary projections include the lateral projection and the posterior oblique projection.

2.3.1 PA Hand

Technique

The forearm is pronated and the hand rests on the cassette (Fig. 11). The ulnar styloid and radial styloid should lie equidistant from the tabletop. The centering point is the third metacarpal head. This projection should include the whole of the fingers (phalanges), metacarpals, carpus together with distal ends of the radius and ulna.

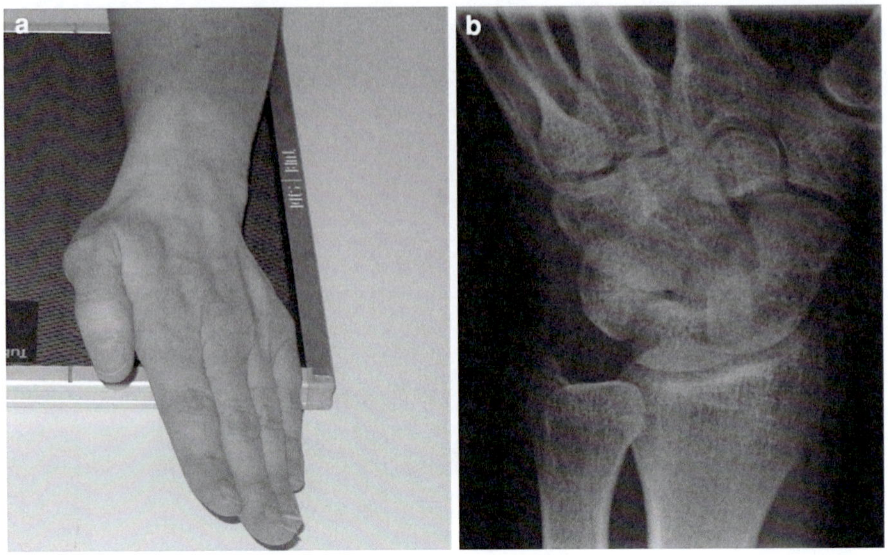

Fig. 8 **a** Patient positioning for anterior oblique of the carpus. **b** Anterior oblique radiograph of the carpus

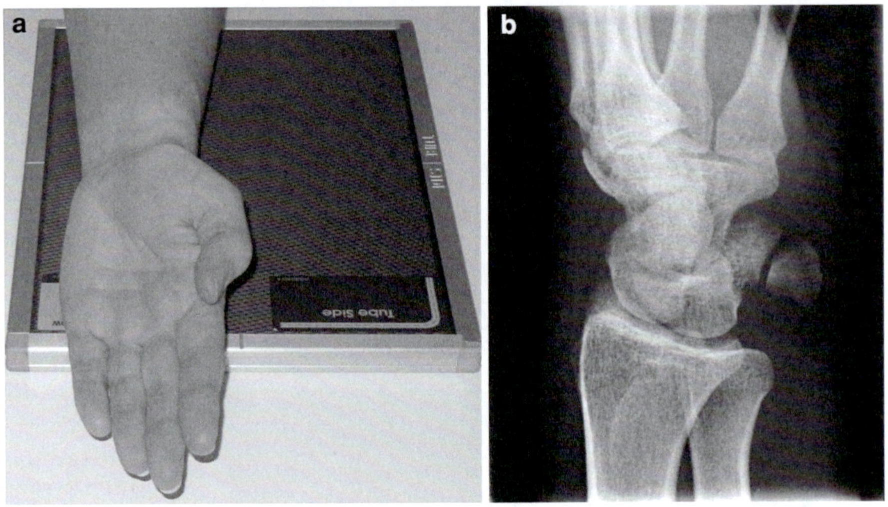

Fig. 9 **a** Patient positioning for posterior oblique of carpus. **b** Posterior oblique radiograph of carpus

Evaluation

The PA hand projection should demonstrate all of the joints of the hand, carpus and wrist (Fig. 11). The joint spaces should be symmetrical and parallel. This projection is used in the evaluation of trauma, arthropathy and a range of miscellaneous conditions. The carpo-metacarpal joint may be evaluated with a line drawn between the distal articular surfaces of the trapezoid, capitate and hamate and the parallel articular surfaces of the second-fifth metacarpals (Fig. 12) (Fisher and Rogers 1983). Discontinuity of this line should raise a suspicion of fracture and or dislocation.

2.3.2 PA Anterior Oblique Hand

Technique

The hand is externally rotated by 45° from the PA projection (Fig. 13). The fingers should be extended and separated. The film is centered over the third metacarpal head.

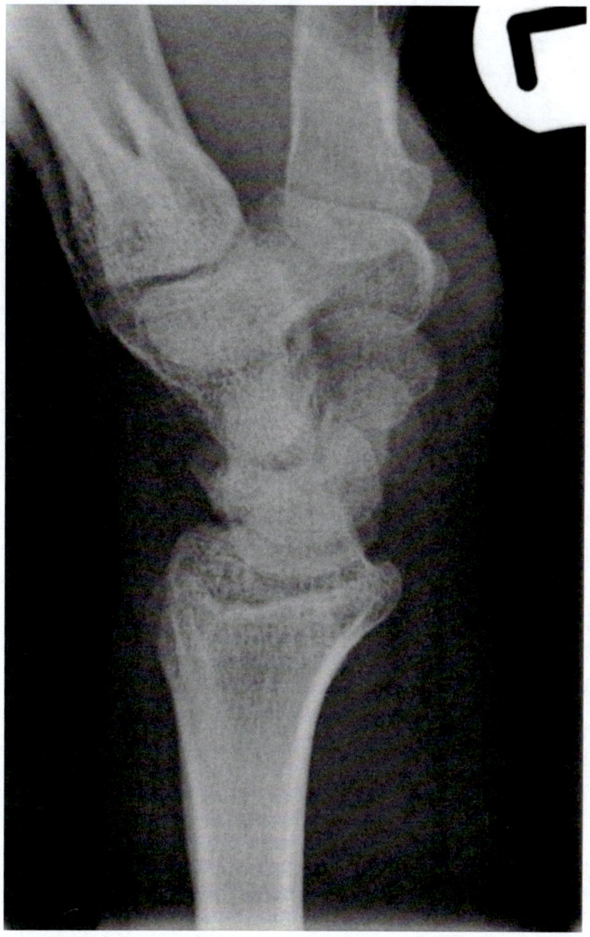

Fig. 10 Lateral radiograph of carpus

Evaluation

This projection is very useful for evaluating the shafts and necks of the metacarpals (Fig. 13). The phalanges are seen in an oblique plane. The first and second metacarpals are usually separated whilst there is an overlap of the fourth and fifth metacarpals.

2.3.3 Lateral Hand

Technique

The hand is placed in the lateral position on the cassette with the medial border of the wrist and hand resting on the cassette. The fingers are extended. The thumb is also extended and placed clear of the rest of the hand (Fig. 14). The centering point is the head of the second metacarpal.

Evaluation

This projection (Fig. 14) is useful for evaluating the carpal metacarpal region for dislocation. It is helpful in evaluating the fifth metacarpal shaft fractures. This projection is also used for foreign body assessment.

2.3.4 Posterior Oblique of Both Hands

Technique

Both hands are placed on the cassette. They should lie symmetrically. Both forearms are supinated with 45° of rotation. The radial styloid is elevated from the cassette on both sides. The centering point is midway between the hands at the level of the fifth metacarpal head.

Evaluation

The metacarpal heads should all be clearly seen and separated (Fig. 15). The purpose of this projection is to evaluate the metacarpal heads for bone erosion. This projection has also been termed the Norgaard view or 'ball catcher's' view. The obliquity of the projection enables a different part of the metacarpal head to be shown in profile. It is considered that this improves the visualisation of bone erosions from rheumatoid disease as more of the beam is tangential to the bare area of the metacarpal head, the area susceptible to erosions. This is when compared with the conventional PA projection. However, two studies have demonstrated that there is limited additional information with this projection (De Smet and Martin 1981; Edwards and Edwards 1983).

2.4 Radiographic Projections of the Phalanges

The standard projections are PA and lateral. Supplementary oblique views either of individual phalanges or as part of a PA oblique hand examination may also be undertaken. The oblique projection does not substitute for the lateral view which is an essential projection when evaluating trauma.

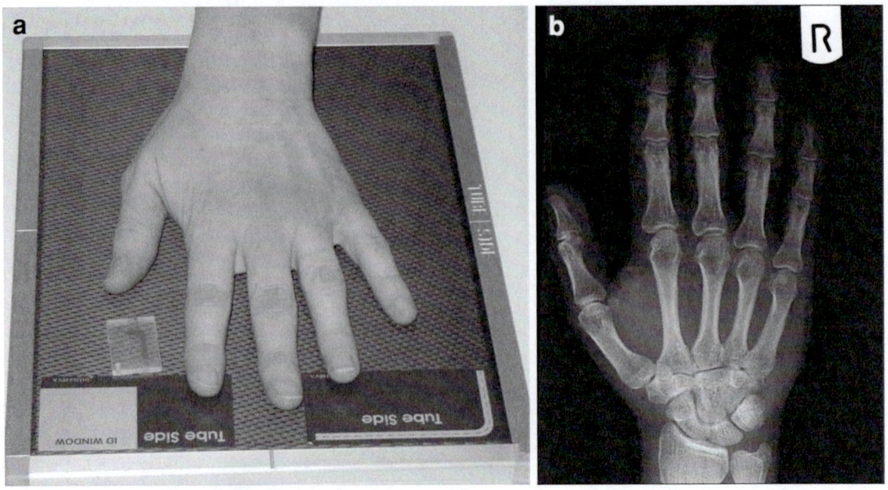

Fig. 11 **a** Patient positioning for PA hand. **b** Radiograph of PA hand

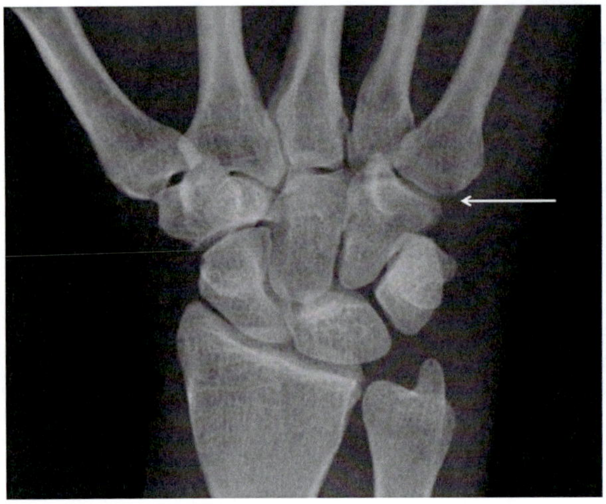

Fig. 12 PA hand radiograph showing level for assessment of parallelism across carpo–metacarpal joint (*white arrow*)

2.4.1 PA Phalanges

Technique

The phalanges may be X-rayed individually or in pairs. For example, the second and third phalanges are imaged together or the fourth and fifth are imaged together. The fingers are placed on the cassette with a hand in the neutral PA position (Fig. 16). The centering is over the PIP joint of the relevant finger. The X-ray should include the distal third of the metacarpal as far as the soft tissue of the fingertip.

Evaluation

The joint spaces should be uniform and parallel (Fig. 16).

2.4.2 Lateral Phalanges

Technique

The phalanges may be X-rayed individually or in pairs. Typically, the second and third are imaged together or the fourth and fifth phalanges. The phalanges are extended and separated so that both are visible on the film. The centering point is the proximal interphalangeal joint of the affected finger (Fig. 17).

Evaluation

The lateral view is especially important in the evaluation of volar plate injuries and extends or extensor avulsion injuries. The phalanx must be X-rayed in the true lateral position (Fig. 17).

2.5 Radiographic Evaluation of the Thumb

The conventional projections of the thumb are AP and lateral. They are performed separately from the examination of the hand. The PA projection may be substituted for the AP projection when there is pain or difficulty in achieving the appropriate position.

2.5.1 AP Thumb

Technique

The forearm is over-pronated such that the thumb lies on the cassette (Fig. 18). The centering point is the base of the first metacarpal.

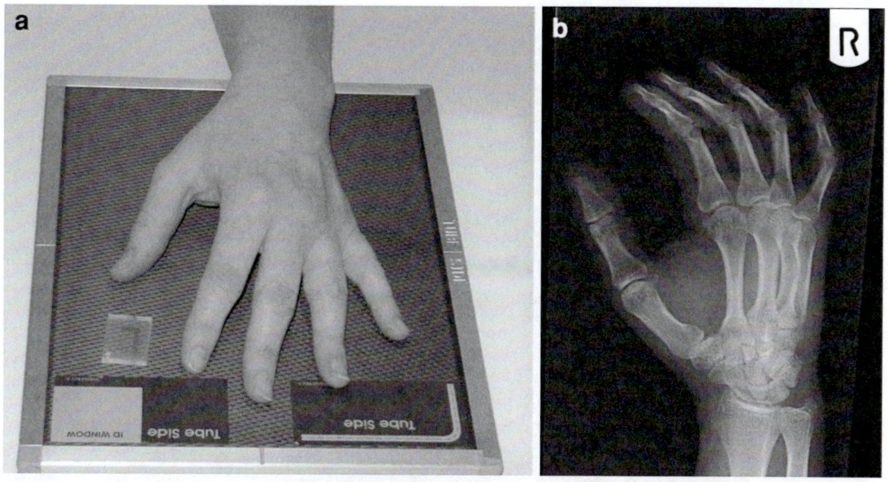

Fig. 13 **a** Patient positioning for PA anterior oblique of hand. **b** Radiograph of PA anterior oblique of hand

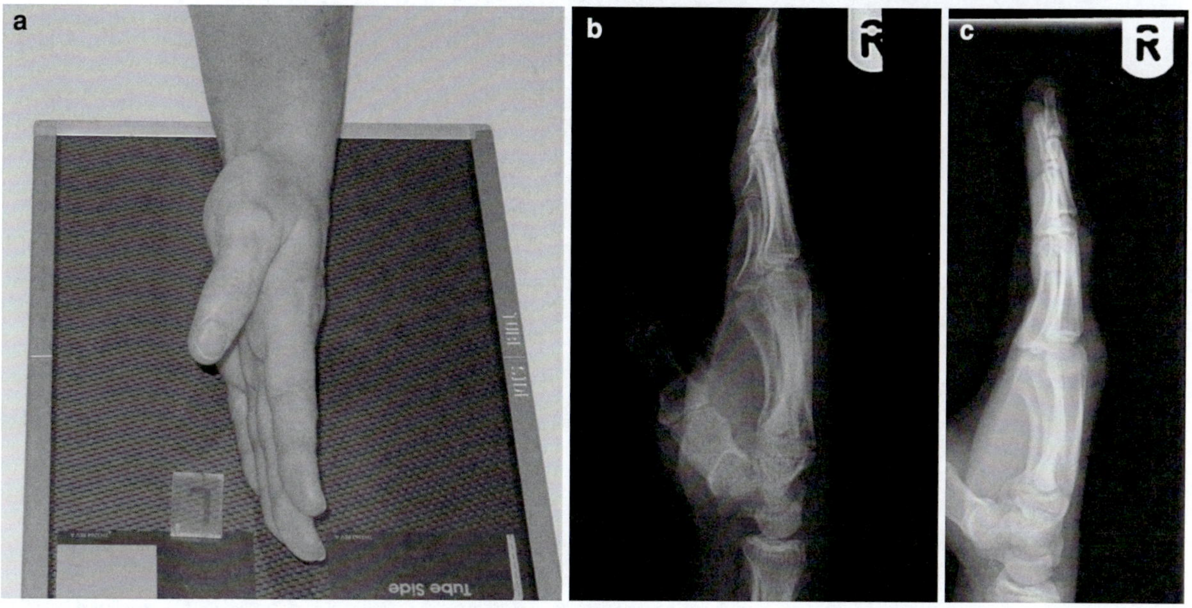

Fig. 14 **a** Patient positioning for lateral radiograph of hand. **b** Lateral radiograph of hand. **c** Soft tissue lateral radiograph of hand

Evaluation

The base of the first metacarpal and the base of the proximal phalanx of the thumb are well demonstrated and can be assessed for fracture (Fig. 18).

2.5.2 Lateral Thumb

Technique

The thumb is rested on the cassette in the lateral position. The palm of the hand is slightly rotated to bring thumb into it through lateral profile. The centering point is the metacarpo–phalangeal joint (Fig. 19).

Evaluation

This projection is important for evaluation of the base of the first metacarpal for fracture (Fig. 19).

2.5.3 PA Thumb

Technique

The medial border of the hand is rested on the cassette. The hand is rotated forwards with the thumb extended until a PA view of the thumb is obtained (Fig. 20). It is important that the thumb is extended, otherwise there is overlap at the metacarpal phalangeal joint. This projection is used when it is not

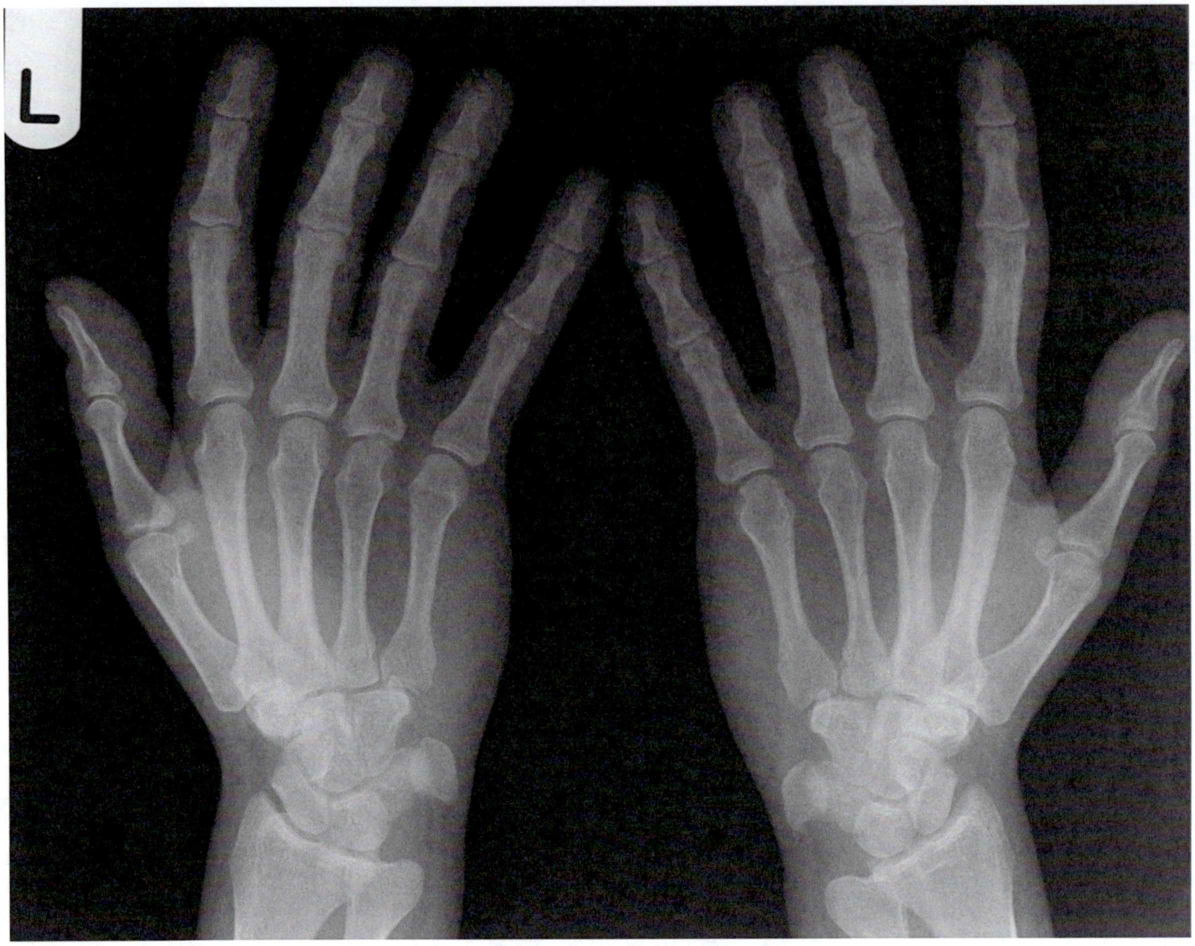

Fig. 15 Posterior-oblique (ball-catcher's) radiograph of the hands

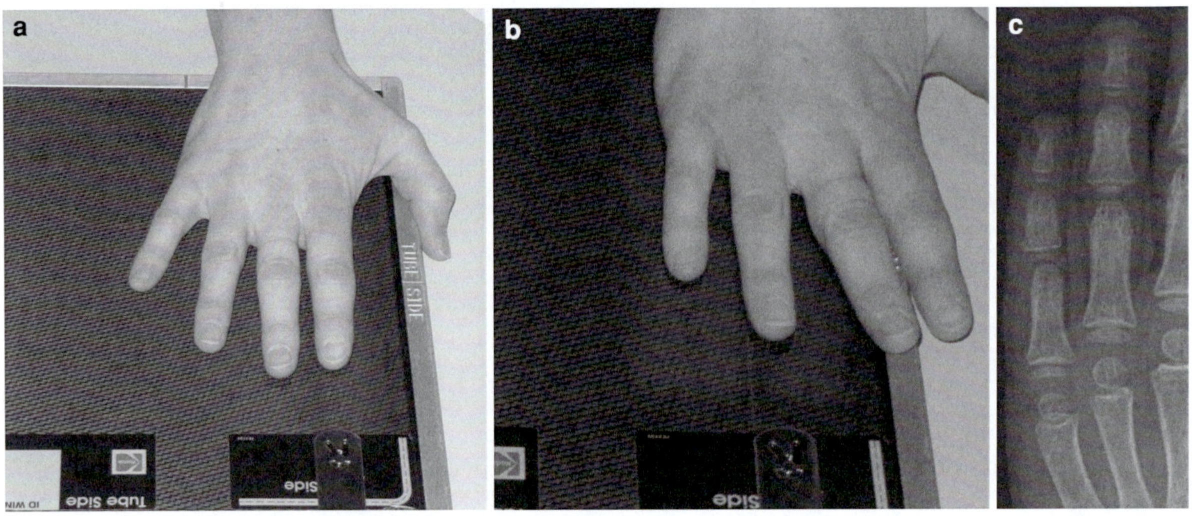

Fig. 16 **a** Patient positioning for PA second and third fingers. **b** Patient positioning for PA fourth and fifth fingers. **c** Radiograph of PA fingers

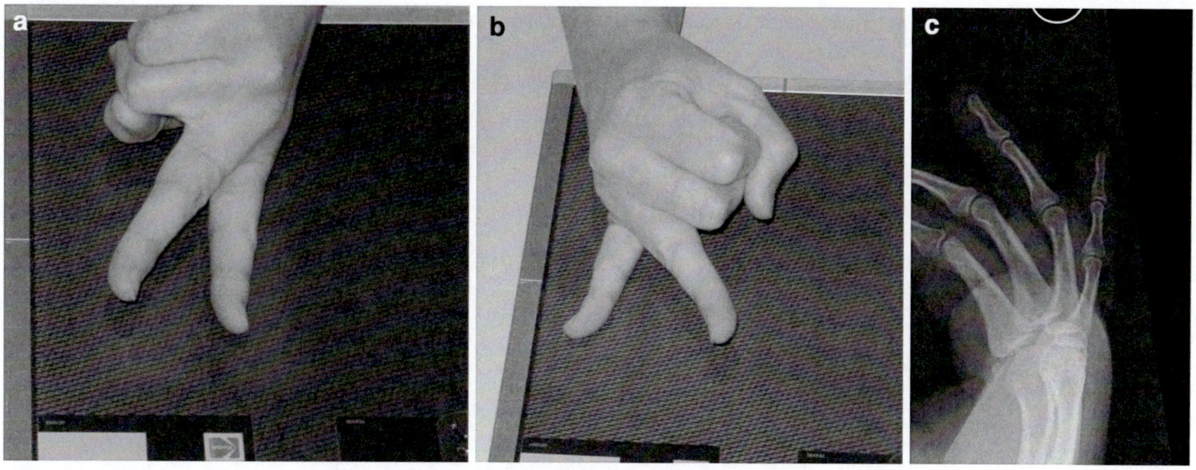

Fig. 17 **a** Patient positioning for lateral of second and third fingers. **b** Patient positioning for lateral of fourth and fifth fingers. **c** Lateral radiograph of fingers

Fig. 18 **a** Patient positioning for AP thumb. **b** AP radiograph of thumb

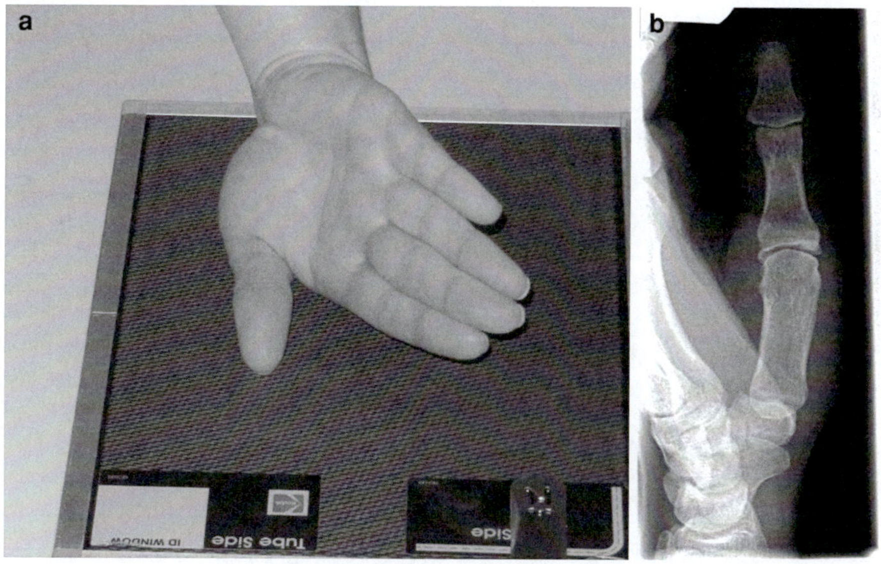

possible for the patient to achieve the over-pronation of the forearm required for the AP projection.

Evaluation

Care must be taken to obtain a good PA view and to assess for parallelism at the metacarpal–phalangeal joint.

3 Radiographic Technique

Film screen technique has been the standard methodology used for plain film radiographic examination for many years. With the advent of digital radiography and the growth in picture archiving and storage systems, new techniques have been introduced which are replacing standard film screen radiography. Computed radiography (CR) was the first technique, introduced in the 1980s. Direct digital radiography is a more recent technique introduced in the 1990s.

Imaging may be thought of in four separate steps: generation, processing, archiving and presentation. Image generation commences when X-rays having passed through the object under examination reach the detector. In the case of film screen radiography, this will be the film. The interaction of X-ray photons with the film results in a latent image which is then processed to

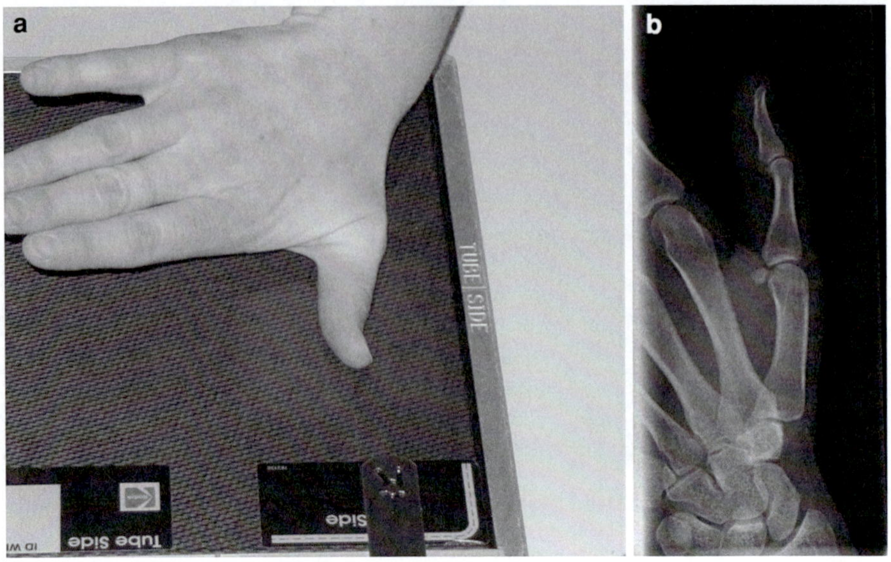

Fig. 19 **a** Patient positioning for lateral thumb. **b** Lateral radiograph of thumb

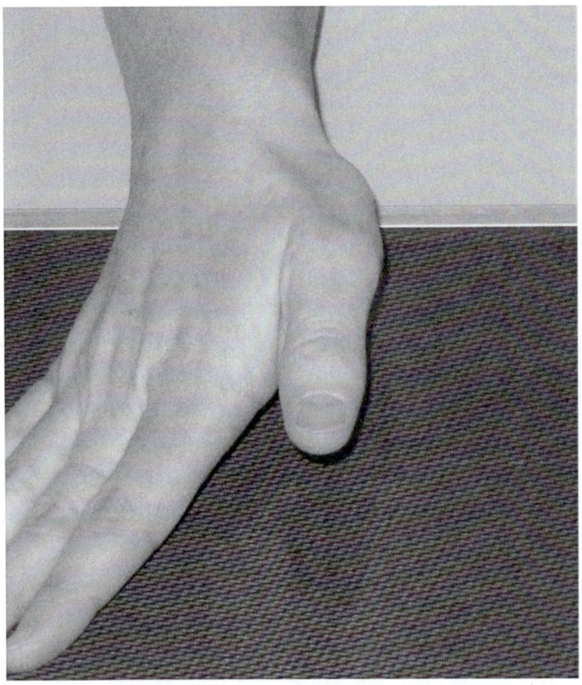

Fig. 20 Patient positioning for PA thumb

produce the real image which is 'stored' on the film. In the case of film-screen radiography, all the four steps are performed on the film. In the case of digital imaging, these steps are separated. CR differs from direct radiography (DR) in the content of these steps. Modern digital imaging produces images of the same quality as conventional film-screen radiography.

3.1 Computed Radiography (CR)

CR uses a cassette-based detector plate comprising photostimulable phosphor. Photons interacting with the phosphor elevate the energy levels of electrons within the phosphor crystals, and this comprises the latent image. The cassette is then taken to a processor. The processor (image plate reader) scans the plate with a helium–neon laser, releasing the energy from the excited electrons. Light is emitted which is converted by photomultiplier tubes into an analog signal which may then be digitised. Specific processing algorithms are then applied to this information resulting in the image for transfer and display. Images are displayed on computers or may be printed out on laser film. The plate is then exposed to intense light to completely erase the latent image and enable a further exposure with the same plate.

The processing algorithms which are used are specific to the body part and the suspected pathology. A key strength of digital imaging is its latitude and ability to display both bone and soft tissue detail with great clarity. It is necessary to optimise the image processing to the body part. Therefore, for example, the processing algorithm for a hip X-ray will be different to the knee and different again to the hand. Also a soft tissue foreign body film will be processed differently to a skeletal film for a fracture. The raw data may be reprocessed as required. A limitation of CR is that the resolution is of the order of 2.5–5 lines per mm. This contrasts with film screen radiography of 2.5–15 lines per mm. However, 2.5 lines per mm is acceptable for standard skeletal radiography.

Whereas overexposure with film screen radiography produces a black film, the processing of an overexposed CR phosphor plate can result in an image which has a normal appearance. The risk of the overexposure is that the radiographer is less able to make a judgment regarding standard exposures. It is easy for there to be an upward creep in exposure factors over a period of time. Thus, careful quality control mechanisms are required. A useful but imperfect guide is the 'exposure index'. Underexposure results in increasing graininess of the image.

For certain applications, high-resolution CR plates have been produced. In general, they would be limited to paediatric applications but may also be used for detailed extremity skeletal work.

3.2 Direct Radiography (DR)

DR produces high-quality digital images. DR has a major impact upon workflow in the radiology department as the image is produced very quickly after exposure. An image is produced 10–40 s after exposure. This enables a rapid decision with regard to the adequacy of the image (exposure, positioning and collimation). With DR the generation and processing occur in the same device which may be placed in, or replace the standard Bucky tray. DR is based upon solid-state, flat panel, digital radiography detectors. These detectors use a very thin layer of amorphous silicon.

The typical DR detector used in skeletal work uses indirect conversion. The detector comprises a combination of a layer of X-ray fluorescent material and the amorphous silicon active matrix read-out array. X-ray photon energy interacts with thallium-activated caesium iodide releasing light photons which are detected in a 2D array of amorphous silicon diodes. An electronic signal is produced which is then digitised. The caesium thallium is applied onto the hydrogenated amorphous silicon. Each pixel in the active matrix array comprises a light-sensitive element (photodiode) together with an associated switching component. The switching component is either in the form of a thin film diode switch or a thin film transistor switch. The charge pattern resulting from the exposure is read out amplified and digitised.

With both CR and DR, an anti-scatter grid is required. The dynamic range of DR is approaching 10,000:1. As a result of this, DR detectors have wide dose latitude. As with CR, this enables good quality images of both bone and soft tissue. DR also suffers from the potential weakness of incremental exposure drift or 'creep' as described above.

Active development of both DR and CR detectors continues with the aim of further refinements to produce improved quality images. In the case of DR, alternative manufacturing methods for large amorphous silicon active matrix arrays are a subject of research. Improvement in X-ray absorption materials for both CR and DR is an important area of development.

Digital imaging has provided the opportunity for immense workflow improvement and image storage with picture archiving and communications systems (PACS). In many centres, PACS has replaced conventional film imaging. The advantages are numerous. Importantly they include the ability to view images at multiple locations simultaneously; storage and retrieval efficiency; and image manipulation and interrogation. Advanced digital imaging techniques take advantage of the improved processing power leading to the development of tomosynthesis, dual energies subtraction and temporal subtraction imaging.

4 Additional Projections and Fluoroscopy

The radiographic evaluation of carpal instability includes a static series and dynamic fluoroscopy. The objective of these examinations is to demonstrate malalignment of the carpal bones either in a static position or alternatively as part of a dynamic examination. The dynamic examination also provides the opportunity to assess for dysynchronous movement between the carpal bones. Malalignment or dysynchronous movement is likely to be a consequence of ligament disruption. Of particular importance in this regard are the scapholunate and lunotriquetral

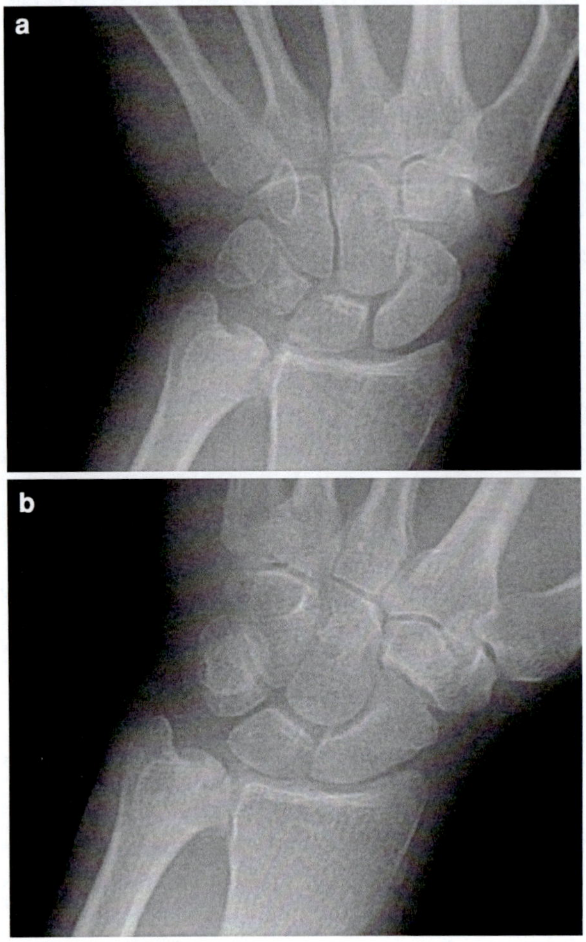

Fig. 21 Fluoroscopy images of PA wrist **a** ulna deviation and **b** radial deviation

ligaments. Both have strong anterior and posterior components with a thin 'membranous' central portion.

4.1 Carpal Instability Series—Static Evaluation

4.1.1 Technique

The standard series would include the following projections (Gilula et al. 1984). Initially, the wrist is placed in the neutral PA position. From this, the wrist is deviated in the ulnar and then radial directions (Fig. 21). Images are taken in all three positions. Following this, this series is repeated with the fist clenched. In some cases, the technique may be conducted with the fist clenched around a pencil or a tennis ball (Schmitt and Froehner 2006). Then three further views are performed with the wrist in the lateral position: neutral, full extension and full flexion (Fig. 22). An additional view which is performed for evaluation of the piso-triquetral joint is the 30° supinated view of the wrist.

4.1.2 Evaluation

The integrity of the carpal arcs is assessed. Congruency of the intercarpal joints and the width of these joints is also assessed. Of particular importance with regard to the proximal carpal row is the relationship of the lunate relative to the radius (Schernberg 1990). The proximal surface of the lunate should not move more than half of its width on the distal surface of the radius (Fig. 21).

4.2 Dynamic Evaluation—Fluoroscopy

4.2.1 Technique

A dynamic study (Gilula et al. 1984; Braunstein and Louis 1985) provides a further opportunity to assess for carpal instability in the situation where the static views are negative. Essentially, the static series are repeated with movement. Therefore, from the PA neutral position the wrist is deviated in the ulnar direction and then back through the neutral position to the radial position. This movement is repeated. From the lateral position the wrist is fully flexed and then fully extended. This is also repeated as required. A further, non-standard part of the study follows enquiry of the patient with regard to the movement causing symptoms. The patient undertakes this movement which is recorded with fluoroscopy. This study may be recorded and therefore replayed at normal and reduced speeds.

4.2.2 Evaluation

The alignment of the carpal bones in all the positions is evaluated. In addition, careful viewing of the relative movements within each carpal row and then between carpal rows is important. For the proximal carpal joint, the movement of the lunate relative to the distal radius is important. For the metacarpal joint, the movement of the hamate relative to the lunate is important.

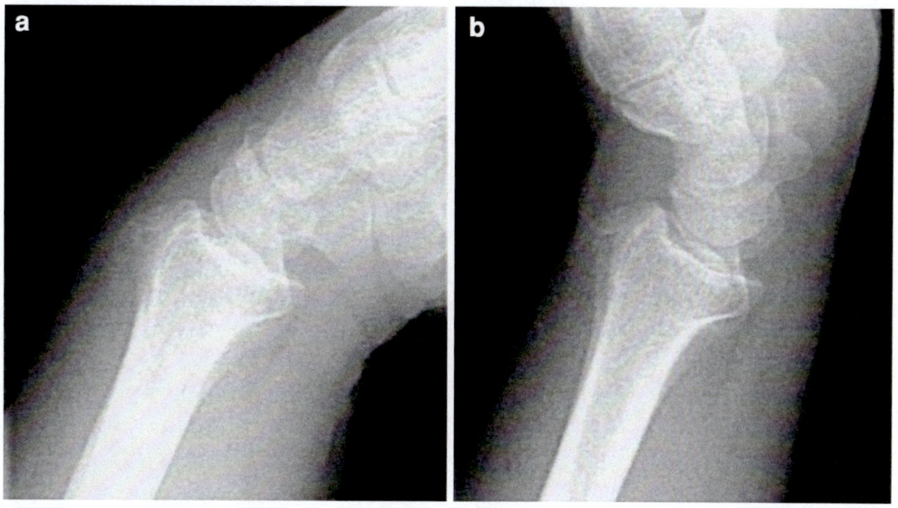

Fig. 22 Fluoroscopy images of lateral wrist in **a** flexion and **b** extension

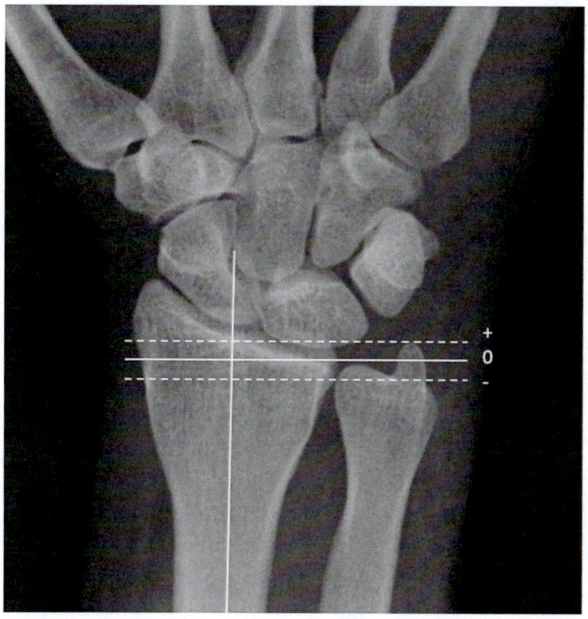

Fig. 23 Measurement of ulna variance. Solid line is ulna neutral (normal). + is positive ulna variance and – represents negative ulna variance

5 Measurements

There are a number of measurements which are useful in the assessment of the wrist which can be performed on plain radiographs (Mann and Wilson 1992; Goldfarb and Yin 2001; Rosner and Zlatkin 2004; Loredo and Sorge 2005). Ulna variance is useful in a range of conditions including assessment following fracture and ulna-sided wrist pain. Distal radial measurements include radial inclination, radial length, and palmar tilt. These are all useful in the assessment of distal radial fractures. The scapholunate and capitate–lunate angles are calculated when carpal instability is suspected. Finally, carpal height is measured when collapse of the carpus is suspected, for example, as a consequence of carpal instability or previous fracture.

5.1 Ulna Variance

Ulna variance is the difference in length between the distal radius and the distal ulna. This measurement is relevant in a number of carpal disorders including fracture assessment and abnormalities of the proximal carpal row such as chondromalacia of the lunate. The wrist is assessed in a neutral PA position. A technique for the assessment of ulna variance involves first, identifying the long axis of the radius at 2.0 and 5.0 cm from the distal radial cortex. A perpendicular running tangential to the most ulna portion of the distal radial articular cortex is then drawn to this line. Second, the line is drawn tangential to the distal ulna and parallel to the line described above (Mann and Wilson 1992; Loredo and Sorge 2005) (Fig. 23). In negative ulna variance (ulna minus), the ulna is shorter than the radius. In positive ulna variance (ulna plus), the ulna is longer than the radius. Normally, the radius and ulna are of the same length or there is mild negative ulna variance.

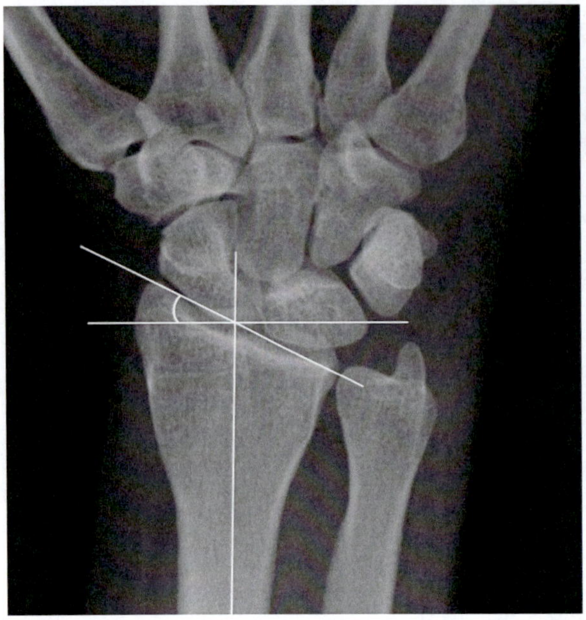

Fig. 24 Measurement of radial inclination. Normal inclination is 21–25°

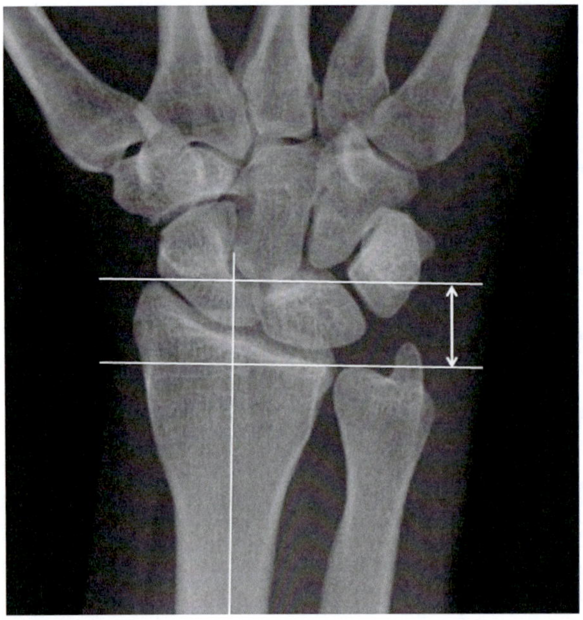

Fig. 25 Measurement of radial length. Normal measurement is 10–13 mm

5.2 Radial Inclination

Radial inclination describes the slope of the radius between the tip of the radial styloid and the ulnar border of the radius in the frontal or PA plane. Its assessment is important following distal radial fractures (Mann and Wilson 1992; Loredo and Sorge 2005). The technique for obtaining the measurement is first to identify the long axis of the radius as described above (Sect. 5.1). Second, a line is drawn from the tip of the radial styloid to the ulnar border of the distal radius. The third line is drawn through the intersection of these lines, perpendicular to the long axis of the radius (Goldfarb and Yin 2001). The radial inclination is the angle between the perpendicular and the line running tangential to the radial styloid and ulnar border of radius (Fig. 24). The normal inclination is 23° (21–25°) (Goldfarb and Yin 2001).

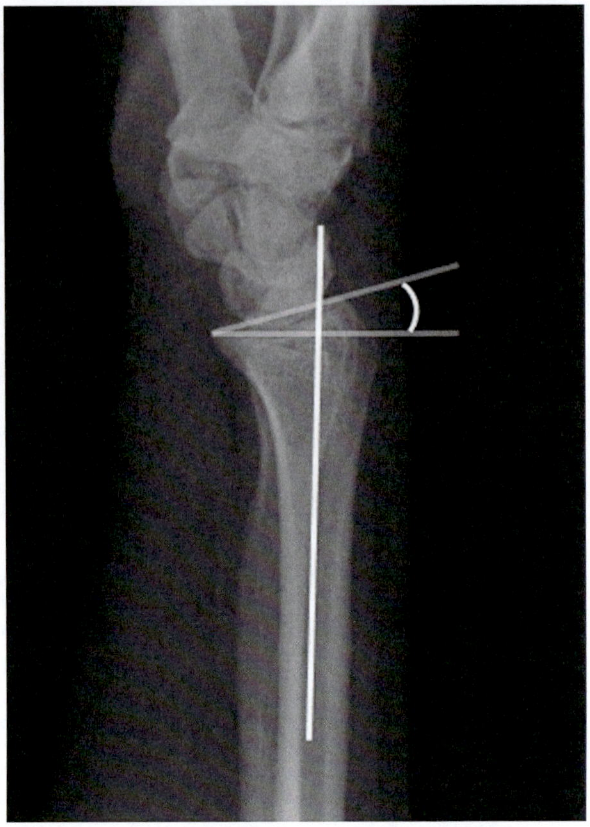

Fig. 26 Measurement of palmar tilt (volar inclination). Normal value 0–22°

5.3 Radial Length (Radial Height)

Radial length (radial height) is a method for assessing shortening of the radius, for example, following a fracture. The measurement involves identification of the

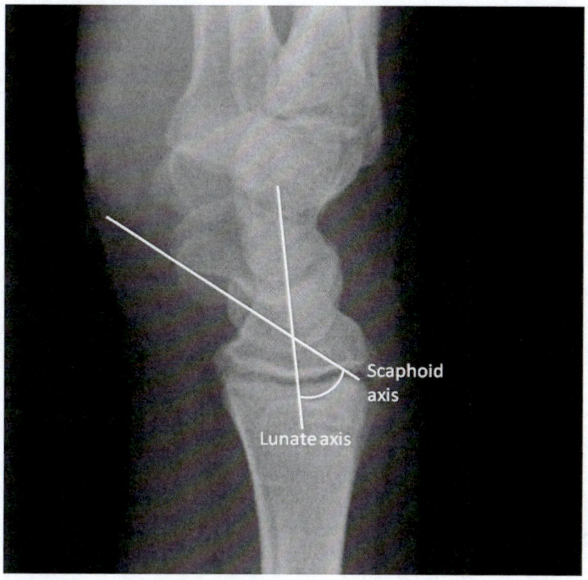

Fig. 27 Scapholunate angle. White lines represent long axis of scaphoid and lunate. Normal range is 30–60°

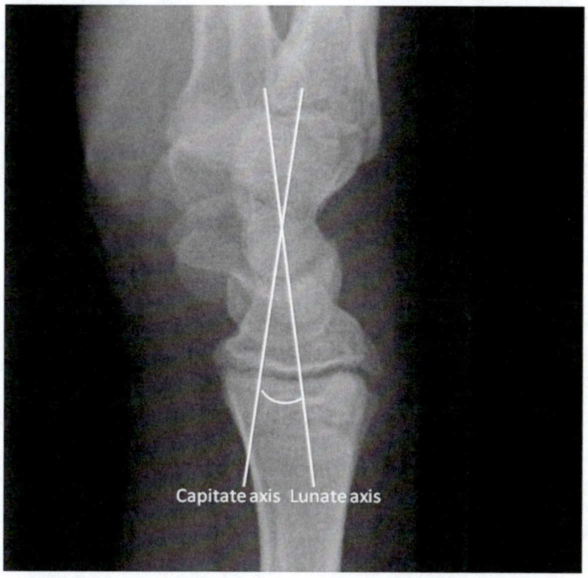

Fig. 28 Capitolunate angle. White lines represent long axis of lunate and capitate. Normal range is 0–30°

long axis of the radius. Two lines perpendicular to this are then constructed. Firstly, tangential to the tip of the radial styloid and secondly tangential to the ulnar border of the distal radius (Fig. 25). The distance between these two lines is the radial length (Goldfarb and Yin 2001). A normal value of 10–13 mm is expected.

5.4 Palmar Tilt (Volar Tilt or Volar Inclination)

This measurement assesses the tilt of the distal radius at the radiocarpal joint. The central axis of the radius is identified in the lateral plane using points at 2 and 5 cm from the midpoint of the distal articular surface. A perpendicular is drawn to this line at the articular surface. A third line is drawn from the dorsal lip of the distal radius to the volar lip of the distal radius. The palmar tilt is the angle between the third line and the perpendicular (Fig. 26). It is normally between 0–22° (Mann and Wilson 1992; Goldfarb and Yin 2001). This is an important measurement in the assessment of distal radial fractures.

5.5 Scapholunate Angle

This angle is calculated when carpal instability is suspected (Goldfarb and Yin 2001). It is particularly pertinent in the assessment of dorsal intercalated instability (DISI). The angle is measured from the lateral view of the wrist. The angle is calculated by drawing two lines (Timins and Jahnke 1995). A line is drawn through the proximal and distal volar convexities of the scaphoid. This defines the scaphoid axis. The lunate axis is perpendicular to a line drawn between the distal poles of the lunate. The normal scapholunate angle lies between 30–60° (Fig. 27).

5.6 Capitate–Lunate Angle

This angle is calculated when the volar instability pattern (VISI) of carpal instability is suspected. The angle is measured from the lateral view of the wrist. The long axis of the lunate is drawn as described above (Sect. 5.5). The long axis of the capitate is drawn from the centre of its distal articular surface to the centre of the proximal articular surface (Timins and Jahnke 1995). The normal capitate–lunate angle lies between 0 and 30° (Fig. 28).

5.7 Carpal height

Carpal height provides quantification of the degree of carpal collapse e.g. in scapholunate advanced collapse

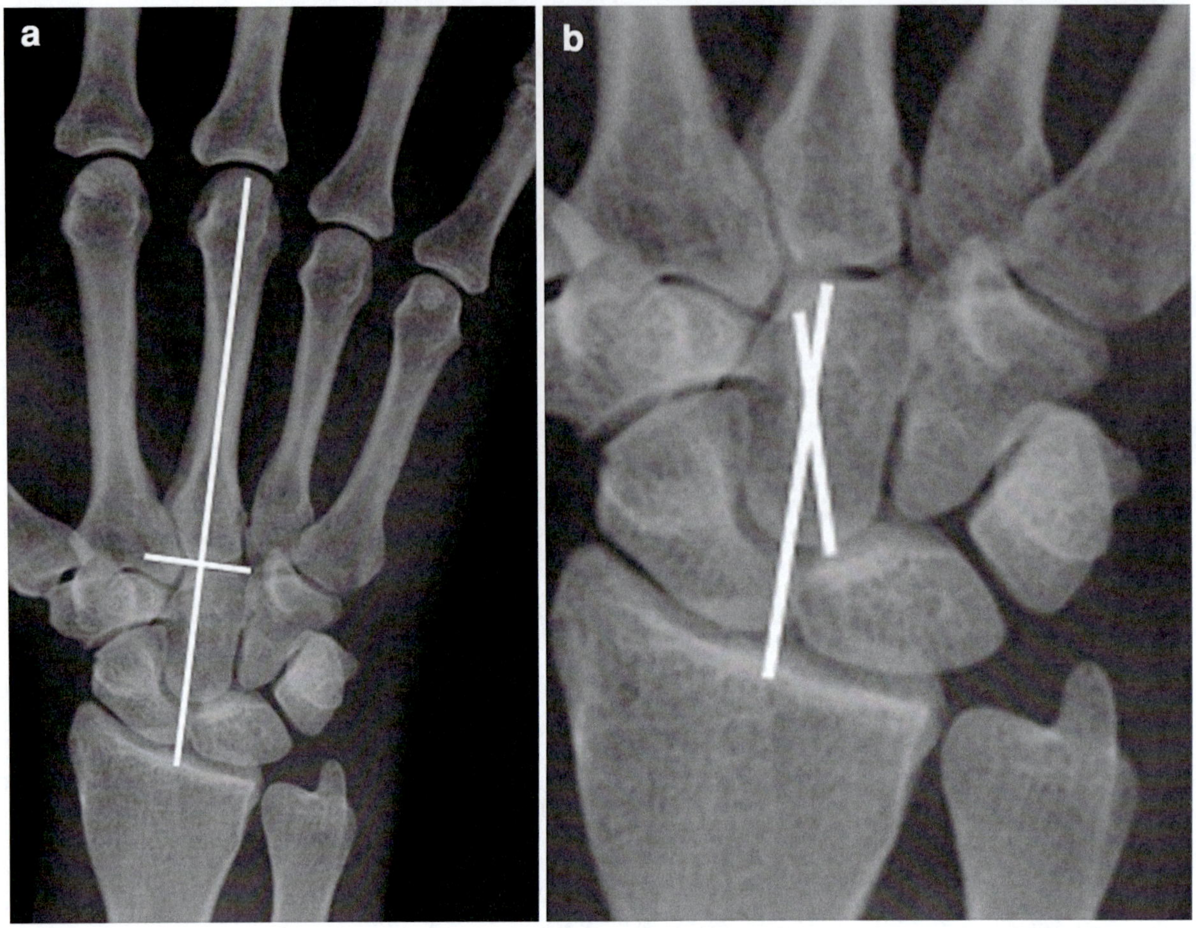

Fig. 29 Measurement of carpal height **a** method 1 and **b** method 2

(SLAC). Two methods have been described. The first method describes a ratio between the distance from the base of the third metacarpal to the proximal articular surface of the radius and the length of the third metacarpal. The line drawn extends from the long axis of the third metacarpal (Fig. 29a). With this method, the normal carpal height ratio is 0.54 (Mann and Wilson 1992).

The second method divides the carpal height (distance from base of the third metacarpal to proximal articular surface of radius) by the capitate length. The capitate length is calculated from the distal angular articular surface of the capitate (between the bases of the second and third metacarpals) and the centre of the proximal articular surface of the capitate (Fig. 29). The normal figure is 1.57 (Mann and Wilson 1992).

A carpal height index is obtained by dividing the carpal height of the diseased wrist with the normal wrist (Loredo and Sorge 2005). This index may be followed with time as a marker of disease progression.

6 Arthrography

Arthrography of the wrist is performed in the assessment of interosseous wrist ligaments and the triangular fibrocartilage complex. Specifically, it is performed for assessment of the scapholunate and luno-triquetral ligaments in addition to the triangular fibrocartilage complex. With the advent of cross-sectional imaging techniques, it is most frequently undertaken now as part of an MRI or CT arthrographic study. The basic technique is that of a proximal row or radiocarpal injection. A more complex study will involve injection of two or three wrist compartments.

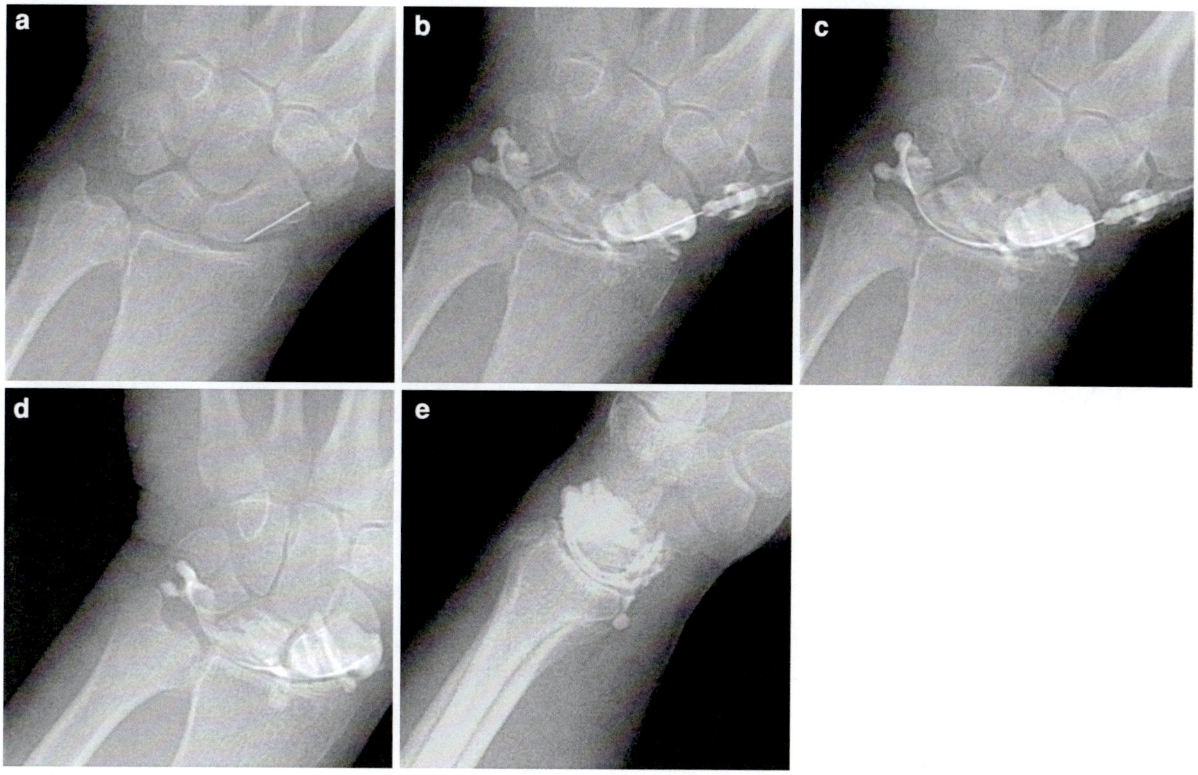

Fig. 30 Fluoroscopy images from radiocarpal arthrogram **a** needle position **b** early filling with contrast **c** mid-filling phase **d** late-filling phase (complete) **e** lateral view post exercise

Unicompartmental injection to the radiocarpal (Fransson 1993) may be undertaken by injection at two different points. The first is a dorsal approach to the junction between the scaphoid and lunate just proximal to the scapholunate ligament. The second is between the scaphoid and distal radius. The wrist is gently flexed and a 22G needle introduced under fluoroscopic guidance. Care must be taken not to damage the scapholunate ligament. Note should be taken of the normal radial inclination and allowance made for the dorsal lip of the radius when introducing the needle.

Contrast is injected into the radiocarpal space. The usual filling volume is between 2 and 4 ml. The end of the injection is signified by gentle resistance to further filling and distribution of contrast across the radiocarpal joint. Generally, contrast of 240 IU/l is sufficient for good radiographic imaging. The mixture injected will alter for CT arthrography and MRI arthrography as is described in subsequent chapters.

Contrast should be injected slowly, carefully observing the filling of the radiocarpal space and looking for contrast tracking into the scapholunate space, lunate triquetral space, or distal radio–ulnar joint. Spot films are taken during injection (Fig. 30). At the end of the injection when there is good filling of the radiocarpal space, a further series of films is taken following gentle exercise of the wrist. A typical series of films would include PA in the neutral, ulnar deviation, and radial deviation positions followed by a lateral view. It is commonplace to have performed a static and dynamic instability series (as outlined earlier in the chapter) prior to injection of contrast.

Fluoroscopy and videotaping the procedure enabled further retrospective analysis (Gilula and Totty 1983).

The normal pattern of filling (Fig. 30) outlines the radiocarpal joint (Resnick 1995). Age-related degenerate perforations of the central portion of the scapholunate and lunate triquetral ligaments are well recognized (Linkous and Pierce 2000). Similarly age-related degenerate perforations of the radial side of the triangular fibrocartilage complex with filling of the distal radio-ulnar joint may also be observed. Small volar outpouchings (radial recesses) of the capsule are well recognized (Fig. 30). On the ulnar

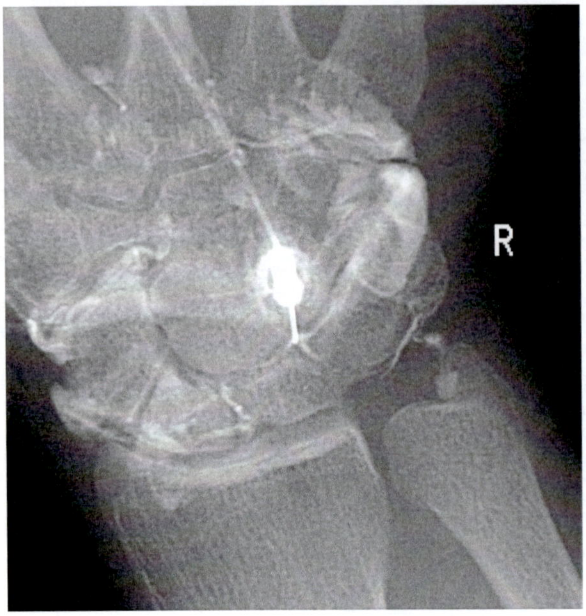

Fig. 31 Fluoroscopy image from midcarpal arthrogram demonstrating needle position and filling of radiocarpal space

side there is a small pre-styloid recess above which the meniscus homologue and a further collection of contrast may be identified. Filling of the piso-triquetral space is a normal variant.

Midcarpal injection has been described by Tirman and Weber (1985). The wrist is gently flexed. The midcarpal joint is injected between the distal scaphoid and capitate (Linkous and Pierce 2000) (Fig. 31). Careful injection with fluoroscopic guidance is undertaken until good filling of the space has been obtained. Careful observation of the scapholunate and lunotriquetral spaces is undertaken, looking for evidence of filling of these spaces. Tirman regarded this as an easier method for establishing the integrity of the scapholunate and lunotriquetral ligaments. A static and dynamic instability series would be obtained.

Triple compartment arthrography (Levinsohn and Palmer 1987; Levinsohn and Rosen 1991) was introduced by Levisnohn and regarded as being of superior diagnostic quality. However, Steinbach and Palmer (2002) preferred single joint injection into the radiocarpal space. This has the advantage of single as opposed to multiple injections, whilst still providing the opportunity to evaluate the scapholunate ligament, lunotriquetral ligament, and triangular fibrocartilage complex. It also avoids the time-consuming wait between each of the three compartment injections whilst awaiting absorption of contrast.

However, the diagnostic yield is greater with a midcarpal injection based on an analysis of unidirectional joint communications (Wilson and Gilula 1991). It was proposed that if a scapholunate or lunotriquetral ligament disruption was suspected then a midcarpal injection should be performed first. If a triangular fibrocartilage complex disruption was suspected, then a radiocarpal injection should be performed first.

Full triple compartment arthrography also involves injecting the distal radio–ulnar joint looking for communication with the proximal carpal joint.

Digital subtraction imaging was introduced to improve visualisation of scapholunate or lunotriquetral space filling when multiple compartments were injected (Quinn and Pittman 1988) without the normal three-hour delay between injections waiting for the contrast to be absorbed.

In current radiological practice, the arthrogram is usually performed in conjunction with an MRI arthrogram or CT arthrogram. Whilst 3T MR without arthrography is producing very high-quality images of the wrist (Saupe 2009) and its associated ligaments, MRI arthrography is preferred for evaluation of the ligamentous structures of the wrist (Magee 2009; Sofka and Pavlov 2009).

References

Braunstein EM, Louis DS (1985) Fluoroscopic and arthrographic evaluation of carpal instability. AJR Am J Roentgenol 144(6):1259–1262

De Smet AA, Martin NL (1981) Radiographic projections for the diagnosis of arthritis of the hands and wrists. Radiology 139(3):577–581

Edwards JC, Edwards SE (1983) The value of radiography in the management of rheumatoid arthritis. Clin Radiol 34(4):413–416

Fisher MR, Rogers LF (1983) Systematic approach to identifying fourth and fifth carpometacarpal joint dislocations. AJR Am J Roentgenol 140(2):319–324

Fransson SG (1993) Wrist arthrography. Acta Radiol 34(2):111–116

Gilula LA (1979) Carpal injuries: analytic approach and case exercises. AJR Am J Roentgenol 133(3):503–517

Gilula LA, Totty WG (1983) Wrist arthrography. The value of fluoroscopic spot viewing. Radiology 146(2):555–556

Gilula LA, Destouet JM et al (1984) Roentgenographic diagnosis of the painful wrist. Clin Orthop Relat Res 187:52–64

Goldfarb CA, Yin Y (2001) Wrist fractures: what the clinician wants to know. Radiology 219(1):11–28
Levinsohn EM, Palmer AK (1987) Wrist arthrography: the value of the three compartment injection technique. Skeletal Radiol 16(7):539–544
Levinsohn EM, Rosen ID (1991) Wrist arthrography: value of the three-compartment injection method. Radiology 179(1):231–239
Linkous MD, Pierce SD (2000) Scapholunate ligamentous communicating defects in symptomatic and asymptomatic wrists: characteristics 1. Radiology 216(3):846–850
Loredo RA, Sorge DG (2005) Radiographic evaluation of the wrist: a vanishing art. Semin Roentgenol 40(3):248–289
Magee T (2009) Comparison of 3-T MRI and arthroscopy of intrinsic wrist ligament and TFCC tears. AJR Am J Roentgenol 192(1):80–85
Mann FA, Wilson AJ (1992) Radiographic evaluation of the wrist: what does the hand surgeon want to know? Radiology 184(1):15–24
Quinn SF, Pittman CC (1988) Digital subtraction wrist arthrography: evaluation of the multiple-compartment technique. AJR Am J Roentgenol 151(6):1173–1174
Resnick D (ed) (1995) Diagnosis of bone and joint disorders. W.B. Saunders, Philadelphia
Resnik CS (2000) Wrist and hand injuries. Semin Musculoskelet Radiol 4(2):193–204
Rosner JL, Zlatkin MB (2004) Imaging of athletic wrist and hand injuries. Semin Musculoskelet Radiol 8(1):57–79
Saupe N (2009) 3-Tesla high-resolution MR imaging of the wrist. Semin Musculoskelet Radiol 13(1):29–38
Schernberg F (1990) Roentgenographic examination of the wrist: a systematic study of the normal, lax and injured wrist. Part 1: the standard and positional views. J Hand Surg Br 15(2):210–219
Schmitt R, Froehner S (2006) Carpal instability. Eur Radiol 16(10):2161–2178
Sofka CM, Pavlov H (2009) The history of clinical musculoskeletal radiology. Radiol Clin North Am 47(3):349–356
Steinbach LS, Palmer WE (2002) Special focus session. Radiographics 22(5):1223–1246
Timins ME, Jahnke JP (1995) MR imaging of the major carpal stabilizing ligaments: normal anatomy and clinical examples. Radiographics 15(3):575–587
Tirman RM, Weber ER (1985) Midcarpal wrist arthrography for detection of tears of the scapholunate and lunotriquetral ligaments. AJR Am J Roentgenol 144(1):107–108
Whitley AS (2005) Clark's positioning in radiography. Hodder Arnold, London
Wilson AJ, Gilula LA (1991) Unidirectional joint communications in wrist arthrography: an evaluation of 250 cases. AJR Am J Roentgenol 157(1):105–109
Yang Z, Mann FA (1997) Scaphopisocapitate alignment: criterion to establish a neutral lateral view of the wrist. Radiology 205(3):865–869

Computed Tomography of Hand and Wrist

Sri Priya Suresh and Tishi Ninan

Contents

Sri P. Suresh (✉) · T. Ninan
Imaging Directorate, Department of Radiology,
Plymouth Hospitals NHS Trust, Derriford Road,
Crownhill, Devon, PL6 8DH, UK
e-mail: sureshpriya2000@yahoo.com

Abstract

The use of computed tomography (CT) in imaging has expanded radically in the last four decades since its invention. Aided by advances in computing and engineering, it has grown from being an object of curiosity in research institutions to the main modality of medical imaging across the world. Although at present, the most common use of computed tomography with respect to imaging of the hand and wrist is in trauma; easy availability, high spatial resolution and recent innovations are helping it to break new ground in assessment of soft tissue structures and dynamic imaging.

1 Introduction

Computed tomography is becoming the mainstay of medical imaging. Several studies have validated this claim including the most recent report from National Council of radiation protection (NRCP) in the USA which stated that the number of CT studies has increased by 10 % per year from 1993 to 2006. Easy availability, very short scanning times and high spatial resolution are currently the main strengths of CT scanning. Modern advances in computing capability and digital image processing enabling instantaneous display of multi-planar reformats has helped to fuel the increase in demand in CT imaging for acute and chronic disorders. Moving on from diagnosis, CT is widely used for treatment planning and assessment of prognosis. Newer operating techniques and equipment enabling surgeons to operate on more complex injuries improving patient outcome also contributed

A. M. Davis et al. (eds.), *Imaging of the Hand and Wrist*, Medical Radiology. Diagnostic Imaging,
DOI: 10.1007/174_2012_754,

to increase use of CT for identification of even subtle injuries.

CT is pivotal in the imaging of hand and wrist. The unique configuration of the carpus, which involves complex articulation between multiple bones with different degrees of rotation and translation between them, makes accurate diagnosis of fractures and dislocations on two-dimensional images provided by plain radiograph problematic. For timely management of injuries and patient comfort, CT scan is the primary imaging modality of the wrist.

Modern multi detector row CT scans have the ability to produce slices that are a fraction of a millimeter thick thus providing spatial resolution capable of identifying non displaced fractures and tiny fracture fragments. CT can also be used to diagnose ligament injuries and arthritis especially in patients where MRI is difficult or contra-indicated.

2 Computed Tomography Techniques

2.1 Patient Positioning

For CT scans of the wrist and hand, the patient is asked to lie prone with the affected arm stretched out above his or her head with the hand and wrist placed with the palm facing down. This is often described as the 'Superman' position and it helps to reduce the dose delivered to the more radiosensitive parts of the body like cornea, breasts, mediastinum and abdominal organs. It also helps to reduce artifacts due to beam hardening that can occur if the hand is placed over the chest or by the side of the body for the scan.

2.2 Technique

Multiple rows of detectors are not essential for CT imaging of wrist trauma but they afford higher spatial and temporal resolution. Parameters like kV, mA, pitch and field of view are adjusted based on factors such as patient's body mass index, presence or absence of cast and the indication for imaging. Radiation dose will be lower while imaging without a cast but in cases of unstable comminuted fractures or open injures, cast and dressing can be left on. The patient is scanned in the "superman" position with the wrist is in the middle of the gantry. The upper arm should be fully extended to counteract radial or ulnar deviation of the wrist. Excessive dorsal flexion of the wrist should also be avoided.

Technical parameters are set to achieve the highest spatial resolution but mindful of the radiation penalty. Newer dose and noise reduction techniques marketed by different manufacturers like Adaptive Statistical Iterative Reconstruction (ASiR) (GE) iDose (Philips), Adaptive Iterative dose Reduction (AIDR) (Toshiba) and Iterative Reconstruction in Image Space (IRIS) (Siemens) can be used according to local protocol.

Isotropic acquisition allows optimal reformation in multiple planes. Corrected transverse, sagittal, and coronal reformatted images are routinely obtained along the axis of the capitate bone.

Maximum bone detail is obtained by using high-resolution bone algorithms most of which involve edge enhancement.

2.3 CT Arthrogram

CT scanning of the wrist after injection of contrast is sometimes performed for better assessment of ligaments and joints in certain situations. Techniques and indications for this are discussed later in this chapter.

3 Clinical Applications

3.1 Acute Trauma

CT is now becoming the primary modality of cross sectional wrist imaging for trauma in several centres. Many centres still use MR as the preferred modality. In this chapter we shall consider the use of CT in various hand and wrist fractures.

3.1.1 Fractures of Distal Radius and Ulna

Fractures of the distal radius generate a high interest amongst orthopaedic and hand surgeons probably due to the fact that it is one of the most frequently encountered fractures in the emergency department. Treatment options have come a long way since the days of Colles' landmark article on distal radius fractures where the main advice was to treat most patients non-operatively (Sternbach 1985). These days surgeons have more operative options and

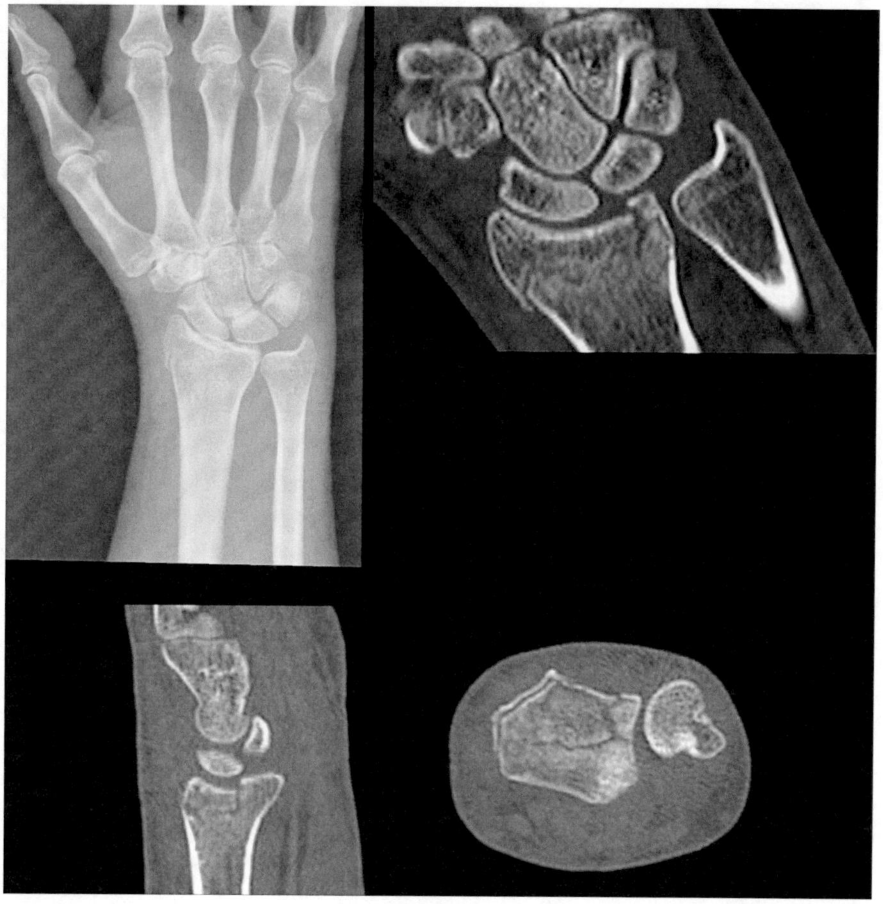

Fig. 1 Radiograph of wrist demonstrating an intra-articular fracture at top left hand corner and clockwise images show coronal, transverse and sagittal CT reconstructions in the same patient. The degree of comminution and extent of articular depression is difficult to appreciate on the plain radiograph. Transverse section also demonstrates subluxation of the Distal radio ulnar joint (DRUJ) is difficult to appreciate on plain radiograph

expect information about fracture configuration, angulation and comminution to make decision about further management. The imaging parameters to be considered while evaluating distal radius fractures include radial inclination, radial shortening, radial tilt, articular incongruity and degree of comminution of fragments. Most of these parameters can be better identified on CT scans compared to plain radiographs. Although operative management of isolated distal ulnar fractures is less common, CT scan is occasionally indicated in badly comminuted, shortened fractures (Fig. 1).

3.2 Fractures of Carpal Bones

Wrist fractures are notoriously difficult to diagnose on initial radiographs. Various modalities including bone scintigraphy and MR imaging have been used in different institutions. There is a wide variation of practice in the world in imaging of acute wrist injury. An international survey published in 2006 (Groves et al. 2006) of hospital practices revealed marked inconsistency in acute wrist fracture imaging protocols, which the authors believe are likely to be multifactorial but also probably reflected a deficiency in scientific evidence regarding the best practice for imaging occult wrist fractures. Moreover, practices will vary according to local expertise and availability of the different modalities operating within the constraints of individual healthcare local resources. In our institution we use CT scan to detect occult fractures if the second plain radiograph after 10–14 days of injury has been negative. Criteria for a bone fracture on CT images are the presence of a sharp lucent line within the trabecular bone, a break in the continuity of the cortex, a sharp step in the cortex, or a dislocation of bone fragments. Trabecular fractures on CT (without cortical disruption) can be difficult to differentiate from nutrient vessel. Soft tissue and

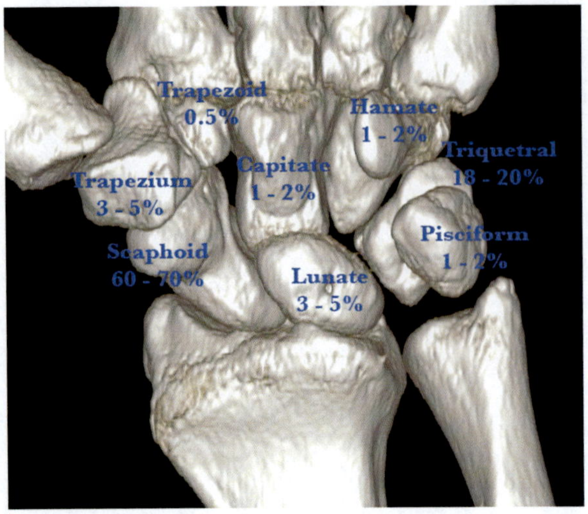

Fig. 2 Illustrates the relative frequency of fractures in the different carpal bones quoted by various sources

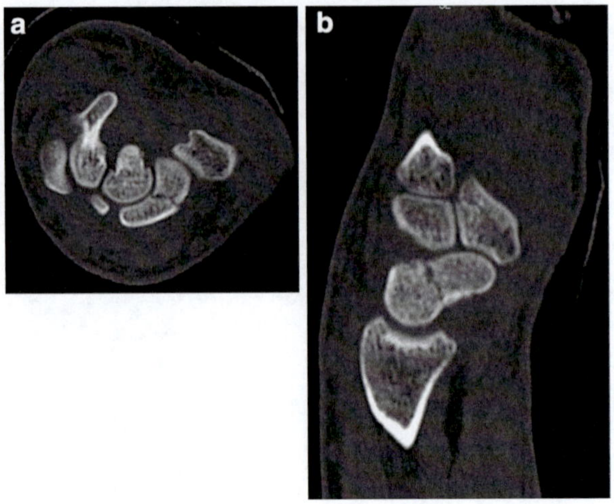

Fig. 3 **a** Transverse CT section through scaphoid demonstrating fracture of the scaphoid waist. **b** Sagittal CT section through scaphoid demonstrating fracture of the scaphoid waist

ligamentous injury on non-contrast CT cannot be accurately diagnosed (Adey et al. 2007). On MR imaging, one can more reliably identify trabecular fracture, and differentiation from a vessel can be done with much more confidence. In addition, bone bruising and ligamentous injuries can be more reliably identified on MRI and not CT. A recent meta-analysis (Yin et al. 2010) examined various studies performed in detecting occult scaphoid fracture comparing between bone scintigraphy, CT and MRI. MRI was shown to be more sensitive (96 %) than CT (93 %). but the specificity of both modalities remains the same (99 %). The meta-analysis also acknowledged that due to low numbers, there was lack of robust evidence to support one modality over another. (Fig. 2).

3.2.1 Scaphoid Fractures

The scaphoid is the largest bone of the proximal carpal row and provides an important link between the proximal and distal carpal row. It is also the most commonly fractured carpal bone accounting for about 70 % of wrist bone fractures (Welling et al. 2008). Waist of the scaphoid is the most common site of fracture.

Choice of imaging is dependent on local availability and as explained above, between MRI and CT, there is no clear winner. MRI is better in the diagnosis of trabecular fractures but CT is better in diagnosis of cortical fractures. MRI is more sensitive in early diagnosis of fractures but there is no clear evidence that it is significantly better than CT (Yin et al. 2010).

The most commonly reported cause of scaphoid fracture is a fall on outstretched hand with forced dorsiflexion of the wrist. Compression or avulsion of the tuberosity is also seen occasionally. Proximal pole avulsion fractures can occur due to traction on the scapho-lunate ligament (Fig. 3).

3.2.2 Lunate Fractures

Lunate fractures account for about 4 % of all carpal fractures. Lunate occupies a central position in the proximal carpal row. Like the scaphoid, late diagnosis or non-diagnosis can result in carpal instability, nonunion and avascular necrosis. Isolated lunate fracture is often difficult to diagnose as lunate overlaps with other carpal bones on radiographs. CT imaging can demonstrate all patterns of fracture. Fracture pattern of the lunate is described according to anatomical location namely body (Fig. 4), dorsal pole and volar pole and also orientation of fracture line namely transverse and sagittal. Isolated fractures in the coronal plane are extremely rare.

3.2.3 Triquetral Fractures

Triquetral fractures are the second most common carpal fractures with a prevalence of about 20 %. Dorsal ridge fractures are the commonest and occur at the dorsal aspect due to impaction of ulnar styloid process against the dorsal surface during wrist

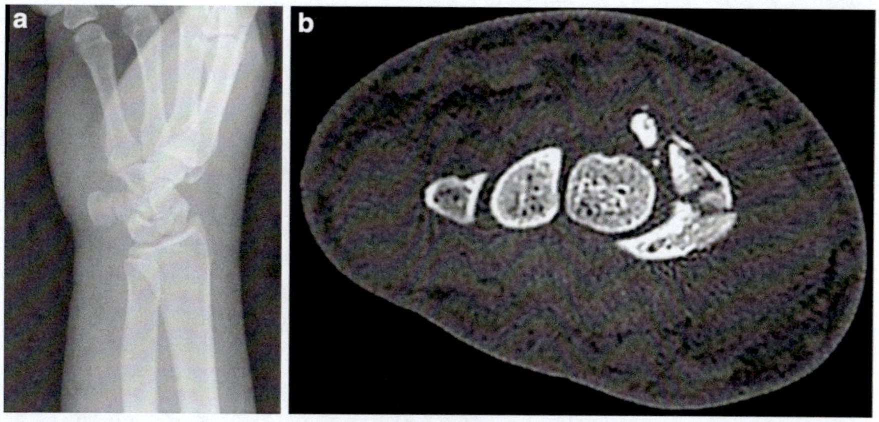

Fig. 4 **a** Plain radiograph that demonstrates a fracture of the lunate. **b** CT transverse section through the lunate in the same patient that demonstrates comminution that is difficult to appreciate on the plain radiograph

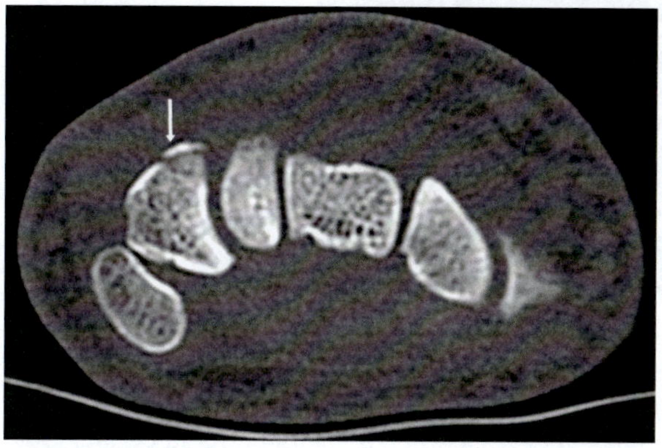

Fig. 5 CT transverse section through the triquetral demonstrating a dorsal ridge fracture (*arrow*) that was occult on the initial plain radiograph

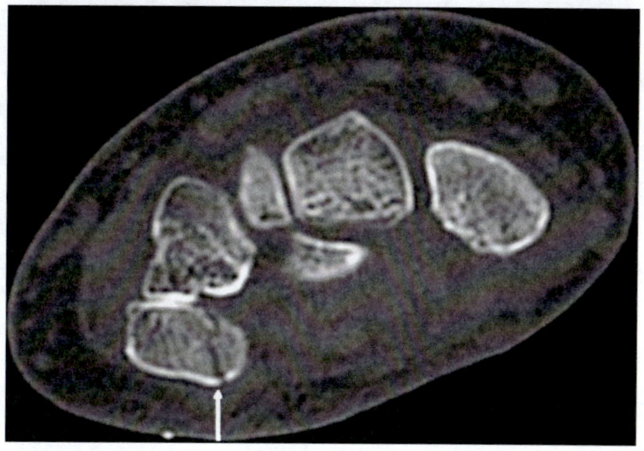

Fig. 6 CT transverse section demonstrating a minimally displaced fracture of the pisiform

hyperextension and ulnar deviation. Alternatively, dorsal ridge fractures may occur in hyperextension that results in ligamentous avulsion from the dorsal surface of the triquetrum. These fractures can be easily picked up on plain radiographs and CT is seldom indicated unless other associated injuries are present.

Fracture of the triquetral body is not very common and occurs in conjunction with perilunate dislocation and CT will be frequently indicated to assess the extent of the injury (Fig. 5).

3.2.4 Pisiform Fractures

The incidence of Pisiform fractures is about 2 %. Pisiform fracture results from a direct blow. Presence of multiple ossification centres and overlap of other bones can make diagnosis of fracture on plain radiograph difficult and CT may be useful to explain the cause of symptoms (Fig. 6).

3.2.5 Trapezium and Trapezoid Fractures

The trapezium is the most mobile bone of the distal carpal row. Trapezial ridge, a vertical prominence on the volar aspect of the trapezium where ligaments and the flexor retinaculum insert, is the most commonly fractured part of trapezium. It might be due to direct blow or avulsion.

Trapezoid is the least commonly fractured carpal bone and accounts for about 0.5 % of carpal fractures. Mechanism is usually high energy impact and fractures can be associated with fractures of other bones. Even though fractures cannot be visualised on plain radiographs, they are frequently picked up on CT (Fig. 7).

3.2.6 Capitate Fractures

The capitate is the largest carpal bone. Injuries are usually caused by high-energy impact. The proximal third of the capitate is almost completely covered by

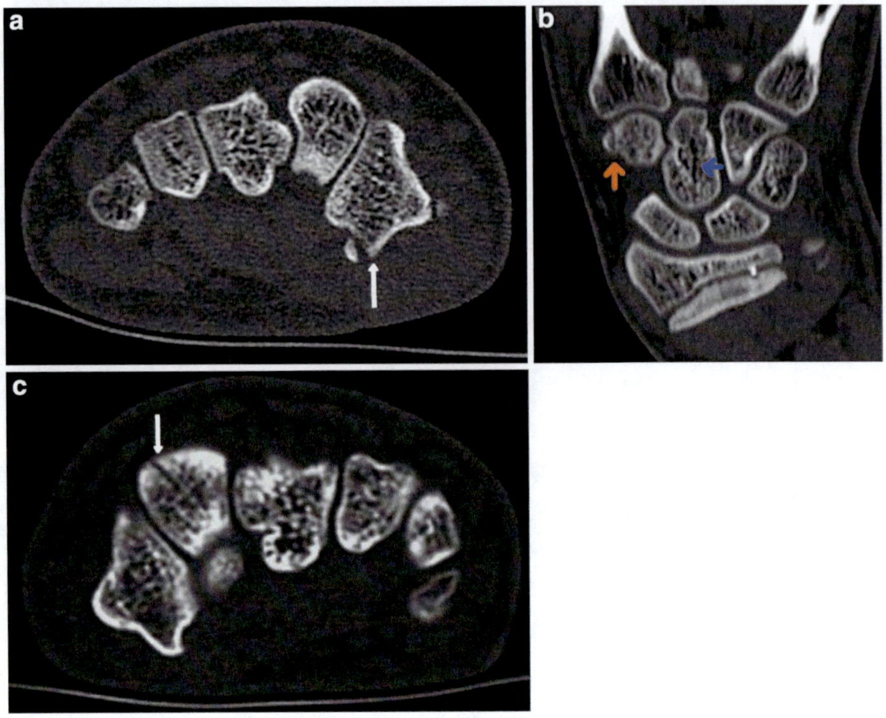

Fig. 7 **a** CT transverse section through the trapezium demonstrating a flake fracture (*arrow*). **b** CT coronal section demonstrating an undisplaced fracture of the trapezoid and a lucent line through the capitate representing a nutrient artery. **c** CT transverse section demonstrating a trapezoid fracture

articular cartilage and CT is frequently used to assess the involvement of the articular surface. Due to poor vascular supply, fractures of the capitate take longer to heal and CT is used to assess healing and look for signs of avascular necrosis (Fig. 8).

3.2.7 Hamate Fractures

Hamate fractures are frequently seen in sporting injuries in individuals using clubs or racquets e.g: Golf and Tennis. These fractures are usually subtle (particularly if they are though the hook of hamate) and are caused by direct trauma from the handle of the club or racquet and can be missed on the plain radiograph. Delayed diagnosis or malunion of the fracture can lead to ulnar nerve palsy and CT is helpful in this scenario (Fig. 9).

3.3 Fractures of Metacarpals

Although metacarpal shaft fractures are easily diagnosed on plain radiographs, fractures and fracture dislocations of the bases of metacarpals can be easily missed and lead to delayed diagnoses and increased morbidity in young patients. Even with views plain radiographs can underestimate the comminution and angulation. Hence CT is used in diagnosis and operative planning of fractures of the metacarpal bones, especially comminuted fractures and those involving the articular surface. Fractures of the base of first metacarpal, even though relatively easier to see on plain radiographs frequently warrant further imaging to assess fragmentation and articular surface. These fractures, if not treated appropriately can lead to early osteoarthritis and disability (Fig. 10).

3.4 Dislocations

Dislocations of the carpal bones can be grossly classified into lunate dislocations, perilunate dislocations or mid-carpal dislocations based on the relative positions of the distal radius articular surface and the carpal bones. (Gilula and Minnie 1979).

In lunate dislocations, the lunate is displaced relative to the distal radius but the rest of the carpal bones (localized by the capitate) are centered over the distal radius. In peri-lunate dislocation, the lunate is centered over the distal radius but the rest of the carpal bones are displaced. If both lunate and capitate

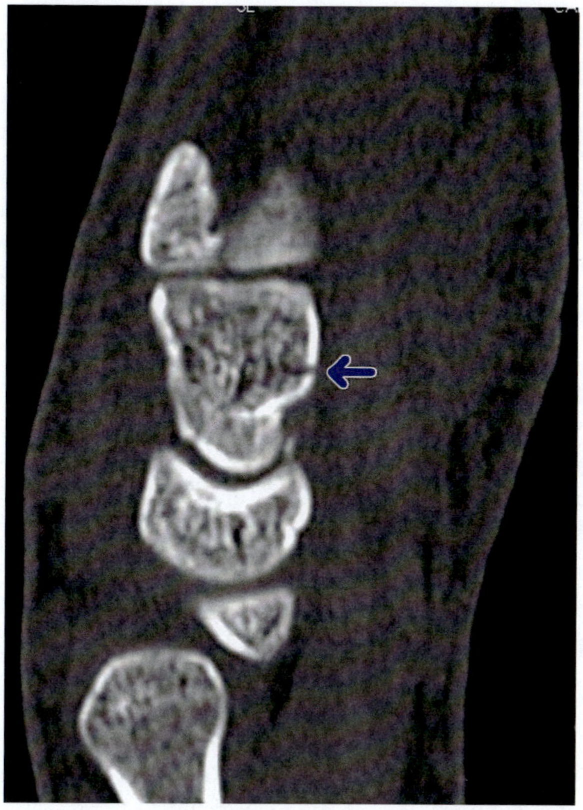

Fig. 8 CT sagittal section through the Capitate demonstrating a fracture line in an oblique plain. (*blue arrow*) Compared with Fig. 7b, note that the line passes through two cortices indicating a fracture as opposed to a nutrient artery which seldom involves two cortices

are dislocated relative to the distal radius, the term mid-carpal dislocation is used.

CT scan is frequently used to assess collateral damage caused by lunate or perilunate dislocations. As stated earlier, CT is able to identify small flake fragments representing avulsion injuries and comminution, especially of articular surfaces although MR imaging is better at assessing ligament injuries. It is not uncommon to use both imaging modalities in conjunction in cases of significant trauma.

The most common dislocation is the perilunate dislocation. These are caused by high energy impact resulting in wrist hyper-extension and ulnar deviation. They are a broad continuum of injuries ranging from minor ligament strains to complete dislocation of the carpus. Perilunate dislocations are generally associated with carpal instabilities. On application of stress, ligamentous failure occurs from ulnar side to radius (Fig. 11).

3.5 Fracture Union

As early as 1987, Bush et al. (1987) concluded that CT was much better than plain radiographs in the assessment of fracture union. CT is better fracture gaps, bony bridges and callus. Although literature has described use of MR and Ultrasound in assessing fracture union CT remains the test of choice in assessment of fracture healing, malunion and non union. Newer techniques discussed at the end of this chapter have improved the visualisation of cortical and cancellous bone even in the presence of metal work.

3.5.1 Sequelae of Trauma (Scapho Lunate Advanced Collapse and Scaphoid Non Union Advanced Collapse)

Degenerative changes in the joint are the most common sequelae of trauma.

Scapholunate Advanced collapse (SLAC) is caused by injury to the scapho lunate (SL) ligament, especially the dorsal component which is the most critical scapholunate stabiliser. The ligament can be injured in isolation or as part of perilunate dislocation.

When the SL ligament is injured, lunate tends to dorsiflex and scaphoid tends to rotate into a palmar flexed position. Capitate tends to follow the lunate into a dorsiflexed position and also migrates proximally. These spectrum of changes lead to a dorsal intercalated segmental instability (DISI) which in turn leads to degenerative changes commonly referred to as SLAC wrist.

Similar changes can also occur with nonunion of scaphoid fracture. The scapholunate ligament is usually intact but the biomechanics are similar to that described above. The degenerative changes in this case are usually referred to as Scaphoid Nonunion Advanced Collapse (SNAC). Pattern of degenerative changes can help to diagnose these conditions. Although MR arthrography is the preferred mode of investigation in several centres for this sort of injury, CT arthography as described in the next section is almost as sensitive and can be used in places where MR arthrography is contraindicated or difficult to access.

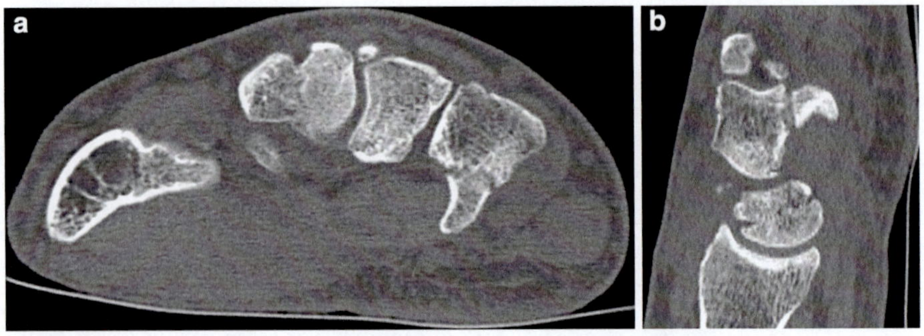

Fig. 9 **a** and **b** Transverse and sagittal reconstructions demonstrating a fracture of the hook of the hamate

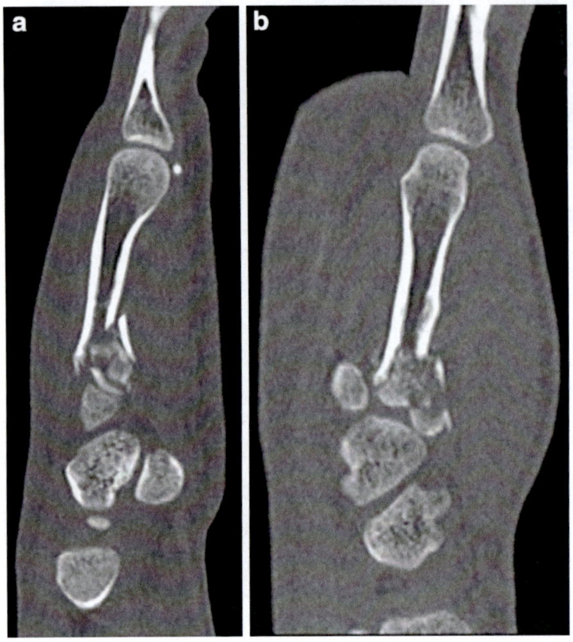

Fig. 10 Base of metacarpal fracture

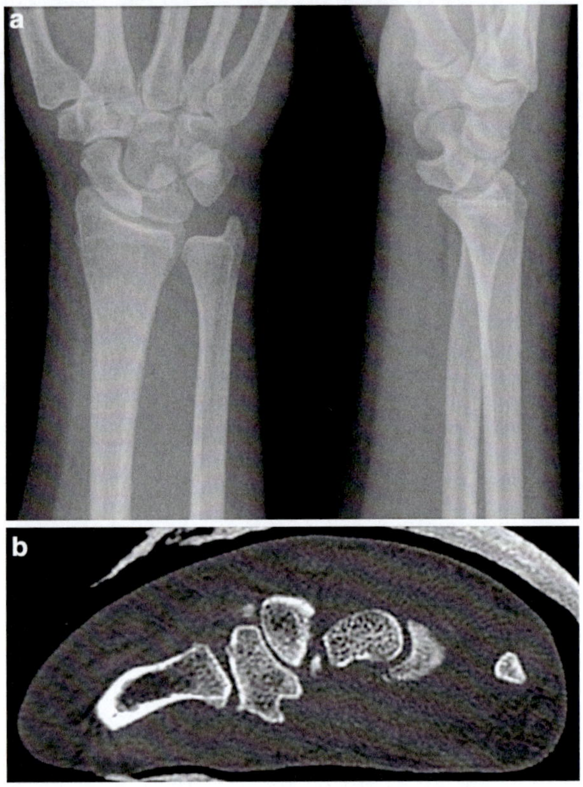

Fig. 11 Lunate dislocation with multiple small avulsion fractures better appreciated on CT scan

First stage involves degenerative changes in the joint between radial styloid and the scaphoid. In the second stage degenerative changes progress to the whole radio-scaphoid joint. In the third stage, changes are seen in scaphocapitate or capitolunate joints (Fig. 12).

3.6 Ligament Injury: CT Arthrography

As alluded to before the wrist joint is one of the most complex joints in the body. For simplification it can be divided into three compartments. The distal radio-ulnar joint, the radiocarpal joint and the midcarpal joint.

The proximal carpal row is very important in the wrist movements as it acts as the intercalated segment (Kauer 1980). The carpal bones in the proximal row are held together by the scapholunate (SL) and the lunotriquetral (LT) ligaments. Both these ligaments are horseshoe shaped, with the palmar and dorsal segments thicker (more important biomechanically) than the central segment (also known as proximal or membranous segment) (Boabighi et al. 1993) (Fig. 13).

They merge anteriorly and posteriorly with the articular capsule, and seal off the radiocarpal and midcarpal compartments (Berger 1996). Another

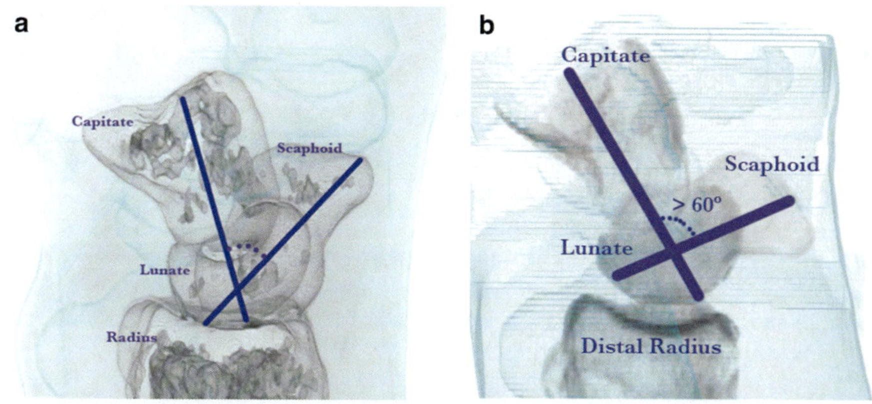

Fig. 12 **a** Demonstration of the normal SL angle(between 30 °–60 °). **b** DISI deformity with dorsal tilt of lunate and SL angle >60 °

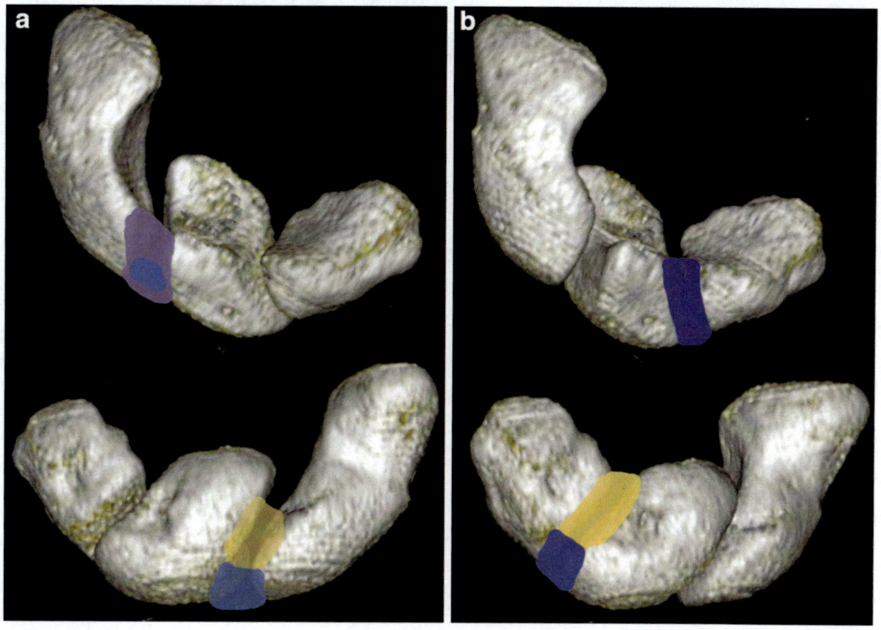

Fig. 13 Demonstration of intrinsic ligaments of the wrist. *Purple*: Volar scapho-lunate and luno triquetral ligaments. *Blue*: Proximal scapho-lunate and luno triquetral ligaments. *Yellow*: Dorsal scapho-lunate and luno triquetral ligaments

important structure is the Triangular Fibro Cartilage Complex (TFCC). It includes the extensor carpi ulnaris tendon sheath, the dorsal radioulnar ligament, the triangular fibrocartilage proper, the volar radio-ulnar ligament, the ulnocarpal ligaments, the ulnar collateral ligament, and the meniscus homologue. The TFCC is the key stabilizer of the DRUJ and it seals off the DRUJ from the radiocarpal joint. The capsular ligaments between the carpal bones form the secondary stabilizers of the wrist joint. These have been described in detail in literature. (Viegas 2001).

These intrinsic ligaments of the wrist can be depicted with several imaging modalities, including conventional arthrography, MR imaging (with and without intraarticular contrast agent administration), and CT arthrography. The development of dynamic multislice CT studies allows a diagnostic approach that combines dynamic information and the accurate assessment of ligaments and the TFC complex.

Technique: Firstly the wrist is positioned horizontally under vertical fluoroscopic guidance. Then under aseptic conditions, using a 24-gauge needle, puncture is made on the dorsal aspect of the wrist (as demonstrated in Fig 14a). On average, a total of 5 mL of iodinated contrast medium is injected. The concentration should be lower than 300 mg of iodine per milliliter to avoid beam-hardening artifacts with MDCT. After the injection the patient is immediately directed to the MDCT to avoid excessive dilution of contrast medium.

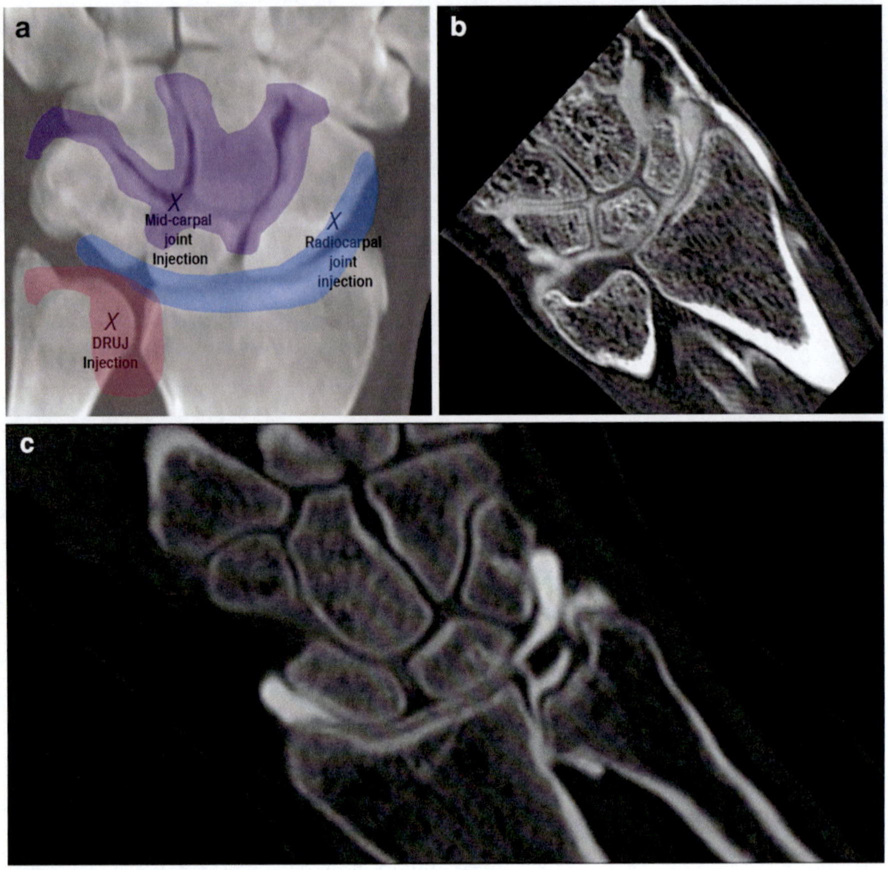

Fig. 14 **a** Image representing the various joint capsules and sites for injection. *Purple*: mid carpal joint with injection site between the carpals *Blue*: Radiocarpal joint with preferred injection site being over the proximal articular surface of scaphoid. *Pink*: Distal radio-ulnar joint with preferred injection site over the distal ulna. **b** Contrast injected into radiocarpal joint was seen within the Distal radio ulnar joint (DRUJ) indicating a perforation of the Triangular fibro cartialge complex (TFCC). **c** Contrast is replacing the normal and LT ligaments indicating a full thickness tear in this young patient who had recent trauma

CT scan is then acquired as described in the previous section.

Coronal images provide a practical overview of the wrist joint. The central (proximal) parts of SL and LT ligaments are best seen on the coronal reformats and are usually meniscoid and insert onto cartilage. The transverse images are essential for appreciating the functionally important dorsal and volar portions of the SL and LT ligaments which are flat and insert onto the bones. Sagittal images provide a good analysis of the TFCC.

Ligament tears: These can be traumatic or degenerative. The traumatic tears are usually after fall on an outstretched hand and may be associated with carpal bone dislocations or fractures. Classification of ligament tears helps differentiate full-thickness (usually communicating) tears from partial-thickness (non-communicating) tears (Fig. 14b). For MDCT arthrography, a ligament tear is defined as communication of intraarticular contrast material through any segment of the ligament. TFCC tears (Fig. 14c) are routinely classified according to the system developed by (Palmer 1989).

In the literature the sensitivity and specificity of CT arthrography has been described as high as 100 % for detecting SL ligament tears and 85 and 100 %, respectively, for LT ligament tears (Theumann et al. 2001; Schmid et al. 2005).

The advantages of CT are small field of view, excellent spatial resolution and quick scan time which virtually eliminates movement artifact.

3.7 Arthropathies

The commonest site of osteoarthritis (OA) in the hand is the first carpometacarpal (CMC) joint followed by distal interphalangeal joints. OA affecting the CMC joint is often debilitating, most commonly affecting postmenopausal women. The first CMC joint is the most commonly operated site in the hand for arthritis (Arnett et al. 1988). CT is useful in

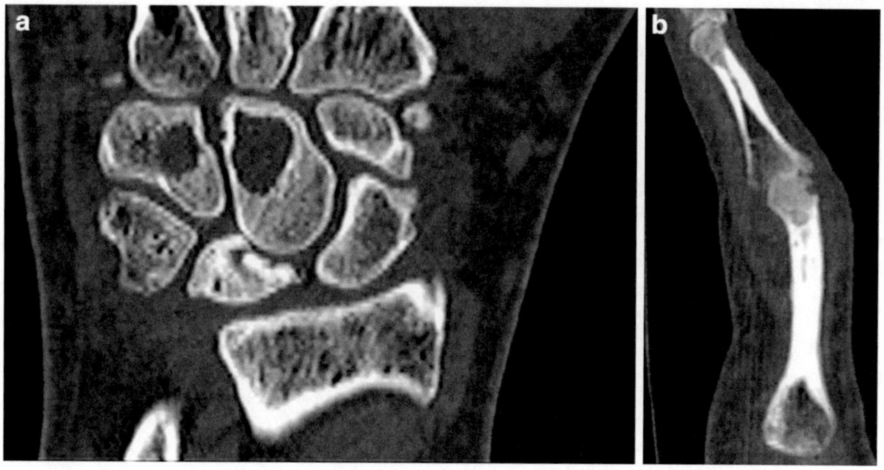

Fig. 15 **a** Cyst within Capitate. Note the clarity of the intact cortical outline. **b** Erosion, tip of proximal phalanx. Due to the size of the erosion, it would have been difficult to illustrate on MR

operative planning and postoperative follow up if required.

Rheumatoid arthritis (RA) is a chronic inflammatory arthropathy of unknown etiology affecting a large cohort of the population. The success of disease modifying antirheumatic drugs (DMARD) and more recently the advent of biologic response-modifying drugs has increased the interest in the imaging modalities for evaluating the disease progression. These drugs are not only very expensive but are also potentially toxic necessitating their judicious use. The presence of erosions in early disease serves as a diagnostic marker for RA and is a sign of poor prognosis, signaling potentially aggressive disease (Van der Heijde et al. 1992).

Plain Radiographs, Doppler Ultrasound, Computerized Tomography (CT), Magnetic Resonance Imaging (MRI) and scintigraphy have been used for evaluation and diagnosis of the erosions. (Østergaard et al. 2003).

In CT cortical bone, being very dense, is readily visible, as is the interface with adjacent soft tissues. Thus, CT is capable of clearly delineating the borders of erosions and differentiating bone (whether edematous or not) from inflamed synovium. While plain radiography has traditionally been used as the gold standard for imaging erosions, the main disadvantage is that there are many regions such as the carpal bones where complex three-dimensional anatomy is very inadequately depicted using a two-dimensional modality. This problem is circumvented by multi-detector helical CT (MDCT), which offers the benefits of multiplanar capability, similar to MRI, with the enhanced cortical definition intrinsic to plain radiography. Erosions on CT were defined as focal areas of loss of cortex with sharply defined margins, seen in two planes, with cortical break seen in at least one plane (Perry et al. 2005).

The main advantages of CT are that it is less expensive and faster than MR. The quick scan time is very useful in patients with concurrent shoulder disease, who have to be lying in the superman position for the scan. Another disadvantage of MR may be the conventional 3 mm slice thickness which can lead to partial volume artifacts on MR. This may lead to misinterpretation of small erosions. MDCT has the advantage of capability of acquiring images of 0.5 mm slice thickness thus reducing this artifact. Bone sclerosis can mask erosions on the MRI, but MDCT is capable of detecting erosions in the presence of extensive sclerosis. MRI does have the advantage that it allows imaging of inflammatory change within the joint, including synovitis, bone edema, and the "activity status" of erosions. None of these can be detected using CT (Perry et al. 2005). These modalities should therefore be regarded as complementary to each other in the detection of disease activity in rheumatoid patients (Fig. 15).

3.8 Tumor Imaging

Role of CT in evaluation of tumours can be complimentary to MR, which is the main modality used for local tumor staging. If a lesion is suspected or discovered, the diagnostic work-up should begin with plain radiographs of the area of interest. If the tumor characterization with radiography is sufficient and in

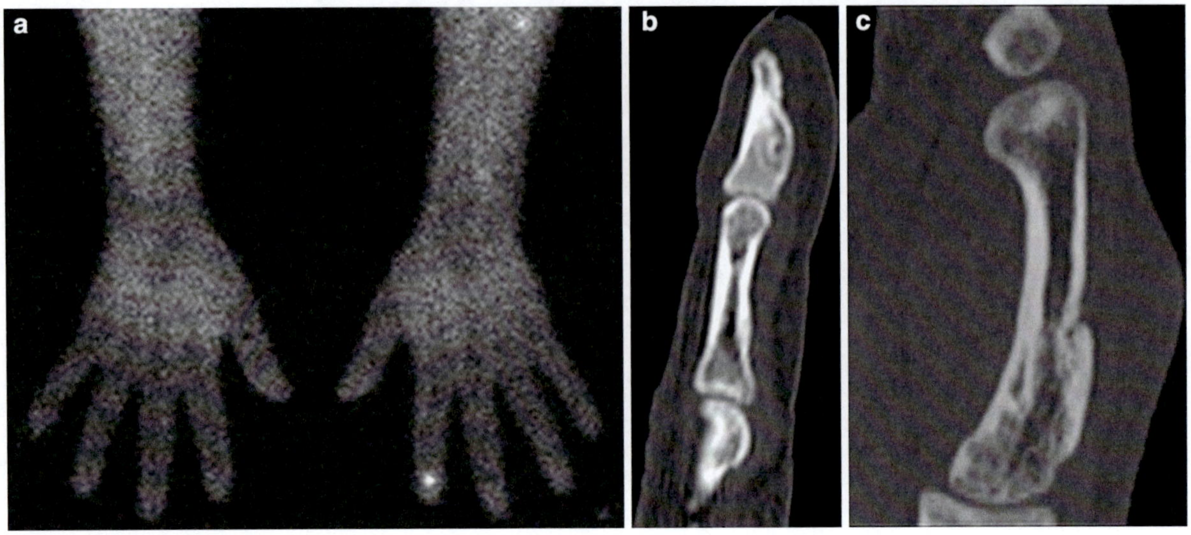

Fig. 16 **a** Bone scintigraphy demonstrating a 'hot spot' which on subsequent CT. **b** was shown to be an osteoid osteoma with smooth round margins and central nidus. Contrast with **c** where cortical break and irregularity of margins is demonstrated in keeping with a more aggressive lesion; in this case osteomyelitis

an adult metastatic disease is suspected then a bone scan to look for multiple metastatic lesions followed by a CT scan of the thorax, abdomen and pelvis is usually recommended. But if a primary bone tumor is suspected then work-up should proceed with MR imaging to evaluate the intra and extraosseous extent of tumor. Where it may be difficult to discern the pattern of bone destruction, it is recommended that CT be performed following radiography. This will help determine the pattern of bone destruction and periosteal new bone formation and to assess for the presence of matrix mineralization.

Osteoid osteoma is a benign bone tumor representing approximately 10 % of all benign bone tumors. It is more common in the lower limbs. Localization in the hand occurs with an incidence of 8 % of all reported cases (Allieu and Lussiez 1988). The phalanges are the most frequent sites in the hand (Ambrosia et al. 1987) followed by the carpal bones. Lesions in the hand may display less reactive sclerosis, a finding that can be misleading. Because of the proximity of the bones in the hands and feet, an inflammatory reaction that originates from one carpal or tarsal lesion often spreads to adjacent bones and joints. Moreover, soft-tissue swelling may be prominent in osteoid osteomas of the hands and feet, a finding that may resemble infection or inflammatory arthritis.

Many studies have shown CT is more useful than MR in illustrating the nidus. (Assoun et al. 1994) CT demonstrates the nidus as a round or oval well defined area with low attenuation. An area of high attenuation may be seen centrally, a finding that represents mineralized osteoid (Gamba et al. 1984) At radiography, it is very difficult to differentiate an intracortical abscess with a sequestrum and an osteoid osteoma with a calcified nidus. However, it is easier to differentiate between the two conditions on CT. In osteoid osteoma, the inner side of the nidus is smooth, and a round calcification is seen in the center of the nidus. In an intracortical abscess, the inner margin is irregular, and an irregularly shaped sequestrum is seen eccentrically (Chai et al. 2010) (Fig. 16).

4 Modern Advances

The limitations of CT scanning traditionally have been high radiation dose, low temporal resolution and artefacts due to metals. Another criticism has been that the anatomical images produced using a CT scanner are a 'snapshot in time' that do not show the dynamic interaction between the various structures which would be useful in guiding treatment. This is especially true of complex joints like the wrist.

Newer generation scanners have several features that help to overcome these limitations.

Various dose reduction techniques have been introduced by different CT manufacturers. With the increase in computing power, statistical and model based iterative reconstruction algorithms are being used for image manipulation. Research work being carried out in various hospitals including our institution have shown that extremity CT scans with good quality diagnostic images can be produced at doses comparable to plain radiography. If proven to work safely and accurately in a clinical setting, CT scans could replace plain radiography in the initial evaluation of trauma.

Modern scanners have high temporal resolution which can be utilised to perform dynamic imaging. Dynamic CT scan of the wrist has been performed in an experimental setting using cadaveric hand by Leng et al. (2011). This is possible due to the high temporal resolution offered by newer generation scanners. In the experimental setting, joint stability and relative motion of the carpal bones could be assessed. This is useful in early SLAC and SNAC wrist before the degenerative changes set in.

Artifacts due to metal can be reduced significantly by newer noise reduction techniques. Better receptors and high definition scanning modes also help to reduce metal artifacts. Another feature that is available in newer scanners is dual energy tubes. By using X-rays at two different energies (e.g 80 and 140 kV) metal prosthesis can be digitally subtracted to assess fracture healing, periprosthetic fractures and joint integrity.

Dual energy CT scanners have found application in characterisation of crystals in joints especially in patients suffering from Gout. Glazebrook et al. (2011) have demonstrated that Dual energy CT can successfully characterize uric acid crystals. Although in most clinical settings, it is difficult to justify irradiating the patient rather than aspirating easily accessible joints like the wrist, it can be used in special circumstances where aspiration is difficult or contra indicated.

5 Conclusion

In the four decades since its invention, the use of CT has rocketed. At the same time advances have placed it at the forefront of medical imaging. This progress looks set to continue and CT is more likely to become the modality of choice in the imaging of trauma. Modern advances look promising and CT could encroach into the domain of other modalities like MR imaging and plain radiography.

References

Adey L et al (2007) Computed tomography of suspected scaphoid fractures. J Hand Surg 32(1): 61–66. Available at http://www.ncbi.nlm.nih.gov/pubmed/18780093

Allieu Y, Lussiez B (1988) Osteoid osteoma of the hand. Apropos of 46 cases. Ann Chir Main 7:298–304

Ambrosia JM, Wold LE, Amadio PC (1987) Osteoid osteoma of the hand and wrist. J Hand Surg (Am) 12:794–800

Arnett FC et al (1988) The American Rheumatism Association 1987 revised criteria for the classification of rheumatoid arthritis. Arthr Rheum 31(3):315–324. Available at http://www.ncbi.nlm.nih.gov/pubmed/3358796

Assoun J, Richardi G, Railhac JJ et al (1994) Osteoid osteoma: MR imaging versus CT. Radiology 191(1):217–223

Berger RA (1996) The gross and histologic anatomy of the scapholunate interosseous ligament. J Hand Surg 21(2):170–178. Available at http://www.ncbi.nlm.nih.gov/pubmed/8683042

Boabighi A, Kuhlmann JN, Kenesi C (1993) The distal ligamentous complex of the scaphoid and the scapho-lunate ligament. An anatomic, histological and biomechanical study. J Hand Surg Edinburgh Scotland 18(1):65–69

Bush CH, Gillespy T, Dell PC (1987) High-resolution CT of the wrist: initial experience with scaphoid disorders and surgical fusions. Am J Roentgenol 149(4):757–760

Chai JW, Hong SH, Choi JY et al (2010) Radiologic diagnosis of osteoid osteoma: from simple to challenging findings. RadioGraphics 30:737

Gamba JL, Martinez S, Apple J, Harrelson JM, Nunley JA (1984) Computed tomography of axial skeletal osteoid osteomas. Am J Roentgenol 142(4):769–772

Gilula LA, Minnie A (1979) Review carpal injuries: analytic approach and case exercises. Am J Roentgenol 133: 503–517

Glazebrook KN et al (2011) Identification of intraarticular and periarticular uric acid crystals with dual-energy CT: initial evaluation. Radiology 261(2):516–524. Available at http://www.ncbi.nlm.nih.gov/pubmed/21926378

Groves AM et al (2006) An international survey of hospital practice in the imaging of acute scaphoid trauma. Am J Roentgenol 187(6):1453–1456. Available at http://www.ncbi.nlm.nih.gov/pubmed/17114536. Accessed 29 Jan 2012

Kauer JM (1980) The functional anatomy of body mass. In: Damuth J, MacFadden BJ (eds) Clin Orthop Relat Res 149(149):9–20. Available at http://www.ncbi.nlm.nih.gov/pubmed/11824284

Leng S et al (2011) Dynamic CT technique for assessment of wrist joint instabilities. Med Phys 38(S1):S50. Available at http://link.aip.org/link/MPHYA6/v38/iS1/pS50/s1&Agg=doi

Østergaard M et al. (2003) New radiographic bone erosions in the wrists of patients with rheumatoid arthritis are detectable with magnetic resonance imaging a median of two years earlier. Available at http://www.ncbi.nlm.nih.gov/pubmed/12905465

Palmer AK (1989) Triangular fibrocartilage complex lesions: a classification. J Hand Surg 14(4):594–606. Available at http://www.ncbi.nlm.nih.gov/pubmed/2666492

Perry D et al (2005) Detection of erosions in the rheumatoid hand; a comparative study of multidetector computerized tomography versus magnetic resonance scanning. J Rheumatol 32(2):256–267. Available at http://www.jrheum.org/content/32/2/256.abstract

Schmid MR et al (2005) Interosseous ligament tears of the wrist: comparison of multi-detector row CT arthrography and MR imaging. Radiology 237(3):1008–1013. Available at http://www.ncbi.nlm.nih.gov/pubmed/16304116

Sternbach G (1985) Abraham Colles: fracture of the carpal extremity of the radius. J Emerg Med 2(6):447–450

Theumann N et al (2001) Wrist ligament injuries: value of post-arthrography computed tomography. Skelet Radiol 30(2):88–93. Available at http://dx.doi.org/10.1007/s002560000302

Van Der Heijde DM et al (1992) Prognostic factors for radiographic damage and physical disability in early rheumatoid arthritis. A prospective follow-up study of 147 patients. Br J Rheumatol 31(8):519–525. Available at http://research.bmn.com/medline/search/results?uid=MDLN.92353764

Viegas SF (2001) The dorsal ligaments of the wrist. Hand Clin 17(1):65–75, vi. Available at http://www.ncbi.nlm.nih.gov/entrez/query.fcgi?cmd=Retrieve&db=PubMed&dopt=Citation&list_uids=11280160

Welling RD et al (2008) MDCT and radiography of wrist fractures: radiographic sensitivity and fracture patterns. Am J Roentgenol 190(1):10–16. Available at http://www.ncbi.nlm.nih.gov/pubmed/18094287

Yin Z-G et al (2010) Diagnosing suspected scaphoid fractures: a systematic review and meta-analysis. Clin Orthop Relat Res 468(3):723–734. Available at http://www.pubmedcentral.nih.gov/articlerender.fcgi?artid=2816764&tool=pmcentrez&rendertype=abstract

MRI and MR Arthrography

Emma L. Rowbotham and Andrew J. Grainger

Contents

E. L. Rowbotham (✉)
Royal United Hospital, Bath, UK
e-mail: emmarowbotham@doctors.org.uk

A. J. Grainger
Department of Musculoskeletal Radiology,
Chapel Allerton Orthopaedic Centre,
Leeds, LS7 4SA, UK
e-mail: andrew.grainger@leedsth.nhs.uk

Abstract

The complex anatomical nature of the hand and wrist brings about diagnostic challenges both for the Clinician and the Radiologist when considering pathology in this region. MR is a proven, widely employed imaging modality used in the detection, assessment and follow-up of disorders of both the hand and the wrist. Optimisation of both sequences and protocols are essential in order to provide good quality images which allow high sensitivity and specificity for detection of pathology. High field strength units are usually used in hand and wrist imaging alongside dedicated extremity coils. Even then, there are numerous artefacts which may be encountered including movement, pulsation, truncation, magic angle and chemical shift. These phenomena will be discussed in this chapter in addition to a brief outline of sequences and their potential uses. Pathology relating to osseous structures, tendons, TFCC and both intrinsic and extrinsic ligaments are all readily assessed on MR imaging and the optimal planes for imaging are discussed alongside common pathologies and potential pitfalls in image interpretation. MR arthrography is also discussed with particular reference to both TFCC and intrinsic ligament pathology. Recent advances in technology, including the advent of 7T units, have led to improvements in the assessment of articular cartilage at the wrist and techniques of biological imaging, which continue to evolve.

A. M. Davis et al. (eds.), *Imaging of the Hand and Wrist*, Medical Radiology. Diagnostic Imaging,
DOI: 10.1007/174_2012_700,

1 Introduction

The complex anatomical nature of the hand and wrist brings about diagnostic challenges both for the Clinician and the Radiologist when considering pathology in this region. However, advances in imaging techniques have allowed increasingly accurate diagnostic performance and MR imaging is a proven, widely employed imaging modality for the detection, assessment and follow-up of disorders of the hand and wrist. The radiologist requires a detailed knowledge of the anatomy and range of pathological conditions affecting the hand and wrist. However, a knowledge of the clinical information and careful consideration of the available and most appropriate imaging modalities are essential in determining the relevant technique and sequence protocols.

There are many potential pitfalls when imaging the hand and wrist, an incorrect sequence or misinterpretation of an anatomical variant may lead to inaccurate diagnosis particularly of both TFCC and intrinsic ligament pathology. This chapter will provide a review of technical considerations and MR protocols followed by discussion of the most common and most relevant clinical applications.

2 Technical Considerations

In general terms, the higher the magnetic field strength used in MR imaging the greater both the signal-to-noise ratio (SNR) and the contrast-to-noise ratio (CNR) achieved. An increased SNR allows thinner slice thickness which in turn allows greater spatial resolution and also shorter acquisition times, thereby reducing the likelihood of patient movement. Thin and contiguous slices are needed in order to accurately image the intrinsic structures of the wrist many of which are no greater than a few millimetres thick.

A high field strength magnet (1.0T or higher) is usually preferred for optimal imaging of the fine architecture of the hand and wrist; in addition a local or surface coil is necessary to ensure sufficient signal-to-noise ratio. However, for applications which rely on contrast resolution as opposed to spatial resolution—for example evaluation of radiographically occult fractures or osteonecrosis of the carpus—lower field strength extremity units (0.1–0.6T) in either open or extremity units may suffice to answer a specific clinical question. However, in this situation cartilage lesions and subtle pathology of the tendons, ligaments and fibrocartilage will not be as readily identified. These low field strength scanners may be useful where there is limited space available within a department and for patients who are either claustrophobic or obese.

The majority of studies comparing the sensitivity and specificity of low field strength versus high field strength units in the upper limb have focussed on shoulder imaging, often with conflicting outcomes. Currently, most centres performing regular hand and wrist imaging will use at least a 1.5T unit and increasingly 3T units are becoming the norm. Thinner slices are possible with 3T imaging and CNR may be increased by a magnitude of 2.0–2.9 times that of 1.5T if all other parameters are kept constant (Saupe et al. 2005). Studies have shown the higher SNR and CNR obtained with 3T units allow significantly improved visualisation of the small anatomical structures of the hand and wrist including the scapholunate and lunotriquetral ligaments (Saupe et al. 2005). Although direct comparisons have not been undertaken, findings suggest that 3T imaging may have improved sensitivity and specificity compared to 1.5T imaging for detection of both TFCC tears and scapholunate tears (Magee 2009). Improved visualisation of the median and ulnar nerves at high field strengths imaging has also been documented (Farooki et al. 2002).

Coil selection is also vitally important in hand and wrist imaging and receiver coils with high signal-to-noise ratio capability and uniformity are needed. Surface array coils are used to provide high SNR and an extended field-of-view (Roemer et al. 1990). Studies have also shown that phased array coils and adapted birdcage head coils may be used to provide both high SNR and image uniformity (Kocharian et al. 2002). Coils continue to improve with greater numbers of elements, but the optimising coils for hand and wrist imaging remains an engineering challenge.

2.1 Positioning

In high field strength systems, there are two main options for patient positioning; the patient may lie prone within the scanner, with their symptomatic arm stretched out above the head and the wrist positioned

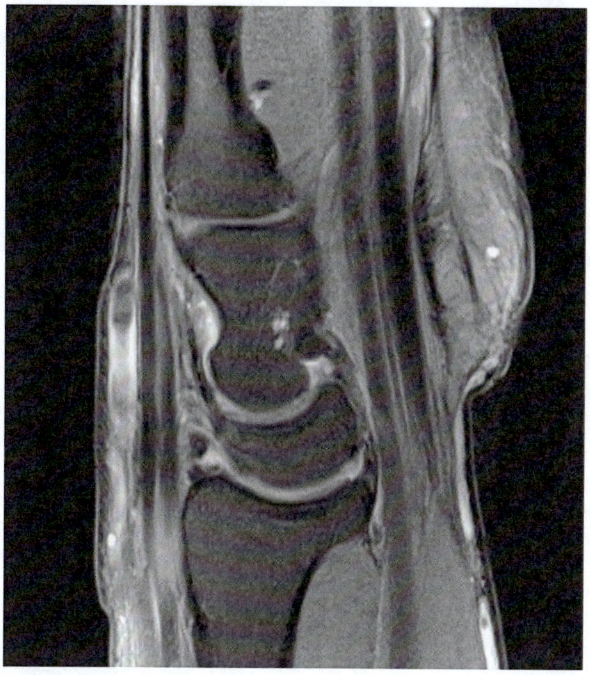

Fig. 1 Sagittal T2W FS image with the wrist in ulnar deviation. The lunate shows slight dorsal tilt but the long axis of the capitate remains aligned with the long axis of the radius—indicating that this appearance is due to physiological positioning

within the isocentre of the magnet, thereby allowing for homogenous fat suppression, or alternatively they may lie supine with the hand and wrist at the side of the body. The latter position may prove to be more comfortable for the patient but can lead to inhomogeneous fat suppression given the wrist and hand are not central within the magnet. Motion artefact can be a significant problem and it may be more important to optimise patient comfort and accept suboptimal positioning. Motion artefact is minimised by using restraints such as foam cushions and wedges. In order that positioning abnormalities are not incorrectly diagnosed as carpal instability syndromes it is important to eliminate significant radial or ulnar deviation at the wrist. However, even correctly positioned wrists may occasionally simulate a dorsal intercalated segment instability and correlation with both clinical findings and a lateral radiograph may be helpful in this situation. It is also useful to note that the long axis of the capitate will remain centred on the long axis of the radius when the lunate undergoes physiological extension, while in a true DISI deformity there will be dorsal translation of the long axis of the capitate (Fig. 1).

The degree of pronation and supination of the wrist will influence the appearances of the distal radioulnar joint (DRUJ). Ideally, MRI is obtained with the wrist in a neutral position as pronation and supination can mimic dorsal and volar subluxation of the ulnar at the DRUJ. It is important to consider wrist positioning before diagnosis of DRUJ subluxation is made (Fig. 2a, b). Pronation and supination also influence the appearance of the relative length of the radius and ulnar. The ulnar appears longer relative to the radius in pronation.

For imaging of the fingers, both supine (with the arm at the side of the body) and prone (with the arm above the head) positions are described in the literature and are accepted techniques for producing good image quality (Blackband et al. 1994). As with wrist imaging positioning within the centre of the magnetic field is vitally important in imaging the fingers. Generally, the fingers are imaged when fully extended, however the flexed position (around 45 degrees), may be of value in evaluating possible pulley lesions as well as collateral ligament injury (Hauger et al. 2000).

For imaging individual finger joints a surface microscopy coil may be useful (Tan et al. 2005). If both hands or both wrists are to be imaged on the same patient then a larger extremity coil may be used to image both sides at one time thereby decreasing the scan time required. The hands and wrists can be placed palm together with the arms above the head both within the coil.

2.2 Imaging Planes

Typically protocols for the hand and wrist include images acquired in all three orthogonal planes. Imaging the thumb presents particular difficulties for alignment of planes as it does not lie in an orthogonal plain relative to the hand and wrist. In this situation, sagittal and coronal imaging is aligned relative to the thumb metacarpal from an axial image.

2.2.1 Axial

Axial imaging is usually performed first as these sequences are then used to set up the coronal and sagittal sequences. The plane should be determined as

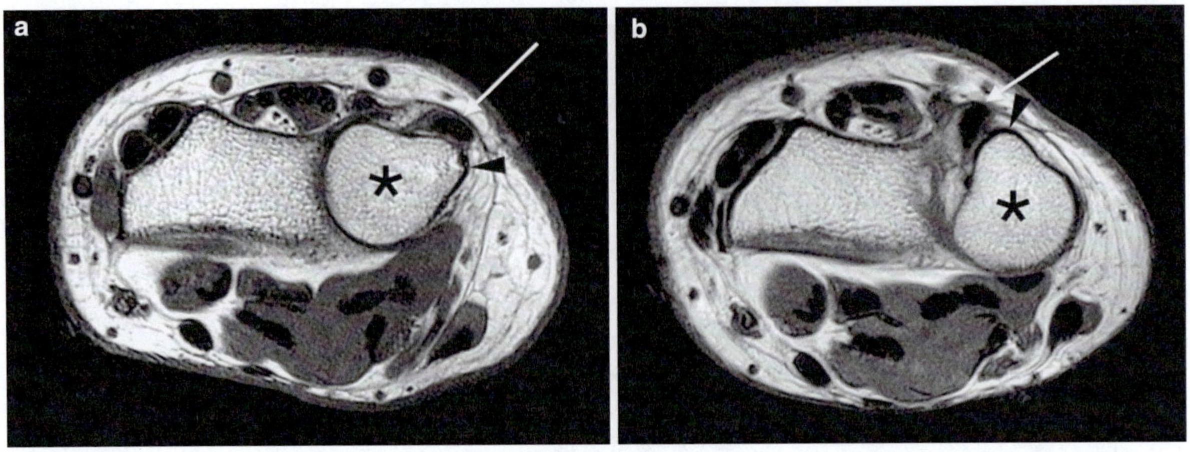

Fig. 2 **a** and **b**—Axial imaging in the same asymptomatic patient with the wrist in **a** pronation and **b** supination. With the wrist in supination appearances suggest volar subluxation of the ulnar (*asterix*) and in pronation there is dorsal subluxation of the ulnar (*asterix*). There is also a marked change in position of the Extensor carpi ulnaris tendon (*white arrow*) between these two wrist positions. To eliminate these apparently abnormal findings it is important to image the wrist in a neutral position

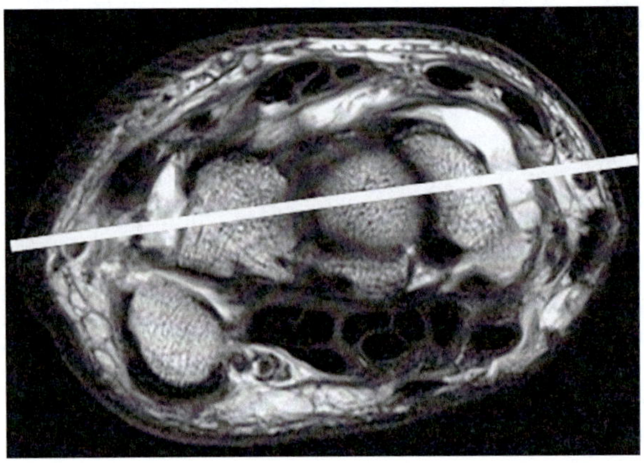

Fig. 3 The coronal plane is determined by a line bisecting the scaphoid, lunate and capitate (*yellow line*) on an axial image through the proximal carpal row

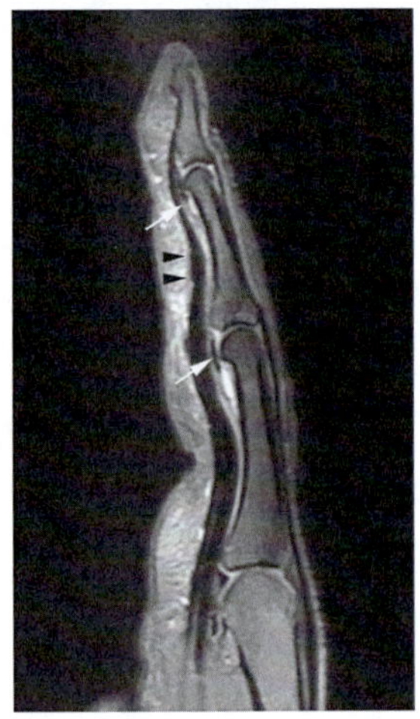

Fig. 4 Sagittal T2 FS image of the index finger shows both the flexor and extensor tendons as low signal structures inserting into the distal phalanx. This plane may be used to assess continuity of the tendons as well as alignment within the digit. The tendon is concave towards the proximal and middle phalanges (*black arrow*) as a result of the action of the associated pulleys at these levels. The volar plate is also demonstrated in this plane (*white arrows*)

being parallel to the distal radius. For imaging of the wrist coverage should include the region between the distal radius/ulnar metaphysis proximally, extending to the proximal metacarpal shafts distally.

2.2.2 Coronal

The correct plane is crucial for coronal imaging and should be derived from an axial image through the proximal carpal row. The plane of section should bisect the scaphoid, lunate and capitate (Fig. 3). The TFCC is best demonstrated on coronal sequences, and this plane may also be used to assess both the intrinsic and extrinsic ligaments of the wrist. For imaging of the fingers the coronal plane will be determined as being parallel to the anterior volar cortex of the metacarpal heads.

2.2.3 Sagittal

The sagittal plane should be perpendicular to the coronal plane and for wrist imaging should include all soft tissues to either side of the radius and ulnar. Sagittal images are useful in determining carpal alignment and carpal instability and in the fingers the flexor and extensor tendons are best evaluated in this plane (Fig. 4).

2.3 Sequences

The exact protocols for imaging the hand and wrist will vary between institutions depending on radiologist and clinician preferences and on the scanning unit involved.

2.3.1 T1 Weighted Imaging

T1 weighted imaging is ideal for detecting marrow infiltration and is also helpful in distinguishing areas of red marrow reconversion from pathological area of change and should be included in a routine wrist protocol in at least one plane without fat saturation.

2.3.2 Fast Spin Echo

Fast Spin Echo (FSE) sequences also referred to as Turbo Spin Echo (TSE) were originally introduced in order to speed up image acquisition through the simultaneous acquisition of multiple echoes. The advantage over spin echo sequences (SE) is the reduction in acquisition time, for long TR sequences. This reduces examination time but also helps to minimise movement artefact whilst maintaining the same SNR. FSE imaging forms the basis of proton density and T2 weighted imaging widely used in clinical hand and wrist MRI. Frequency selective fat suppression will be often applied to these sequences. In addition to improving their sensitivity to water, particularly in fatty bone marrow, fat suppression will also improve contrast between bone and articular cartilage. Fat suppressed proton density FSE imaging is particularly good for imaging articular cartilage. Recently, 3D fast SE became available from some manufacturers giving the potential for thin slice contiguous images and multiplanar reconstructions. Their use is still being evaluated and evidence would suggest they are not yet suitable to replace 2D FSE imaging (Stevens et al. 2011).

2.3.3 Short T1 Inversion Recovery

Short T1 Inversion Recovery (STIR) sequences provide an alternative means to achieve fat suppression. Where a relatively short inversion time is used to null the fat signal whilst maintaining water and soft tissue signal. This technique is particularly helpful where field inhomogeneities prevent uniform fat suppression. This can be a particular problem with hand and wrist imaging if it is not possible to position the area of interest in the isocentre of the magnet. STIR sequences are particularly useful in the detection of bone marrow abnormalities in the hand and wrist such as occult fractures. In addition the TFCC and intrinsic ligaments are often well visualised on STIR sequences. STIR images show high contrast but suffer from a low signal to noise ratio. STIR is not specific to fat and tissues with a similar T1 signal to fat will also be suppressed—this includes structures which have shown enhancement following gadolinium administration.

2.3.4 Gradient Echo

Gradient Echo images provide a high degree of spatial resolution but at the expense of relatively poor contrast resolution. In addition, 3D T1 weighted gradient echo images may be used to allow thin slice multiplanar reconstructions. These sequences show increased susceptibility artefact and therefore are of little use in the presence of metalwork, such as following surgery.

2.3.5 Typical Protocols

As already stated protocols will vary depending on preference, indication of the examination and MRI equipment. Typically, a routine wrist MRI protocol will include axial coronal and sagittal imaging using a combination of FSE proton density and T2 imaging. Fat suppressed imaging is helpful for demonstrating cartilage and improving sensitivity to fluid in bone and will usually be applied in at least two planes. It is important to include at least one non-fat suppressed T1 weighted sequence. The authors also make frequent use of thin slice 3D gradient echo sequences (GE), particularly for the evaluation of subtle bony erosions in the wrist and hand joints.

In some situations a far more limited protocol can be utilised. For instance to identify radiographically occult bone injury, particularly possible scaphoid fracture, T1 and T2 imaging in the coronal and sagittal plane may suffice.

The use of iodinated contrast may be required in some situations such as the evaluation of scaphoid non-union/avascular necrosis or for identifying synovitis (and distinguishing it from effusion) in arthritis imaging.

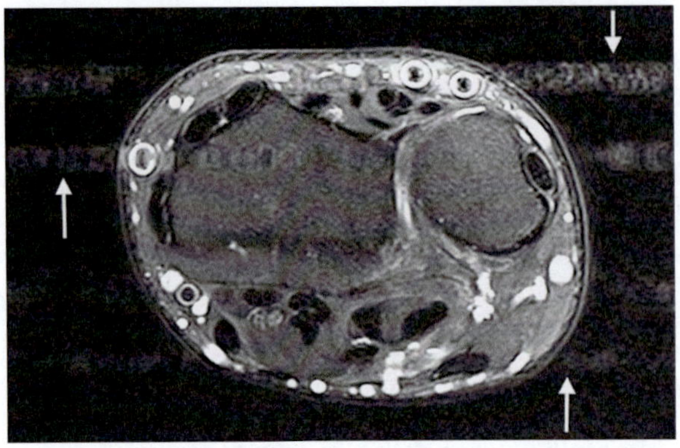

Fig. 5 T2 FSE axial image which shows several areas of flow artefact which manifests as ghosting of the vessels perpendicular to the blood flow in the direction of the phase-encoding gradient (*white arrows*)

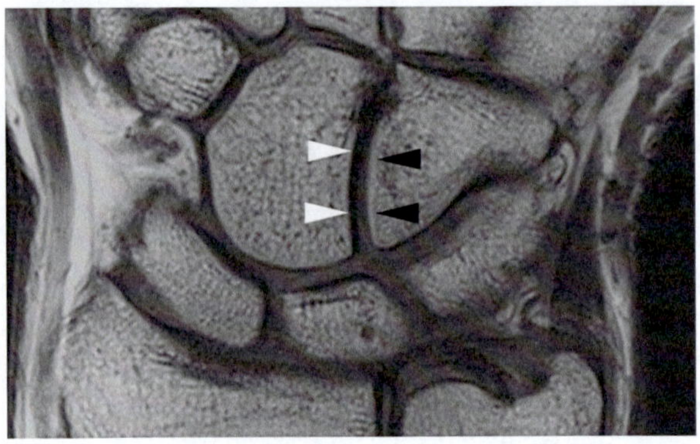

Fig. 6 Chemical shift artefact—Coronal image of the wrist which shows chemical shift artefact between the capitate and hamate. This occurs in the direction of the frequency encoding gradient and manifests as a low signal intensity band adjacent to the subchondral plate of the capitate (appearing as a thickened subchondral plate) (*white arrowheads*) and a corresponding high intensity band along the subchondral bone of the opposing articular surface of the hamate (*black arrowheads*). The effect is to give an apparent asymmetry to the thickness of the articular cartilage on the two surfaces

2.4 Artefacts

2.4.1 Motion Artefact

Motion artefact will manifest as blurring or ghosting of the images. In the hand and wrist patient movement is a common cause however pulsation artefact from vessels may also occur.

2.4.2 Pulsation Artefact

Pulsation artefact results from blood flow and can be minimised by saturation bands perpendicular to blood vessels. The effect can also be minimised by planning the phase encoding direction to cast the artefact away from anatomical structures that need to be evaluated (Fig. 5).

2.4.3 Chemical Shift Phenomena

Chemical shift phenomena are usually apparent at water–fat interfaces due to a difference in resonance frequency between fat and water; fat resonates at a slightly lower frequency than water (Larmor frequency). Both SE and GE may demonstrate chemical shift artefact which appears as a hypointense band, one to several pixels in width, towards the lower part of the gradient field, and as a hyperintense band towards the higher part of the readout gradient field. This phenomenon is more pronounced at higher field strengths and lower gradient strength. In MR imaging of the wrist, chemical shift artefact is most frequently appreciated at the cartilage–bone marrow interface (Fig. 6), and may lead to overestimation or underestimation of the cartilage thickness.

2.4.4 Susceptibility Artefact

Susceptibility artefact is related to the internal magnetisation induced in tissues by the external magnetic field and refers to the focal loss of signal intensity and distortion of the magnetic field secondary to low proton structures such as air or metal. This form of artefact is encountered frequently in musculoskeletal imaging due to the presence of surgical hardware or clips (Fig. 7). The metallic objects produce T2 and $T2^*$ shortening which results in signal loss and geometrical distortion. This effect increases exponentially with high field strength and is one of the disadvantages when imaging at 3T and higher. Approaches to reducing susceptibility artefact include: increasing the band width and/or decreasing the TE, parallel imaging, decreasing the voxel size, or lengthening the echo train length.

2.4.5 Truncation Artefacts

Truncation artefacts may occur at interfaces between high and low signal intensity structures and appear as rings at boundaries such as bone–tissue interfaces. This artefact is related to the finite number of steps used by the Fourier transform to reconstruct an image and is reduced by utilising more frequency encoding steps.

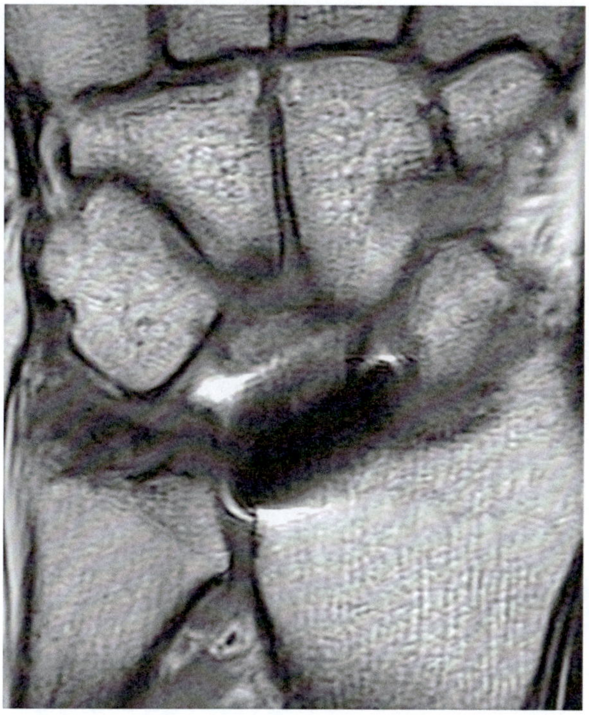

Fig. 7 Susceptibility artefact—Coronal image of the wrist joint in a patient who had previously undergone scapholunate ligament repair. A low signal area is seen in the region of the repair secondary to susceptibility artefact arising from a metallic anchor

2.4.6 Magic Angle Effect

Magic angle effect may be seen in any structure containing collagen fibres and is seen as a result of the dipole interaction between the applied external magnetic field (Bo) and the collagen fibres. This effect results in regions of artefactually increased signal intensity within the structure being imaged on short TE (T1 and proton density) sequences. The phenomenon is maximised when the relative angular orientation of the collagen fibres to the static magnetic field is approximately 55 degrees. Tendons, hyaline cartilage and menisci may all be affected by the magic angle effect which should not be misinterpreted as tendinopathic change or tearing (Fig. 8). Repositioning of the patient in a different orientation to the applied magnetic field or by using sequences with a long echo time (T2-weighted sequences) will eliminate the artefact. When magic angle effect is suspected it is useful to compare the short TE images with the same area on T2 weighted imaging.

2.4.7 Aliasing or Wraparound Artefact

Aliasing or wraparound artefact is seen where an image of tissue from outside the field-of-view (FOV) appears superimposed on images of the area of interest. This may be from a different body part positioned adjacent to the area of interest or the result of parts of the hand or wrist outside the field-of-view being superimposed on the area of interest (Fig. 9). The former is most usually seen when the hand or wrist is positioned by the side of the patient while the latter is particularly common with the small FOV imaging usually employed in hand and wrist imaging. In this case, images of adjacent body parts may be superimposed on the FOV. In both cases the resultant image resembles a double exposure photograph.

All frequency related artefacts are more pronounced at 3T imaging compared with 1.5T imaging (Barth et al. 2007). This includes metal related signal voids and other types of susceptibility artefact related to hemosiderin deposition and at air tissue interfaces as well chemical shift artefact. However, at 3T imaging the increased SNR can be employed to compensate for these artefacts more effectively whilst still maintaining a high degree of spatial resolution.

3 Imaging Findings

3.1 Osseous Structures

T1 weighted images demonstrate osseous anatomy well and are particularly useful for the detection of fracture lines and bone marrow oedema (appearing as a low signal change within the medullary cavity). However, fat suppressed T2 imaging is also sensitive to marrow signal change [seen as increased (fluid) signal] although anatomical definition may be less clearly shown. In cases of non-specific wrist pain, focal bone oedema has been shown to be present in approximately one-third of all cases on MR imaging (Alam et al. 1999); in this study, the causes demonstrated included arthritis, fracture and avascular necrosis.

MR imaging has been proven to be useful post trauma in the context of negative radiographs with particular reference to identifying occult scaphoid fractures (Breitenseher et al. 1997; Hunter et al. 1997). Early confirmation of the diagnosis is possible

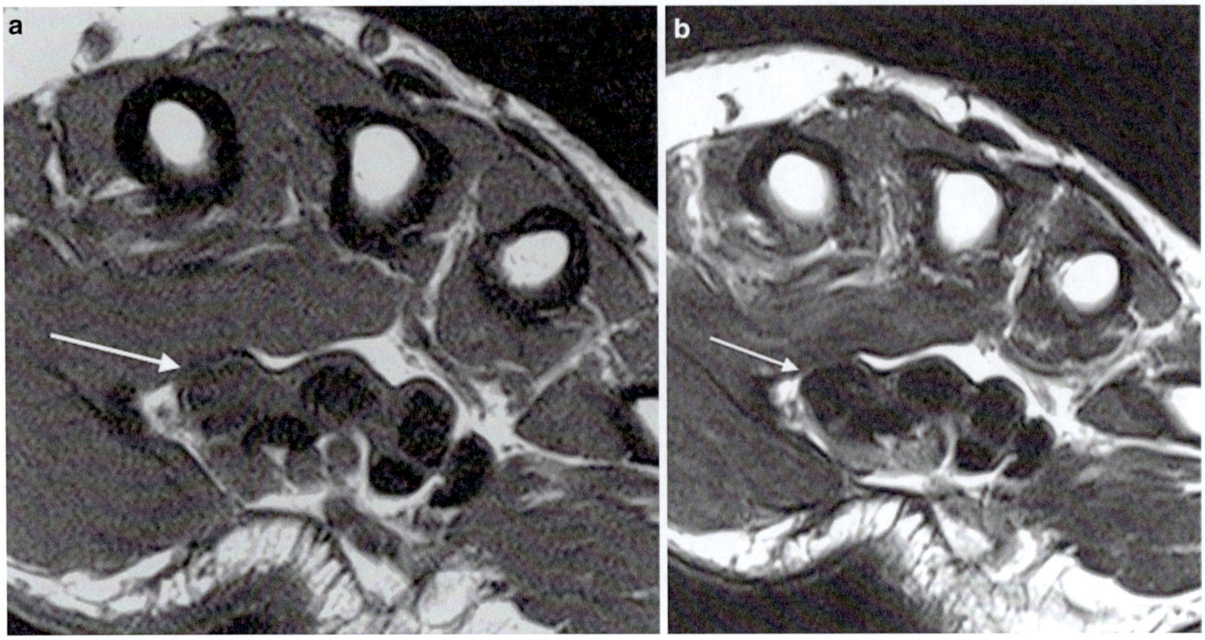

Fig. 8 **a** T1 axial image of the hand distal to the carpal tunnel. There is low signal change seen within the Flexor Pollicis Longus tendon due to magic angle phenomenon (*arrow*). **b** axial image of the same patient but with altered parameters—this sequence has a long TE value and the magic angle phenomenon is abolished (*arrow*)

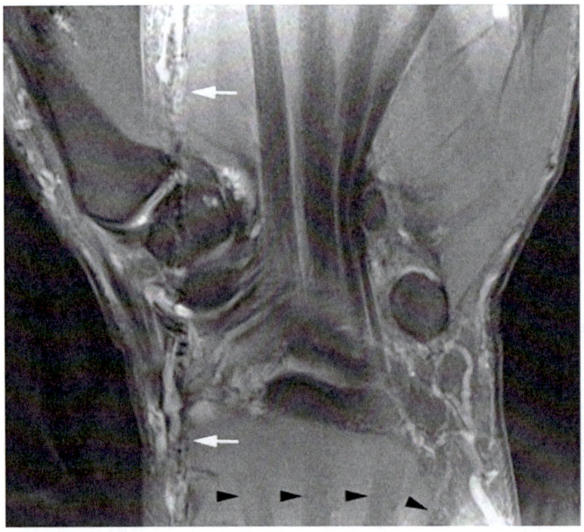

Fig. 9 Wraparound artefact—Superimposed ghosting of the splaying flexor tendons is seen at the periphery of the image as a result of wraparound artefact. In addition, there is a ghost image of the thumb to the *left* of the image

with MR imaging as opposed to the previously accepted method of repeating plain radiographs 7–10 days following the initial presentation. MR imaging is also useful for demonstrating the early stages of avascular necrosis when plain film images appear normal. This is most commonly seen following fracture to the scaphoid in association with non-union. An indicator of developing non-union is sclerosis around the fracture site without evidence of bridging bone. In the advanced stages of the condition findings also include articular surface collapse and fragmentation of the involved bone. Gadolinium sequences are used to assess for the presence of vascularity within the scaphoid where there is concern for avascular necrosis—in this case T1 weighted images show uniform low signal within a necrotic segment and there is no enhancement in a non-viable segment following administration of IV gadolinium.

3.2 Tendons

The extensor tendons situated on the volar aspect of the wrist are divided into six numbered compartments by vertical septae and the extensor retinaculum (Table 1). On the volar aspect of the wrist the eight digital flexor tendons are divided into superficial and deep groups which—along with the flexor pollicis longus tendon which inserts into the distal phalanx of the thumb, pass through the carpal tunnel. The digital flexors share a

Table 1 Extensor tendon compartments

I	Abductor pollicis longus, Extensor pollicis brevis
II	Extensor carpi radialis longus, Extensor carpi radialis brevis
III	Extensor pollicis longus
IV	Extensor digitorum longus
V	Extensor digiti minimi
VI	Extensor carpi ulnaris

common flexor tendon sheath apart from the flexor pollicis longus which has its own sheath. At the level of the carpal tunnel the flexor digitorum superficialis (FDS) tendons lie superficial to the flexor digitorum profundus (FDP) tendons. Each superficial tendon then splits at the level of the proximal phalanx passing either side of the profundus tendon to insert into the middle phalanx. The flexor digitorum profundus continues to insert onto the distal phalanx.

The flexor and extensor tendons of the hand and wrist are best evaluated in an axial plane; normal tendons should appear as homogenously low signal structures regardless of the imaging sequence used (Fig. 10). Both proton density and T2 weighted sequences in the axial plane are usually sufficient to assess the intrinsic signal characteristics of the tendons and assess for any surrounding fluid. The tendons are susceptible to magic angle effect and the T2 sequence is helpful to rule this out where high signal is seen in tendons on the shorter TE sequence (Fig. 8). A small amount of fluid may be seen within the tendon sheath in normal asymptomatic patients and when seen warrants careful correlation with clinical findings before it is reported as abnormal. Tendinopathy is characterised by high signal change within the tendon. The tendon is frequently also thickened. Tenosynovitis is characterised by circumferential high signal fluid within the tendon sheath (Fig. 11). The tendons which are most frequently affected by tendinosis are those of the first and sixth extensor compartments, namely the abductor pollicis longus and the extensor pollicis brevis (involved in De Quervain's tenosynovitis) and the extensor carpi ulnaris respectively. The latter is particularly frequently affected in rheumatoid arthritis. De Quervain's tenosynovitis is typically associated with thickening of the tendons themselves. In the acute phase fluid may be seen in the tendon

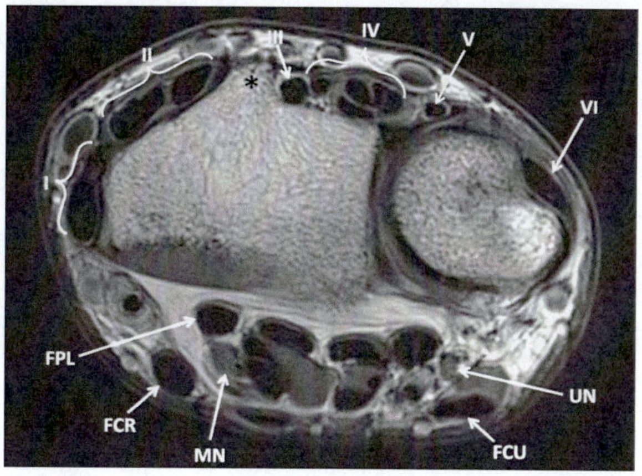

Fig. 10 Axial normal wrist—Axial PD image of the wrist. The tendons appears as homogenously low signal oval structures. The six extensor compartments are labelled on the volar aspect of the wrist. Listers tubercle (*asterix*) is a useful landmark on the distal radius which separates compartments II and III

sheath but in the chronic situation thickening of the soft tissue around the compartment (the extensor retinaculum) will be seen. Tenosynovitis of the digital flexors is commonly related to chronic injury, repetitive microtrauma and inflammatory arthropathy. Flexor tendon tenosynovitis is a common cause of carpal tunnel syndrome due to the close anatomical proximity of these tendons to the median nerve.

Coronal sequences of the flexor and extensor tendons are rarely useful owing to partial volume effects which occur in this plane. Sagittal sequences are of most value when assessing abnormalities of the finger flexor and extensor tendons.

3.3 Triangular Fibrocartilage Complex

The TFCC is a fibrocartilage ligament complex which overlies the distal ulna and is not only an important stabiliser of the distal radioulnar joint but also acts as a soft tissue cushion between the distal ulna and the carpus. This complex comprises five components: the triangular fibrocartilage, dorsal and volar radioulnar ligaments, ulnolunate and ulnotriquetral ligaments, the meniscal homologue and the extensor carpi ulnaris (ECU) tendon sheath (Fig. 12). The thickness of the TFCC varies from 2 to 5 mm and depends upon the configuration of the joint space—negative ulnar variance will lead to a thicker TFCC and conversely positive variance will lead to

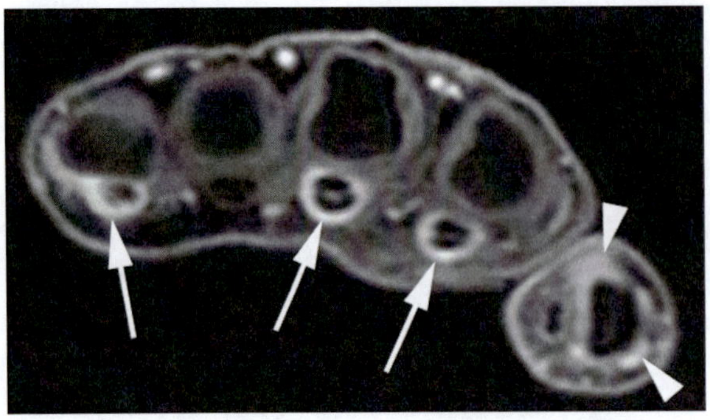

Fig. 11 Tenosynovitis—Axial T1W imaging post gadolinium administration in a patient with rheumatoid arthritis shows circumferential enhancing soft tissue within the flexor tendon sheath of the little, middle and index fingers separating the deep and superficial flexor tendons and representing tenosynovitis. In addition, there is marked enhancing synovitis seen thumb MCP joint (*arrowheads*)

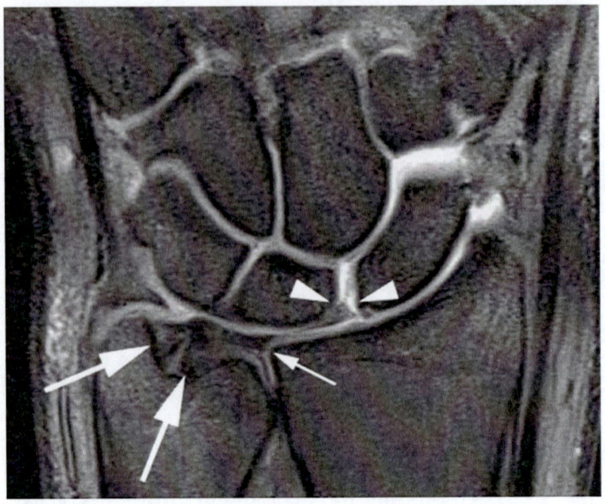

Fig. 12 Normal TFCC anatomy—coronal T2 FS image shows a normal TFCC. The bifid ulnar attachment (*white arrows*) may be seen here as well as the radial attachment. At the radial attachment hyaline cartilage is seen interposed between the TFCC and the bone (*black arrow*)—this appearance should not be misinterpreted as a TFCC tear. In this case, there is a tear of the scapholunate ligament with consequent widening of the scapho-lunate distance (*arrowheads*)

a thinner structure. Its radial attachment is to the articular cartilage of the sigmoid notch of the radius. There are two distinct ulnar attachments, the first to the ulnar fovea at the styloid base and the second to the styloid process of the ulnar. Separating these two areas of insertion is an area of connective tissue known as the ligamentum subcruentum (Nakamura et al. 1996). The blood supply to the TFCC comes from three sources: the ulnar artery and both the palmar and dorsal branches of the anterior interosseous artery. These vessels penetrate the peripheral aspect of the TFCC however the central and radial portions are avascular. Consequently, the peripheral portion has the potential to heal following repair whereas the central and radial portions do not.

Assessment of the integrity, thickness and signal characteristics of the TFCC is optimal in the coronal plane where the articular disc, the meniscal homologue, triangular ligament and ulnotriquetral ligament are all well visualised. The dual attachment of the TFCC to the ulnar is also best appreciated in this plane, where insertion into both the ulnar styloid tip and the fovea are seen. It is important not to mistake this bifid attachment for a tear. In addition the axial plane will better demonstrate the volar and dorsal radioulnar ligaments. The sagittal plane is also useful in visualising the ulnar foveal attachment (Amrami and Felmlee 2008).

The articular disc of the TFCC is seen on high resolution MR imaging as a low to intermediate signal intensity band with slightly higher signal characteristics seen within the ulnar attachment on proton density and T2 star weighted images. Perforations or tears of the TFCC structure are seen as discrete areas of high signal intensity coursing through the substance of the articular disc. Degenerative change will manifest as an area of high signal intensity within the articular disc but without extension to the articular surface (Fig. 13). The radial attachment of the triangular fibrocartilage is onto hyaline cartilage and on conventional MRI this will appear as relatively high signal between the cortical bone and fibrocartilage, an important pitfall when diagnosing radial attachment tears.

Several studies have confirmed the role of MR imaging in diagnosing TFCC pathology. However, the performance of standard MRI in the diagnostic work-up of TFCC tears is highly dependent upon the location of the lesion. Studies have demonstrated that for central and radial sided TFCC tears sensitivity and specificity is in the region of 90 % when compared with arthroscopy. However, for peripheral attachment tears sensitivity and specificity are much lower. The relatively low yield of MRI for peripheral tears is primarily attributed to the false positive results induced by the high signal of the ligamentum

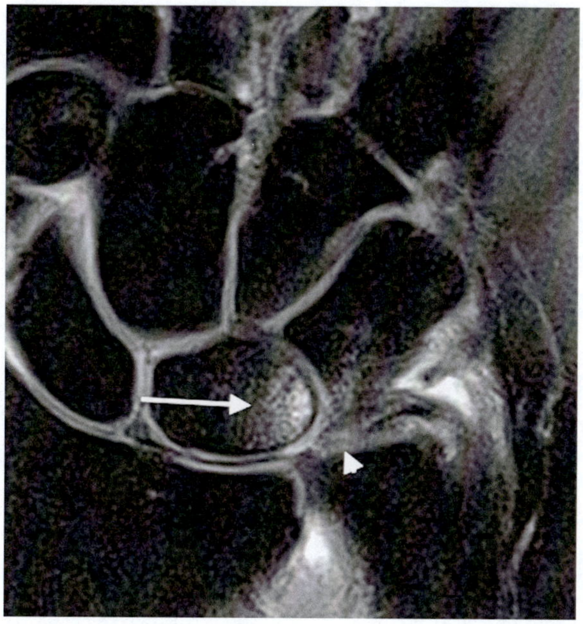

Fig. 13 Degenerative TFCC—PD FS coronal image shows. This case shows a patient with ulnar lunate abutment syndrome. There is bone oedema seen with the proximal aspect of the lunate (*white arrow*) and diffuse intrinsic high signal is seen within the radial central portion of the TFCC representing degenerative change within the fibrocartilage (*arrowhead*). This high signal does not extend to the articular surface and should not be misinterpreted as a tear

subcruentum on T2-weighted sequences along with the abnormal signal that may stem from degenerative changes of fibrocartilage. Tears affecting the central portion of the articular disc are generally felt to have a degenerative aetiology and are often asymptomatic. Asymptomatic perforations are a frequent finding in the triangular fibrocartilage even in young patients, one study reporting 51 % of asymptomatic wrists showing perforations (Brown et al. 1994). Peripheral tears tend to be traumatic in nature, often symptomatic and necessitate surgical intervention.

In view of the limitations of conventional MRI, MR arthrography is frequently advocated as the investigation of choice for the assessment of TFCC injury (Fig. 14). Proponents of conventional MRI suggest the use of 3D volumetric acquired gradient recalled sequences for evaluating the TFCC and have shown sensitivity of 100 %, specificity of 90 % and an accuracy of 97 % when using arthroscopy as the gold standard (Potter et al. 1997).

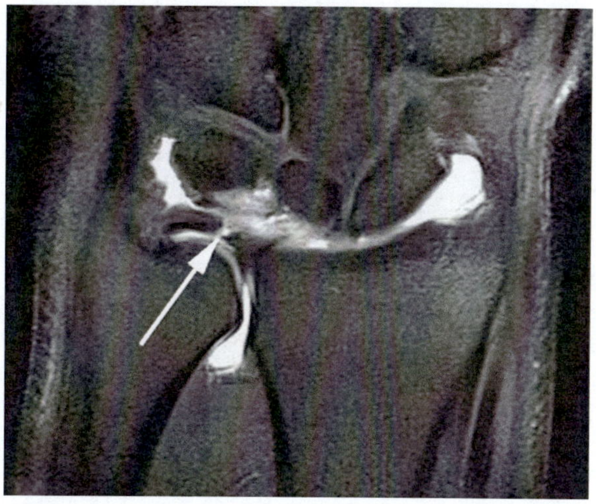

Fig. 14 Full thickness TFC tear. Coronal T1 fat suppressed image from MR arthrogram. Iodinated contrast injected into the radiocarpal joint at the time of the arthrogram was seen on fluoroscopy to pass into the distal radioulnar joint so only a single injection was undertaken. MRI shows the full thickness perforation through the triangular fibrocartilage (*arrow*) representing a full thickness tear and the passage through which contrast has passed between the two compartments. This is traumatic Palmer type 1A tear

3.4 Ligaments

3.4.1 The Intrinsic Ligaments

The intrinsic ligaments of the wrist are crucial to the intrinsic stability of the joint. These ligaments pass between the carpal bones without attachment to the radius or ulnar. The scapholunate ligament and the lunotriquetral ligament are clinically the most important and imaging is often integral in determining the extent of pathology related to these structures. The two ligaments are responsible for the stabilisation of the bones of the proximal carpal row and their disruption is an important component of dissociative carpal instability. Both the ligaments have three distinct components, namely the dorsal, volar and proximal. The scapholunate ligament is C shaped whereas the lunotriquetral ligament appears V shaped. The proximal portions of both these ligaments are thin fibrocartilaginous membranes with no stabilizing role. However, the fibrous volar and dorsal components act as true ligaments preventing independent flexion and extension of the proximal carpal bones so the entire unit at as an intercalated segment (Fig. 15).

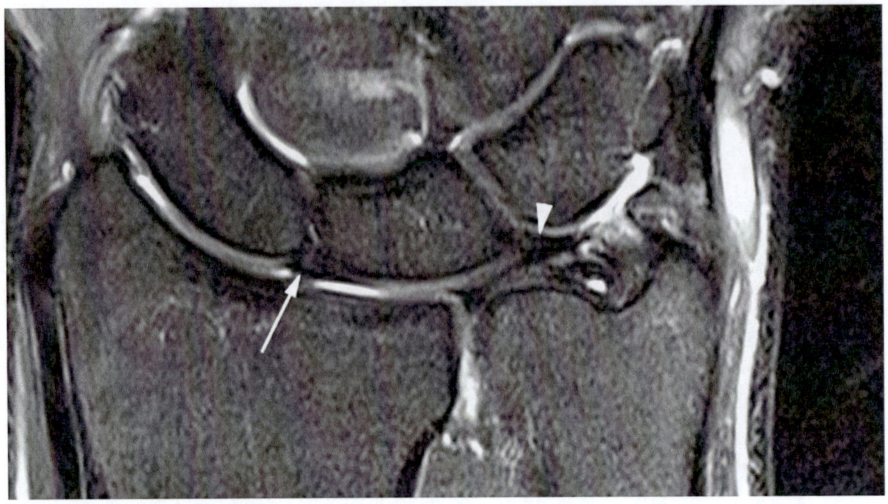

Fig. 15 Normal Intrinsic ligaments—T2 FS coronal image of the wrist shows both the scapholunate (*white arrow*) and lunate-triquetral (*black arrow*) ligaments

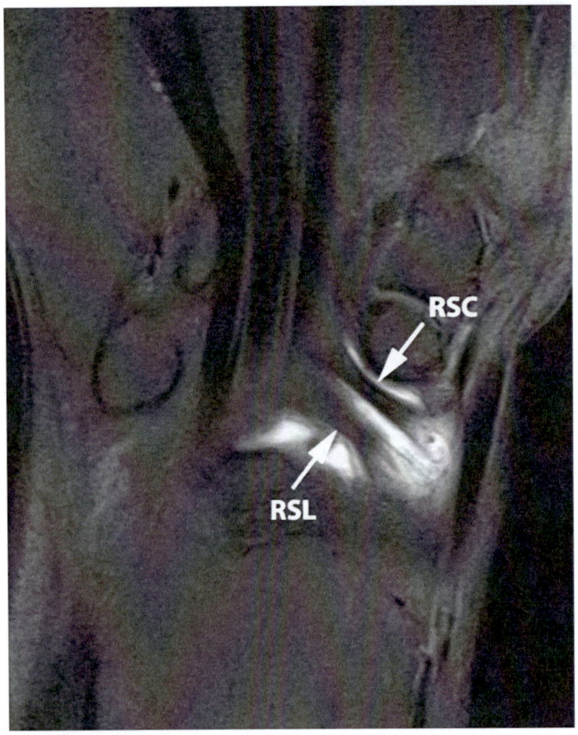

Fig. 16 Normal Extrinsic Ligaments. Coronal image from an arthrographic study shows part of the radioscapholunate and radioscaphocapitate extrinsic ligaments on the volar aspect of the wrist

Although scapholunate ligament injuries are usually assessed on conventional radiographic imaging in the first instance, MR imaging, and particularly MR arthrography plays an increasingly important role in diagnosing injuries of the intrinsic ligaments. Conventional radiographs will only show abnormality where there is either an increased scapholunate gap or alteration in alignment between bones of the proximal carpal row.

Both CT and MR arthrography are more sensitive than standard MR imaging in the detection of scapholunate tears, particularly for more subtle injuries (Cerezal et al. 2005). The use of MR arthrography may allow more accurate delineation of the exact location of a tear allowing differentiation between lesions which are degenerate in nature and predominantly affecting the membranous portion of the ligament from acute injuries which involve either or both of the dorsal or volar components.

3.4.2 The Extrinsic Ligaments

The extrinsic ligaments are classified as either volar or dorsal; the volar ligaments are considered to be important stabilisers of the wrist whereas the dorsal ligaments are thought to be less crucial for stability (Theumann et al. 2003). The volar ligaments on the radial aspect of the wrist comprise the radioscaphocapitate, the radiolunatotriquetral and the radioscapholunate ligaments. On the ulnar aspect of the wrist there are two main volar ligaments which also form part of the triangulofibrocartilage (TFCC) complex, namely the ulnolunate and the ulnotriquetral ligaments. On the dorsal aspect of the wrist the extrinsic ligaments form a V shape centred over the dorsal aspect of the triquetrum. These ligaments are areas of focal thickening within the joint capsule and are often difficult to visualise with both MR and MR arthrography (Fig. 16).

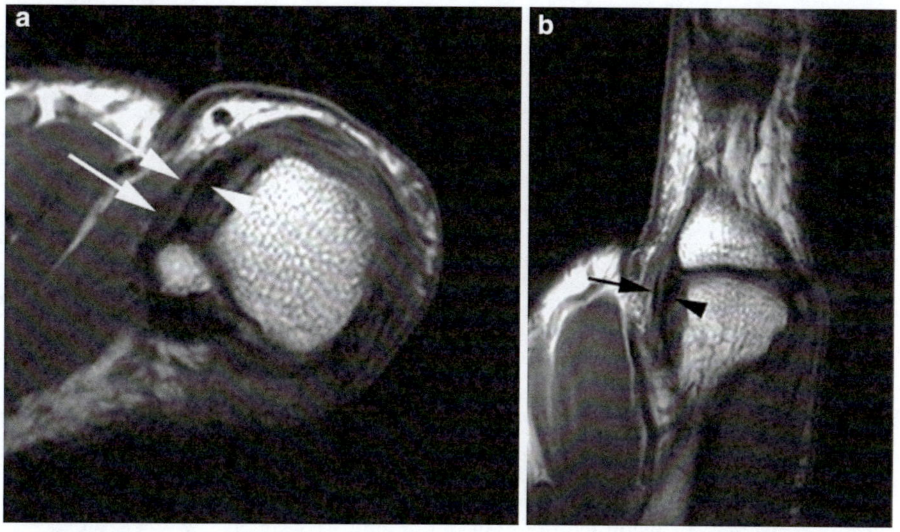

Fig. 17 Ulnar collateral ligament of the thumb—**a** and **b** shows axial and coronal imaging of a normal UCL in the thumb. Both the ulnar collateral ligament (*white arrow*) itself and the overlying adductor aponeurosis are shown (*arrowheads*)

An avulsion injury of these extrinsic ligaments from their triquetral attachment is the cause of the triquetral fracture best appreciated on a lateral wrist radiograph.

3.4.3 The Ulnar Collateral Ligament of the Thumb

The Ulnar Collateral Ligament of the Thumb is also generally assessed with MRI, although ultrasound can also usefully image this frequently injured ligament. Overlying the normal ligament a thin adductor aponeurosis is identified (Fig. 17a, b). The ulnar collateral ligament stabilises the thumb metacarpophalangeal joint against radial deviation and its injury is frequently termed gamekeepers skiers thumb. When torn the adductor aponeurosis may interpose itself between the torn ends of the ligament, known as a Stener lesion, preventing healing without intervention. Failure of the torn ligament to heal results in instability and ultimately early osteoarthritis at the joint.

3.5 Hyaline Cartilage

Despite their marked clinical impact, cartilage lesions of the radiocarpal and intercarpal joints are frequently underestimated with MRI and MR arthrography possibly due to their small and subtle nature. High spatial resolution and tissue contrast is needed to detect these subtle changes. At 3T, the SNR is sufficient but interpretation is complicated by the increased chemical shift artefact at the articular cartilage–bone interface (Fig. 6). Arthroscopy has been shown to be superior to both these imaging methods in the assessment of cartilage damage (Mutimer et al. 2008).

Much of the work regarding cartilage assessment has focussed on imaging of the knee. Various different protocols have been evaluated in this context including fat suppressed 3D spoiled GE, fast SE and direct arthrography (Gold et al. 2003). Three-dimensional GE are useful in cartilage evaluation as a high signal-to-noise ratio is afforded and allows thin slices to be produced, in addition the image may be reconstructed in different planes. These properties have not been shown to easily transfer to imaging of the cartilage within the wrist (Haims et al. 2004). This is thought in part to be due to the thickness of the cartilage at the wrist as well as the other potential difficulties with wrist imaging such as field inhomogeneity and patient movement. Therefore, an optimum method for cartilage evaluation at the wrist remains elusive at present.

4 MR Arthrography

MR arthrography is primarily indicated for the following suspected pathologies:

- Triangular fibrocartilage complex tears
- Scapho-lunate or lunate-triquetral ligament tears

- Suspected cartilage damage/intra-articular body

Communication, and therefore passage of contrast, between the radiocarpal joint and other compartments has been described in asymptomatic patients and findings therefore need to be carefully correlated with the clinical situation. A communication between the radiocarpal and midcarpal compartments has been described in 13–47 % of the population and between the radiocarpal and distal radioulnar compartments in 7–35 % of the population (Manaster 1991; Wilson et al. 1991; Cantor et al. 1994).

4.1 Protocols

As is the case with standard MR, imaging protocols for arthrographic imaging will vary between institutions. However, T1 weighted imaging will form the basis of the study showing the gadolinium arthrographic contrast as high signal. While T1 fat suppressed imaging has advantages in increasing contrast and also clarifying high signal due to contrast as opposed to fat, it is important to include at least one T1 weighted sequence without fat suppression for bony detail. It is also helpful to include a water sensitive (T2 fat suppressed) sequence to look for soft tissue pathology outside the joint itself and also for demonstrating oedematous change in bone marrow. The authors employ this sequence in the coronal plane.

4.2 Injection of Contrast

Since the first description of wrist arthrography by Kessler and Silberman (1961), many different methods, protocols and injection techniques have been described. Intra-articular injection of contrast material for the purposes of performing an MR arthrogram is usually performed under fluoroscopic guidance, although ultrasound guided injection may be used. The advantage of using fluoroscopic guidance is that a dynamic assessment for carpal instability can be made at the same time, and also fluoroscopic screening during contrast injection may demonstrate passage of contrast into adjacent compartments through ligament or fibrocartilage tears.

Single, double and triple compartment injection techniques have been described (Cerezal et al. 2005; Malfair 2008). The single compartment technique involves injection into the radiocarpal joint usually via a dorsal approach. However, a lateral approach has also been described (Medverd et al. 2011). Because of the dorsal lip which overlies the radiocarpal joint on an AP image slight proximal angulation of the image intensifier will allow improved visualisation of the joint.

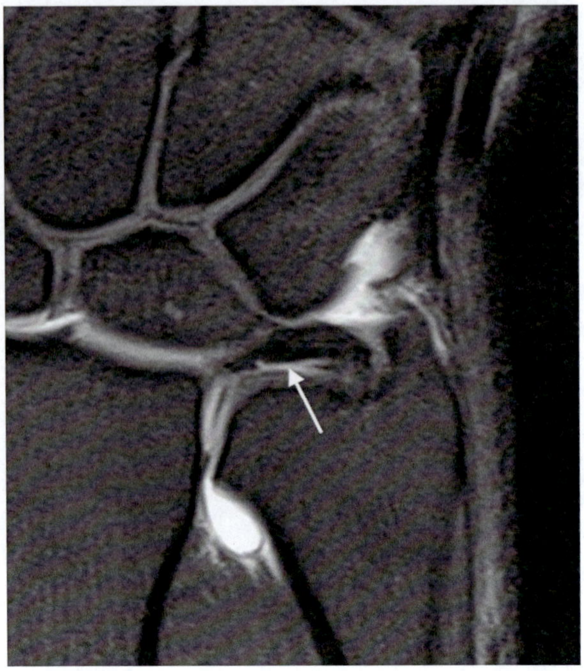

Fig. 18 Undersurface Flap tear of the TFCC—In this case the DRUJ was injected with contrast as well as the radiocarpal joint. This coronal image shows a partial thickness undersurface tear of the TFCC (*white arrow*) outlined by contrast injected into the DRUJ. This tear may not have been appreciated with a single radiocarpal joint injection

When investigating possible TFCC injury a double compartment technique is useful with a second injection into the DRUJ to outline the proximal (undersurface) of the triangular fibrocartilage (Fig. 18). This technique is useful for demonstrating partial ulnar attachment tears which are frequently non-communicating and may only be seen at the proximal attachment which may not be visible when contrast is only injected into the radiocarpal joint (Ruegger et al. 2007; Burns et al. 2011).

In the normal situation intact scapholunate and lunatetriquetral ligaments should prevent flow of contrast passage of contrast into the midcarpal joint from the radiocarpal joint and such passage will indicate a perforation or tear (which may be asymptomatic) through one of these ligaments. Conventional arthrographic studies have indicated that flow may be one way through tears in these ligaments and there may be an advantage to injecting the midcarpal joint (Levinsohn et al. 1987, 1991; Wilson et al. 1991). However, with the direct visualisation of the intrinsic ligaments afforded by MRI it is not clear that a midcarpal joint injection offers any advantages when arthrography is combined with MRI.

4.3 Artefacts

Besides artefacts seen using conventional MRI and described in 2.4 there are additional artefacts which need to be considered in arthrography. These primarily relate to the injectate and injection technique. Injected air bubbles may mimic intra-articular bodies and care should be taken to eliminate any air bubbles from the injected system wherever possible. Injectate or local anaesthetic which has been inadvertently injected into muscle or surrounding soft tissue may be confused for oedematous change or contusion.

4.4 Indirect Arthrography

Indirect arthrography is also advocated to improve the diagnostic accuracy of standard MR sequences and is considered less invasive than direct arthrography. In this technique, intravenous contrast diffuses into the joint in a concentration high enough that an arthrographic effect may be achieved on T1 weighted images, although clearly the joint is not distended as with direct arthrography. Studies have reported the increased sensitivity in evaluation of the scapholunate ligament using indirect arthrography when compared with unenhanced MRI of the wrist but this has not been shown to be the case in evaluation of the lunatetriquetral ligament (Haims et al. 2003).

4.5 Alternative Modalities

Other imaging modalities should also of course be considered and recent studies have shown Multidetector CT (MDCT) arthrography to be more accurate than both 1.5T MR imaging and MR arthrography for the detection of partial tears of the scapholunate and lunatotriquetral ligaments (Schmid et al. 2005; Moser et al. 2007). CT arthrography offers advantages in terms of spatial resolution despite the absence of soft tissue contrast. An extremely small pilot study has shown similar performance for direct MR arthrography and CT arthrography for the depiction of the triangular fibrocartilage although no attempt was made to evaluate the accuracy of these techniques for diagnosing tears (Omlor et al. 2009).

5 7T Imaging

7T imaging is a technique which is potentially particularly useful in the hand and wrist owing to its superior signal to noise ratio which allows higher spatial resolution; a quality which would allow even more detailed imaging of the fine anatomical structures of the hand and wrist, particularly the TFCC, intrinsic ligaments and articular cartilage. At present, this technique is limited to research purposes and presents many technical difficulties. These include the need for specialised RF coils which are currently not commercially widely available and the increasing chemical shift artefact encountered with increasing field strength. A potential future direction will be the opportunities 7T imaging offers for enhancing biological imaging techniques such as spectroscopy, sodium imaging and delayed gadolinium-enhanced MRI of cartilage (dGEMRIC) which will benefit significantly from the signal-to-noise gains at increased field strengths with particular advantages when applied to the smaller structures of the hand and wrist.

References

Alam F, Schweitzer ME, Li XX, Malat J, Hussain SM (1999) Frequency and spectrum of abnormalities in the bone marrow of the wrist: MR imaging findings. Skeletal Radiol 28(6):312–317

Amrami KK, Felmlee JP (2008) 3-Tesla imaging of the wrist and hand: techniques and applications. Semin musculoskelet radiol 12(3):223–237

Barth MM, Smith MP, Pedrosa I, Lenkinski RE, Rofsky NM (2007) Body MR imaging at 3.0 T: understanding the opportunities and challenges. Radiographics 27(5): 1445–1462 discussion 1462–1444

Blackband SJ, Chakrabarti I, Gibbs P, Buckley DL, Horsman A (1994) Fingers: three-dimensional MR imaging and angiography with a local gradient coil. Radiology 190(3): 895–899

Breitenseher MJ, Metz VM, Gilula LA, Gaebler C, Kukla C, Fleischmann D et al (1997) Radiographically occult scaphoid fractures: value of MR imaging in detection. Radiology 203(1):245–250

Brown JA, Janzen DL, Adler BD, Stothers K, Favero KJ, Gropper PT et al (1994) Arthrography of the contralateral, asymptomatic wrist in patients with unilateral wrist pain. Can Assoc Radiol J 45(4):292–296

Burns JE, Tanaka T, Ueno T, Nakamura T, Yoshioka H (2011) Pitfalls that may mimic injuries of the triangular fibrocartilage and proximal intrinsic wrist ligaments at MR imaging. Radiographics : a review publication of the Radiological Society of North America 31(1):63–78

Cantor RM, Stern PJ, Wyrick JD, Michaels SE (1994) The relevance of ligament tears or perforations in the diagnosis of wrist pain: an arthrographic study. J Hand Surg 19(6):945–953

Cerezal L, Abascal F, Garcia-Valtuille R, Del Pinal F (2005) Wrist MR arthrography: how, why, when. Radiologic clin N Am 43(4):709–731

Farooki S, Ashman CJ, Yu JS, Abduljalil A, Chakeres D (2002) In vivo high-resolution MR imaging of the carpal tunnel at 8.0 tesla. Skeletal Radiol 31(8):445–450

Gold GE, McCauley TR, Gray ML, Disler DG (2003) What's new in cartilage? Radiographics : a review publication of the Radiological Society of North America 23(5): 1227–1242

Haims AH, Moore AE, Schweitzer ME, Morrison WB, Deely D, Culp RW et al (2004) MRI in the diagnosis of cartilage injury in the wrist. AJR Am J Roentgenol 182(5):1267–1270

Haims AH, Schweitzer ME, Morrison WB, Deely D, Lange RC, Osterman AL et al (2003) Internal derangement of the wrist: indirect MR arthrography versus unenhanced MR imaging. Radiology 227(3):701–707

Hauger O, Chung CB, Lektrakul N, Botte MJ, Trudell D, Boutin RD et al (2000) Pulley system in the fingers: normal anatomy and simulated lesions in cadavers at MR imaging, CT, and US with and without contrast material distention of the tendon sheath. Radiology 217(1):201–212

Hunter JC, Escobedo EM, Wilson AJ, Hanel DP, Zink-Brody GC, Mann FA (1997) MR imaging of clinically suspected scaphoid fractures. AJR Am J Roentgenol 168(5):1287–1293

Kessler I, Silberman Z (1961) An experimental study of the radiocarpal joint by arthrography. Surg Gynecol Obstet 112:33–40

Kocharian A, Adkins MC, Amrami KK, McGee KP, Rouleau PA, Wenger DE et al (2002) Wrist: improved MR imaging with optimized transmit-receive coil design. Radiology 223(3): 870–876

Levinsohn EM, Palmer AK, Coren AB, Zinberg E (1987) Wrist arthrography: the value of the three compartment injection technique. Skeletal Radiol 16(7):539–544

Levinsohn EM, Rosen ID, Palmer AK (1991) Wrist arthrography: value of the three-compartment injection method. Radiology 179(1):231–239

Magee T (2009) Comparison of 3-T MRI and arthroscopy of intrinsic wrist ligament and TFCC tears. AJR Am J Roentgenol 192(1):80–85

Malfair D (2008) Therapeutic and diagnostic joint injections. Radiologic Clin N Am 46(3):439–453

Manaster BJ (1991) The clinical efficacy of triple-injection wrist arthrography. Radiology 178(1):267–270

Medverd JR, Pugsley JM, Harley JD, Bhargava P (2011) Lateral approach for radiocarpal wrist arthrography. AJR Am J Roentgenol 196(1):W58–W60

Moser T, Dosch JC, Moussaoui A, Dietemann JL (2007) Wrist ligament tears: evaluation of MRI and combined MDCT and MR arthrography. AJR Am J Roentgenol 188(5): 1278–1286

Mutimer J, Green J, Field J (2008) Comparison of MRI and wrist arthroscopy for assessment of wrist cartilage. J Hand Surg 33(3):380–382

Nakamura T, Yabe Y, Horiuchi Y (1996) Functional anatomy of the triangular fibrocartilage complex. J Hand Surg 21(5):581–586

Omlor G, Jung M, Grieser T, Ludwig K (2009) Depiction of the triangular fibro-cartilage in patients with ulnar-sided wrist pain: comparison of direct multi-slice CT arthrography and direct MR arthrography. Eur Radiol 19(1):147–151

Potter HG, Asnis-Ernberg L, Weiland AJ, Hotchkiss RN, Peterson MG, McCormack RR Jr (1997) The utility of high-resolution magnetic resonance imaging in the evaluation of the triangular fibrocartilage complex of the wrist. J Bone Joint Surg 79(11):1675–1684

Roemer PB, Edelstein WA, Hayes CE, Souza SP, Mueller OM (1990) The NMR phased array. MRM: official journal of the society of magnetic resonance in medicine/society of magnetic resonance in medicine 16(2):192–225

Ruegger C, Schmid MR, Pfirrmann CW, Nagy L, Gilula LA, Zanetti M (2007) Peripheral tear of the triangular fibrocartilage: depiction with MR arthrography of the distal radioulnar joint. AJR Am J Roentgenol 188(1):187–192

Saupe N, Prussmann KP, Luechinger R, Bosiger P, Marincek B, Weishaupt D (2005) MR imaging of the wrist: comparison between 1.5- and 3-T MR imaging–preliminary experience. Radiology 234(1):256–264

Schmid MR, Schertler T, Pfirrmann CW, Saupe N, Manestar M, Wildermuth S et al (2005) Interosseous ligament tears of the wrist: comparison of multi-detector row CT arthrography and MR imaging. Radiology 237(3):1008–1013

Stevens KJ, Wallace CG, Chen W, Rosenberg JK, Gold GE (2011) Imaging of the wrist at 1.5 Tesla using isotropic three-dimensional fast spin echo cube. JMRI 33(4):908–915

Tan AL, Grainger AJ, Tanner SF, Shelley DM, Pease C, Emery P et al (2005) High-resolution magnetic resonance imaging for the assessment of hand osteoarthritis. Arthritis Rheum 52(8):2355–2365

Theumann NH, Pfirrmann CW, Antonio GE, Chung CB, Gilula LA, Trudell DJ et al (2003) Extrinsic carpal ligaments: normal MR arthrographic appearance in cadavers. Radiology 226(1): 171–179

Wilson AJ, Gilula LA, Mann FA (1991) Unidirectional joint communications in wrist arthrography: an evaluation of 250 cases. AJR Am J Roentgenol 157(1):105–109

Radionuclide Imaging of the Hand and Wrist

Gopinath Gnanasegaran, Nicola J. R. Mulholland, Bo Povlsen, and Ignac Fogelman

Contents

G. Gnanasegaran (✉) · I. Fogelman
Consultant Physician in Nuclear Medicine,
Department of Nuclear Medicine,
St Thomas' Hospital Guy's and St Thomas' Hospital NHS Foundation Trust, Lambeth Palace Road, London, SE1 7EH, UK
e-mail: gopinath.gnanasegaran@gstt.nhs.uk

N. J. R. Mulholland
Department of Nuclear Medicine and Radiology,
Kings College Hospital, London, UK

B. Povlsen
Department of Orthopedics,
Guy's and St Thomas Hospital NHS Foundation Trust,
London, UK

Abstract

Nuclear medicine techniques continue to play a role in the diagnosis and management of hand, and wrist disorders, despite the advent of other cross-sectional imaging techniques such as MRI and CT. This chapter reviews the techniques available, concentrating on specific applications in the hand and wrist.

1 Introduction

Nuclear medicine techniques continue to play a role in the diagnosis and management of hand, and wrist disorders, despite the advent of other cross-sectional imaging techniques such as MRI and CT. This chapter reviews the techniques available, concentrating on specific applications in the hand and wrist.

The anatomy of the wrist is complex and the diagnosis, and management of hand and wrist injuries is difficult and challenging. In general, radiological techniques such as plain X-rays, computed tomography (CT), magnetic resonance imaging (MRI), and ultrasound (US) form the basis of investigations, but additional information may be provided with bone scintigraphy.

Two phase radionuclide bone scanning with ^{99} ^{m}Tc-MDP (Technetium 99 m labelled methylene diphosphonate) or ^{99} ^{m}Tc-HDP (Technetium 99 m labelled hydroxymethylene diphosphonate) is reported to be useful in imaging the hand and wrist, in both acute and chronic conditions. Bone scintigraphy is sensitive for the detection and diagnosis of occult

A. M. Davis et al. (eds.), *Imaging of the Hand and Wrist*, Medical Radiology. Diagnostic Imaging,
DOI: 10.1007/174_2010_143,

fractures, malunion, and osteonecrosis. In centres where the availability of MRI or CT is limited, radionuclide bone scanning has a correspondingly increased role to play. The advantage of a radionuclide bone scan is its high sensitivity; however, its specificity is relatively low (78%). A significant problem with bone scintigraphy is the accurate localization and characterization of lesions which can be difficult due to the relatively low spatial resolution of the technique (Hawkes et al. 1991; Mohamed et al. 1997). This is particularly true in the wrist where the small carpal bones lie close together, and new techniques are evolving to better localize areas of increased tracer uptake.

2 Techniques

2.1 Bone Scintigraphy

The most common nuclear medicine technique used for assessing the hand and wrist is bone scintigraphy, making use of $^{99\,m}$Tc-MDP or similar compound. This compound binds to bone matrix by poorly understood mechanisms and emits gamma rays which can be detected by gamma cameras. A typical radiation dose following injection of 400 MBq $^{99\,m}$Tc-MDP would be 2.3 mSv. Typical amounts of activity administered to adults undergoing bone scintigraphy are in the order of 555–750 MBq.

When imaging the hand and wrist, injection of the isotope should be undertaken in the contralateral arm to that being examined or ideally into the foot, so a direct comparison between the two upper limbs can be made.

A two-phase bone scan is generally undertaken with an early blood pool phase (at approximately 5 min) obtained to provide information relating to the vascular and extra-vascular distribution of the radiopharmaceutical. This gives an indication of vascularity. Subsequently bone uptake is assessed 3–4 h following injection. Here uptake will relate to the level of bone turnover (Fig. 1).

Generally, both hands/wrists are imaged, enabling comparison between the two sides to be made. The hand and wrists are positioned symmetrically, with the palms facing down on the gamma camera.

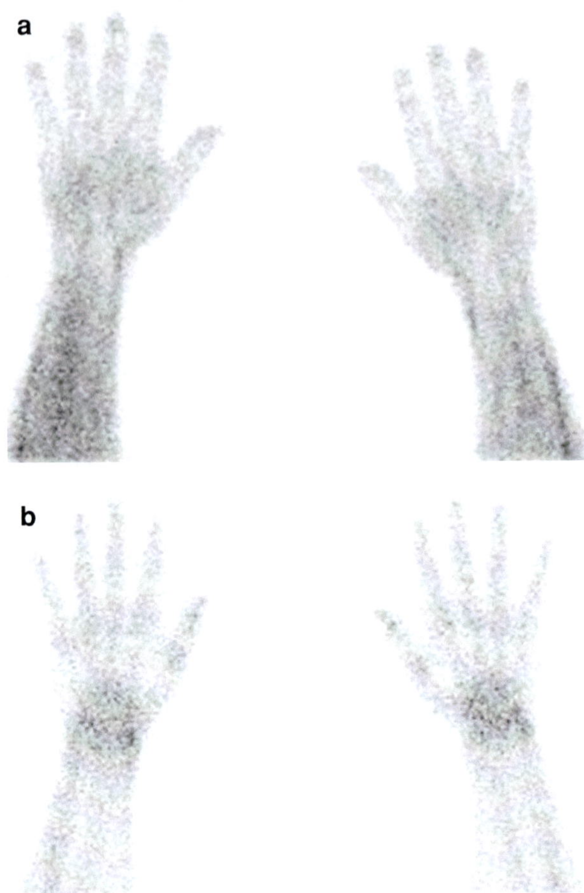

Fig. 1 Normal two-phase bone scintigraphy with **a** early (vascular) and **b** late phases. Note the poor spatial resolution of the study

2.2 Conventional 2 Phase Bone Scan With X-ray Registration

Wrist registration scintigraphy is used as a method to overcome the inherent low spatial resolution of the bone scan by co-registration with a radiograph (Fig. 2) (Hawkes et al. 1991; Mohamed et al. 1997). The addition of registration of the bone scan with X-ray has been shown to improve the localization of lesions to individual bones or joints (Hawkes et al. 1991; Mohamed et al. 1997; Vande Streek et al. 1998; Wraight et al. 1997). The techniques employed for X-ray registration of bone scans vary and are relatively cumbersome. This may involve the production of a custom cast with metallic markers and corresponding radioisotope markers. The hand is placed in the cast

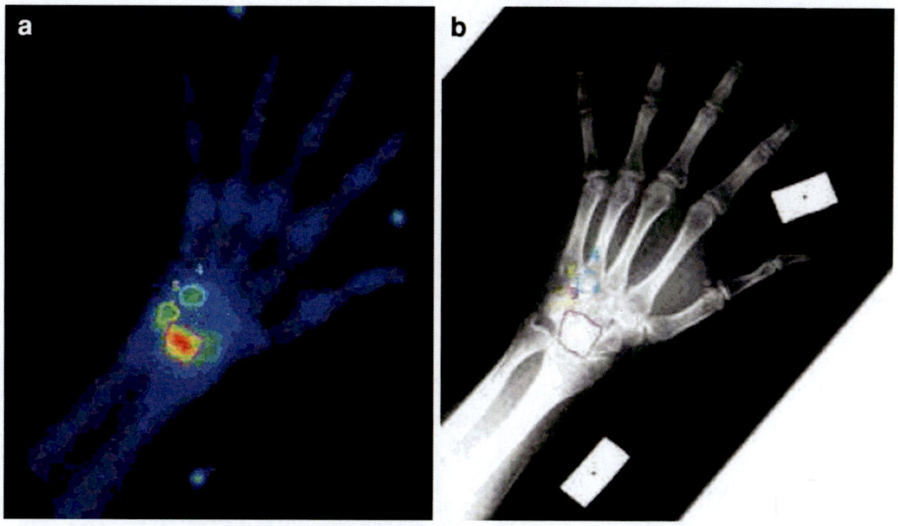

Fig. 2 Avascular necrosis of lunate: **a** registered bone scan and **b** X-ray of the hand: The region of interest is drawn around the intense bone scan lesion, and the tracer uptake is located in the region of the metabolically active avascular necrosis of lunate bone

for conventional radiography and scintigraphy, and the two images are registered by means of the markers.

2.3 Multislice SPECT/CT

The integration of SPECT and CT provides precise localization and may enable characterization of abnormalities, identified on planar or SPECT imaging by providing additional structural information from CT.

The wrist multislice SPECT/CT offers the advantage of distinguishing individual carpal bones unlike conventional bone scans, which traditionally do not have sufficient spatial resolution to localize and characterize the site of abnormality, accurately.

The principle of SPECT/CT is to integrate/fuse SPECT and CT images accurately, and provide precise localization and characterization of metabolically active abnormalities, identified either on a planar or SPECT imaging by providing structural information from CT.

2.3.1 SPECT/CT Imaging Protocol

Dual-phase bone scans are obtained following injection of 750 MBq 99 m Tc-MDP, followed by CT, and finally SPECT imaging.

2.3.1.1 Two Phase Planar Wrist Scintigraphy

Following injection, both hands are positioned (palm down) on the camera face and static image for 5 min are acquired using a 256 × 256 matrix. Delayed imaging is performed at 3–4 h post injection with both the hands placed on the camera face, palms down, and static images in the anterior position are acquired.

2.3.1.2 Patient Positioning for SPECT/CT

The patient lies prone with one or both arms stretched out above their head towards the centre of the couch (Superman position). It is important to get the patient as comfortable, as possible. Supporting polycarbonate blocks are placed under the hands and wrists, which are taped firmly to the blocks. If needed, pillows or foam blocks are placed under the arms to provide further support. The patient's head is turned towards one side, so that they lie as flat as possible, allowing minimal distance from the gamma head.

2.3.1.3 CT Imaging

Once the patient is comfortably placed in the required position, a scout view is carried out to define the CT field. A low dose CT is used for both hands. Localization CT is then carried out with voltage settings of 120 keV, current setting of 100 mAs/slice, with slice thickness of 1.5 mm and increment of 0.75 mm. (CT imaging takes approximately 40–60 s).

For single wrist, a diagnostic CT is carried out using the following setting of 140 keV, 150 mAs/slice, slice thickness of 0.8 mm and increment of 0.4 mm. Diagnostic CT of a single wrist is performed because the single wrist is placed in the center of the couch, and hence in the center of the FOV.

2.3.1.4 SPECT Imaging

Once the CT scan is completed, a SPECT study is performed using the following parameters; Low energy high-resolution, parallel hole collimator, number of projections; 128 with 20 s time per

Fig. 3 Triquetral fracture: on dual-phase planar bone scan, there is increased blood pool (**a**) and increased tracer uptake (**b**) in the carpal bones on the ulnar side of the left hand. On the SPECT/CT images, the tracer uptake localizes to the triquetral fragment (fracture), and triquetral-Pisiform articulation (**c**–**e**)

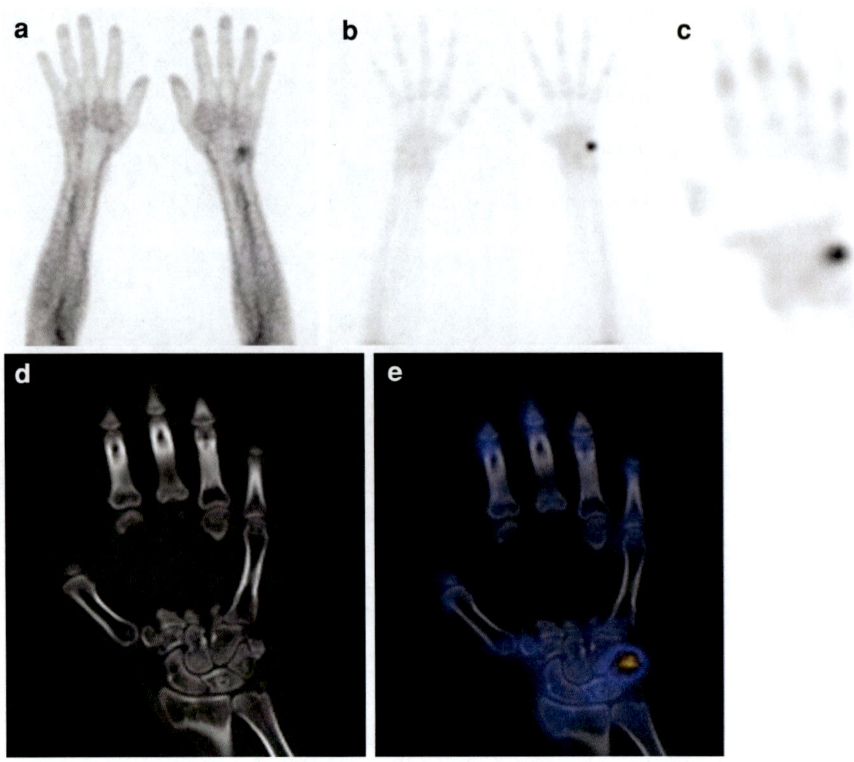

projection and matrix size equivalent to 128 × 128. The SPECT procedure is the same for both wrists, as well as for single wrist.

2.3.1.5 Image Processing

The raw data from the SPECT study is processed and transaxial slices are co-registered with the CT (Fig. 3).

2.4 Other Nuclear Medicine Techniques

Although $^{99\,m}$Tc-MDP scintigraphy is the common nuclear medicine investigation undertaken for the hand and wrist, other techniques exist. These include the use of labelled leucocytes for the investigation of infection. ^{111}In-Chloride and ^{67}Ga-Citrate have also been used as markers for inflammation. However, not commonly used for the evaluation of the peripheral small joints (Tumeh 1996).

Labelled antibodies can be used in the investigation of arthritis. Techniques include the labelling of human polyclonal immunoglobulin G (IgG) with ^{111}In or $^{99\,m}$Tc, or labelled anti-E-selectin monoclonal antibody (Tumeh 1996; Jamar et al. 1995, 1997). More recently it has been shown possible to label anti-TNF monoclonal antibodies with $^{99\,m}$Tc, demonstrating activity in synovitis in patients with rheumatoid arthritis which shows a close relationship to disease activity (Barrera et al. 2003).

Currently, increasing roles for the use of ^{18}F-fluorodeoxyglucose positron emission tomography (FDG-PET) are being found in nuclear medicine. Although specific clinical applications for the technique in the hand and wrist are yet to evolve, there is evidence that disease activity of rheumatoid arthritis can be assessed using the FDG-PET scanning of the wrist (Palmer et al. 1995).

3 Clinical Applications

3.1 Acute Fractures

Radionuclide bone scintigraphy is highly sensitive in the assessment of carpal fractures when radiographs are normal in the clinical context of trauma. Fractures of any of the carpal bones may be detected, although scaphoid fractures are the most common (Maurer 1991; Patel et al. 1992) (Figs. 3, 4 and 5). In general, radionuclide wrist registration with X-ray combines the sensitivity of scintigraphy to detect fractures, with a rapid and inexpensive method to aid fracture localization. Such registration techniques have been shown to improve reporter confidence and influence management (Mohamed et al. 1997; Wraight et al. 1997). When assessing fractures, it is suggested that scintigraphy is more reliable if delayed at least 48 h following trauma (Rolfe et al. 1981). However, in practical terms most wrist and hand fractures are hot essentially immediately. Importantly, scintigraphic uptake often precedes radiological changes in occult fractures, the latter may still be equivocal at 2–3 weeks (Dias et al. 1990). A recent study by Groves evaluated the use of 16 slicemultislice CT versus skeletal scintigraphy in suspected scaphoid injuries. They recorded 23 scintigraphically positive bone scans for fracture with only 16 fractures visible on CT the same day (Groves et al. 2005a, b). In their study, all patients with discordant CT findings had significantly lower MDP uptake to background activity ratios, than those with CT proven fracture. They postulate that the scintigraphic findings of fracture may be mimicked by bone bruising (micro-fractures of the trabeculae) and this should be considered when reporting. Such trabecular bone injury does not have the same deleterious sequelae seen with fractures, such as avascular necrosis.

SPECT/CT may be helpful in the assessment of complicated fractures, where the injury may be relatively difficult to localize and characterize (Figs. 3 and 6). SPECT/CT scanning has a further advantage that it can be performed in a single sitting, providing early, and accurate diagnosis.

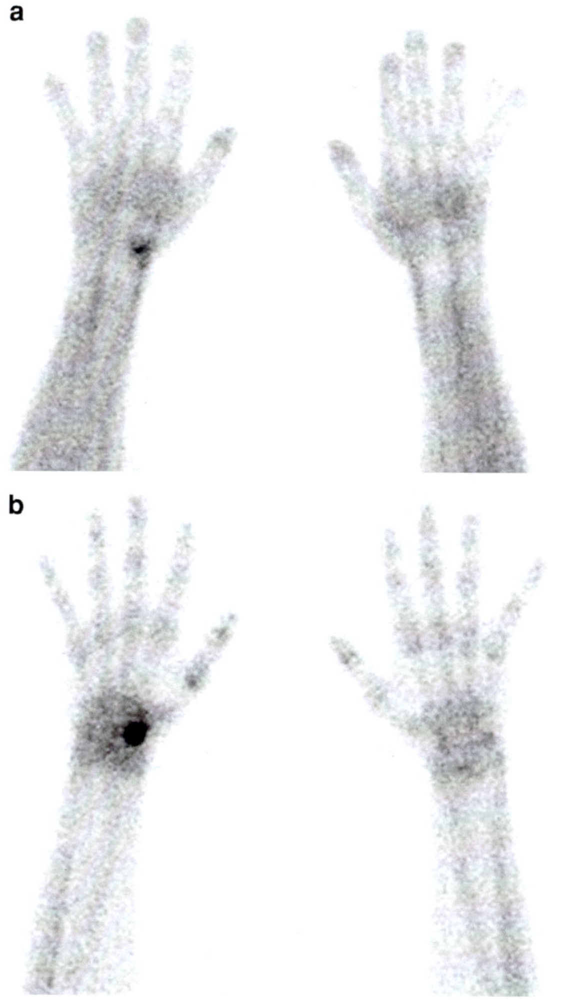

Fig. 4 Scaphoid fracture: **a** early and **b** delayed phase scanning, shows intense uptake in the scaphoid at the site of fracture. Courtesy of Dr. R. Bury, Department of Radiology, Leeds Teaching Hospitals, Leeds, UK

3.2 Fractures of Uncertain Age

The most common carpal fracture is that of the scaphoid. It is also the most common fracture to be misdiagnosed as a simple sprain and may become surprisingly pain free despite absence of union in the fracture. A number of such non-unions will later present with secondary degenerative arthritis. The wrist may then become symptomatic after an acute re-injury. A relatively common diagnostic problem is establishing why there is now persistent pain, particularly if only the non-union is visible on the radiograph, without obvious degenerative change. In these situations, the choice may be to undertake MRI or even wrist arthroscopy, to establish whether or not there has been a loss of articular cartilage at the radio-scaphoid facet. This will help determine whether surgical treatment of the non-union is likely to improve the patient's symptoms. SPECT/CT may also clarify this in a non-invasive manner, at the same time, identifying any other carpal fracture, which may be difficult to localize on the conventional planar bone scan.

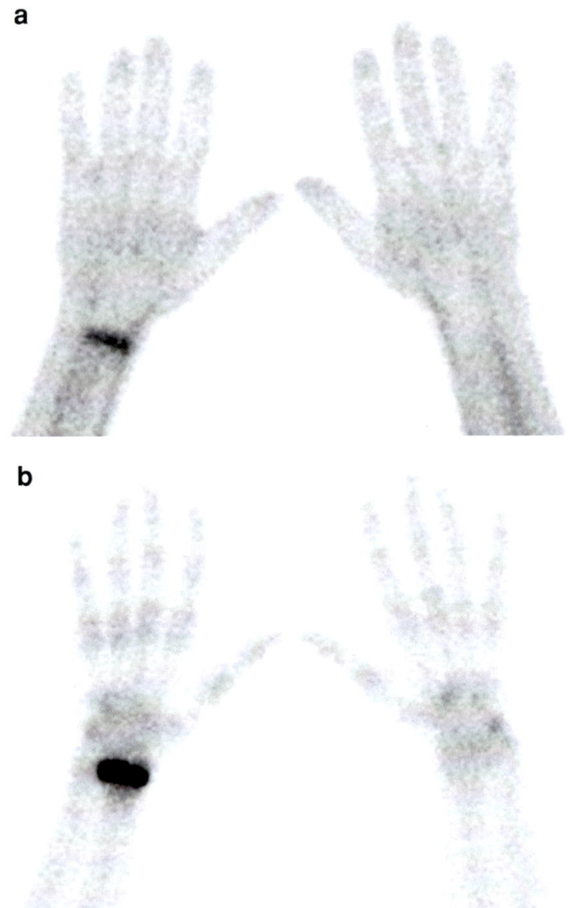

Fig. 5 Radial Fracture. This patient with normal plain films was suspected of having a scaphoid fracture. However, **a** early and **b** delayed phase scanning shows intense uptake in the distal radius representing a distal radius fracture. Courtesy of Dr. R. Bury, Department of Radiology, Leeds Teaching Hospitals, Leeds, UK

3.3 Arthritis

3.3.1 Osteoarthritis

While bone scanning alone is sensitive, its lack of resolution may prevent precise localization of arthritic change. Furthermore, its inherent lack of specificity means it has a limited role in the diagnosis and management of the disease. Bone scintigraphy is not a routine investigation in osteoarthritis (OA), but it should be recognized that the condition is a cause of increased radiopharmaceutical uptake, which may be important when interpreting studies undertaken for other indications. OA is a common condition which may be frequently encountered either as a primary disease process, typically affecting the proximal and distal interphalangeal joints and thumb base (first carpometacarpal and scaphoid–trapezial–trapezoid (STT) joints) or as a secondary condition, such as may be seen in the wrist as a consequence of trauma. The improved localization and characterisation of SPECT/CT, pin points the site of uptake and may help in clarifying the cause of uptake by localizing the disease process (Figs. 7 and 8).

3.3.2 Inflammatory Arthritis

The inflammatory arthritides are commonly associated with synovitis and show increased uptake on both, the blood pool and delayed images of the dual-phase bone scintigraph. The appearance of increased activity is non-specific, but the distribution, for instance wrist, MCP, and PIP joint involvement in rheumatoid arthritis or DIP involvement in psoriatic arthritis may be helpful in identifying the underlying arthritis (Fig. 9). The accuracy of US and MRI in identifying synovitis and erosions, in the hand and wrist, means isolated hand and wrist scintigraphy has only a minor role to play in investigating inflammatory arthritis. However, whole-body scintigraphy may still be undertaken (to include the hands and wrists) in a technique to identify sites of inflammation throughout the body. The technique of scintigraphy may also be helpful in identifying a monoarthritis from a polyarthritis, thereby changing the differential diagnosis. As has been outlined in Sect. 2.4, other nuclear medicine techniques have become available for the assessment of inflammatory arthritis. Techniques such as scanning with ^{111}In-Chloride show good specificity for the disease, and disease activity in some joints, but uptake in the small joints of the hand is relatively weak with lower accuracy, than was seen in large joints (Sewell et al. 1993). Work using labelled IgG found the intensity of uptake, correlates well with clinical markers of inflammatory activity (de Bois et al. 1992). This study showed no correlation with radiographic measures of joint destruction.

Intraosseous cysts and erosions may be seen in combination with arthritides, or degeneration. Such processes may include intraosseous ganglion formation, typically within the lunate. Inflammatory change associated with such bony lesions may be seen as areas of increased uptake on the bone scan. The findings on the bone scan are non-specific and may

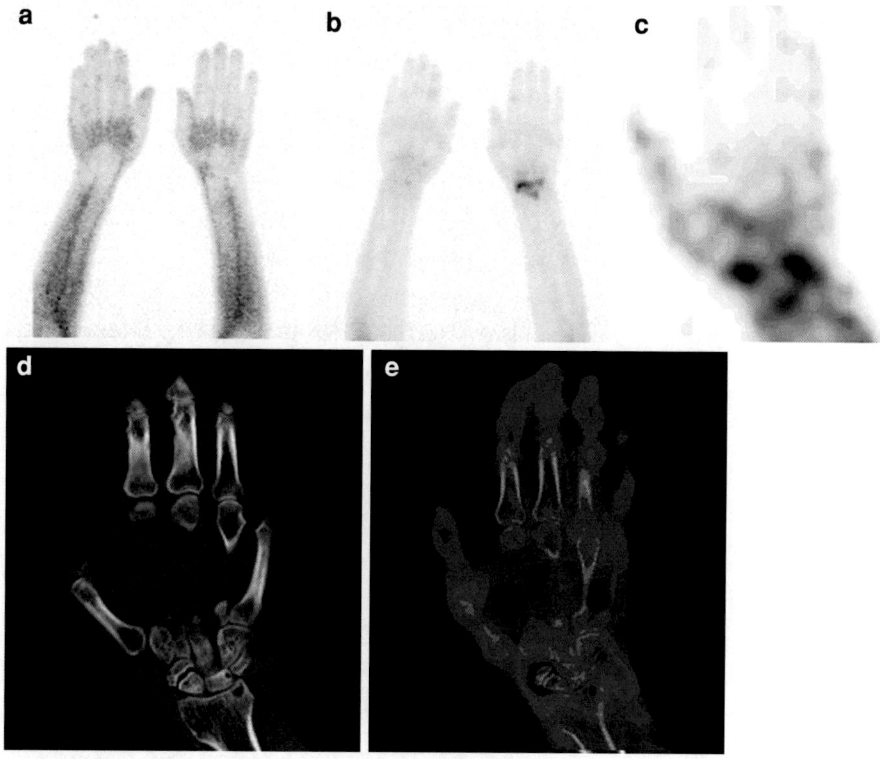

Fig. 6 Non-union scaphoid fracture: The delayed phase planar image shows, increased tracer uptake within the lateral aspect of the left wrist joint (**b**) with very subtle, increased blood on the early blood pool images (**a**). On the SPECT/CT images, the increased uptake localizes to the non-united fracture of the Scaphoid (**c**–**e**)

include multiple differentials. However, with localization techniques such as SPECT/CT the area of increased tracer uptake can be identified and characterized on the CT component of the study (Fig. 10).

3.3.3 Infection

Early differentiation of soft tissue infection from osteomyelitis is critical to ensure appropriate management. Osteomyelitis will commonly require a protracted course of antibiotics and sometimes debridement. Plain radiographic changes of osteomyelitis are often not present in early disease, and scintigraphy can be used to determine bony involvement. Typically, the bone scan is hyperaemic in the blood pool and delayed-phase within 48–72 h of onset (Maurer et al. 1981). Although an uncommon appearance, a photon deficiency may also be appreciated at a site of osteomyelitis (Barron and Dhekne 1984). The use of ^{111}In labelled white cells or ^{67}Ga-Citrate improves specificity for infection assessment, but there is a corresponding increase in radiation dose, and resolution is generally poorer. The use of SPECT/CT aids localization and characterization. SPECT/CT may be useful in differentiating soft tissue and bone infection, and can be useful to assess the extent of disease particularly when planning debridement (Fig. 11).

3.3.4 Avascular Necrosis

Avascular necrosis is a serious and frequent complication of carpal fractures, especially of the scaphoid and lunate. Idiopathic avascular necrosis may also be seen in the carpal bones as in Keinboch's disease, affecting the lunate. Bone scintigraphy can be used to identify established AVN. In its early stages, AVN may show a photon deficiency and this may be seen at a stage where the plain radiographs are unremarkable. With time, an osteoblastic response develops in the bone leading to increased uptake of tracer on delayed scanning (Fig. 2). Typically, scintigraphy is undertaken in the subacute phase by which time the hypervascular response has occurred along with the osteoblastic response. By this stage, changes may be evident on the conventional radiographs. MRI will detect the changes at both stages. In more advanced stages of avascular necrosis, there may be involvement of other carpal bones; with degenerative changes developing in the mid-carpal joints (Bain and Begg 2006).

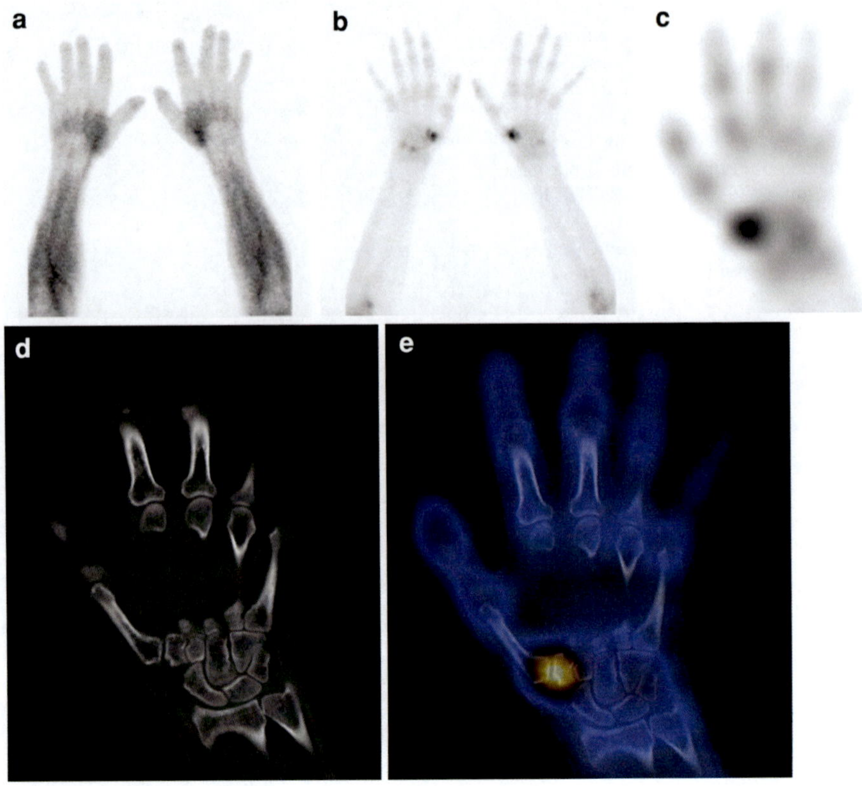

Fig. 7 Degenerative first carpo-metacarpal joint: Dual-phase bone scan shows increased vascularity (**a**) and tracer uptake (**b**) in the distal carpal bones of the radial side of the wrist bilaterally. On SPECT/CT images, the area of increased uptake localises to the first carpo-metacarpal joint (**c**–**e**)

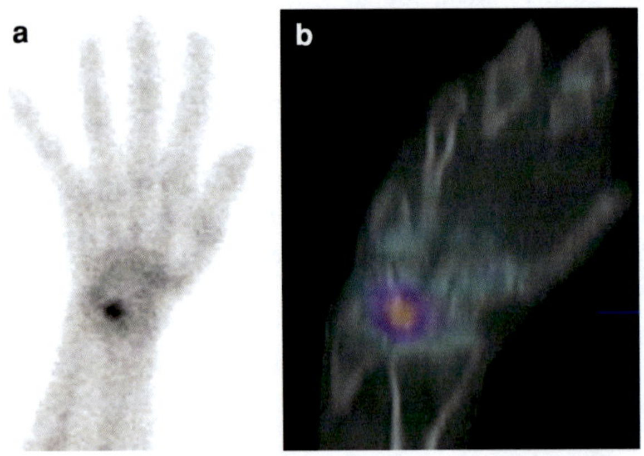

Fig. 8 Lunate-triquetral osteoarthritis: **a** planar scintigraphy shows increased tracer uptake associated with the proximal carpal row and **b** SPECT-CT identifies the site of activity as the lunate-triquetral joint. Courtesy of Drs. R. Cooper and S. Allwright, Department of Nuclear Medicine, Mater Hospital and Dee Why Nuclear Medicine, Sydney, Australia

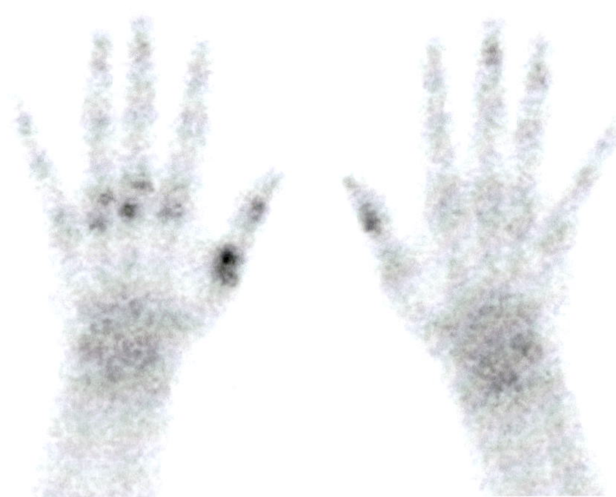

Fig. 9 Rheumatoid arthritis. Late-phase scintigram shows uptake at the MCP joints on the right hand and both thumb interphalangeal joints. The MCP involvement is typical for rheumatoid arthritis

The improved localization using SPECT/CT may provide valuable information not only regarding vascular supply, but also the degree of surrounding secondary OA, when evaluating avascular necrosis of the lunate, which we have found, can be used to guide the hand surgeon to the most appropriate surgery.

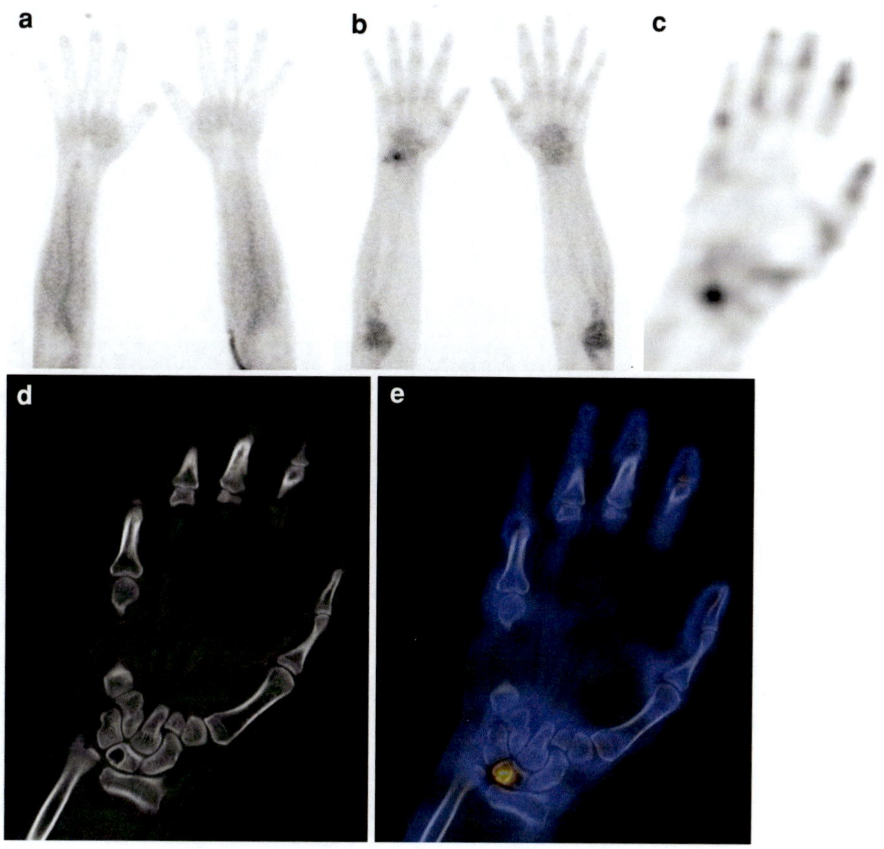

Fig. 10 Lunate cyst with degenerative disease. The dual-phase planar imaging shows increased tracer uptake (**b**) in the distal ulnar region. The early blood pool images are unmarkable (**a**). On the SPECT/CT image, the increased tracer uptake is localized to the lunate cyst (**c–e**)

3.3.5 Miscellaneous

3.3.5.1 Wrist Impaction Syndromes

There are a various causes for impaction syndromes associated with ulnar-sided wrist pain with the commonest being the ulnar impaction syndrome (Cerezal et al. 2002; Friedman and Palmer 1991). Less common causes include conditions such as ulnar impingement syndrome, ulnar styloid impaction syndrome, ulnocarpal impaction, and hamatolunate impingement syndrome. Ulnar impaction syndrome is also known as ulnar abutment, and is reported to be a degenerative condition characterized by ulnar wrist pain associated with swelling, and limitation of movement across the ulnar aspect of the wrist (Cerezal et al. 2002; Friedman and Palmer 1991; Escobedo et al. 1995; Hodge et al. 1996; Imaeda et al. 1996). MRI is a useful investigation to assess the structural abnormalities that contribute to ulnocarpal instability and pain. Scintigraphy can be useful to localize the site of intense metabolic activity and guide MRI, but localization is most accurately achieved using registration techniques such as CT/SPECT.

3.3.5.2 Bone Tumours

Isolated peripheral skeletal metastases in the hand/wrist are relatively unusual but may occur, particularly from bronchogenic, thyroid, renal cell or malignant melanoma primaries. Hypertrophic pulmonary osteoarthropathy (HPOA) may also be detected with bone scintigraphy as increased uptake at the wrists.

Benign bone tumours include osteoid osteoma, and one study would suggest around 8% of these lesions occur in the hand and wrist (Cohen et al. 1983). When these lesions do occur in this location they seem to be most frequently seen in the proximal phalanges, and metacarpals, with a relatively low incidence in the intermediate and terminal phalanges and the carpal bones (Carroll 1953). Bone scintigraphy will classically show a double density sign with increased uptake in the surrounding sclerotic bone, but very intense uptake at the site of the nidus (Helms 1987).

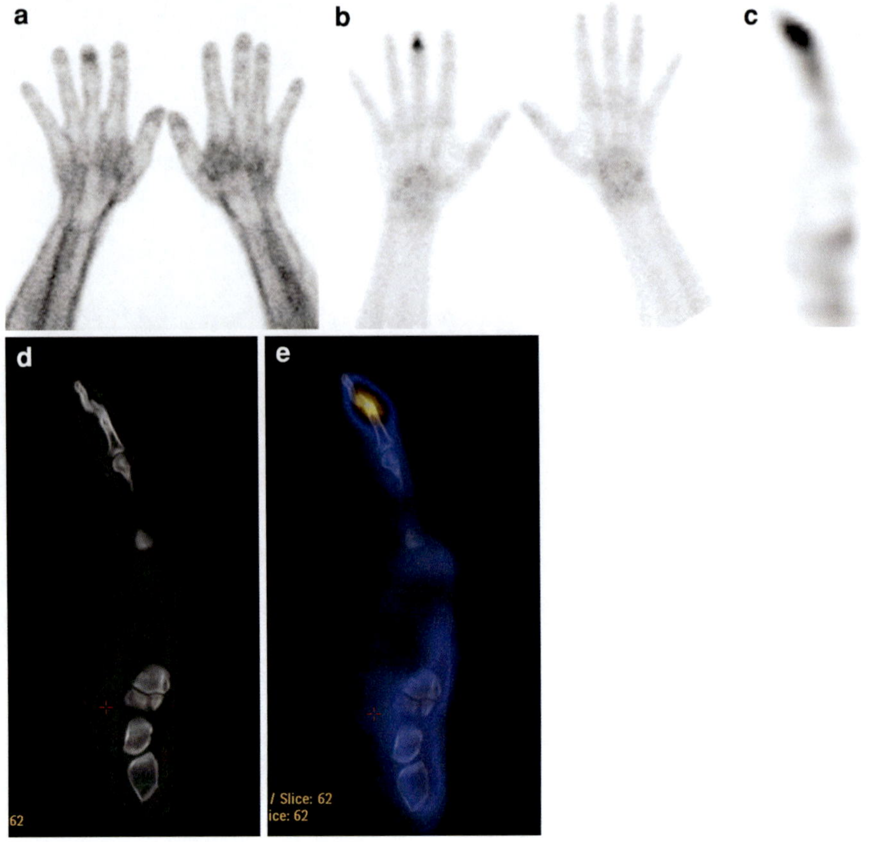

Fig. 11 Septic arthritis and osteomyelitis. The planar images show increased blood pool (**a**) and increased tracer uptake around the distal phalanx of the middle finger (**b**). On the SPECT/CT images the increased tracer uptake localizes to the distal inter-phalangeal joint of the middle finger consistent with known infection at this site (**c**–**e**)

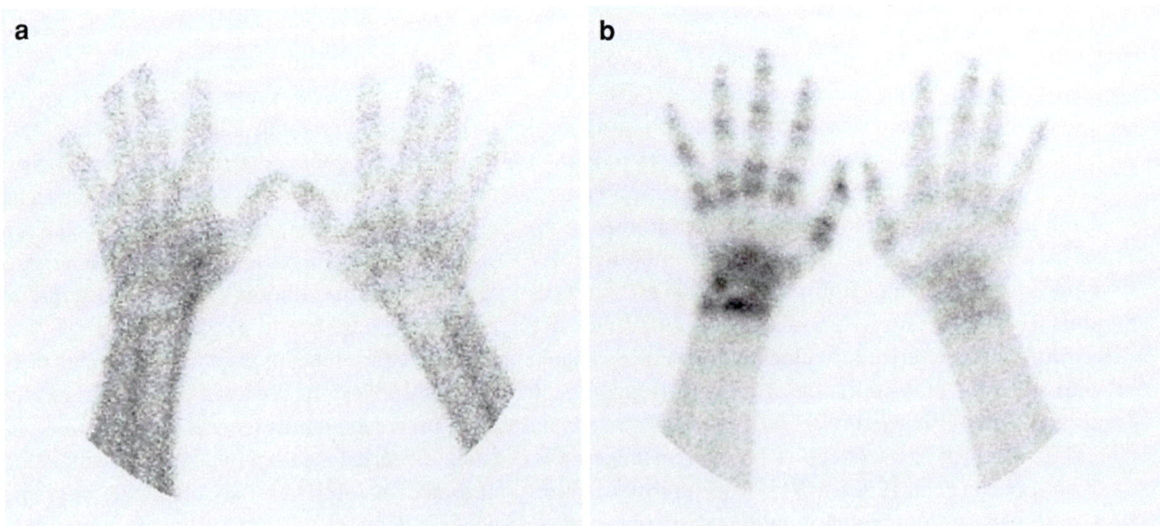

Fig. 12 Reflex sympathetic dystrophy. There is increased tracer activity in the right hand and wrist, on early phase scanning (**a**). Late phase scanning (**b**) shows increased activity in a typical periarticular distribution throughout the hand and wrist. Courtesy of Drs R Cooper and S Allwright, Department of Nuclear Medicine, Mater Hospital and Dee Why Nuclear Medicine, Sydney, Australia

Increasingly these lesions are being treated with percutaneous ablation, but the use of an intraoperative nuclear medicine probe, following administration of radioactive tracer can be used by surgeon to help localize osteoid osteoma and ensure excision of the nidus. The most common benign bone tumour seen in the hand is an enchondroma which shows relatively low uptake on bone scanning (Vande Streek et al. 1994). Bone scintigraphy cannot reliably distinguish between benign and malignant chondroid tumours.

3.3.5.3 Reflex Sympathetic Dystrophy

Reflex sympathetic dystrophy is a poorly understood condition presenting with severe limb pain. The syndrome comprises intense pain, soft tissue swelling and discolouration, alteration in skin temperature, and limitation of movement. In many cases there is no antecedent event, but there is frequently a history of minor trauma or recent surgery. While the diagnosis may be obvious on clinical examination, it can be difficult. Bone scintigraphy typically shows abnormality on both vascular and delayed phase imaging with increased uptake, classically a periarticular distribution (Fig. 12). Clearly this pattern of uptake is not specific and must be viewed in the clinical context. Published studies show variable sensitivity and specificity for the diagnosis using Bone scintigraphy (Genant et al. 1975; Holder and Mackinnon 1984; Kozin et al. 1981).

4 Conclusion

Inevitably, newer cross-sectional imaging modalities such as MRI and CT are useful in the diagnosis of hand and wrist disorders. However, new registration techniques such as CT/SPECT have improved the ability of bone scintigraphy to accurately localize the site pathology. While bone scintigraphy has many applications it continues to play an important role in many centres for the identification of occult fractures.

References

Bain GI, Begg M (2006) Arthroscopic assessment and classification of Kienbock's disease. Tech Hand Up Extrem Surg 10:8–13

Barron BJ, Dhekne RD (1984) Cold osteomyelitis. Radionuclide bone scan findings. Clin Nucl Med 9:392–393

Barrera P, Oyen WJ, Boerman OC, van Riel PL (2003) Scintigraphic detection of tumour necrosis factor in patients with rheumatoid arthritis. Ann Rheum Dis 62:825–828

Carroll RE (1953) Osteoid osteoma in the hand. J Bone Joint Surg Am 35-A:888–893

Cerezal L, del Pinal F, Abascal F, Garcia-Valtuille R, Pereda T, Canga A (2002) Imaging findings in ulnar-sided wrist impaction syndromes. Radiographics 22:105–121

Cohen MD, Harrington TM, Ginsburg WW (1983) Osteoid osteoma: 95 cases and a review of the literature. Semin Arthritis Rheum 12:265–281

de Bois MH, Arndt JW, van der Velde EA, van der Lubbe PA, Westedt ML, Pauwels EK et al (1992) 99mTc human immunoglobulin scintigraphy—a reliable method to detect joint activity in rheumatoid arthritis. J Rheumatol 19:1371–1376

Dias JJ, Thompson J, Barton NJ, Gregg PJ (1990) Suspected scaphoid fractures. The value of radiographs. J Bone Joint Surg Br 72:98–101

Escobedo EM, Bergman AG, Hunter JC (1995) MR imaging of ulnar impaction. Skelet Radiol 24:85–90

Friedman SL, Palmer AK (1991) The ulnar impaction syndrome. Hand Clin 7:295–310

Genant HK, Kozin F, Bekerman C, McCarty DJ, Sims J (1975) The reflex sympathetic dystrophy syndrome. A comprehensive analysis using fine-detail radiography, photon absorptiometry, and bone and joint scintigraphy. Radiology 117:21–32

Groves AM, Cheow HK, Balan KK, Bearcroft PW, Dixon AK (2005a) 16 detector multislice CT versus skeletal scintigraphy in the diagnosis of wrist fractures: value of quantification of 99Tcm-MDP uptake. Br J Radiol 78:791–795

Groves AM, Cheow H, Balan K, Courtney H, Bearcroft P, Dixon A (2005b) 16-MDCT in the detection of occult wrist fractures: a comparison with skeletal scintigraphy. AJR Am J Roentgenol 184:1470–1474

Hawkes DJ, Robinson L, Crossman JE, Sayman HB, Mistry R, Maisey MN et al (1991) Registration and display of the combined bone scan and radiograph in the diagnosis and management of wrist injuries. Eur J Nucl Med 18:752–756

Helms CA (1987) Osteoid osteoma. The double density sign. Clin Orthop Relat Res 222:167–173

Hodge JC, Yin Y, Gilula LA (1996) Miscellaneous conditions of the wrist. In: Gilula LA, Yin Y (eds) Imaging of the wrist and hand. Saunders, Philadelphia, pp 523–546

Holder LE, Mackinnon SE (1984) Reflex sympathetic dystrophy in the hands: clinical and scintigraphic criteria. Radiology 152:517–522

Imaeda T, Nakamura R, Shionoya K, Makino N (1996) Ulnar impaction syndrome: MR imaging findings. Radiology 201:495–500

Jamar F, Manicourt DH, Leners N, Vanden Berghe M, Beckers C (1995) Evaluation of disease activity in rheumatoid arthritis and other arthritides using 99mtechnetium labeled nonspecific human immunoglobulin. J Rheumatol 22:850–854

Jamar F, Chapman PT, Manicourt DH, Glass DM, Haskard DO, Peters AM (1997) A comparison between ^{111}In-anti-E-selectin mAb and ^{99}Tcm-labelled human non-specific immunoglobulin in radionuclide imaging of rheumatoid arthritis. Br J Radiol 70:473–481

Kozin F, Soin JS, Ryan LM, Carrera GF, Wortmann RL (1981) Bone scintigraphy in the reflex sympathetic dystrophy syndrome. Radiology 138:437–443

Maurer AH (1991) Nuclear medicine in evaluation of the hand and wrist. Hand Clin 7:183–200

Maurer AH, Chen DC, Camargo EE, Wong DF, Wagner HN Jr, Alderson PO (1981) Utility of three-phase skeletal scintigraphy in suspected osteomyelitis: concise communication. J Nucl Med 22:941–949

Mohamed A, Ryan P, Lewis M, Jarosz JM, Fogelman I, Spencer JD et al (1997) Registration bone scan in the evaluation of wrist pain. J Hand Surg Br 22:161–166

Palmer WE, Rosenthal DI, Schoenberg OI, Fischman AJ, Simon LS, Rubin RH et al (1995) Quantification of inflammation in the wrist with gadolinium-enhanced MR imaging and PET with 2-[F-18]-fluoro-2-deoxy-D-glucose. Radiology 196:647–655

Patel N, Collier BD, Carrera GF, Hanel DP, Sanger JR, Matloub HS et al (1992) High-resolution bone scintigraphy of the adult wrist. Clin Nucl Med 17:449–453

Rolfe EB, Garvie NW, Khan MA, Ackery DM (1981) Isotope bone imaging in suspected scaphoid trauma. Br J Radiol 54:762–767

Sewell KL, Ruthazer R, Parker JA (1993) The correlation of indium-111 joint scans with clinical synovitis in rheumatoid arthritis. J Rheumatol 20:2015–2019

Tumeh SS (1996) Scintigraphy in the evaluation of arthropathy. Radiol Clin North Am 34:215–231

Vande Streek PR, Carretta RF, Weiland FL (1994) Nuclear medicine approaches to musculoskeletal disease. Current status. Radiol Clin North Am 32:227–253

Vande Streek P, Carretta RF, Weiland FL, Shelton DK (1998) Upper extremity radionuclide bone imaging: the wrist and hand. Semin Nucl Med 28:14–24

Wraight AP, Bird N, Screaton N (1997) The clinical impact of accurate co-registration of bone scintigrams and radiographs. Nuc Med Commun 18:291 (Abstract)

Ultrasound Imaging Techniques and Procedures

Stefano Bianchi, René de Gautard, Giorgio Tamborrini, and Stefan Mariacher

Contents

S. Bianchi (✉) · R. de Gautard
CIM SA Cabinet Imagerie Medicale,
Route de Malagnou 40, 1208 Geneva, Switzerland
e-mail: stefanobianchi@bluewin.ch

G. Tamborrini
Rheumaklinik, Universitäts-Spital Zürich,
Rämi-Strasse 100, 8091 Zürich, Switzerland

S. Mariacher
Chefarzt und stv. Vorsitzender der Klinikleitung,
aarReha Schinznach, Badstrasse 55P,
5116 Schinznach-Bad, Switzerland

S. Bianchi
Clinique des Grangettes, Chemin de Grangettes 7, 1224
Geneva, Switzerland

Abstract

The role of ultrasound (US) in the assessment of musculoskeletal disorders is persistently increasing. Recent developments in hardware and software of US equipments and in particular use of small-size, high-frequency transducers have allowed accurate assessment of a wide variety of hand and wrist disorders.

1 Introduction

The role of ultrasound (US) in the assessment of musculoskeletal disorders is persistently increasing (Van Holsbeeck and Introcaso 2001; Mc Nally 2004; Brasseur and Tardieu 2006; Bianchi and Martinoli 2007). Recent developments in hardware and software of US equipments and in particular use of small-size, high-frequency transducers have allowed accurate assessment of a wide variety of hand and wrist disorders. The main advantages of US are its low cost, readiness, non invasivity and possibility to perform a dynamic examination. The main disadvantage is the impossibility to detect and assess deep structures, located behind bones. In addition, US is a highly operator-dependent technique and has a long learning curve. US has been used in the assessment of wrist and hand traumatic, degenerative and infective disorders, as well as in evaluating local masses (Read et al. 1996; Ferrara and Marcelis 1997; Bianchi et al. 1999, 2001, 2003; Teefey et al. 2000; Milbradt et al. 1990; Chiou et al. 2001; Moschilla and Breidahl 2002). Additional studies have stressed its role in the evaluation of inflammatory arthritis (Koski 1992; Grassi et al. 1993).

A. M. Davis et al. (eds.), *Imaging of the Hand and Wrist*, Medical Radiology. Diagnostic Imaging,
DOI: 10.1007/174_2010_109,

Quantification of inflammation and of structural damage is mandatory in the assessment, management and monitoring of rheumatoid arthritis (RA). Without appropriate treatment (e.g. DMARD's, biologics), RA inflammation can progress and result in joint dysfunction and deformity. An early diagnosis can lead to early instauration of a successful treatment. Standard radiographs have an important role to identify changes such as osteopenia, joint space reduction or erosions in patients with advanced arthritis. US is a useful tool in the assessment and follow-up of early to established RA (Wakefield et al. 2000, Szkudlarek et al. Szkudlarek et al. 2004a, b) and can efficiently guide local procedures such as aspiration of effusions or therapeutic injection (Karim et al. 2001). In RA US can detect different pathologic changes including synovitis, cartilage and bone changes, tenosynovitis and tendon tears, bursitis, rheumatoid nodules or secondary nerve entrapment (e.g. carpal tunnel syndrome). Clinical studies have shown that US is as effective or even more effective in detecting inflammatory changes as clinical examination. Sensitivity and specificity of US in assessment of joints changes in RA is comparable to MR imaging (Backhaus et al. 1999; Backhaus et al. 2002; Szkudlarek et al. 2004a, b; Scheel et al. 2006). Power Doppler and Colour Doppler US detects active synovial inflammation associated with hypervascularisation and neoangiogenesis. In the presence of an active synovitis, there is an increase in signal activity, which is correlated to the degree of inflammatory activity. Therefore, the use of color and power Doppler US facilitates a differentiation between active and inactive synovitis. Furthermore, numerous studies have shown a good correlation between activity of synovitis at power Doppler and inflammatory changes evident at MRI and at histopathology studies (Walther et al. 2001; Terslev et al. 2003). Echo-contrast-enhanced US has shown an improvement in the measurement of synovial thickness and activity of synovial processes in patients with rheumatoid arthritis and allows better differentiation between effusion and synovial proliferation (Goldberg et al. 1994; Blomley et al. 2001). Besides assessment of the synovium, US can evaluate pathological changes of cartilages and bones if performed using high-resolution ultrasound probes. Bone erosions are a pathophysiological hallmark of RA. US can provide a more accurate and comprehensive assessment of bone erosions than plain radiography. The size of erosions can be monitored to evaluate disease progression.

Accurate knowledge of the normal anatomy, technique of US examination and of the US appearance of the hand and wrist are definite pre-requisites for a successful US examination. The target of this chapter is to present the technique of the US examination and the normal US anatomy of the hand and wrist.

2 Technique of Examination and Normal US Appearance

Before starting the US examination, any previous imaging studies and blood tests, if available, are reviewed. Every effort must be made to obtain a recent radiographic examination, in at least two perpendicular views, since this allows a good analysis of joints and bones and is complementary to US that permit an excellent assessment of most soft tissues. A brief clinical evaluation is always obtained since it helps in pointing the attention of the examiner to a specific area, thus shortening the time of examination and allowing a more detailed local assessment. The patient is asked for duration of symptoms, type and rhythm of pain (mechanic or inflammatory), presence of tingling, numbness or morning stiffness. If pain is the main symptom, its location and modification during muscle contraction or joint movements can often orient toward the correct diagnosis. In De Quervain tenosynovitis, for example, a sharp, acute pain located over the radial styloid and worsened by ulnar deviation of the wrist with the thumb flexed is highly suggestive of the diagnosis. The distribution of peripheral tingling can indicate the injured nerve (radial, ulnar or median). A brief regional physical examination including assessment of any local or diffuse swelling, warm or reddens follows. The joint range of motion and local tenderness are also briefly assessed.

Schematically, there are two main kinds of performing a US examination of the wrist and hand. A *focused examination* generally performed in patients suffering from disorders affecting the periarticular tissues and a *systemic examination* mostly directed to the joints. The first is a shorter examination concentrated on a specific region, selected by the sonologist according to the data available from the physician's US request, type of symptoms and results of the brief clinical examination described earlier. We perform this type of examination in the vast majority of our patients. To give an example in a patient presenting with a painless lump at the dorsum of the wrist suspected to be a ganglion by the referring physician, the US examination can be limited to the dorsal aspect of the wrist. A time-consuming, detailed examination of all metacarpophalangeal and interphalangeal joints is not necessary and useless in such a patient. The second type of US examination is a more time-consuming, systematic examination usually obtained only in patients with a clinical suspicion or diagnosis of systemic arthritis. In both cases, a scrupulous technique of realization of the US examination, including images obtained in several planes and dynamic test, must be deployed (Creteur and Peetrons 2000; Middleton et al. 2001; Lee and Healy 2005; Tagliafico et al. 2007).

For didactic purposes, we first describe the basic anatomy of the main structures amenable to US assessment followed by description of the US technique of examination and of the normal US anatomy. We will follow an anatomic pattern, starting with the dorsal aspect of the wrist and the hand followed by the palmar aspect.

For optimal US examination of the wrist and hand, the patient sat facing the examiner with the forearm resting on the examination bed. We routinely start the examination by scanning the dorsal aspect of the wrist followed by the hand through transverse and sagittal sonograms. Then, the patient is asked to supinate the hand that now lies on its dorsal aspect, to allow examination of its palmar aspect. Again transverse sonograms are followed by longitudinal images. Color Doppler is routinely obtained. Dynamic scanning allows identification of each extensor and flexor tendon of the fingers and, most importantly, allows optimal judgement of tendons' gliding and eventual impingement inside osteofibrous tunnels. This is very useful in judging presence of tendons adhesions. Application of variable pressure with the transducer permits obtaining additional data. A firm pressure helps in eliciting local pain and thus in focalizing the examination. It also assists in judging consistency of masses facilitating for example the diagnosis of soft tissue lipoma. On the contrary, large amount of gel must be used in assessing fluid collections in order to lessen local pressure trough the probe and avoid inadvertent displacement of the fluid that can result in a negative examination. In assessing presence of vessels with color Doppler, excessive pressure can result in squeezing of vessels resulting in impossibility to accurately detect local hypervascular changes. In testing the permeability of subcutaneous veins, color Doppler is obtained during squeezing of the soft tissues distal to the site of examination performed with the contralateral hand of the examiner. This allows a temporary increase in venous blood velocity and its easier detection at color Doppler. On the contrary, blocking the venous drainage at the forearm causes dilatation of the distal vein and results in stagnation of blood inside venous masses. As previously discussed, palpation under US guidance can be realized through the transducer when a large mass is evaluated. When the mass is small, US-guided palpation is better performed by using an opened paper clip. Once placed between the transducer and the skin, this can be followed under real-time scanning thanks to its typical posterior comet tail artifact. This technique works well in cutaneous marking of soft tissue foreign bodies as well as in accurate localization of small neuromas.

3 Dorsal Aspect

US allows an accurate evaluation of the dorsal aspect of wrist and hand (Figs. 1, 2, 3, 4, 5, 6, 7, 8). Accessory muscles can be found at the dorsal face of the wrist (Muncibì et al. 2008) as anatomic variants mimicking local tumors. They show at US the typical internal muscle structure made by alternating hypoechoic (muscle fibers) and hyperechoic (fibroadipose septa) bands. Dynamic examination during resisted contraction shows contraction of the accessory muscle thus confirming the diagnosis. Located under the skin and subcutaneous tissues, a thin fascia covers the extensor tendons (ET). These tendons origin from the miotendineous junctions, located in the forearm at different level for each muscle, run distally between the joint plane and the subcutaneous tissue, to finally insert into the bone of the wrist and hand. Since all ET change their course before joining their insertion, they are prone to instability during changes of position of the wrist and hand joints. To avoid instability, the ET run inside fibrosseous tunnels. These are made by the surface of bones covered by periosteum (the floor) and by superficial fibrous bands named retinacula (the ceiling). To further increase tendons stability, the bone surface is not flat but made by grooves, sulci or protuberances. A synovial sheath composed by a visceral and parietal

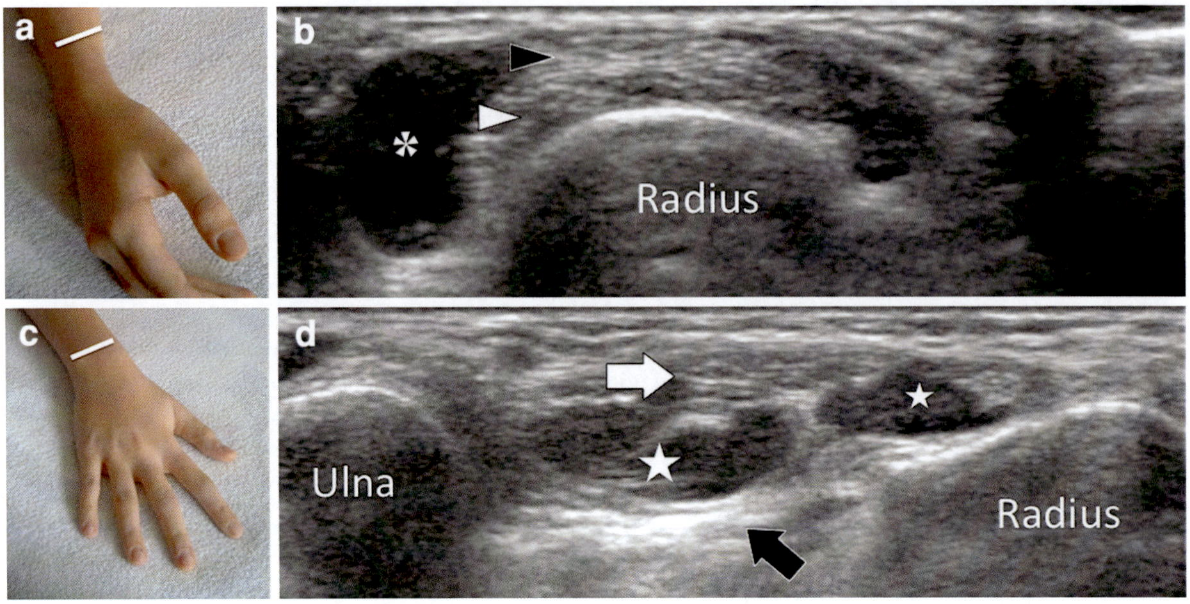

Fig. 1 Dorsal aspect. **a**, **c** Probe positioning for transverse examination. **b** Sonogram obtained as shown in a. US shows the crossing of the tendon of the first extensor compartment (*black arrowhead*) over those of the second compartment (*white arrowhead*). *Asterisk* distal part of the muscle of the first extensor compartment. **d** Sonogram obtained as shown in c. US shows the miotendineous junctions of the extensor pollicis longus (*small star*) and extensor indicis proprius (*large star*). The extensor digitorum communis tendons (*white arrow*) are located more superficially. Note the interosseous membrane (*black arrow*) appearing as a hyrechogenic structure connecting the ulna and the radius

Fig. 2 Dorsal aspect. **a**, **c**, **e** Probe positioning for transverse examination. **b**, **d**, **f** corresponding sonograms. **b** *White arrowhead* extensor digitorum communis tendons, *black arrowhead* extensor pollicis longus tendon. **d** *White arrowhead* extensor digitorum communis tendons, *arrow* extensor carpi ulnaris tendon. **f** *Black arrowhead* extensor pollicis longus tendon, *stars* extensor carpi radialis tendons

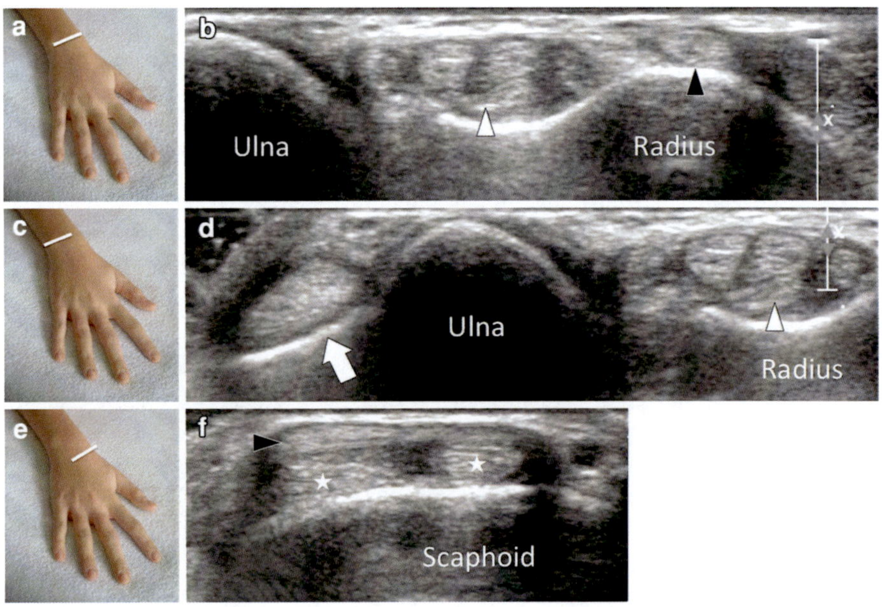

layer, gliding one over the other, surrounds the tendons and reduces local frictions during gliding. The visceral layer is adherent to the tendon and moves with it, while the parietal layer is lax and blends with the retinacula and other peritendineous structures. The layers are separated by a thin amount of synovial fluid. At the level of the distal radius and wrist, the twelve ET run inside six tunnels. The tunnels are numbered from the

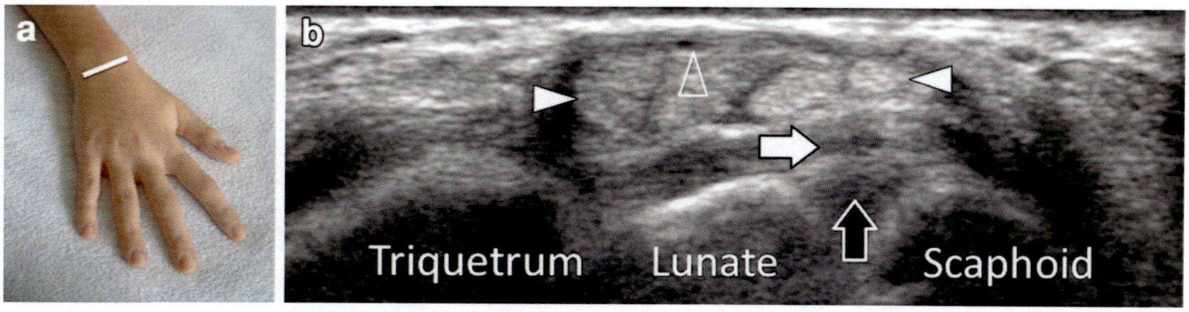

Fig. 3 Dorsal aspect. **a** Probe positioning for transverse examination **b** corresponding sonogram. *White arrowheads* extensor digitorum communis tendons, *void arrowhead* retinaculum of the 4th compartment of the extensor tendons. *White arrow* extrinsic dorsal carpal ligaments and radiocarpal synovial space, *black arrow* dorsal band of the scapho-lunate ligament

Fig. 4 Dorsal aspect. **a**, **c** Probe positioning for transverse examination. **b** Sonogram obtained as shown in **a**. *Met* metacarpals, *DIM* dorsal interosseous muscles, *black arrowheads* extensor tendons. **d** Sonogram obtained as shown in **c**. *White arrowheads* extensor indicis proprius and extensor digitorum communis tendon of the index

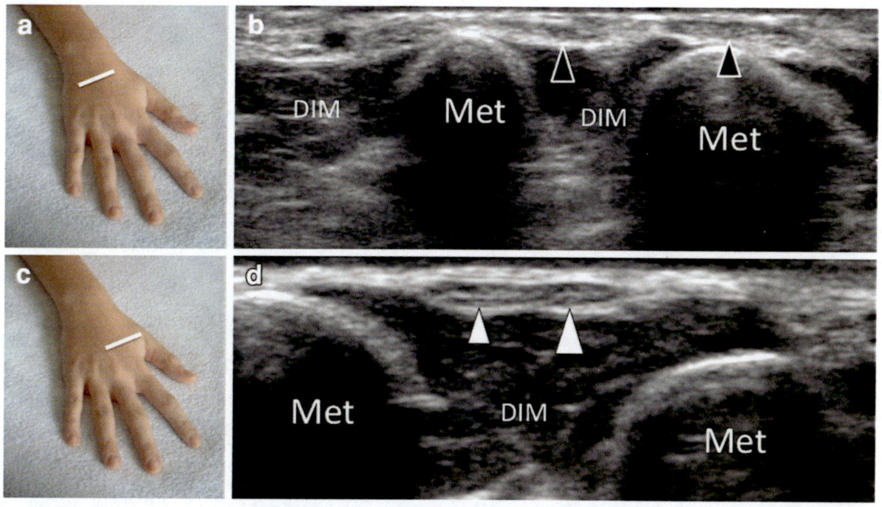

Fig. 5 Dorsal aspect. **a**, **c** Probe positioning for transverse examination. **b** Sonogram obtained as shown in **a**. *Met* metacarpal, *white arrowhead* extensor digitorum tendon, *asterisks* subcutaneous veins. **d** Sonogram obtained as shown in **c**. *White arrowheads* extensor digitorum communis tendons, *black arrowheads* sagittal bands

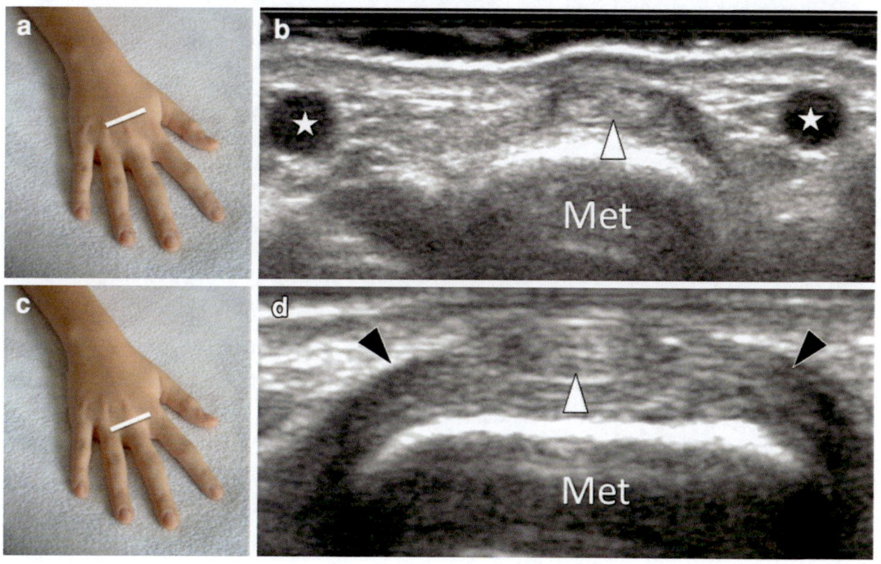

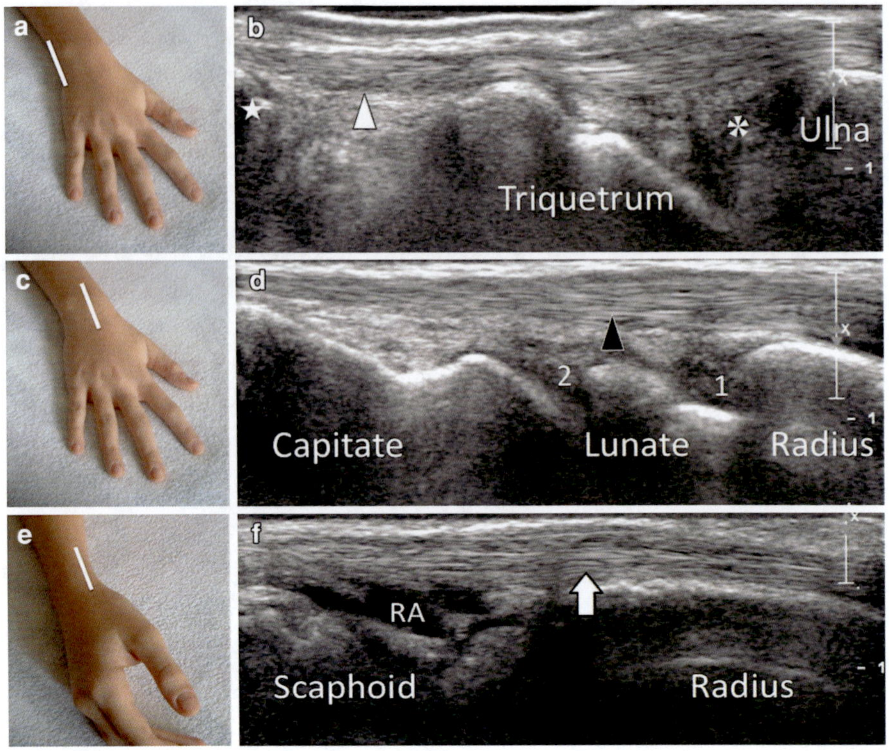

Fig. 6 Dorsal aspect. **a**, **c**, **e** Probe positioning for longitudinal examination. **b**, **d**, **f** corresponding sonograms. **b** *Asterisk* triangular fibrocartilage complex, *white arrowhead* extensor carpi ulnaris tendon, *star* base of the fifth metacarpal. **d** *Black arrowhead* extensor digitorum communis tendons, *1* radiocarpal joint, *2* mediocarpal joint. **f** *Arrow* extensor tendons of the first compartments, *RA* radial artery

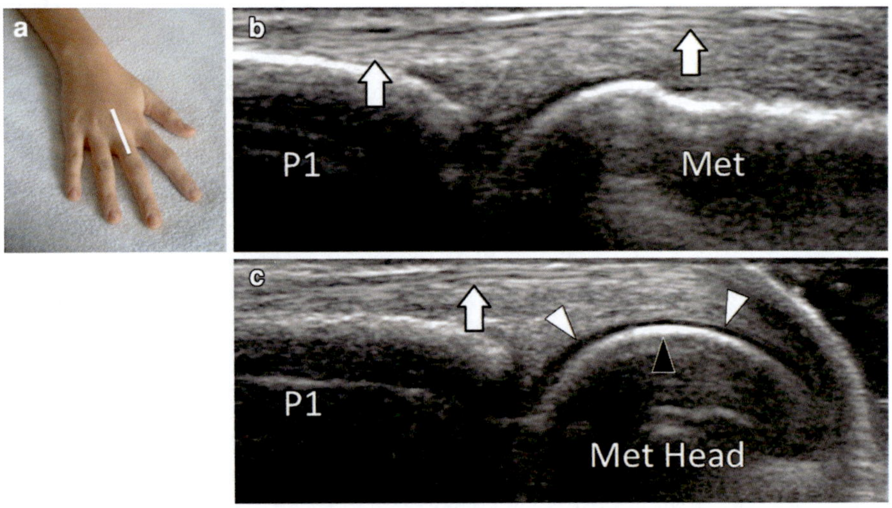

Fig. 7 Dorsal aspect. **a** Probe positioning for longitudinal examination. **b** Sonogram obtained as shown in **a**. **b** *Arrows* extensor digitorum communis tendon, *P1* proximal phalanx. **c** Sonogram obtained with 90° of flexion of the metacarpophalangeal joint. *White arrowheads* articular cartilage, *black arrowhead* subchondral bone plate

most radial to the most ulnar. The first tunnel is located over the radial styloid while the sixth is found at the level of the cubital head. Table 1 resumes the arrangement of the tendons inside the six tunnels.

US shows the ET as hyperechoic, homogeneous structures showing a typical fibrillar structure in the longitudinal sonograms. The borders of normal tendons are regular and well defined. The normal synovial sheath and the tiny amount of fluid contained inside it can't be detected even if high-resolution transducers are used. Retinacula are imaged at US as hyper or hypoechoic structures depending on the incidence of the US bean. They present different thickness depending of the fibroosseous tunnel examined. The retinaculum of the fourth compartment is the thicker and, since it appears mostly

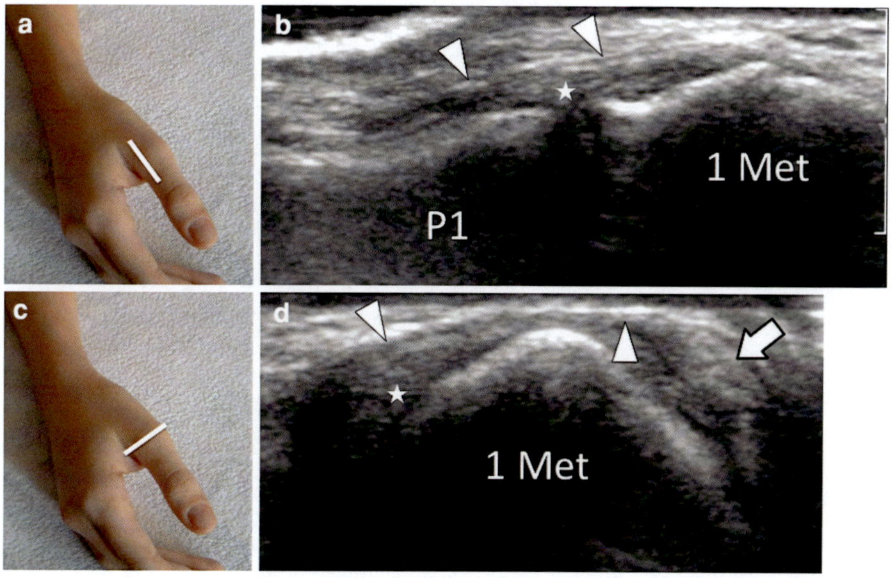

Fig. 8 Dorsal aspect. **a**, **c** Probe positioning for longitudinal and transverse examination. **b** Sonogram obtained as shown in **a**. *1 Met* first metacarpal, *white arrowheads* aponeurosys of the adductor pollicis brevis muscle, *asterisk* ulnar collateral ligament. **d** Sonogram obtained as shown in **c**. *1 Met* first metacarpal, *white arrowheads* aponeurosys of the adductor pollicis brevis muscle, *asterisk* ulnar collateral ligament, *arrow* extensor pollicis longus tendon

Table 1 Extensor tendons

1 Tunnel = abductor pollicis longus
2 Tunnel = extensor pollicis brevis
3 Tunnel = extensor pollicis longus
4 Tunnel = extensor digitorum communis and extensor indicis proprius
5 Tunnel = extensor digiti minimi
6 Tunnel = extensor carpi ulnaris

hypoechoic, can simulate an effusion to unexperienced examiners (Robertson et al. 2007). The mean value or retinaculas' thickness in other tunnels is around 0.3-0.5 mm. In case of suspicion of mild thickening of retinacula, the contralateral side can be scanned to improve diagnostic confidence. In normal conditions, color Doppler does not allow detecting the normal vascularisation of tendons, sheath or retinacula. Any Doppler signals inside these structures must be retained as pathologic. Axial images allow a good analysis of details of different ET. To give an example, the APL is almost always made by multiple thin tendons rather then by a single tendon (De Maeseneer et al. 2009). This normal variation seems to facilitate impingement inside the first osteofibrous tunnel.

Deep to the ET of the third compartment, located close to the lateral aspect of the Lister's tubercle, the distal sensitive branch of the posterior interosseous nerve can be seen running from the forearm to the dorsal aspect of the wrist. At its distal portion, the normal nerve can present a bulbous swelling (Acrel's ganglion) that must not be interpreted as a pathologic neuroma or as evidence of chronic compression. The origin of this fusiform swelling is unknown. Histologically, it is made by normal peripheral nerve structures without any neuronal cell bodies (Tubbs et al. 2007). The term pseudoganglion seems then more appropriate then that of ganglion. In younger subjects, a small artery (distal anterior interosseous artery) can be detected running close to the nerve. The distal radio-ulnar, radiocarpal, mediocarpal and carpo-metacarpal joints can be well imaged and changes related to degenerative or erosive arthropathy detected. US can efficiently guide intraarticular injections (Lohman et al. 2007) under real time control. This helps in avoiding injury to adjacent structures such as nerves and vessels and in confirming the correct site of injection. US allows detection and assessment of several extrinsic articular ligaments as well as of the scapho-lunate ligament (Griffith et al. 2001; Jacobson et al. 2002; Finlay et al. 2004; Boutry et al. 2005; Taljanovic et al. 2008; Bihan et al. 2009; Renoux et al. 2009).

At the level of the dorsum of the hand and of the fingers, the ET can be followed till their distal insertion by US. The EPB is one of the thinnest tendons and inserts into the base of the proximal phalanx of the thumb. The two extensor carpi tendons (ECRB and ECRL) can be followed till their insertion into the base of the second and third metacarpals. The EPL has a more complex course. At the distal radius, it reflects on the medial aspect of the Lister's tubercle, a bony ridge separating the third and the second compartment of the ET. Then, it points to the base of the thumb and overlies the ECRB and ECRL tendons. Finally, it joins the EPB at the level of the head of the first metacarpal to then insert into the base of the distal phalanx of the thumb. The EPL is then subject to local friction at two levels: at the Lister tubercle and when it crosses with the two extensor carpi tendons (De Maeseneer et al. 2005). The index has two extensor tendons, the communis and the indicis proprius, which runs medial to the communis. They have similar size and course. The EIP can be harvested and used as a tendon graft in several surgical procedures. The extensor digitorum communis tendons present a high variable organization at the dorsum of the hand related to presence of the so-called tendinous junctions. These are thin tendons directed obliquely and joining adjacent ET. The dorsal interossei muscles can be seen appreciated lying among the hyperechoic metatarsals.

At the level of the metacarpophalangeal joints, the ET are retained over the dorsal aspect of the joint by the sagittal bands, thin ligaments that prevent palmar displacement of the tendons during flexion of the fingers. These bands appear as thin hyperechoic laminae covering the tendons and inserting into the periphery of the capsule. At the level of the proximal phalanx, the ET of the 2–5 fingers split into a central band and two lateral bands. The central band inserts into the base of the middle phalanx while the lateral bands join into the midline to insert into the distal phalanx. The ET are well assessed by US at the level of the MCP joint. Their distal splitting is sometimes difficult to be appreciated at transverse images. Longitudinal images allow visualization of the insertion of the central band as well as of the distal insertion into the distal phalanx. Details of the insertion of the intrinsic muscles are not detected at US. The metacarpophalangeal and interphalangeal joints can be imaged in the sagittal and axial plane. US allows an accurate assessment of erosive articular changes (McNally 2008). The cartilage of the metacarpal and phalanx head can be judged by using a dorsal and palmar approach in the extended and flexed joint while the cartilage of the bases of the phalanges are not detectable at US. US examination performed during gentle stress of the fingers' joints can help in judging the capsuloligamteous complex. This is most often performed at the level of the MCP of the thumb in the evaluation of tears of the ulnar collateral ligament.

4 Palmar Aspect

The palmar aspect of the wrist houses several tendons, nerves, and vessels (Figs. 9, 10, 11, 12, 13, 14, 15). Abbreviations for these structures are listed in Table 2. The most superficial and thinnest tendon is the PG that runs in the midline of the wrist within the subcutaneous tissue. The PG presents a high anatomic variability. It can be absent or be replaced by a muscle (palmaris inversus). In a deeper position, the flexor tendons of the fingers (FDS, FDP, FPL) run inside the carpal tunnel (CT), a fibroosseous tunnel made by the carpal bones (the floor) and a palmar thick ligament, the transverse carpal ligament (TCL) (the ceiling). Inside the CT, the tendons are surrounded by a common synovial sheath enveloping the FDS and FDP of the 2–5 fingers. This common sheath generally communicates with the digital sheath of the fifth finger. The 2–4 fingers have separate digital sheaths. The FPL has a separate long sheath extending from the CT till to the proximal phalanx of the thumb. The FCR, a strong tendon surrounded by its own synovial sheath, is also located inside the CT but runs in a separate lateral channel. In its distal portion, the FCR overlies the tubercle of the scaphoid and reflects over the palmar aspect of scapho-trapezio-trapezoid joint to deepen and reach its distal insertion into the base of the 2 and 3 metacarpals. The FCU is a straight tendon located at the medial aspect of the anterior face of the wrist that inserts into the proximal pole of the pisiform. Since it has a straight course this tendon is not surrounded by a synovial sheath but by its peritenon, a thin connective tissue lamina that facilitates its gliding. Besides several tendons, the CT houses also the MN, a flat nerve located just under the TCL at the radial aspect of the tunnel. The nerve has a close relation with the FDP and FDS of the index. It innervates the muscles of the thenar eminence as well as the 1st and 2nd lumbrical muscles. The MN is responsible for sensitivity of the first three fingers and radial aspect of the fourth finger. Details of its anatomy and anatomic variations will be discussed in more details in Nerve Entrapment Syndromes. The Guyon's tunnel is a small fibrooseeous tunnel located superficially and medially to the CT. It is delimited by the TCL and the lateral aspect of the pisiform (the roof) and the

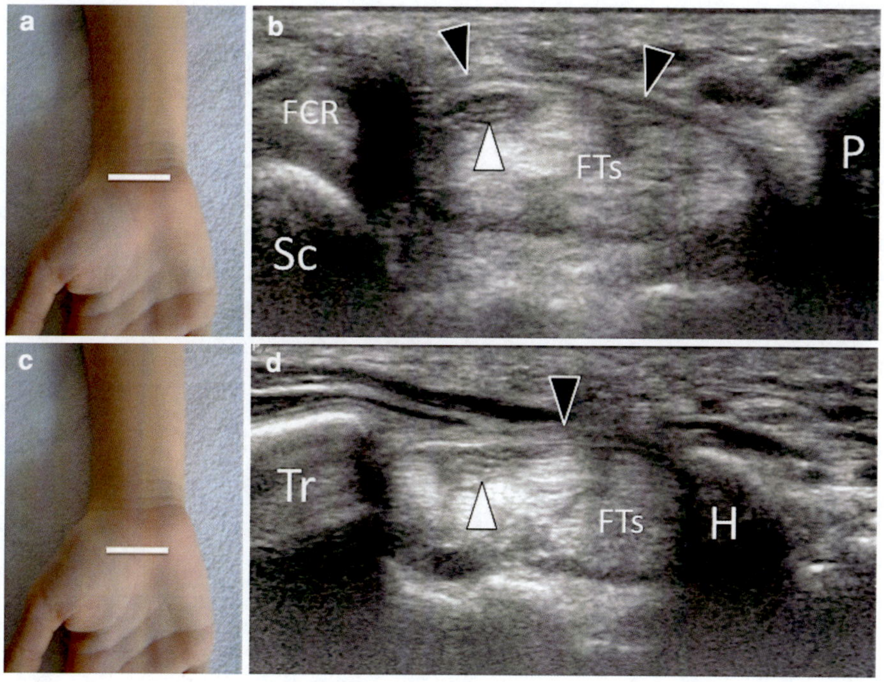

Fig. 9 Palmar aspect. **a**, **c** Probe positioning for transverse examination. **b** Sonogram obtained as shown in **a**. *Sc* scaphoid, *P* pisiform, *FTs* flexor tendons, *white arrowhead* median nerve, *black arrowheads* transverse carpal ligament. **d** Sonogram obtained as shown in **c**. *Tr* trapezium, *H* hook of the hamate, *FTs* flexor tendons, *white arrowhead* median nerve, *black arrowheads* transverse carpal ligament

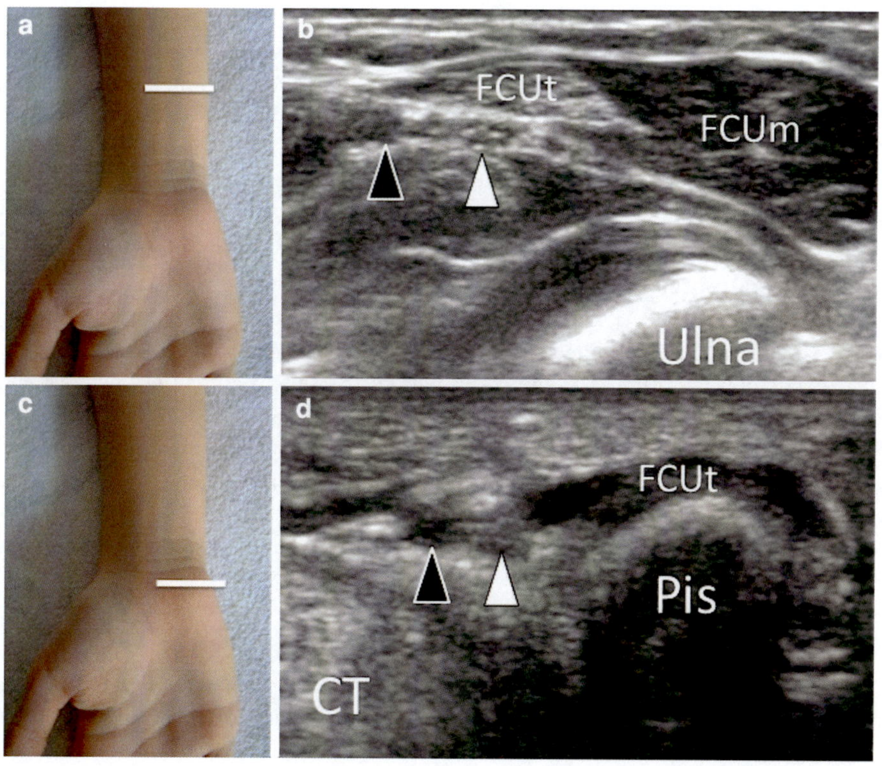

Fig. 10 Palmar aspect. **a**, **c** Probe positioning for transverse examination. **b** Sonogram obtained as shown in **a**. *FCUt* and *FCUm* tendon and muscle of the flexor carpi ulnaris, *white arrowhead* ulnar nerve, *black arrowhead* ulnar artery. **d** Sonogram obtained as shown in **c** (Guyon's tunnel). *Pis* pisiform, *CT* carpal tunnel, *white arrowhead* ulnar nerve, *black arrowhead* ulnar artery

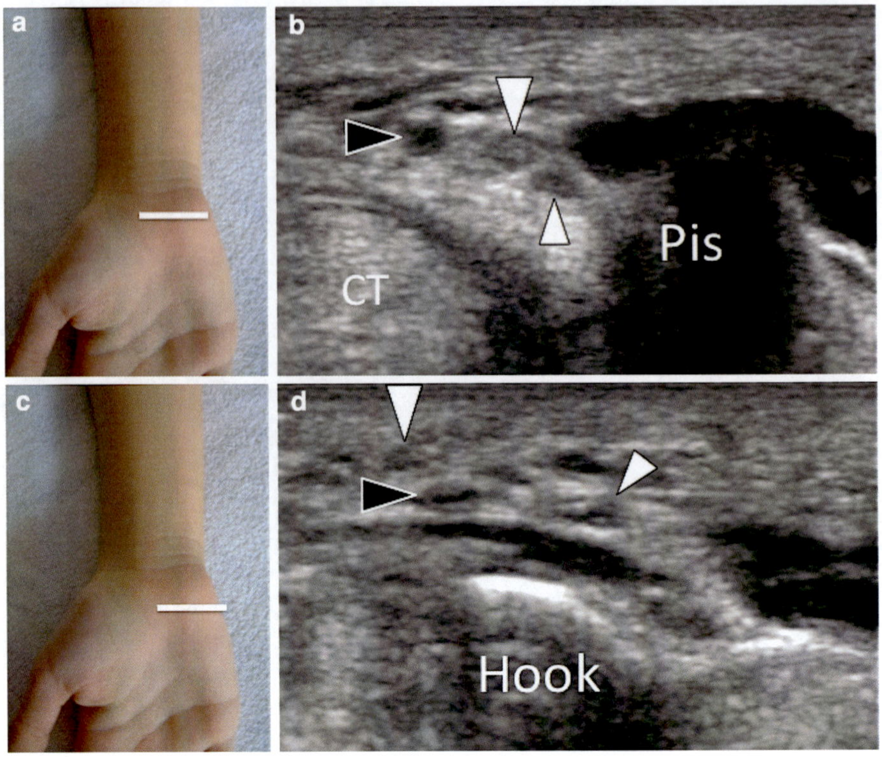

Fig. 11 Palmar aspect. **a**, **c** Probe positioning for transverse examination. **b** Sonogram obtained as shown in **a** (Guyon's tunnel). *Pis* pisiform, *CT* carpal tunnel, *large white arrowhead* superficial branch of the ulnar nerve, *small white arrowhead* deep branch of the ulnar nerve, *black arrowhead* ulnar artery. **d** Sonogram obtained as shown in **c** (Guyon's tunnel), *Hook* hook of the hamate bone, *large white arrowhead* superficial branch of the ulnar nerve, *small white arrowhead* deep branch of the ulnar nerve, *black arrowhead* ulnar artery

palmar carpal ligament (the ceiling). The tunnel houses, embedded by fat, the UN and the UAr surrounded by several UVe. The nerve is located between the artery and the pisiform. At variable level inside the tunnel or immediately distal to it, the UN splits in one motor branch and one or two sensitive branches. A more detailed description of the Guyon's anatomy will be presented in Nerve Entrapment Syndromes. The UN is responsible for sensitivity of the fifth finger and medial aspect of the fourth finger. At the radial aspect of the wrist, the RAr is found running deep to the superficial fascia surrounded by satellite veins. The artery has close relation with the distal part of the sensitive branch of the RN. At the palm of the hand, the FDS and the FDP of the 2–5 fingers run together to join the base of the fingers. Their synovial sheaths are not detectable even when high-frequency transducers are used. The FDP, located just inferior to the FDS, give insertion to the lumbricals muscles. The vessels and the branches of the MN and UN run together located among the lumbricals muscles and the FDS surrounded by fat. More deeply are located the palmar interossei muscles. Utilization of high-frequency probes allows an optimal assessment of the anatomy of the flexor tendons at the fingers. Transverse images show splitting of the FDS at the level of the proximal phalanx. The two tendineous laminae are located from proximal to distal: first superior, then lateral and medial and finally, inferior to the FDP tendon. They insert into the base of the middle phalanx. The FDP presents typically a triangular aspect with the base inferior in proximal scans and superior in more distal images. A frequent anatomic variation is bifidity of the FDP at the level of the distal part of the middle phalanx. This must not be interpreted as a posttraumatic longitudinal split. Longitudinal images are best suited to evaluate the tendons dynamically. When performed at the level of the MCP joint during flexion of the DIP joint, they show selective movements of the FDP tendon. Simultaneous flexion of the IPP joint allows concomitant movements of the FDS tendon. The insertion of the two FDS hemitendons can be imaged at the level of the intermediate phalanx by displacing the transducer medially and laterally. The insertion of the FDP into the base of the P3 is ready evident on sagittal images obtained over the distal phalanx. A variety of pulleys (annular and cruciform) retain the flexor tendons against the palmar aspect of the phalanges thus preventing palmar instability during

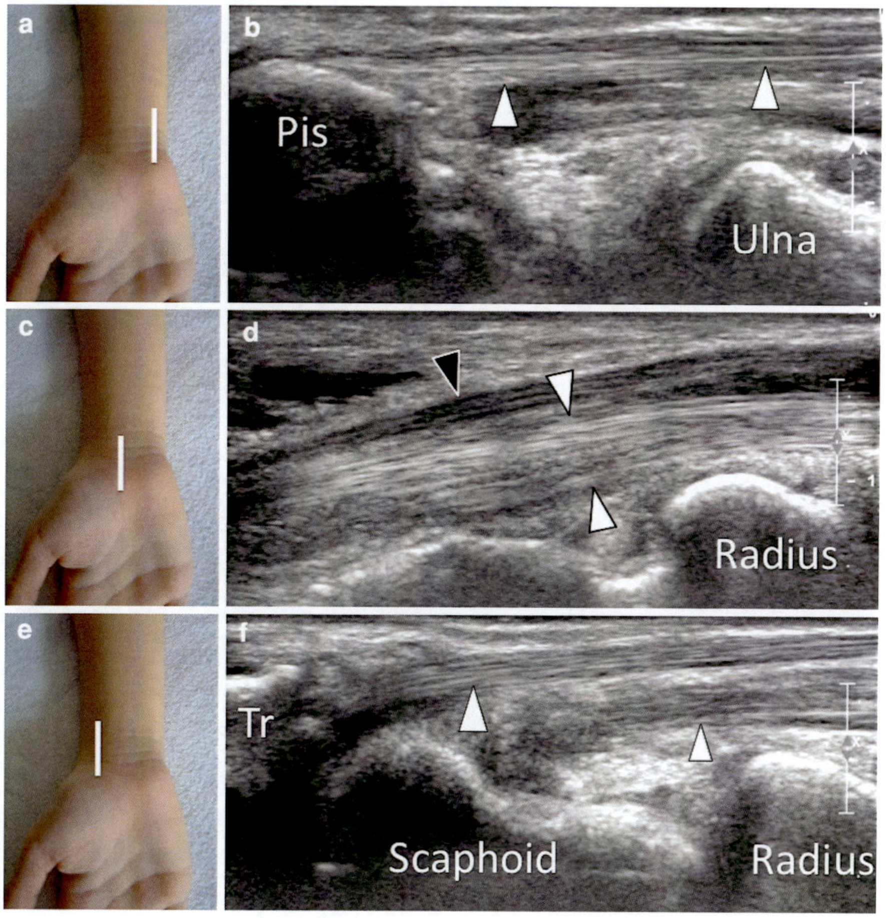

Fig. 12 Palmar aspect. **a**, **c**, **e** Probe positioning for longitudinal examination. **b**, **d**, **f** corresponding sonograms. **b** *Pis* pisiform, *white arrowheads* flexor carpi ulnaris tendon. **d** *Black arrowhead* median nerve, *white arrowheads* flexor digitorum tendons. **f** *Large white arrowhead* flexor carpi radialis tendon, *small white arrowhead* flexor pollicis longus tendon, *Tr* Trapezium

flexion (Bodner et al. 1999; Martinoli et al. 2000). Annular pulleys are quite rigid and are the main structures that prevent tendons bowstringing during flexion. They are numbered from 1 to 5 from proximal to, distal. The A2 and A4 pulleys located, respectively, at the base of P1 and P2 are functionally the most important. The annular pulleys are visualized as thin hyperechoic structures in longitudinal images. They show a normal thickening of their insertion in transverse images. The cruciform pulleys are more lax and located among the annular pulleys. They can be visualized at US only when a significant amount of fluid is present inside the tendon sheath.

The different joints of the fingers can be examined by sagittal and axial sonograms. The palmar plates are well depicted as hyperechoic structures, with homogeneous internal appearance, inserting into the base of the phalanges. Examination performed during gentle hyperextension of the examined joint can help in analysis of local tears or avulsions. The palmar articular synovial recess is ready evident and must be analyzed for local effusion or synovial hypertrophy. Axial sonograms of the digital soft tissues allow assessment of the digital vessels and nerves till the level of the distal interphalangeal joint if high-frequency transducers are used.

5 Key Points

5.1 Advantages of Ultrasound in Wrist and Hand Assessment

- Ready available
- Non invasive
- Inexpensive
- Patient friendly
- Dynamic
- High resolution

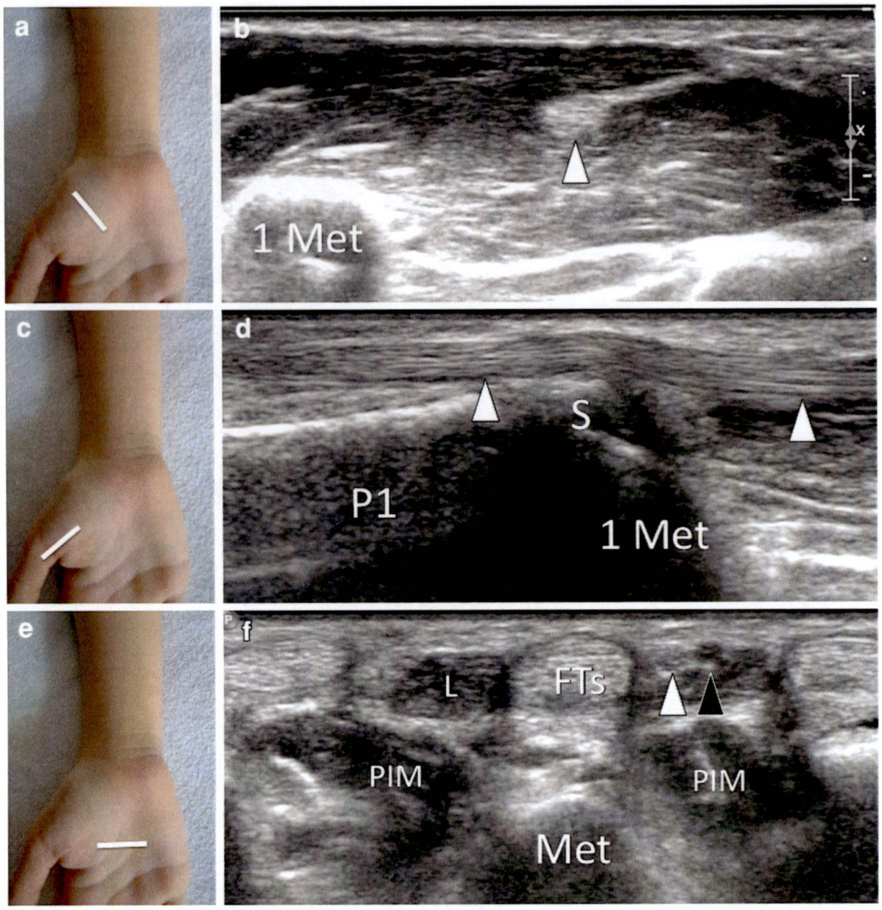

Fig. 13 Palmar aspect. **a**, **c**, **e** Probe positioning. **b**, **d**, **f** Corresponding sonograms. **b** *1 Met* first metacarpal, *white arrowhead* flexor pollicis longus tendon. **d** *P1* proximal phalanx of the thumb, *S* sesamoid bone, *white arrowhead* flexor pollicis longus tendon. *F Fts* flexor tendons, *L* lumbrical muscle, *PIM* palmar interosseous muscles, *Met* metacarpal, *white arrowhead* common palmar digital artery, *black arrowhead* palmar digital nerve

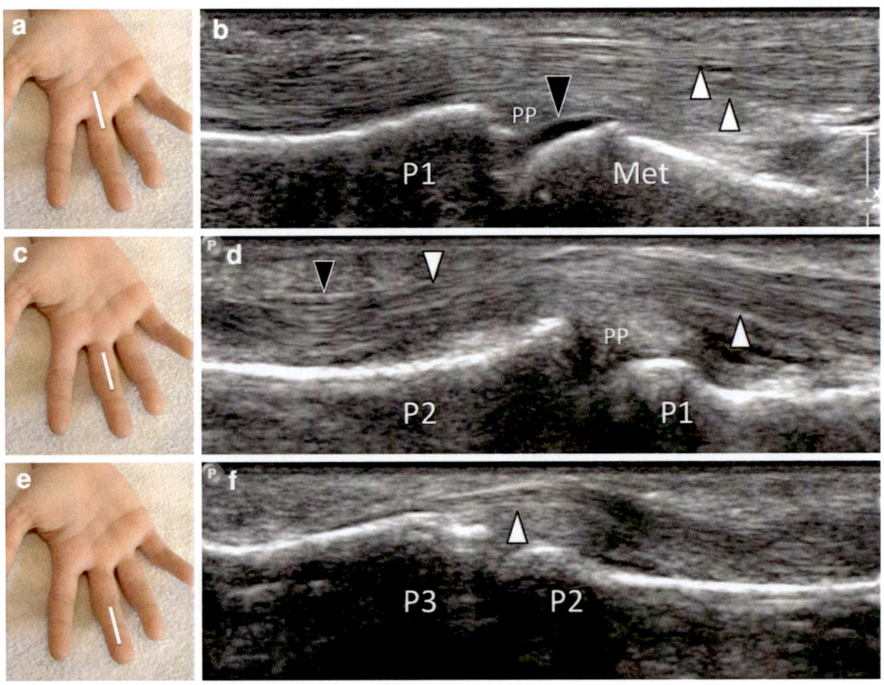

Fig. 14 Palmar aspect. **a**, **c**, **e** Probe positioning for longitudinal examination. **b**, **d**, **f** corresponding sonograms. **b** *Met* metacarpal, *P1* proximal phalanx, *PP* palmar plate, *white arrowheads* flexor digitorum superficialis and profundus tendons, *large black arrowhead* cartilage of the metacarpal head. **d** *P2* middle phalanx, *white arrowheads* flexor digitorum superficialis and profundus tendons, *small black arrowhead* A4 annular pulley. *F P3* distal phalanx, *white arrowhead* flexor digitorum profundus tendon

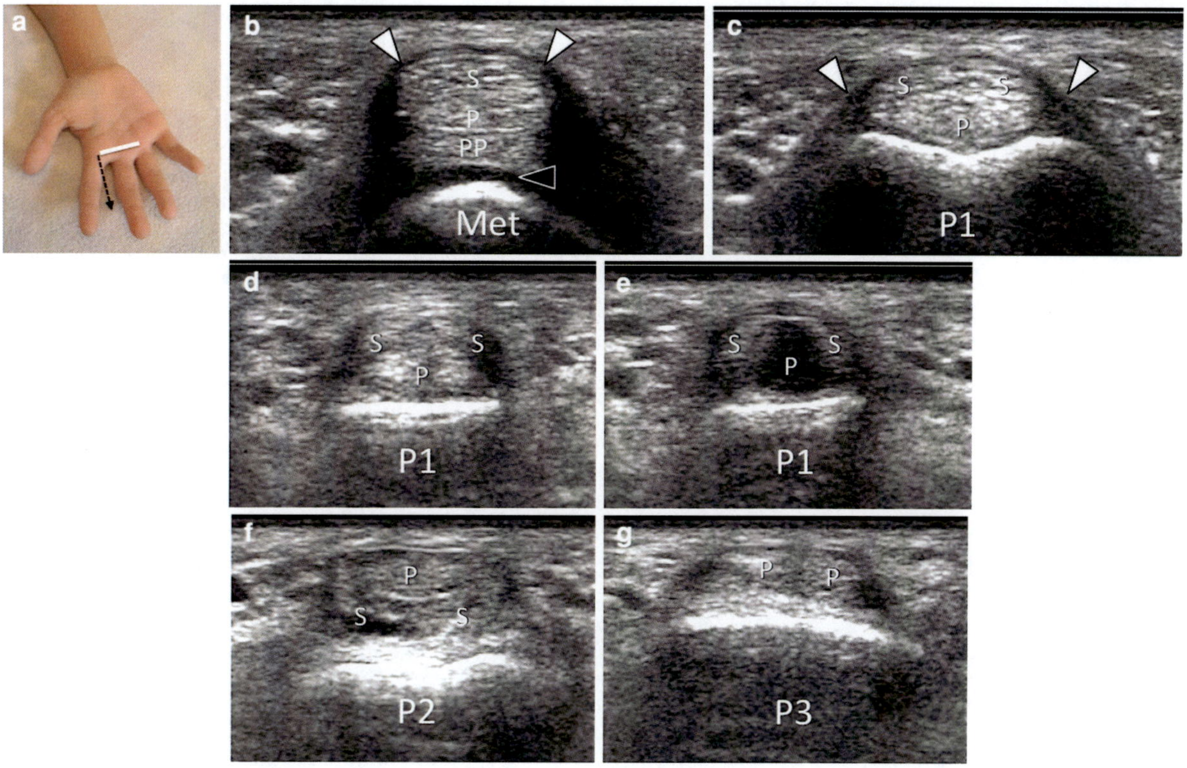

Fig. 15 Palmar aspect. **a** Probe positioning for transverse examination. **b–g** corresponding sonograms obtained from proximal to distal. **b–g** *White arrowheads* Annular pulleys, *S* flexor digitorum superficialis tendon, *P* flexor digitorum profundus tendon, *PP* palmar plate of the metacarpophalangeal joint, *black arrowhead* cartilage of the metacarpal head, *Met* metacarpal, *P1* proximal phalanx, *P2* middle phalanx, *P3* distal phalanx

Table 2 Anatomic structures of the palmar aspect of the wrist

Flexor tendons
PG = palmaris gracilis
FDS = flexor digitorum superficialis
FDP = flexor digitorum profundus
FPL = flexor pollicis longus
FCR = flexor carpi radialis
FCU = flexor carpi ulnaris
Nerves
MN = median nerve
UN = ulnar nerve
RN = radial nerve
Vessels
RAr = radial artery
RVe = radial veins
UAr = ulnar artery
UVe = ulnar veins

5.2 Disadvantages of Ultrasound in Wrist and Hand Assessment

- Long learning curve
- Operator dependent
- Partial assessment of cartilages, ligaments and bones

5.3 Operator Requisites for US Examination in Wrist and Hand Assessment

- Perfect knowledge of the normal anatomy and anatomic variants
- Clinical knowledge of the main disorders affecting the wrist and hand
- Use of accurate and standardized technique of examination

5.4 Basic Principles of US Technique of Examination in Wrist and Hand Assessment

- Perform a basic clinical examination of the affected area and review other imaging studies before starting the US examination
- Focus the examination on the basis of clinical findings
- Analyze the structures using multiple planes of scanning
- Perform dynamic examination and color Doppler examination
- Bilateral examination if required

References

Backhaus M, Kamradt T, Sandrock D et al (1999) Arthritis of the finger joints: a comprehensive approach comparing conventional radiography, scintigraphy, ultrasound, and contrast-enhanced magnetic resonance imaging. Arthritis Rheum 42:1232–1245

Backhaus M, Burmester G-R, Sandrock D et al (2002) Prospective two-year follow-up study comparing novel and conventional imaging procedures in patients with arthritic finger joints. Ann Rheum Dis 61:895–904

Bianchi S, Martinoli C (2007) Ultrasound of the musculoskeletal system. Springer, Heidelberg

Bianchi S, Martinoli C, Abdelwahab IF (1999) High-frequency ultrasound examination of the wrist and hand. Skeletal Radiol 28:121–129

Bianchi S, Martinoli C, Sureda D et al (2001) Ultrasound of the hand. Eur J Ultrasound 14:29–34

Bianchi S, Martinoli C, Montet X et al (2003) Wrist and hand ultrasound. Radiologe 43:831–840

Bihan M, Pesquer L, Meyer P et al (2009) High resolution sonography of the dorsal radiocarpal and intercarpal ligaments: findings in healthy subjects with anatomic correlation to cadaveric wrists. J Radiol 90:813–817

Blomley MJ, Cooke JC, Unger EC et al (2001) Microbubble contrast agents: a new era in ultrasound. BMJ 322:1222–1225

Bodner G, Rudish A, Gabl M et al (1999) Diagnosis of digital flexor tendon annular pulley disruption: comparison of high frequency ultrasound and MRI. Ultraschall Med 20:131–136

Boutry N, Lapegue F, Masi L et al (2005) Ultrasonographic evaluation of normal extrinsic and intrinsic carpal ligaments: preliminary experience. Skeletal Radiol 34:513–521

Brasseur J-L, Tardieu M (2006) Echographie de l'appareil locomoteur. Masson, Paris

Chiou HJ, Chou YH, Chang CY (2001) Ultrasonography of the wrist. Can Assoc Radiol J 5:302–311

Creteur V, Peetrons P (2000) Ultrasonography of the wrist and the hand. J Radiol 81:346–352

De Maeseneer M, Marcelis S, Osteaux M et al (2005) Sonography of a rupture of the tendon of the extensor pollicis longus muscle: initial clinical experience and correlation with findings at cadaveric dissection. AJR Am J Roentgenol 184:175–179

De Maeseneer M, Marcelis S, Jager T et al (2009) Spectrum of normal and pathologic findings in the region of the first extensor compartment of the wrist: sonographic findings and correlations with dissections. J Ultrasound Med 28:779–786

Ferrara MA, Marcelis S (1997) Ultrasound examination of the wrist. J Belge Radiol 80:78–80

Finlay K, Lee R, Friedman L (2004) Ultrasound of intrinsic wrist ligament and triangular fibrocartilage injuries. Skeletal Radiol 33:85–90

Goldberg BB, Liu JB, Forsberg F (1994) Ultrasound contrast agents: a review. Ultrasound Med Biol 20:319–333

Grassi W, Tittarelli E, Pirani O et al (1993) Ultrasound examination of metacarpophalangeal joints in rheumatoid arthritis. Scand J Rheumatol 22:243–247

Griffith JF, Chan DP, Ho PC et al (2001) Sonography of the normal scapholunate ligament and scapholunate joint space. J Clin Ultrasound 29:223–229

Jacobson JA, Oh E, Propeck T et al (2002) Sonography of the scapholunate ligament in four cadaveric wrists: correlation with MR arthrography and anatomy. AJR Am J Roentgenol 179:523–527

Karim Z, Wakefield RJ, Conaghan PG et al (2001) The impact of ultrasonography on diagnosis and management of patients with musculoskeletal conditions. Arthritis Rheum 44:2932–2933

Koski JM (1992) Ultrasonography in the detection of effusion in the radiocarpal and midcarpal joints. Scand J Rheumatol 21:79–81

Lee JC, Healy JC (2005) Normal sonographic anatomy of the wrist and hand. Radiographics 25:1577–1590

Lohman M, Vasenius J, Nieminen O (2007) Ultrasound guidance for puncture and injection in the radiocarpal joint. Acta Radiol 48:744–747

Martinoli C, Bianchi S, Derchi L et al (2000) Sonographic evaluation of digital annular pulleys tears. Skeletal Radiol 29:387–391

McNally E (2004) Practical musculoskeletal ultrasound. Elsevier, Amsterdam

McNally EG (2008) Ultrasound of the small joints of the hands and feet: current status. Skeletal Radiol 37:99–113

Middleton WD, Teefey SA, Boyer MI (2001) Hand and wrist sonography. Ultrasound Q 17:21–36

Milbradt H, Calleja Cancho E, Qaiyumi SA et al (1990) Sonography of the wrist and the hand. Radiologe 30:360–365

Moschilla G, Breidahl W (2002) Sonography of the finger. AJR 178:1451–1457

Muncibì F, Carulli C, Paez DC et al (2008) A case of bilateral extensor digitorum brevis manus. Chir Organi Mov 92:133–135

Read JW, Conolly WB, Lanzetta M et al (1996) Diagnostic ultrasound of the hand and wrist. J Hand Surg 21:1004–1010

Renoux J, Zeitoun-Eiss D, Brasseur JL (2009) Ultrasonographic study of wrist ligaments: review and new perspectives. Semin Musculoskelet Radiol 13:55–65

Robertson BL, Jamadar DA, Jacobson JA et al (2007) Extensor retinaculum of the wrist: sonographic characterization and pseudotenosynovitis appearance. AJR Am J Roentgenol 188:198–202

Scheel AK, Hermann KG, Ohrndorf S et al (2006) Prospective long term follow-up imaging study comparing radiography, ultrasonography and magnetic resonance imaging in rheumatoid arthritis finger joints. Ann Rheum Dis 65:595–600

Szkudlarek M, Narvestad E, Klarlund M et al (2004a) Ultrasonography of the metatarsophalangeal joints in rheumatoid arthritis: comparison with magnetic resonance imaging, conventional radiography, and clinical examination. Arthritis Rheum 50:2103–2112

Szkudlarek M, Narvestad E, Court-Payen M et al (2004b) Ultrasonography of the RA finger joints is more sensitive than conventional radiography for detection of erosions without loss of specificity, with MRI as a reference method. Ann Rheum Dis 63:82–83

Tagliafico A, Rubino M, Autuori A et al (2007) Wrist and hand ultrasound. Semin Musculoskelet Radiol 11:95–104

Taljanovic MS, Sheppard JE, Jones MD et al (2008) Sonography and sonoarthrography of the scapholunate and lunotriquetral ligaments and triangular fibrocartilage disk: initial experience and correlation with arthrography and magnetic resonance arthrography. J Ultrasound Med 27: 179–191

Teefey SA, Middleton WD, Boyer MI (2000) Sonography of the hand and wrist. Semin Ultrasound CT MR 21:192–204

Terslev L, Torp-Pedersen S, Savnik A et al (2003) Doppler ultrasound and magnetic resonance imaging of synovial inflammation of the hand in rheumatoid arthritis: a comparative study. Arthritis Rheum 48:2434–2441

Tubbs RS, Stetler W, Kelly DR et al (2007) Acrel's ganglion. Surg Radiol Anat 29:379–381

Van Holsbeeck M, Introcaso JH (2001) Musculoskeletal ultrasound, 2nd edn. Mosby Co, St Louis

Wakefield RJ, Gibbon WW, Conaghan PG et al (2000) The value of sonography in the detection of bone erosions in patients with rheumatoid arthritis. Arthritis Rheum 43: 2762–2770

Walther M, Harms H, Krenn V et al (2001) Correlation of power Doppler sonography with vascularity of the synovial tissue of the knee joint in patients with osteoarthritis and rheumatoid arthritis. Arthritis Rheum 44:331–829

Skeletal Development and Aging

Jim Carmichael, Lil-Sofie Ording Müller,
and Karen Rosendahl

Contents

K. Rosendahl (✉)
Department of Paediatric Radiology,
Haukeland University Hospital and University of Bergen,
Bergen, Norway
e-mail: karen.rosendahl@helse-bergen.no;
rosenk@gosh.nhs.uk

L.-S. Ording Müller
Section for Paediatric Radiology,
Oslo University Hospital, HF, Ullevål,
Oslo, Norway

J. Carmichael
Department of Paediatric Radiology,
Guys and Thomas'/Evelina Childrens Hospital,
London, UK

Abstract

Growing bone is challenging, as bone structure, shape and size change continuously until skeletal maturity. The numerous normal variants of growth which may mimic pathology have been accurately described radiographically, but little is known on the appearances on other modalities such as magnetic resonance imaging (MRI), computed tomography (CT) and ultrasound. This chapter will take you through fetal and post natal growth of the hand skeleton, and also give an overview of the assessment of bone age.

1 Introduction

The hand and wrist start developing in the early stages of foetal growth, through chondrification and ossification to finally achieve skeletal maturity at the end of adolescence. Skeletal development of the hand proceeds through a complex interplay of growth, biomechanical forces, and reciprocal development of bone shape. These bone changes have been extensively studied by radiograph, and several established methods are used in clinical practice for assessment of bone age.

The advent of magnetic resonance imaging (MRI) has shed light on the pre and post ossification changes of the areas of bone not assessed by radiography. Magnetic resonance imaging data of the hand is sparse for the neonatal period, but increasingly, more information is available for later stages of development (Ording Müller et al. 2011).

A. M. Davis et al. (eds.), *Imaging of the Hand and Wrist*, Medical Radiology. Diagnostic Imaging,
DOI: 10.1007/174_2011_167,

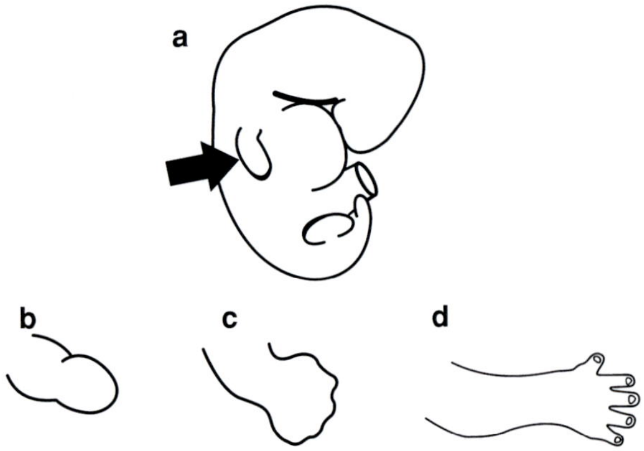

Fig. 1 Embryological development. **a** The upper limb bud appears at 5 weeks (*blackarrow*) and the limb develops, showing separation of the individual rays by 8 weeks (**b–d**)

2 Embryology of the Hand—Foetal Period

The limb buds develop at the end of the fourth gestational week, arising from the ventrolateral body wall under the influence of a thickened area of ectoderm, at the distal end of the limb bud called the apical ectodermal ridge (Fig. 1). The upper limb consists of three layers: lateral mesoderm, somatic mesoderm, and ectoderm. During the fifth week, neuronal tissue grows into the limbs and the hand plates become visible at the distal end of the upper limb. A process of programmed cell death forms the digital rays from the hand plate and individual rays are seen in the sixth week. The bones form as hyaline cartilage models of chondrified condensed mesenchyme, and in the sixth week this chondrification occurs in the distal limb skeleton including the carpal and metacarpal bones. This process continues into week seven, by the end of which all the phalanges are involved. Endochondral ossification is seen by eight weeks and progresses rapidly. Foetal ossification of the radius, ulna, and phalanges is complete by 35–40 weeks (Fig. 2). The ossification of the hand epiphyses and carpals begins in the postnatal period, in proportion with the longitudinal growth of the tubular bones.

3 Postnatal Growth of the Hand Skeleton

Until three months of age there is no ossification of the carpals and hand epiphyses. Skeletal age at this stage is best assessed by views of the lower limb (knee and ankle) to demonstrate ossified nuclei in the proximal tibia, calcaneum, and talus in normal children. After three months of age, the left hand is used in standard assessment. Skeletal development proceeds in the same sequence in both males and females, though faster in females. This accelerated development begins to become apparent after three months of age continuing to puberty.

3.1 Carpus

Enchondral ossification of the carpal bones starts at around three months of age (Fig. 3a) and continues until skeletal maturation at 14–16 (Pyle et al. 1971). In most children, bone growth and modeling follows a specific sequential pattern with a constant ratio between carpal bone volumes (Bull et al. 1999; Canovas et al. 1997). Radiographically, the small spherical ossification centres develop into multifaceted, articulating bones with a well defined cortex. With growth, the bony surface may take a slightly more squared and irregular form, the 3 dimensional nature of which is better appreciated in MR images than radiographically (Ording Müller et al. 2011; Avenarius et al. 2012).

The carpal bones' ossification order is more variable than that seen in the other hand bones. A reliable sequence is *capitate*, *hamate*, *triquetral*, *lunate*, *trapezium*, *trapezoid*, and *pisiform*. The *scaphoid* ossification usually appears before that of the trapezium in boys and either just before or just after in girls, the ossification of both occurs by 3 years (Fig. 3b, c). The *capitate* and *hamate* begin ossification around three months of age gradually enlarging until reciprocal shaping can be seen around one year of age. These bones will begin to overlap at 8y ♂/5y ♀. The bony projection of the hamate—the hamulus—will become visible at 13y ♂/11y ♀ and growth finally completes around age 17y ♂/15y ♀. On T1 weighted MR-images, an increasing number of bony surface depressions can be seen with advancing age in both the capitate and the hamate, from at least 5 years of age until skeletal maturity (Fig. 4a–d). In the capitate, this is typically seen along the radial side. The depressions reflect normal growth, and should not be mistaken for destructive change in children with conditions such as juvenile idiopathic arthritis (JIA). Some of these depressions can be seen on ultrasound examination (Fig. 5).

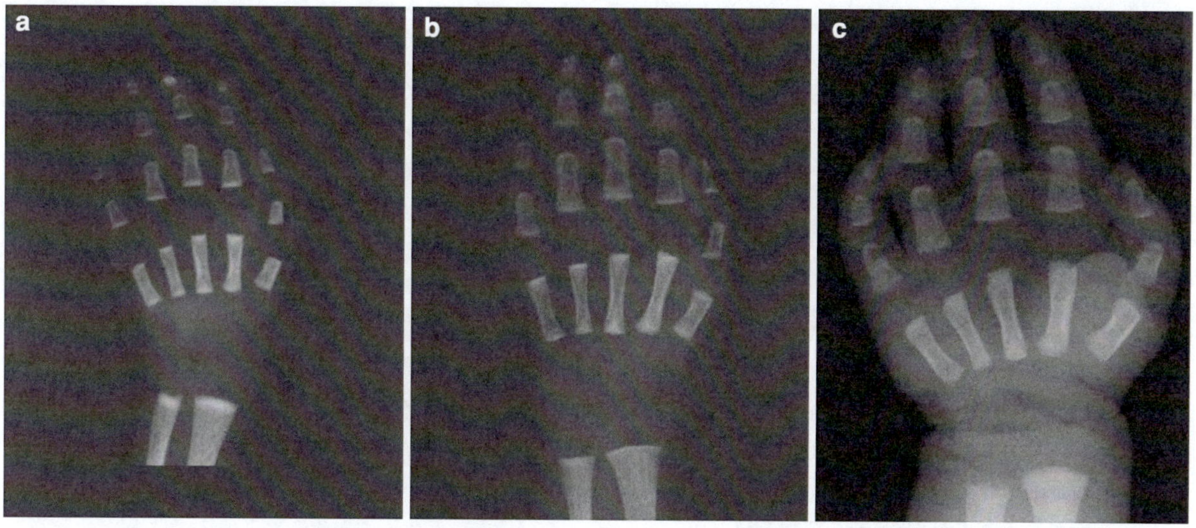

Fig. 2 Embryological development. Images of the developing foetal hand at **a** 20 weeks, **b** 30 weeks and **c** 40 weeks demonstrating gradual development of the bones and thickening of the soft tissues. At 40 weeks there is no ossification of the distal radial and ulnar epiphyses, nor of the carpals

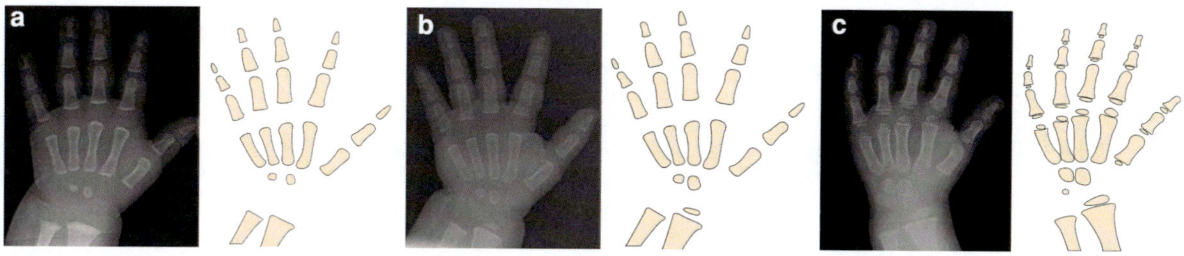

Fig. 3 Skeletal Development to age 3. **a** Development compatible with 3 months. There is flaring of the distal radius and ulna, and flattened bases of the metacarpals. Ossification centers are present in the capitate and hamate. After 3 months differences between the sexes begin to become apparent. **b** Development compatible with 1y 3m ♂/1y ♀. There is ossification of the capitate, hamate, and radial epiphysis. **c** Development compatible with 2y 8m ♂/3y ♀. Ossification continues in the triquetral and 1st metacarpal epiphysis. The distal radial epiphysis has becomes wedge shaped toward the ulna

The *triquetral* begins ossification around 3y ♂/2y ♀. The initial rounded shape develops its mature contour with flattening of the *hamate* and *lunate* facets seen aged 9y ♂/7y ♀. Ossification of the *pisiform* is seen at 11y ♂/9y ♀, growth is complete by 16 years of age.

Lunate ossification begins around 3y ♂/2y 6m ♀, occasionally from two ossification centres. Clear facets are seen at 10y ♂/8y ♀, especially at the *capitate* surface. Growth is complete by 16y ♂/14y ♀. *Scaphoid* ossification begins at 6y ♂/4y ♀. Its characteristic concave capitates surface is seen by 10y ♂/8y ♀. Flattening of the radial surface and alignment with the radial epiphysis can be seen at 13y ♂/11y ♀. Growth is complete by age 16y ♂/14y ♀. On MRI, typical surface irregularities seen in the radial corners (Fig. 5b), are seen in increasing numbers with increasing age (Ording Müller et al. 2011).

The *trapezium* and *trapezoid* begin to ossify after the epiphysis of the thumb, with the trapezium becoming visible by 4y ♂/3y 6m ♀, and the trapezoid by 6y ♂/4y ♀. Overlap between the two bones is seen at 8y ♂/6y ♀ when corresponding flattening of the first and second metacarpal articular surfaces is seen. Concavity of this metacarpal surface begins to be visible by age 9y ♂/7y ♀. The *trapezium* and *trapezoid* attain their adult shapes by 15 ♂/13y ♀.

Bony depressions due to physiological development and ligamentous insertions appear in the carpus and can be occasionally mistaken for pathology

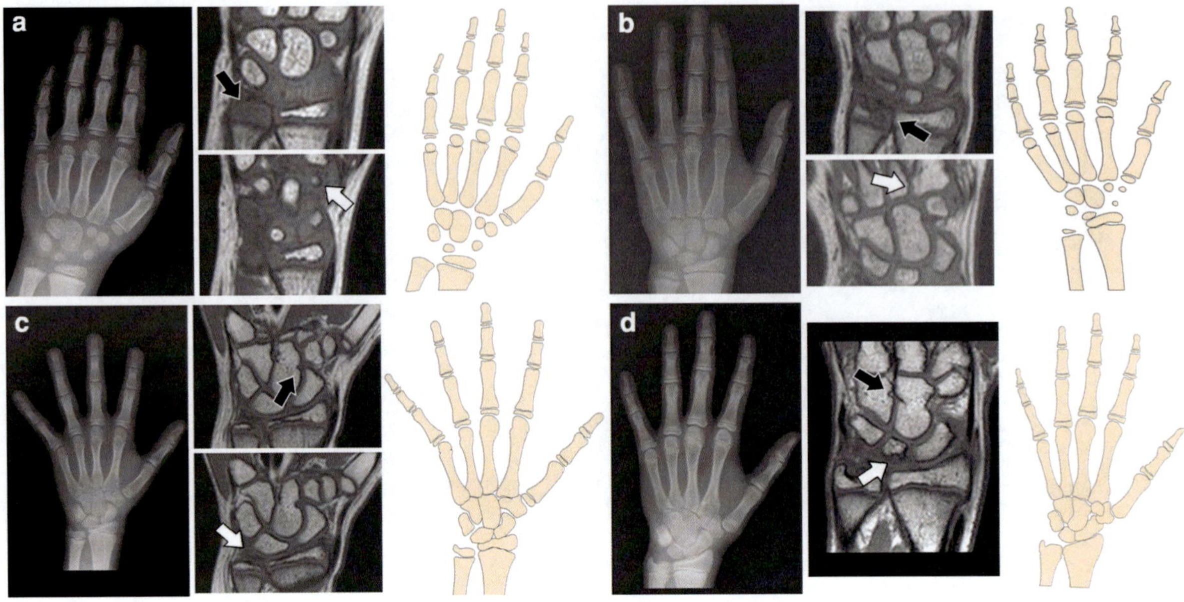

Fig. 4 Development to age 5–14 with MR correlation. **a** Development compatible with 6y ♂/5y ♀. Ongoing carpal ossification with the beginning of reciprocal shaping. MR images show pre-ossified cartilage: ulnar epiphysis and triquetral (*black arrow*) and the emerging rounded ossification center of the trapezoid (*white arrow*). **b** Development compatible with 8y ♂/9y ♀. The carpals are now ossified with reciprocal shaping. The distal phalangeal epiphyses are as wide as their shaft. MR images show developing ulnar ossification (*black arrow*) and emerging carpal and metacarpal indentations (*white arrow*). **c** Development compatible with 11y ♂/9y ♀. The carpals have developed reciprocal contours. The distal phalangeal epiphyses begin to conform to the adjacent middle phalanx. MR images show capitate irregularities not visible on the radiograph (*black arrow*). Ligaments are clearly visible, i.e. scapho-lunate ligament (*white arrow*). **d** Development compatible with 14y ♂/12y ♀. All epiphyses are beginning to cap their shafts and the physes are narrowing. MR images show further carpal irregularities corresponding to ligamentous insertions (*arrows*)

(Ording Müller et al. 2011). The carpal intraosseous ligaments are mostly within the joint capsule, some inserting directly into bone and others attaching to articular surfaces (Schmitt and Lanz 2008). They have complex anatomical relations and a brief overview of these is necessary to understand the development of carpal depressions (Fig. 6). Proximally the scapholunate and lunotriquetral ligaments reinforce the palmar joint capsule. The radioscapholunate ligament extends from the mid-palmar aspect of the radiolunate ligament to the radius, containing neurovascular structures. Distally thick interossious ligaments run between the carpal bones, for example the capitohamate ligament. Two groups of ligaments are present on the palmar aspect of the carpal bones: the 'Proximal Palmar V' comprises of the Radioulnar triquetral, Ulnolunate, and Ulnotriquetral ligaments. The 'Distal Palmer V' comprises of the Radioscaphocapitate ligament and the arcuate complex (triquetrocapitoscaphoid ligament). The dorsal aspect of the carpus also has a 'V' complex: the 'dorsal V' consists of the dorsal radiotriquetral, dorsal intercarpal ligaments, and the extensor reticulum complex.

3.2 Metacarpals

The epiphysis of the first metacarpal develops in conjunction with the trapezium. At birth the proximal aspect is flattened and the adjacent trapezium is not yet ossified. Ossification of the first epiphysis starts at 2y ♂/1y 6m ♀. Enlarging transversely, the epiphysis flattens and begins to conform to the base of its shaft by 4y 6m ♂/3y ♀.

The trapezium surface becomes indented, conforming to the trapezoid by 9y ♂/8y 10m ♀. There is reciprocal shaping of the trapezium to the epiphysis, which is as wide as the shaft of the 1st metacarpal by 13y 6m ♂/11y ♀. Fusion of the first epiphysis begins by 15 years ♂/13y 6m ♀ and the fusion line may persist

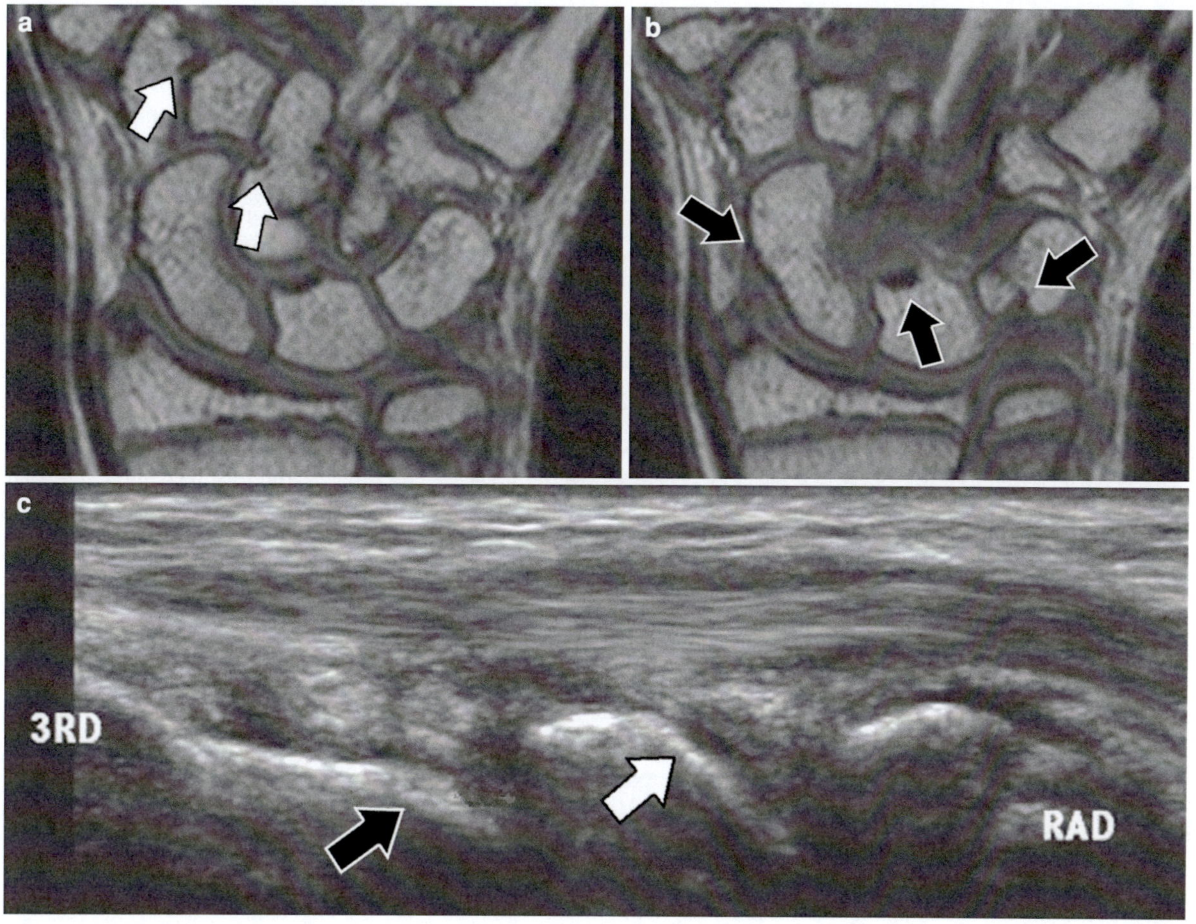

Fig. 5 Ultrasound and MR of carpal depressions. **a** Carpal irregularities in the capitate and trapezium (*white arrow*). **b** Typical surface irregularities of the radial corners of the scaphoid. Further irregularities seen in the lunate and triquetral corresponding to ligamentous insertions. **c** Sagital Ultrasound image from radius (*right*) to third metacarpal (*left*) demonstrating carpal irregularities

for many years. On MRI, there is a typical bony depression at the base of the 2nd metacarpal, which may easily be mistaken for an erosion (Fig. 4b).

The 2nd–5th metacarpal epiphyses develop at a slightly different rate to the first. The 2nd metacarpal epiphysis tends to lead, followed stepwise by the 3rd–5th with the 5th being the last in development. The epiphyses begin to ossify at 1 year ♂/1y 6m ♀. Their oval contour is seen to flatten, adjusting to the distal metacarpal surface by 2y ♂/1y 6m ♀. The epiphysis becomes more cuboidal and is as wide as the metacarpal shaft at 11y 6m ♂/10y ♀. Fusion of the growth plate begins by 15y 6m ♂/13y 6m ♀. On MRI, the basis of the 3rd and 4th metacarpals typically narrows dorsally.

3.3 Phalanges

The growth of the phalanges follows a similar order to the metacarpals, with the 2nd leading, and the 5th slightly behind. At birth the proximal phalanges have flat proximal surfaces and the ossification of the epiphyses appears by 1y 6m ♂/1y ♀. These epiphyses are flattened and disc like, becoming slightly concave as they develop, and are as wide as the diaphysis at 10y ♂/7y 10m ♀. At this age, the distal end of the proximal phalanx also becomes concave. The epiphysis begins to cap its shaft at 13y ♂/10y ♀, and begins fusion at 15y 6m ♂/13y 6m ♀.

The middle phalanges follow similar development to the proximal, with ossification beginning at 2y ♂/

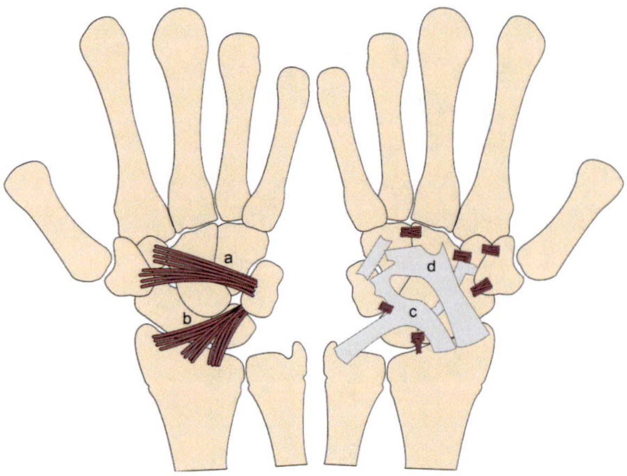

Fig. 6 Major ligamentous groups accounting for carpal depressions. *Leftimage*: Dorsal ligament groups. **a** dorsal intercarpal iligament, **b** dorsal radiotriquetral ligament. *right image*: Palmar ligament groups. *Red* interossious ligaments. *Grey***c** proximal v. **d** distal v

1y 6m ♀. The width of the adjacent metaphysis is obtained by 12y 6m ♂/8y 10m ♀, with capping of the shaft seen by 13y 6m ♂/11y ♀. Fusion of the epiphysis is seen by 15y 6m ♂/13y 6m ♀.

The distal phalanx epiphysis ossifies slightly later than the proximal and middle, becoming visible by 2y 8m ♂/2y ♀. Similar disc shaped growth is seen and the epiphysis is as wide as its shaft by 7y ♂/5y 9m ♀. Capping is seen at 12y 6m ♂/10y ♀, with fusion beginning at 15y ♂/13y 6m ♀. Fusion is usually complete before that of the middle phalangeal physes.

The thumb phalanges develop ahead of the 2nd–5th digits. The proximal phalanx epiphysis begins ossification by 2y 8m ♂/2y ♀. This becomes disc-like and is as wide as its diaphysis by 10y ♂/7y 10m ♀. Capping of the epiphysis is seen by 15y ♂/11y ♀, and ossification of the (smaller flexor) sesamoid is present. Fusion of the epiphysis begins at 16y ♂/14y ♀.

The distal phalanx of the thumb ossifies by 1y 6m ♂/1y 3m ♀, gradually enlarging to cap its shaft by 13y 6m ♂/11y ♀. Fusion begins shortly afterward at 14y ♂/12y ♀.

3.4 Radius and Ulna

At birth, the distal radius and ulna metaphyses are slightly flared, with the ulna slightly more proximal than the radius. The distal ulna may be slightly cupped, not to be mistaken for metabolic bone disease, such as rickets (Fig. 2). Ossification of the distal epiphysis occurs around 15 months in the radius and 6 years in the ulna in both males and females, with both epiphyses being initially rounded and 'pea' like. On MRI, both epiphyses may appear very flat and nearly fragmented (Fig. 4). In the radius the ossification flattens and elongates toward the ulna. The ulnar articular facet is thinner than the styloid aspect of the radial epiphysis, giving a 'wedge shape' seen clearly by 4 years of age. The radial styloid process enlarges and the epiphysis is as wide as the radius by 11 ♂/10y ♀. Capping of the radial metaphysis occurs by 14 ♂/11y ♀. Fusion of the distal radial epiphysis is the last of any in the hand, beginning at around 17 ♂/15y ♀. The ulna ossification proceeds in either of two directions: flat and parallel to the ulna metaphysic or obliquely pointing toward the future site of the ulna styloid process: these patterns will be apparent by 6–7 years of age. A clear ulna styloid process with distal concavity of the adjacent mid-epiphysis should be apparent by 11y 6m ♂/9y ♀. Capping of the ulna and epiphyseal fusion is seen at 14 ♂/11y ♀.

3.5 Maturation of the Bone Marrow

In the neonate all bone marrow is haemopoeitic and the conversion of red haemopoetic marrow to yellow fatty marrow takes place throughout childhood. The process begins in the extremities, progressing through the distal, then proximal long bones and finally in the axial skeleton (Laor and Jaramillo 2009) (Fig. 7). By the age of skeletal maturity, the appendicular bone marrow is almost entirely converted.

MR imaging is a very sensitive tool for the detection of changes in fat composition within bone marrow. Normal haematopoietic marrow contains approximately 40% fat, 40% water and 20% protein, whereas fatty marrow contains approximately 80% fat, 20% water and 5% protein. Due to the fat content of haemopoetic marrow, MR demonstrates apparent conversion in advance of the histological change. Marrow conversion in boys and girls is thought to proceed at the same rate (Moore and Dawson 1990).

Mature fatty bone marrow is hyperintense on spin echo sequences, with intermediate homogenous hypointense signal on fat suppressed gradient echo sequences. No enhancement is seen. Haemopoetic marrow returns a signal similar or higher than muscle

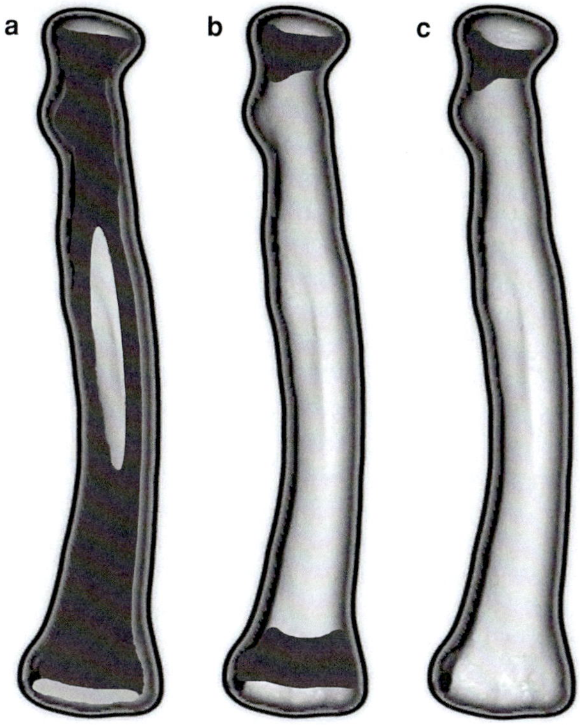

Fig. 7 Conversion of Red marrow. Red marrow conversion begins in the epiphyses (**a**) within 6 months of the development of the secondary ossification centre. Conversion is then seen in the diaphysis, expanding with time towards the metaphyses (**b**). The distal metaphysis converts followed by the proximal (**c**)

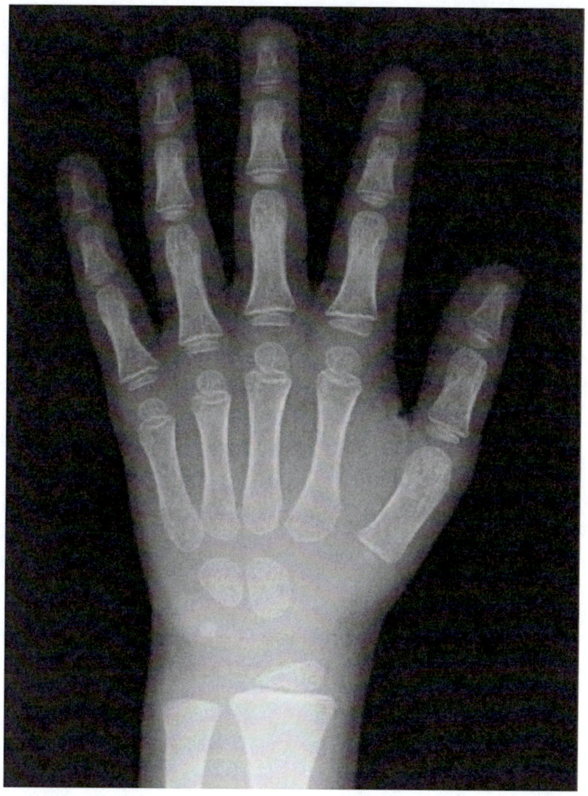

Fig. 8 Individual bones of differing ages. 11y old, healthy male. Assessment of skeletal maturity shows a marked discrepancy between proximal and distal development, with a skeletal age of 10y based on the fingers, and 7y based on the carpal bones. Such variation can be normal, but there are known associations with central causes of growth disturbance

on T1 weighted images, due to the fat content. The higher water content results in high signal on water sensitive sequences such as STIR.

In the infant, epiphyseal cartilage is of homogenous intermediate signal intensity on T1 weighted images and of low signal intensity on water sensitive sequences. As ossification takes place, the signal returned on water sensitive sequences becomes heterogenous. Vascular channels within the cartilage can enhance, often showing a radial arrangement (Moore and Dawson 1990). As ossification begins, the ossification centre develops haemopoetic marrow and the signal intensity becomes rapidly similar to the adjacent metaphysis. Fatty conversion begins in the epiphysis and is seen within six months of the appearances of the secondary ossification centre (Moore and Dawson 1990; Jaramillo et al. 1991). Conversion then continues in the diaphysis, extending to the distal metaphysis and lastly to the proximal metaphysis.

Normal variants seen on MR include residual foci of haemopoetic marrow in otherwise converted bones. These areas will characteristically will have straight 'flame' contours and return increased signal in comparison to adjacent muscle on T1 images. Signal changes suggestive of bone marrow oedema are seen in at least one of the carpals or metacarpal bases in more than half of healthy children aged between 5 and 15 years, with no differences according to sex, age or degree of daily physical activity (Ording Müller et al. 2011). In addition bony depressions, often not appreciated on radiographs, are present in all cases (Figs. 4a–d and 5).

4 Assessment of Bone Age

Assessment of bone age is a complex task: it is prone to intraobserver and interobserver variation and can depend on experience of the method used. A hand of a given age can often contain individual bones of differing maturity (Fig. 8). Variations in skeletal maturation between ethnic groups have been observed, however the cause is a contentious subject. Development is known to take place in a sequence which is identical for both sexes and all ethnicities (Zhang et al. 2009), however, the most robust evidence indicates that variations in the rate of skeletal development are minimally affected by ethnicity, and that socio–economic factors are of much greater significance (Schmeling et al. 2000).

Several methods of bone age assessment have been devised. Atlas methods involve comparison by age and sex matched controls with descriptions of bones, accompanying radiographs are intended primarily as illustrations. Examples include the Atlases of Greulich and Pyle, and Theimann and Nitz, which refer to North Americans of Northern European descent and Central European children of unspecified ethnicity respectively. The Greulich and Pyle age assessment is by comparison with the given reference standards within the given normal variance for age. No variance data was given in the original Theimann and Nitz method (Schmeling et al. 2006). Bone measurement methods include the Tanner and Whitehouse system. This system has gone through several refinements, the latest being the 'TW3' system (Tanner et al. 2001). The developing hand is divided into multiple regions of interest and the development of each region divided into discrete stages. A numerical score is associated with each stage and the total score allows assessment of maturity.

Studies comparing the various methods of assessment must be analysed with the understanding that, as discussed earlier, skeletal maturation is dependent on socio–economic factors. Therefore, methods based on certain populations at certain times may not be comparable with other populations.

Greulich and Pyle, and Theimann and Nitz offer close agreement in assessment, however, the Thiemann and Nitz method may be better for preventing over estimation of skeletal age in populations with high acceleration status (Schmidt et al. 2007). Atlas methods may be subject to greater interobserver variation, but are much less time consuming than measurement methods. The Tanner–Whitehouse system allows a more objective assessment, but is much more time consuming than the atlas methods. Greulich and Pyle, and Tanner and Whitehouse have been compared and found to give clinically significant differences in bone age and therefore only one method should be used in longitudinal assessment (Bull et al. 1999; Schmidt et al. 2008).

Automated computer systems have been developed in an attempt to avoid the difficulties associated with the human mind assigning a discrete age to the essentially continuous changes of bone age. The initial aim was to automatically identify bones by means of comparison with deformable models. Identified bones are then individually assessed for age before conversion into a recognised bone age scale i.e. Greulich and Pyle or TW3. This modern approach has been validated clinically (Thodberg 2009), and future refinements may result in completely automated systems.

As has been seen, MRI shows characteristic changes to the bones of the hand and wrist with development and may provide more accurate means to assess bone age in the future without the disadvantage of exposure to ionising radiation. The technique has already been shown to have some role in assessing skeletal age of adolescent football players, where the use of ionising radiation cannot be justified (Dvorak et al. 2007).

References

Bull RK, Edwards PD, Kemp PM, Fry S, Hughes IA (1999) Bone age assessment: a large scale comparison of the Greulich and Pyle, and Tanner and Whitehouse (TW2) methods. Arch Dis Child 81(2):172–173

Canovas F, Jaeger M, Couture A, Sultan C, Bonnel F (1997) Carpal bone maturation during childhood and adolescence: assessment by quantitative computed tomography. Preliminary results. Surg Radiol Anat 19(6):395–398

Dvorak J, George J, Junge A, Hodler J (2007) Age determination by magnetic resonance imaging of the wrist in adolescent male football players. Br J Sports Med 41:45–52

Jaramillo D, Laor T, Hoffer FA, Zaleske DJ, Cleveland RH, Buchbinder BR et al (1991) Epiphyseal marrow in infancy: MR imaging. Radiology 180(3):809–812

Laor T, Jaramillo D (2009) MR imaging insights into skeletal maturation: What is normal? Radiology 250(1):28–38

Moore SG, Dawson KL (1990) Red and yellow marrow in the femur: age-related changes in appearance at MR imaging. Radiology 175(1):219–223

Ording Müller LS, Avenarius D, Damasio B, Eldevik OP, Malattia C, Lambot-Juhan K, Tanturri L, Owens CM, Rosendahl K (2011) The paediatric wrist revisited: redefining MR findings in healthy children. Ann Rheum Dis 70(4):605-610. Epub 2010 Dec 20

Pyle SI, Waterhouse AM, Greulich WW (1971) Attributes of the radiographic standard of reference for the national health examination survey. Am J Phys Anthropol 35(3):331–337

Schmeling A, Reisinger W, Loreck D, Vendura K, Markus W, Geserick G (2000) Effects of ethnicity on skeletal maturation:

consequences for forensic age estimations. Int J Legal Med 113(5):253–258
Schmeling A, Baumann U, Schmidt S, Wernecke KD, Reisinger W (2006) Reference data for the Thiemann–Nitz method of assessing skeletal age for the purpose of forensic age estimation. Int J Legal Med 120:1–4
Schmidt S, Koch B, Schulz R, Reisinger W, Schmeling A (2007) Comparative analysis of the applicability of the skeletal age determination methods of Greulich–Pyle and Thiemann–Nitz for forensic age estimation in living subjects. Int J Legal Med 121(4):293–296
Schmidt S, Nitz I, Schulz R, Schmeling A (2008) Applicability of the skeletal age determination method of Tanner and Whitehouse for forensic age diagnostics. Int J Legal Med 122(4):309–314
Schmitt R, Lanz U (2008) Diagnostic imaging of the hand. Thieme, Stuttgart
Tanner J, Healy MJR, Golstein H, Cameron N (2001) Assessment of skeletal maturity and prediction of adult height (TW3) method, 3rd edn. Saunders, London
Thodberg HH (2009) Clinical review: an automated method for determination of bone age. J Clin Endocrinol Metab 94(7):2239–2244
Zhang A, Sayre JW, Vachon L, Liu BJ, Huang HK (2009) Racial differences in growth patterns of children assessed on the basis of bone age. Radiology 250(1):228–235

Congenital and Developmental Abnormalities

Emily J. Stenhouse, James J. R. Kirkpatrick, and Greg J. Irwin

Contents

Abstract

Congenital hand differences (CHD) have been estimated to occur in 10% of children born with congenital abnormalities. CHD can be classified according to their pre-dominant abnormality using the Swanson classification. Failure of differentiation represents the most common group. Associated (nonlimb) abnormalities are common and it is important to identify those CHD requiring systemic evaluation. Radiology is important in the diagnosis and management of CHD with plain films providing the mainstay of imaging postnatally. The management of CHD should be within a multi-disciplinary environment.

E. J. Stenhouse (✉)
Consultant Paediatric Radiologist,
Royal Hospital for Sick Children,
Dalnair Street, Glasgow, G3 8SJ, UK
e-mail: Emily.Stenhouse@ggc.scot.nhs.uk

J. J. R. Kirkpatrick,
Consultant Plastic and Hand Surgeon,
Canniesburn Plastic Surgery Unit,
Glasgow Royal Infirmary and Royal Hospital
for Sick Children, Dalnair Street,
Glasgow, G3 8SJ, UK

G. J. Irwin
Consultant Paediatric Radiologist, Diagnostic Imaging,
Royal Hospital for Sick Children,
Dalnair Street, Glasgow, G3 8SJ, Scotland, UK

A. M. Davis et al. (eds.), *Imaging of the Hand and Wrist*, Medical Radiology. Diagnostic Imaging,
DOI: 10.1007/174_2011_205, © Springer-Verlag Berlin Heidelberg 2013

1 Introduction

Of the 1–2% of newborns born with congenital defects, 10% are born with upper limb malformations (McCarroll 2000). The incidence is higher in boys, with pre and post-term births, with multiple pregnancies and with increased maternal age (Giele et al. 2001). Congenital hand abnormalities are now commonly described as congenital hand differences (CHD). The majority (60%) of CHD has an unknown etiology but genetic factors may be attributable in 20% and environmental teratogens in 20% (Netscher and Baumholtz 2007). The embryologic limb bud can be seen at 4 weeks after fertilization, and the existing fetal limb structures continue to grow and develop for 8 weeks after fertilization. Most CHD are thought to arise during this 4-week interval (Kozin 2003).

CHD vary widely in their functional and aesthetic implications. Associated (nonlimb) abnormalities are also common, up to 26.7% in some series (De Smet 2002). It is important to identify those CHD which require further systemic evaluation and to differentiate them from isolated CHD. For example, radial deficiency occurs commonly in a number of syndromes such as the VACTERL association (vertebral abnormalities, ano-rectal and cardiac abnormalities, tracheo-oesophageal fistula, oesophageal atresia, renal defects, radial dysplasia and lower limb abnormalities).

Management must always be conducted in a multidisciplinary environment, involving surgeons, physiotherapists, orthotists, paediatricians, prosthetists, psychologists, anaesthetists, geneticists and radiologists. The purpose of this review is to provide an illustrated classification of congenital hand differences for radiologists, which will also be of interest to the other members of the multi-disciplinary team.

2 Imaging

CHD may be demonstrated by antenatal ultrasound particularly late in the first trimester and in the middle of the second trimester of pregnancy (Rypens et al. 2006) (Fig. 1). Three-dimensional ultrasound may be helpful in defining the abnormality more clearly (Ploeckinger-Ulm et al. 1996). Prenatal classification and characterization may help to identify fetuses that would benefit from more complete prenatal cardiac and karyotypic workup.

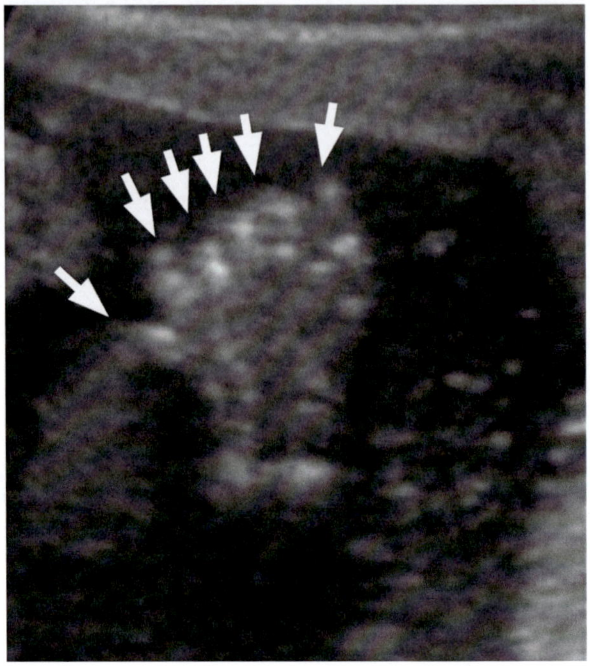

Fig. 1 2D Ultrasound image of a fetal hand of a fetus in the second trimester with trisomy 13 and post-axial polydactyly (Image courtesy of Dr Françoise Rypens)

Postnatally, plain films provide the mainstay of imaging, with ultrasound and magnetic resonance imaging (MRI) providing useful additional characterization in a minority of cases, principally in the clarification of the nature of masses and other causes of overgrowth.

3 Classification

The most widely accepted classification of CHD was proposed by Frantz and O'Rahilly and presented by Swanson (Frantz and O'Rahilly 1961; Swanson 1976). This was subsequently modified by the International Federation of Societies for Surgery of the Hand (IFSSH) in 1983 (Swanson et al. 1983), and further modified by the Japanese Society of Surgery of the Hand (JSSH) in 2000. The major categories are listed in Table 1 and are subsequently discussed.

Table 1 Abbreviated embryologic classification of CHD (adapted from Swanson 1976)

1	Failure of formation
2	Failure of differentiation
3	Duplication
4	Overgrowth
5	Undergrowth
6	Constriction ring syndrome
7	Generalised skeletal abnormalities

The seven categories differentiate the CHD according to the predominant abnormality, and further define the abnormality according to the nature of the embryonic failure during development. Group II (failure of differentiation) represents the most common group.

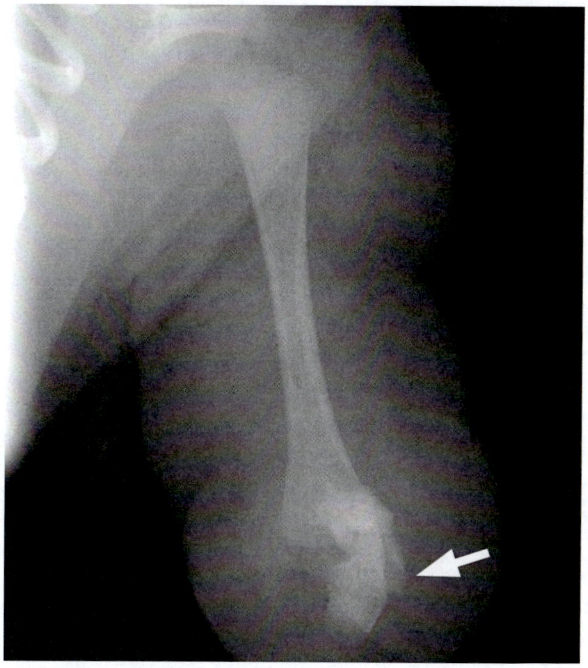

Fig. 2 Commonest level of transverse growth arrest at proximal radius and ulna (*arrow*)

4 Failure of Formation

Failure of formation of parts can be divided into transverse and longitudinal subgroups. Transverse deficiencies occur when growth stops abruptly, resulting in a "congenital amputation" and a shortened or truncated limb. Longitudinal deficiencies occur when structures are hypoplastic or absent along a longitudinal axis of the limb, resulting in abnormal formation and function biased down one 'side' of the limb (either the radial or ulnar sides, or 'centrally' between the two) (Kozin et al. 2004). In reality, most CHD within this group are mixed to some degree.

4.1 Transverse

This is defined according to the bone segment at which the growth arrest occurs (Van Heest 1996). The most common transverse deficiency occurs at the junction of the proximal and middle thirds of the forearm (Fig. 2).

These anomalies are usually unilateral, sporadic, and are rarely associated with other anomalies. Rudimentary "nubbins" or dimpling may be found at the distal end of the congenital amputation (Kozin 2003). This should not be confused with Constriction ring syndrome which may also manifest as an 'amputation' but requires the presence of a constriction ring either affecting the involved extremity or elsewhere (Wiedrich 1998).

4.2 Longitudinal

In this group the radial, central or ulnar side of the limb is abnormal. They may very rarely be characterized by absence of one or more 'segments' ('forearm' versus 'upper arm' versus 'both') of the upper limb (phocomelia), such as those defects attributed to maternal exposure to thalidomide. For example, when both segments are missing ('complete phocomelia'), the hand is attached directly to the shoulder.

4.2.1 Radial

Radial dysplasia is the most common longitudinal deficiency and occurs when structures on the radial side of the arm fail to develop properly. It is frequently bilateral (40–60%) with a male:female ratio of 3:2 (Van Heest 1996). It has been described as "an abnormal hand joined to a poor limb by a bad wrist" (Flatt 1994) (Fig. 3).

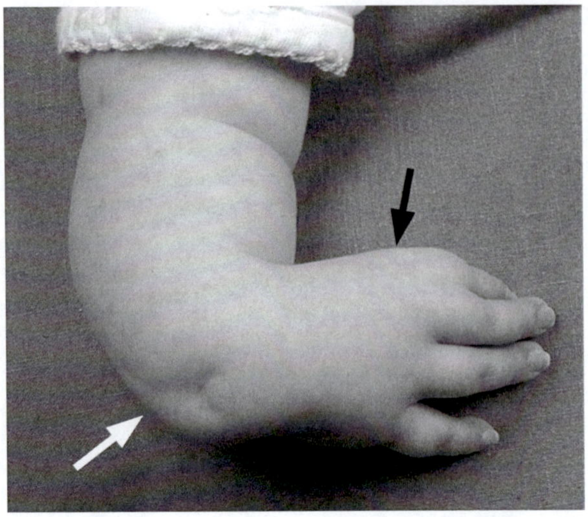

Fig. 3 Radial dysplasia displays an array of upper limb differences, the most striking of which are usually the radially deviated wrist (*white arrow*), absent thumb (*black arrow*), shortened forearm and stiff elbow

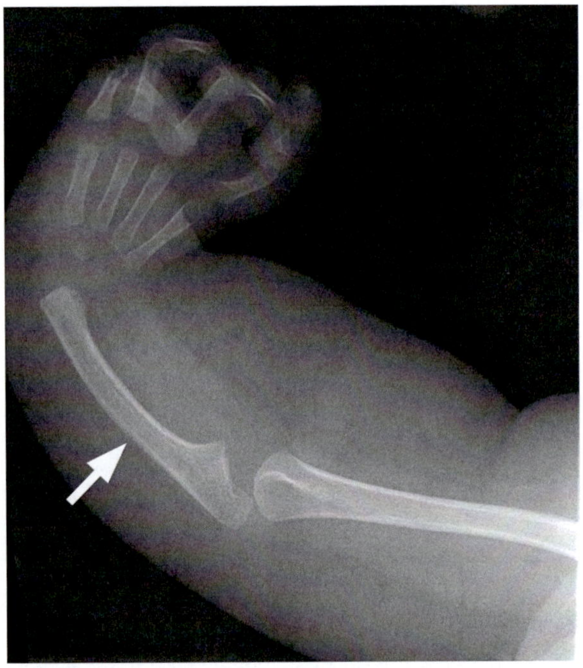

Fig. 4 Radial dysplasia has a spectrum of abnormalities of the radius, the commonest being complete absence of the radius. In such cases the ulna (*arrow*) is relatively hypoplastic also

Radial deficiency can range from mild hypoplasia to complete absence of the radius and thumb (the commonest type) (Fig. 4). The child presents with a hand that is radially deviated at the wrist. In the hand, the thumb is almost always affected and the fingers frequently have limited motion and function, the severity of which decreases from the radial to the ulnar side (James et al. 2004). The ulna is also usually shortened and bowed and may need later osteotomy (Fig. 5a, b).

A classification scheme has been described by Bayne and Klug for radial deficiency with proposed modifications by James et al. (Bayne and Klug 1987; James et al. 1999). For the purposes of imaging, it is useful to divide the deficiency into components and describe the characteristics of each component (James et al. 1999; Kozin 2003).

1. Thumb:
   I. absent
   II. hypoplastic
2. Carpal bones:
   I. normal
   II. absent
   III. hypoplastic
   IV. coalition

(Nb: Ossification centers of the carpal bones appear at a variety of ages ranging from 2 months for the capitate and hamate, to 4 years for the scaphoid, trapezium and trapezoid.)

3. Distal radius
   I. normal
   II. >2 mm shorter than ulna
   III. absent physis
   IV. absent
4. Proximal radius:
   I. normal
   II. radioulnar synostosis
   III. radial head dislocation
   IV. hypoplastic
   V. absent

The elbows are commonly stiff, and the abnormal features frequently extend further proximally (Fig. 6). Recently Goldfarb and colleagues (Goldfarb et al. 2005) proposed a further subtype of proximal radial longitudinal deficiency, involving an abnormal glenoid, an absent proximal humerus (with the distal humerus articulating with the ulna) and radial sided hand abnormalities.

Treatment involves straightening (centralization) of the wrist, currently achieved by initial distraction (Fig. 7a) followed by centralization (Fig. 7b) (both of which require perioperative fluoroscopic

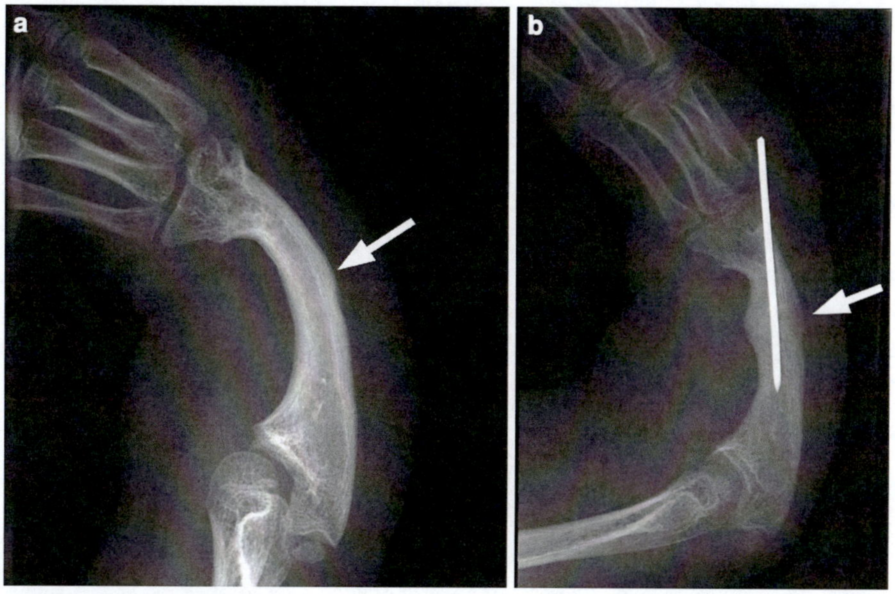

Fig. 5 **a** and **b** In radial dysplasia the ulna is frequently bowed, and may require correction as in this case which had been centralized 10 years previously. The osteotomy site (*arrow*) is secured with a large K-wire, removed at six weeks **a** pre-op **b** post op

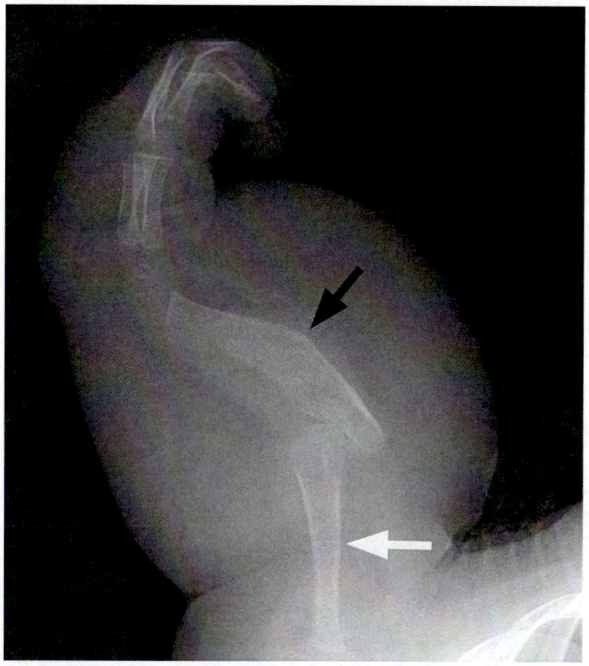

Fig. 6 Radial dysplasia with severe hypoplasia of the ulna (*black arrow*) and humerus (*white arrow*), both of which are shorter than the hand itself

screening), and later pollicisation (shortening and rotation of the index ray on its neurovascular pedicle to the position of the thumb, with tendon and intrinsic muscle rebalancing to create a 'thumb' from the index finger).

Importantly, radial longitudinal deficiencies often present as part of a syndrome. Associations include hematological conditions (e.g., thrombocytopenia-absent radius syndrome and Fanconi's anaemia), cardiac anomalies (e.g., Holt Oram syndrome), the VACTERL syndrome (see Sect. 1) and craniofacial syndromes (e.g., Nager and Duane syndromes) (Lourie and Lins 1998).

Children with radial longitudinal deficiencies should therefore have a thorough multi-disciplinary evaluation at the time of presentation to exclude associated abnormalities, understanding that some of these may not be immediately apparent (e.g., Fanconi's anaemia has a median age of onset of seven years of age) (Kozin 2003).

4.2.2 Central

This involves deficiencies of the central part of the hand and is also known descriptively as 'cleft hand', with traditional terms such as 'split hand' or 'lobster claw hand' having been rightly dropped because of their potentially emotive nature. Two types of cleft hand have been described, formerly known as 'typical' and 'atypical'. Although they may appear similar morphologically, they both have major clinical differences and probably different embryological derivations (Miura and Suzuki 1984; Ogino 1990a).

The typical cleft hand (now known as 'true' cleft hand) has a deep V-shaped defect (Fig. 8a, b). Most commonly the phalanges are missing. The metacarpals may be absent or malpositioned (Fig. 9), but are

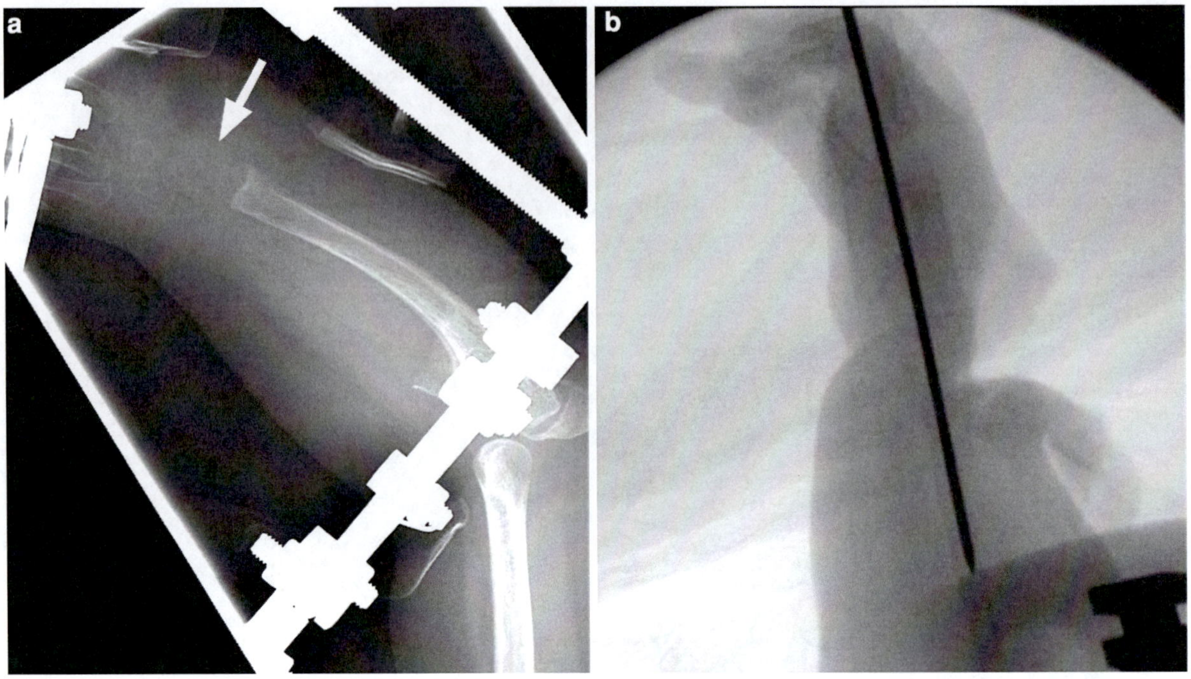

Fig. 7 Treatment of the radially deviated wrist is best achieved by (**a**) initial gradual lengthening of the soft tissues using an external distraction frame to bring the hand in line (*arrow*) over the end of the ulna, followed by (**b**) removal of the frame and formal centralization, with tendon transfers and temporary axial K-wire fixation, requiring intraoperative fluoroscopy

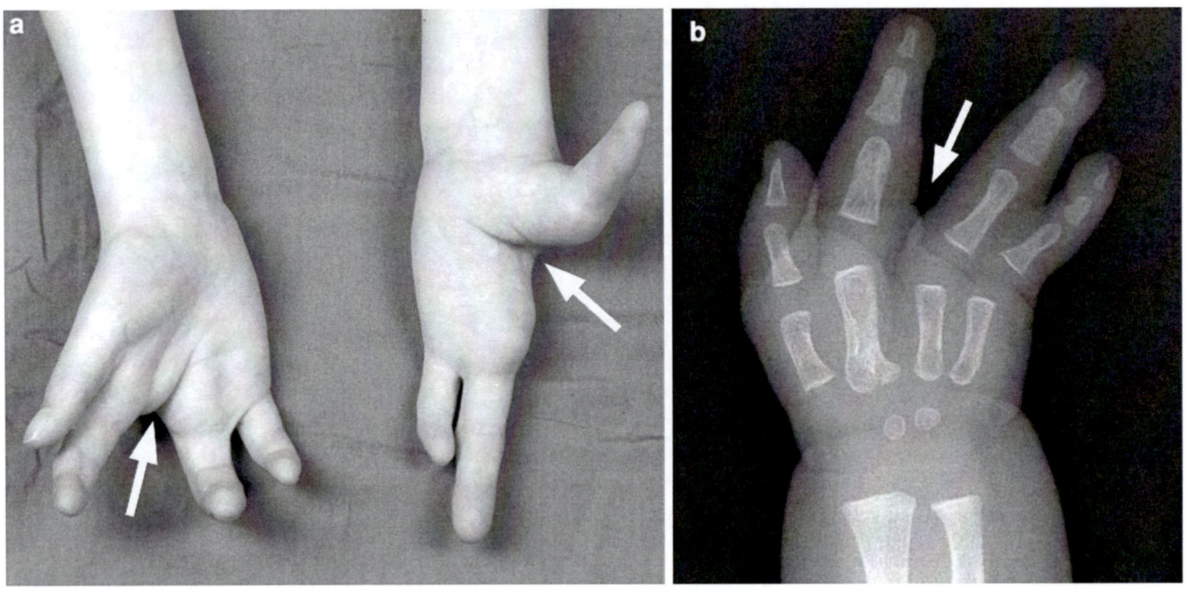

Fig. 8 **a** True cleft hand is usually bilateral, with V-shaped clefts (*arrows*), though the severity may differ between the two hands as in this case. **b** True clefts are usually centered on an absent third ray (*arrow*)

rarely hypoplastic. Joints at the site of the cleft can be very complex (Fig. 10), (Barsky 1964; Ogino 1990). This type of deficiency is often bilateral, and is usually inherited. There may be syndactyly of the ring-small or thumb-index web space, and associated foot involvement is common (Fig. 11). True central

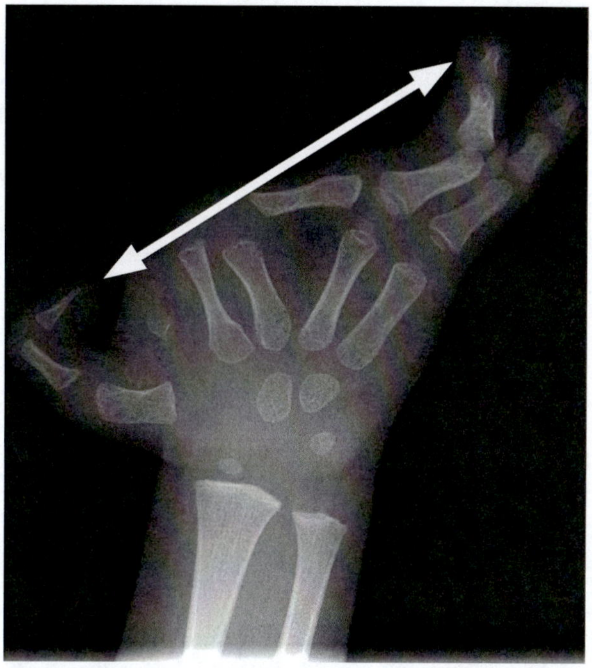

Fig. 9 In true cleft hand a wide spectrum of severity is seen, in which transverse metacarpals can cause progressive widening of the cleft (*arrow*)

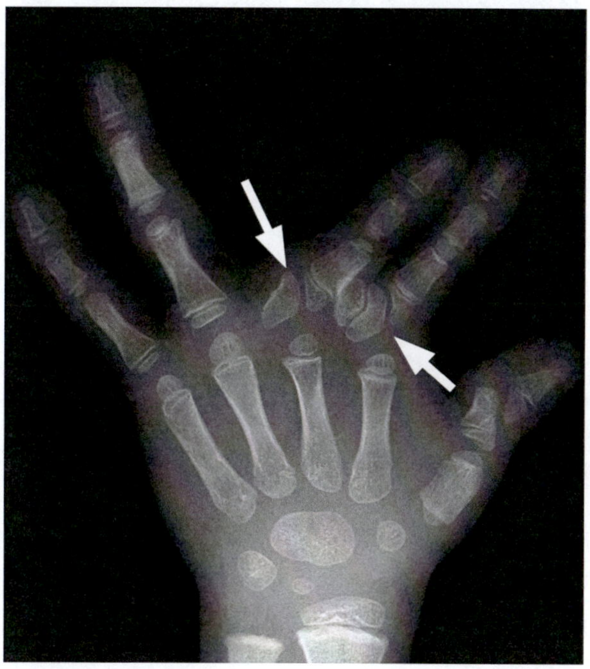

Fig. 10 This unusual variant demonstrates the complex joints (*arrows*) which can exist in cleft hands, requiring vigilance during surgical corrections

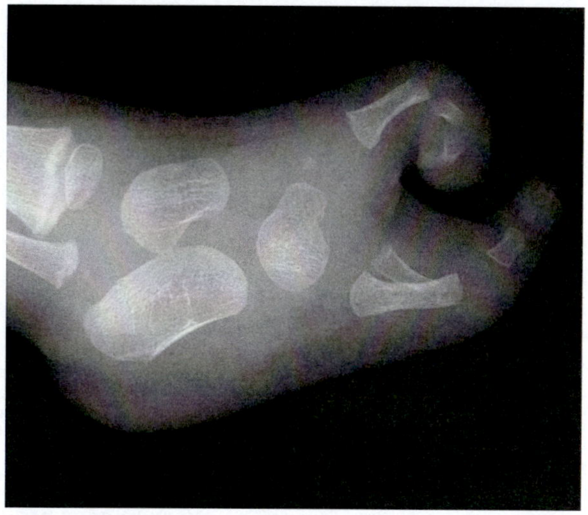

Fig. 11 Foot involvement is common in true cleft hand patients

dysplasia is also associated with cleft lip and palate but not Poland syndrome (Miura and Suzuki 1984; Ogino 1990a).

Atypical cleft hand has a shallower, U-shaped central defect that involves the central three digits (index, long and ring) (Fig. 12a), (Kozin 2003). It is a form of symbrachydactyly (shortened and webbed digits) that can vary in degree from the 'short finger type' (Fig. 12b), to absence of the central three digits (Fig. 12a), to a monodactylous type (thumb only, no fingers) (Fig. 12c, d), to complete absence of all digits, with only very rudimentary 'nubbins' (peromelic type) (Fig. 12e).

Atypical cleft hand is usually unilateral and sporadic. It is not associated with lower limb malformations or cleft lip and palate (Miura and Suzuki 1984; Ogino 1990a) but is associated with Poland syndrome (Fig. 13) (Ireland et al. 1976). The degree of hand deficiency in Poland syndrome does not correlate with that of the chest wall deformity, therefore clinical evaluation of the chest wall is required with all cases of symbrachydactyly (Kozin 2003).

4.2.3 Ulnar

This represents a spectrum of abnormalities along the ulnar surface of the upper limb. It is far less common than radial and central longitudinal deficiency (Miller et al. 1986; Schmidt and Neufield 1988) (Figs. 14a, b; 15; 16a, b).

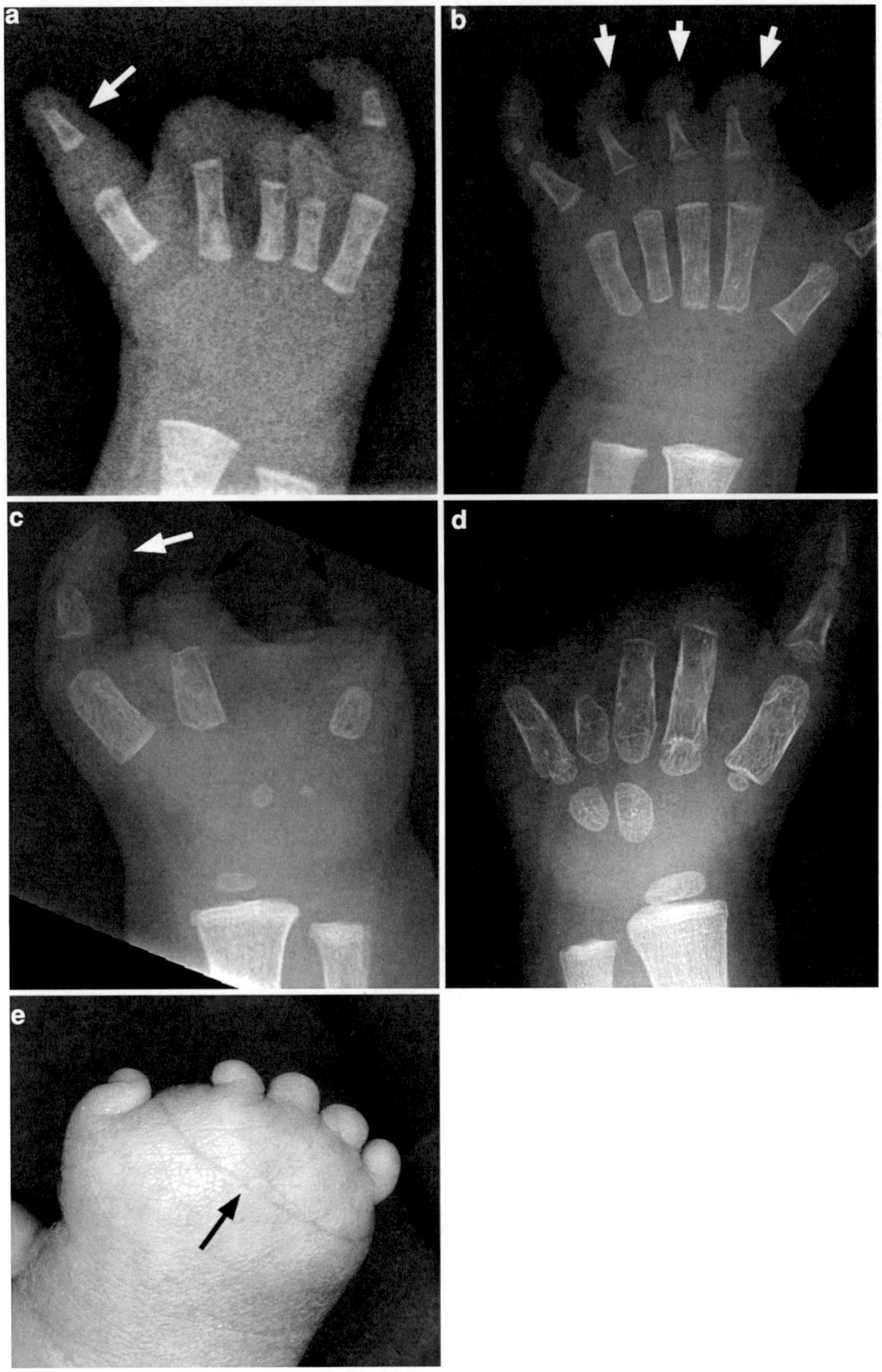

Fig. 12 Symbrachydactyly subtypes **a** Atypical cleft hand also known as'U-shaped cleft hand type' with absence of the central three digits, leaving only the thumb (*arrow*) and little finger, both of which are hypoplastic in this case. **b** Short finger type, with proximal phalanges and reasonable soft tissue envelopes distally (*arrows*) of the central three digits, which could be amenable to augmentation with bone grafts. **c** Monodactylous type, in which only the thumb remains (*white arrow*), but potentially useful soft tissue envelopes to the index and little fingers (*black arrows*). **d** Monodactylous type, with only the thumb, and no distal soft tissue. Function would be greatly improved by free toe transfers, or even custom made prostheses. **e** Peromelic type, with severe attenuation at metacarpal level (*arrow* denotes proximal palmar crease)

Radial sided hand anomalies may co-exist with ulnar longitudinal deficiency and hand abnormalities are present in 68–100% of cases (Miller et al. 1986). Ulnar longitudinal deficiency may be associated with other musculoskeletal anomalies (e.g., scoliosis), but is not associated with the visceral and haemopoetic disorders seen in radial deficiencies.

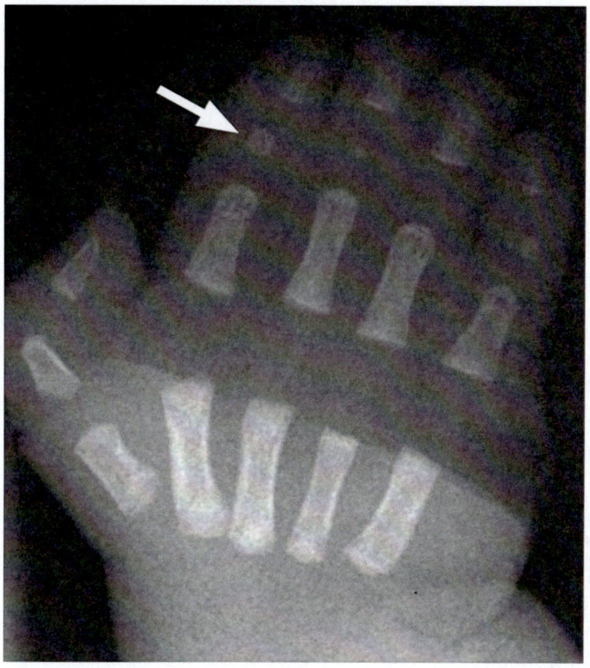

Fig. 13 Poland's syndrome with shortened digits due mostly to attenuation or absence of the middle phalanges (*arrow*), syndactylies and global hypoplasia of the hand, in association with other upper limb and chest deformities

5 Failure of Differentiation

5.1 Syndactyly

Syndactyly is one of the most common hand anomalies and results from incomplete separation of two or more adjacent digits. It has an incidence of 1:2,000 live births (Flatt 1994). The anomaly can be sporadic or familial (a family history is present in 10–40% of cases) and it may be associated with other syndromes including Poland syndrome and craniosynostoses such as Apert's syndrome (Fig. 17) (Kozin 2001).

It is classified as 'complete' if it reaches the distal interphalangeal joint (Fig. 16a), 'incomplete' if proximal to this joint, 'simple' if it involves only skin and soft tissue, and 'complex' if there is a bony fusion (usually distal) (Fig. 16b) (Van Heest 1996). Any combination of web spaces may be involved, but the commonest is an isolated third web-space involvement (between the ring and middle fingers). Syndactyly can also be classified as 'complicated' if it occurs in association with other abnormalities in the affected area, such as duplication (Fig. 18). Syndactyly should be differentiated from. 'Acrosyndactyly' (distal fusion with a proximal fenestration) which occurs in association with Constriction ring syndrome (see Sect. 9).

Radiographs may indicate that separation of syndactyly is not always appropriate (Fig. 19a, b).

5.2 Arthrogryposis

This term has been used to describe conditions that present with congenital joint contractures (Mennen et al. 2005). This clinical entity has also been described by Sheldon as amyoplasia (Sheldon 1932) and most affected children (84%) present with involvement of all four limbs (Sells et al. 1996).

The contractures are thought to be the end result of decreased intra-uterine movement by the fetus which may occur because of neuropathies, myopathies, abnormal connective tissue or decreased intra-uterine space. It is a sporadic condition with an incidence of 1 in 10,000 live births (Hall 1997) (Fig. 20a, b).

5.3 Camptodactyly

This is a painless flexion contracture of the proximal interphalangeal joint (PIPJ) that usually affects the little finger and may be progressive. It is not related to trauma and is estimated to affect just under 1% of the population to some degree (Smith and Kaplan 1968) (Fig. 21). A classification system has been described by Benson with three main types (Benson and Kaplan 1994). Type I presents in infancy and is frequently confined to one or both little fingers, with approximately equal sex incidence. Type II presents in adolescence with females being affected more commonly than males. The deformity worsens with the adolescent growth spurt. Type III is more severe and usually affects multiple digits in both hands (Koman et al. 1990), and may be associated with chromosomal disorders and skeletal abnormalities. Most structures within the finger have been implicated, although abnormalities of the intrinsic lumbrical muscles of the superficial flexor tendon are not uncommon operative findings.

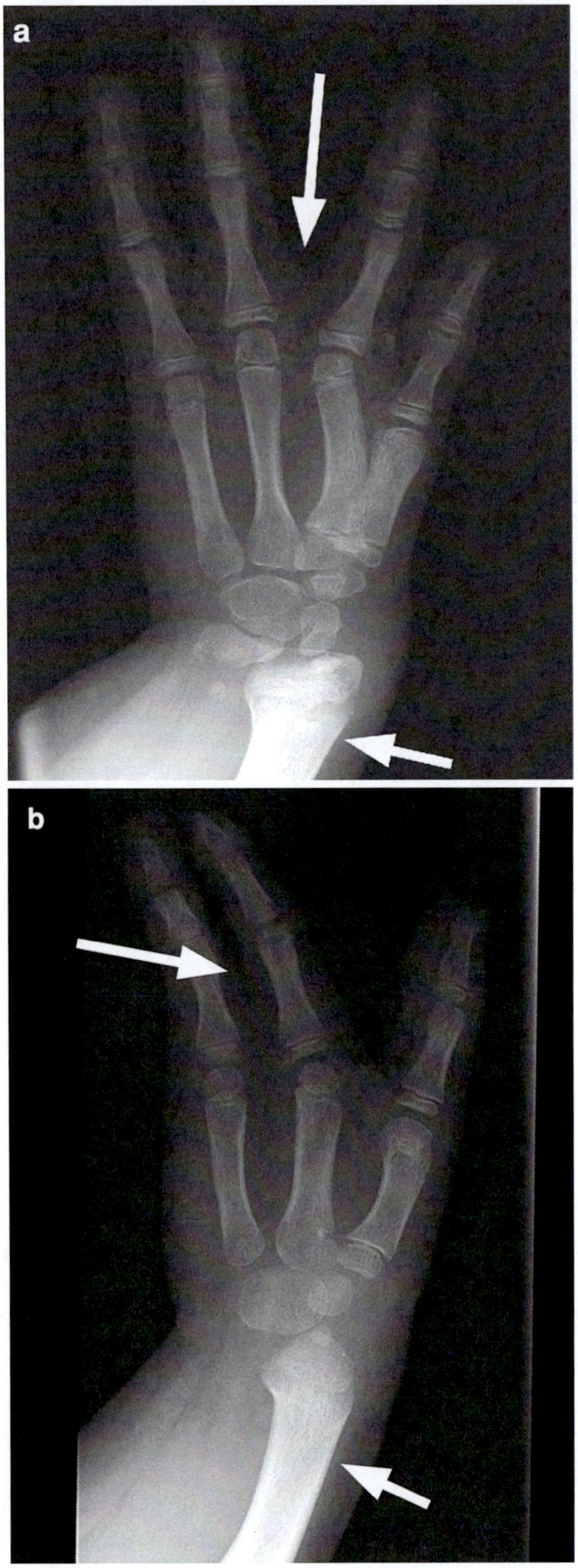

◂**Fig. 14** **a** and **b** Ulnar dysplasia has deficiencies of the ulnar side of the upper limb, with partial or complete absence of the ulna, commonly with the radius providing a one-bone forearm (*short arrows*), loss of ulnar digits, ulnar deviation at the wrist, and syndactylies (*long arrows*)

Plain radiograph assessment is vital, as the presence of classical bony changes around the joint predicts a very poor surgical outcome. These bony changes include flattening of the head of the proximal phalanx, widening of the base of the middle phalanx, and an indentation at the neck of the proximal phalanx (Ty and James 2009) (Fig. 22).

5.4 Clinodactyly

This refers to an abnormal deviation of a finger in the coronal or radioulnar plane which typically affects the middle phalanx of the little finger. The finger deviation is usually directed radially. Minor angulation of <10 degrees is so common that it may be regarded as a normal variant (Ezaki 1999).

Familial clinodactyly with an autosomal dominant pattern of inheritance usually presents bilaterally, and

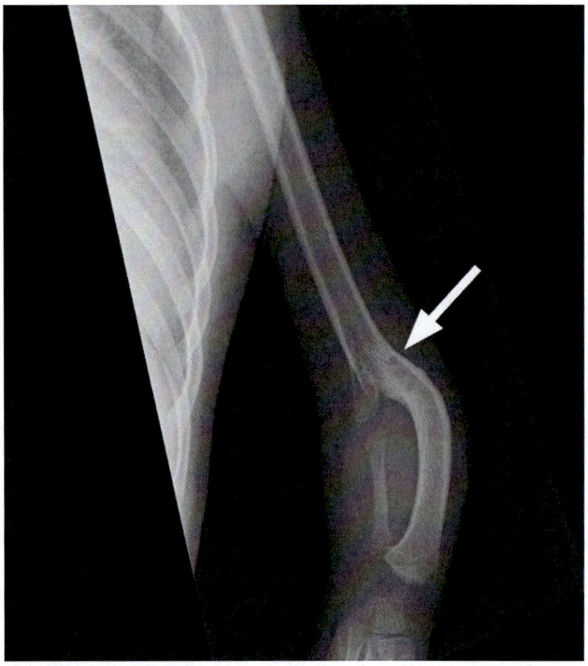

Fig. 15 Radiohumeral synostosis (*arrow*) can be seen in ulnar dysplasia

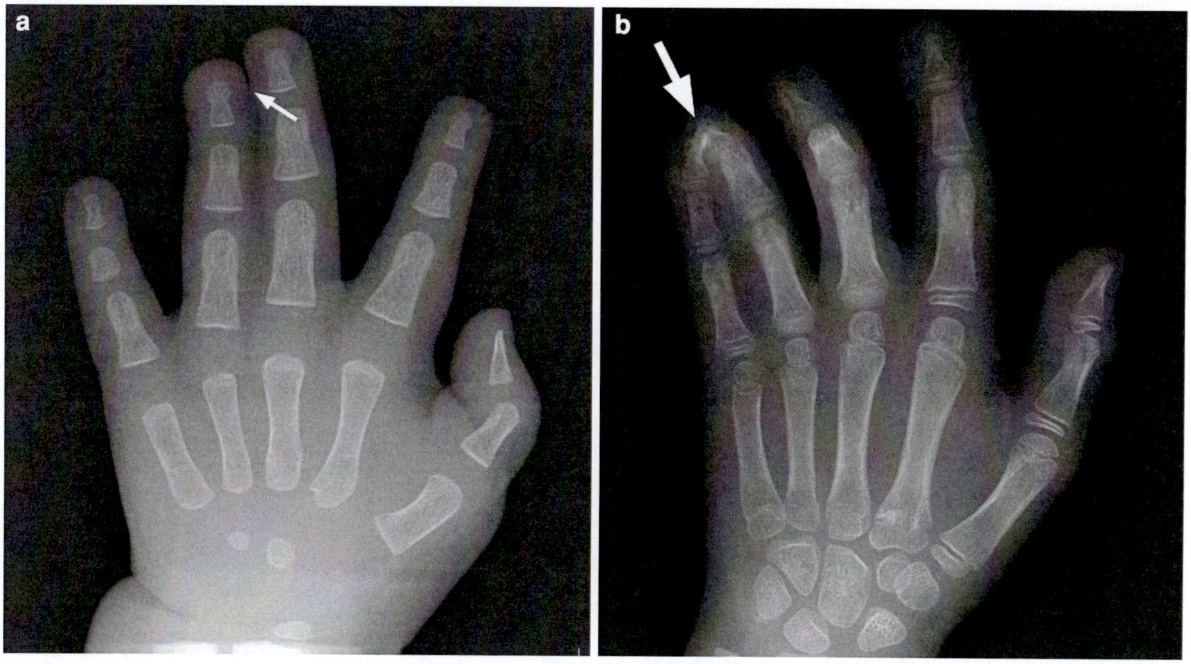

Fig. 16 Syndactyly **a** Simple, complete syndactyly with soft tissue union only, distal-to-distal interphalangeal joint (*arrow*). **b** Complex syndactyly with bony union which is usually at the distal phalangeal level (*arrow*), and requires earlier release than simple syndactyly as bony deformities can occur quickly with growth

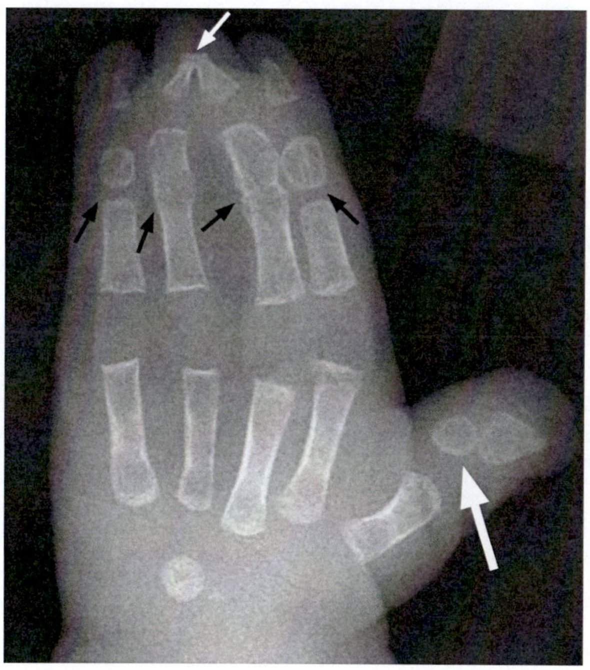

Fig. 17 Apert's hand with complex syndactyly (*short white arrow*), poorly developed or absent proximal interphalangeal joints ('symphalangism' (*black arrows*)), and a shortened deviated thumb caused by a delta phalanx (*large white arrow*)

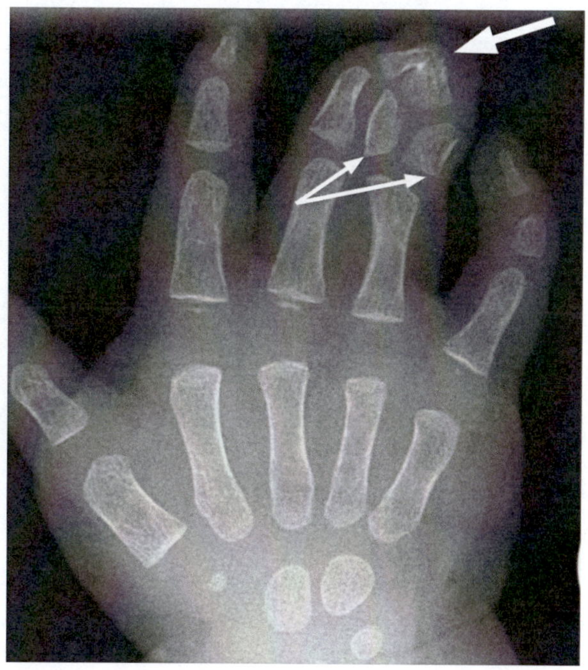

Fig. 18 Complicated syndactyly, with distal bony union (*large arrow*) and unusual duplication of the middle phalanx (*small arrows*)

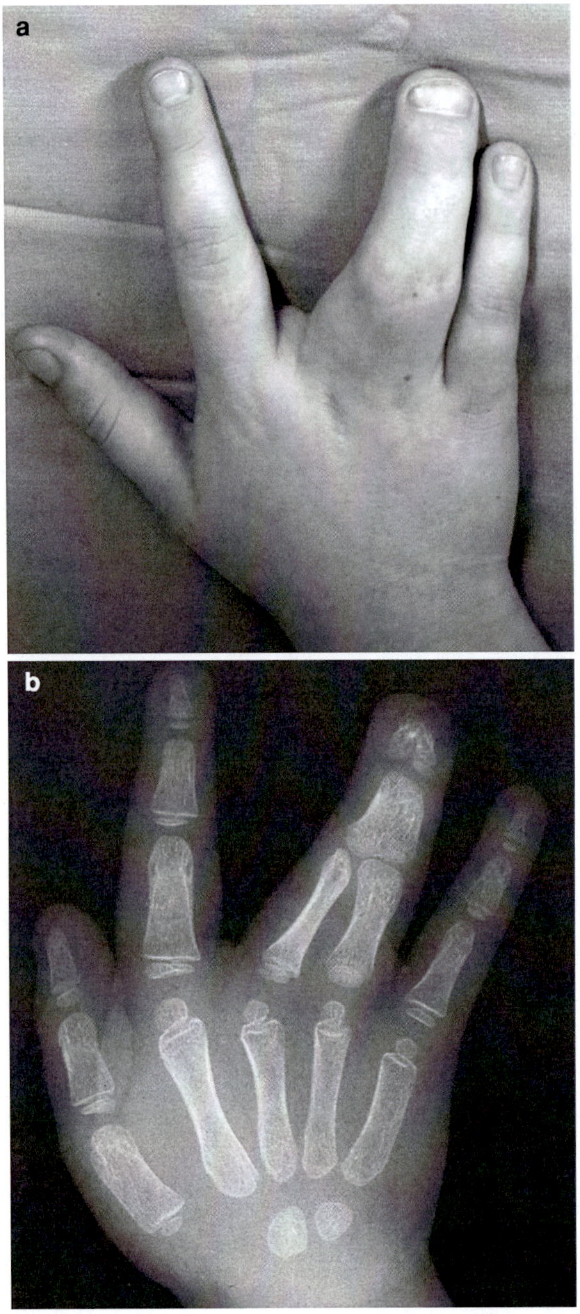

Fig. 19 Syndactyly release is sometimes contraindicated, as X-rays may reveal that the fingers work better together than if they were separated

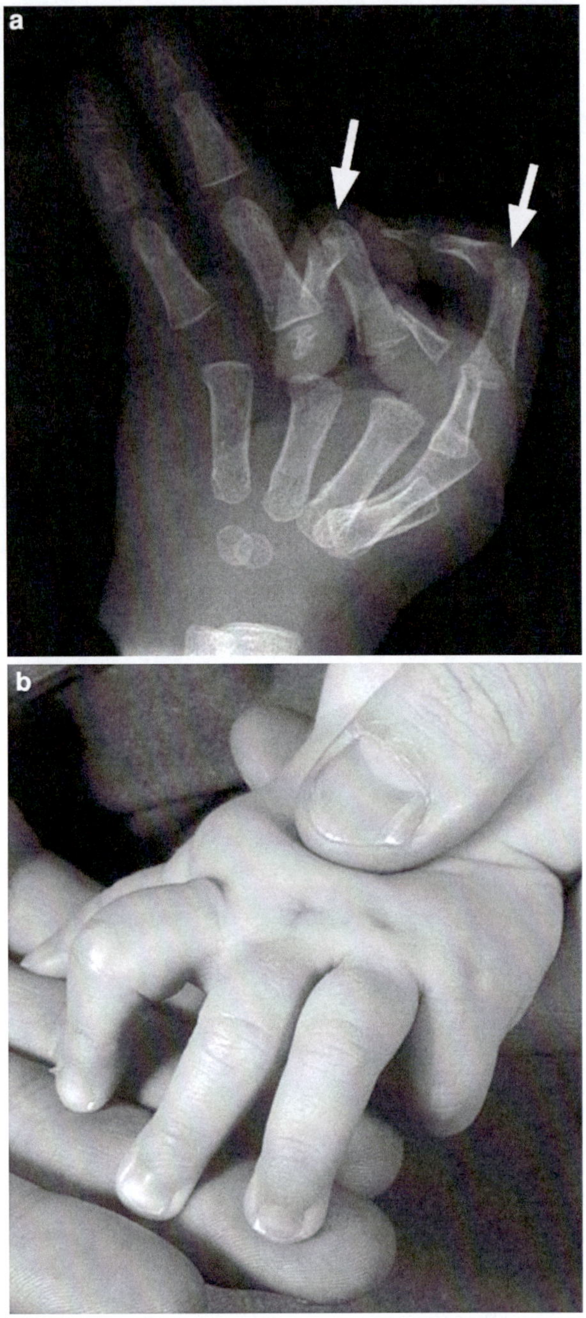

Fig. 20 Arthrogryposis is frequently associated (**a**) with multiple camptodactylies (*arrows*), sometimes affecting all digits (**b**)

is not associated with genetic syndromes. Clinodactyly may also be associated with syndromic and genetic conditions, most notably Down syndrome, in which the prevalence has been estimated at 35–79% (Flatt et al 1994).

The deformity is caused by an abnormally shaped middle phalanx, which may be triangular (a "delta" phalanx) or trapezoidal because of a C-shaped epiphysis (Jones 1964) (Fig. 23). Serial plain radiographs can be useful for objective monitoring of the angle of deviation. If progression occurs despite non-operative treatments

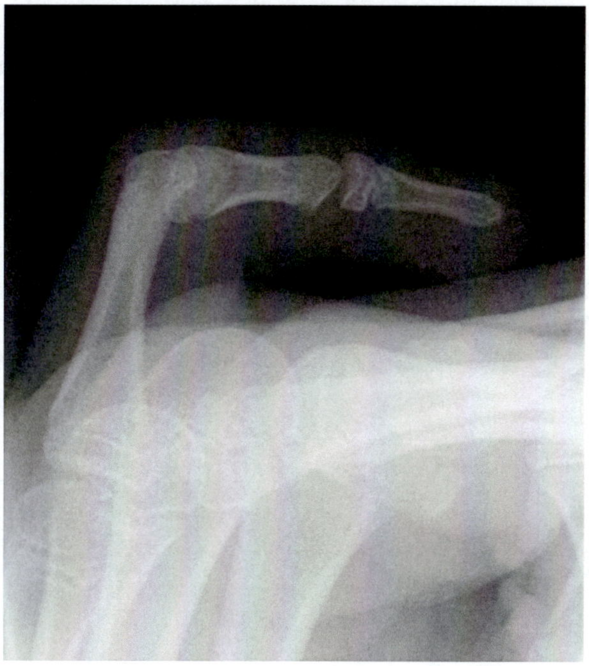

Fig. 21 Camptodactyly most commonly involves the little fingers, with stretching exercises and splintage forming the mainstay of treatment, with surgery often yielding disappointing results

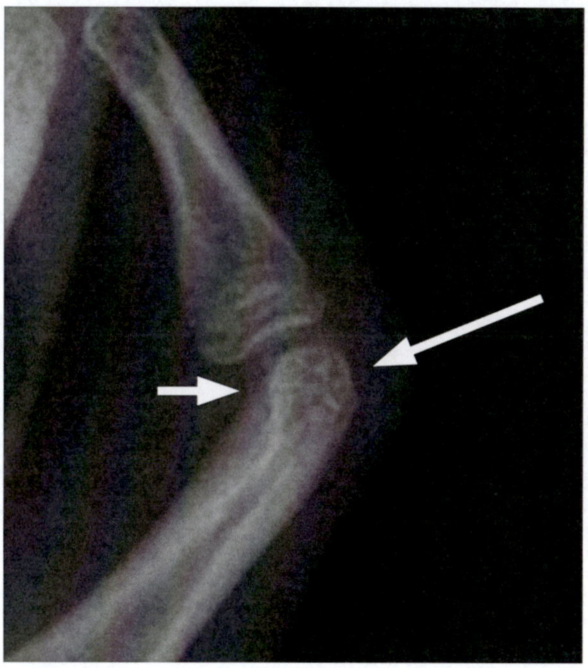

Fig. 22 Bony changes in camptodactyly chisel shaped head of proximal phalanx (*long arrow*), indentation of the neck of the proximal phalanx (*short arrow*), and widening of the base of the middle phalanx augur a poor surgical result

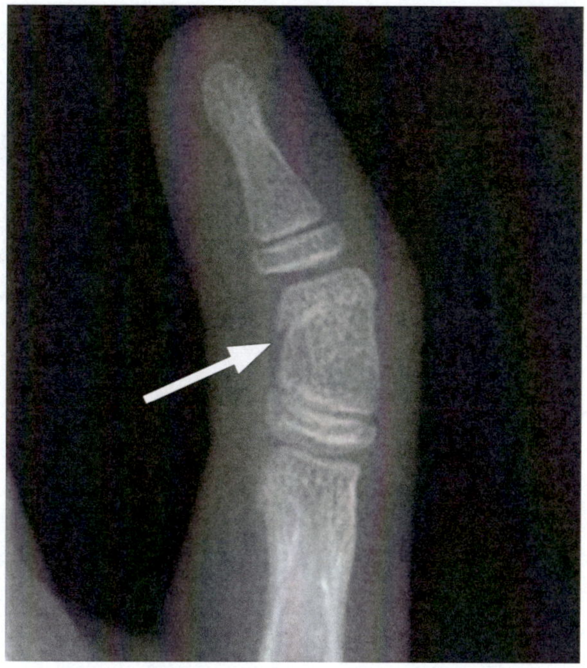

Fig. 23 Clinodactyly showing abnormal C-shaped epiphysis of middle phalanx (*arrow*)

(principally night splintage), surgery in the form of a wedge osteotomy may be required (Fig. 24a, b).

Delta phalanges can occur elsewhere in the hand and are frequently seen in the thumbs of Apert's patients, where they can cause marked deviation (Fig. 25) and often require surgery.

5.5 Congenital Thumb Flexion Deformities

Trigger and clasped thumbs are the two main causes of congenital flexion deformities of the thumb, with flexion, respectively at the interphalangeal and metacarpophalangeal joints. In trigger thumbs, a thickening in the flexor tendon may be felt at the A1 pulley level (clinically at the level of the metacarpophalangeal level).

In clasped thumbs there is a wide spectrum of differences, starting with attenuation then absence of the extensors, and progressing to flexion contractures with global thumb hypoplasias. Clinical evaluation usually suffices, though ultrasound may be useful in assessment of the tendons to aid in treatment planning. Hypoplastic extensors in a clasp thumb may respond to simple splintage whereas aplasias require tendon transfer.

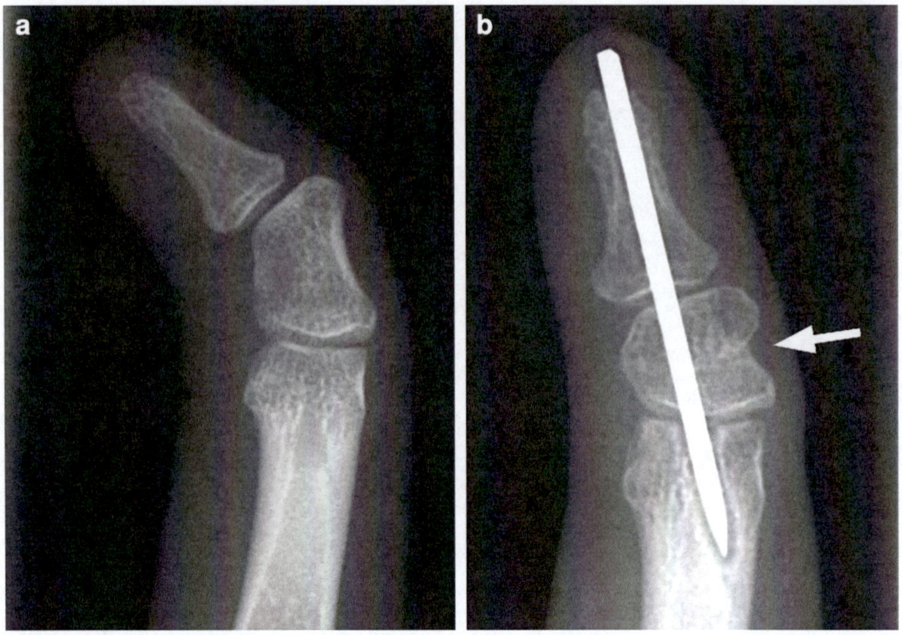

Fig. 24 Clinodactyly showing (**a**) a delta phalanx with fused epiphysis, treated by (**b**) a closing wedge osteotomy (*arrow*) and temporary K-wire

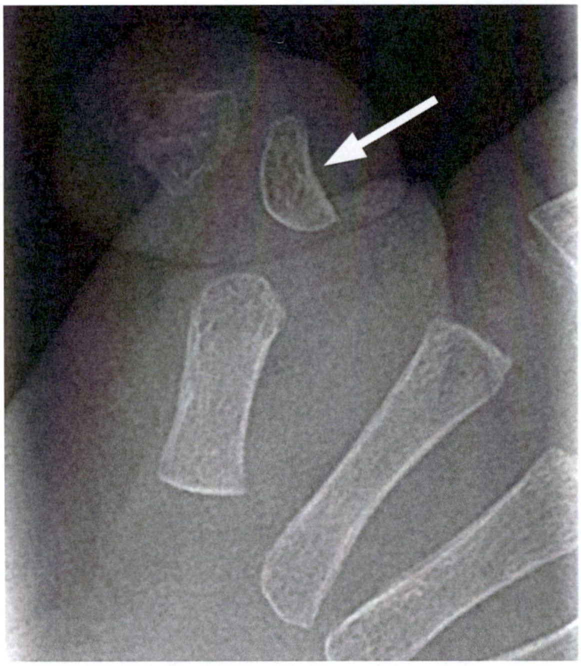

Fig. 25 Apert's thumb delta phalanx (*arrow*), which usually requires surgical correction

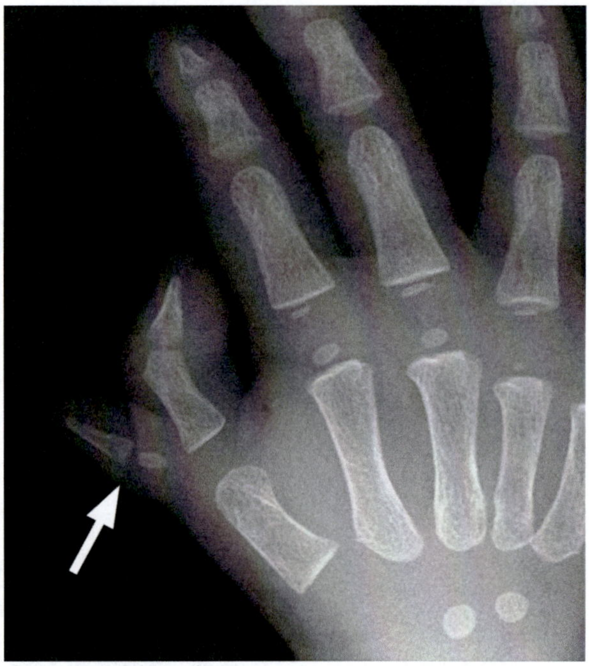

Fig. 26 Rudimentary radial duplicate (*arrow*)

6 Duplication

This probably results from splitting of the original embryonic part rather than a true duplication (Van Heest 1996). Polydactyly may be 'preaxial' (radial i.e., thumb), postaxial (ulnar i.e., little finger) or central.

6.1 Post-Axial Polydactyly

Duplications involving the ulnar aspect of the hand are more common in patients of African descent. The incidence is reported as 1 in 1,339 live births in Caucasians and 1 in 143 live births in African Americans (Watson and Hennrikus 1997).

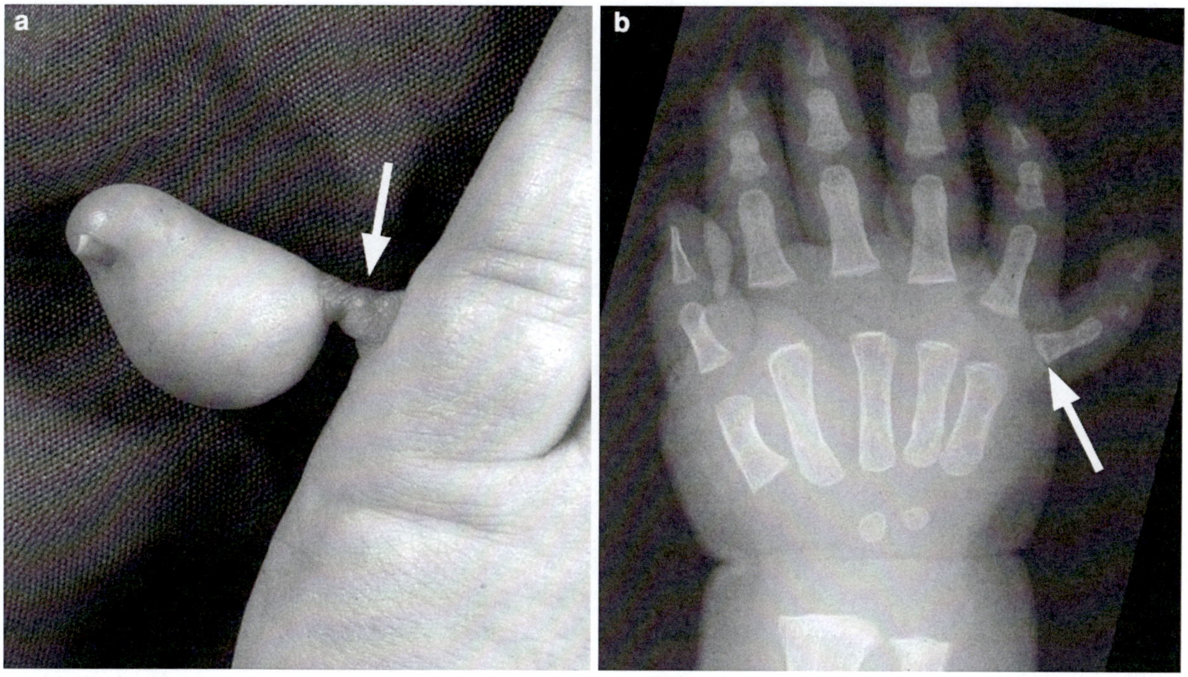

Fig. 27 Ulnar duplication is based on the Stelling classification. **a** *Type 1* skin bridge only (*arrow*) requiring only simple excision. **b** *Type 2* strong bony attachment, requiring preservation and reinsertion of the ulnar collateral ligament from accessory digit to fifth finger (position of insertion marked with *arrow*). *Type 3* is complete duplication of metacarpal

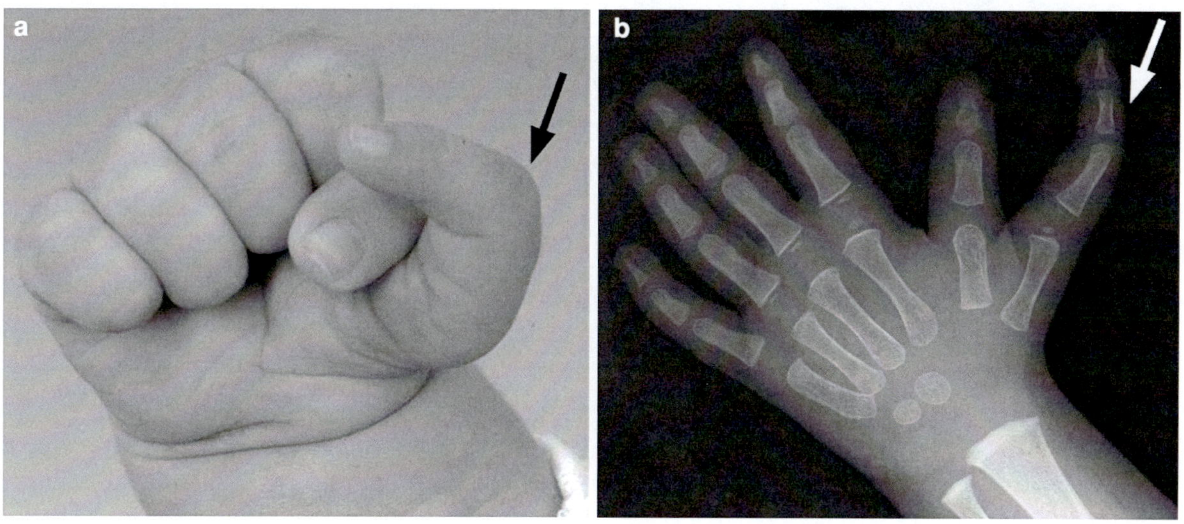

Fig. 28 Triphalangeal thumb (*arrow*)

Although it is commonly an isolated finding with autosomal dominant transmission and a favorable prognosis, it may also be associated with various syndromes. The presence of post-axial polydactyly in Caucasians is more suggestive of an underlying syndrome and merits systemic evaluation. Syndromes

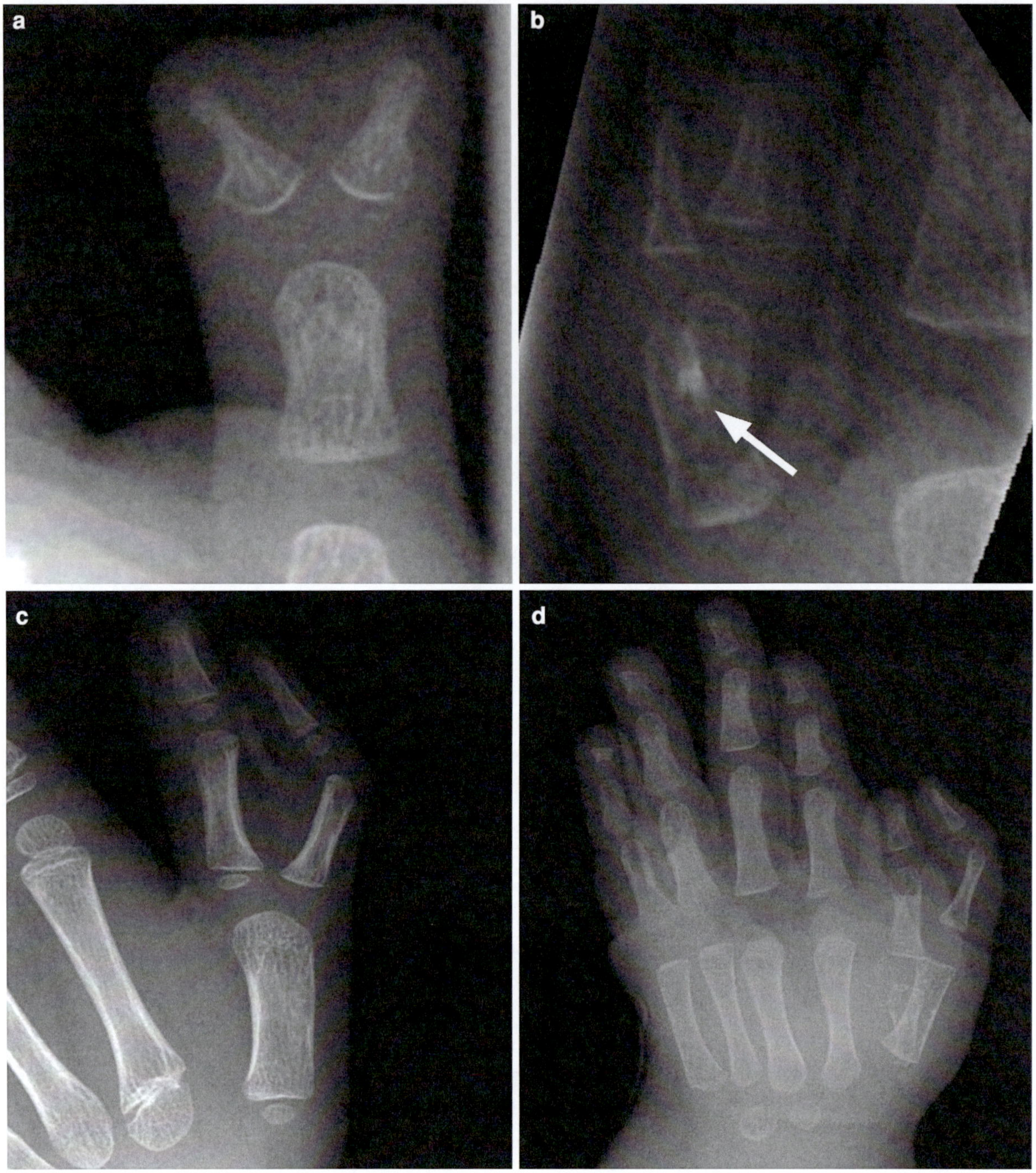

Fig. 29 The Wassel classification divides radial duplication into seven subtypes. **a** *Type 2* duplicated distal phalanx. **b** *Type 3* bifid proximal phalanx. **c** *Type 4* duplicated proximal phalanx. **d** *Type 6* duplicated metacarpal. *Type 1* is a bifid distal phalanx, *type 5* is a bifid metacarpal, and any duplication with a triphalangeal element is classified as a Wassel *type 7*

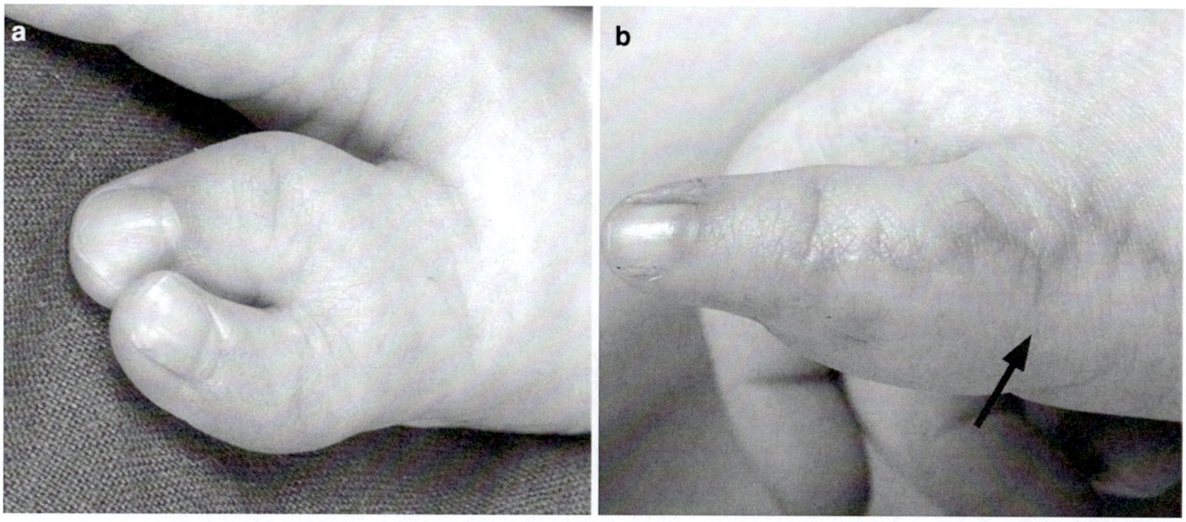

Fig. 30 Wassel 4 duplication at the metacarpophalangeal level is the commonest subtype (50%). **a** Well-matched duplicates, which would require skeletal amalgamation. **b** Post-amalgamation procedure of Wassel 4 duplication in which the radial duplicate was relatively hypoplastic, but which still requires preservation of soft tissues (*arrow*) from radial duplicate (radial collateral ligament, thenar muscle insertions and almost all of the skin), and reinsertion into the dominant ulnar duplicate. Only the hypoplastic skeleton, pulp and nail complex has been discarded

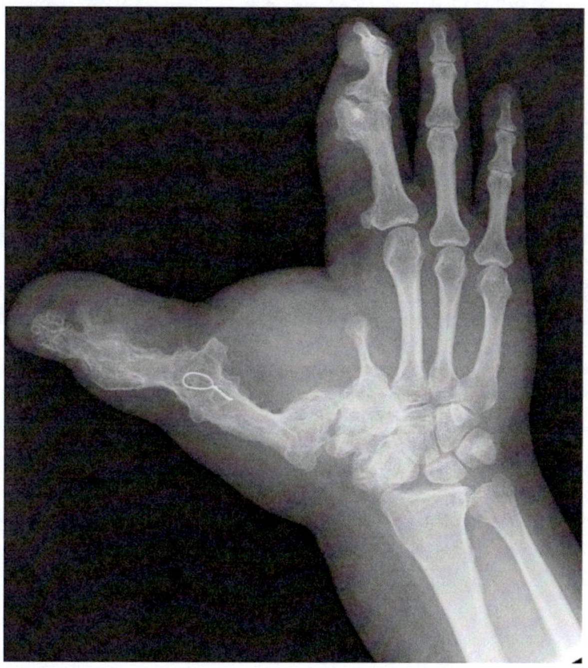

Fig. 31 Proteus syndrome

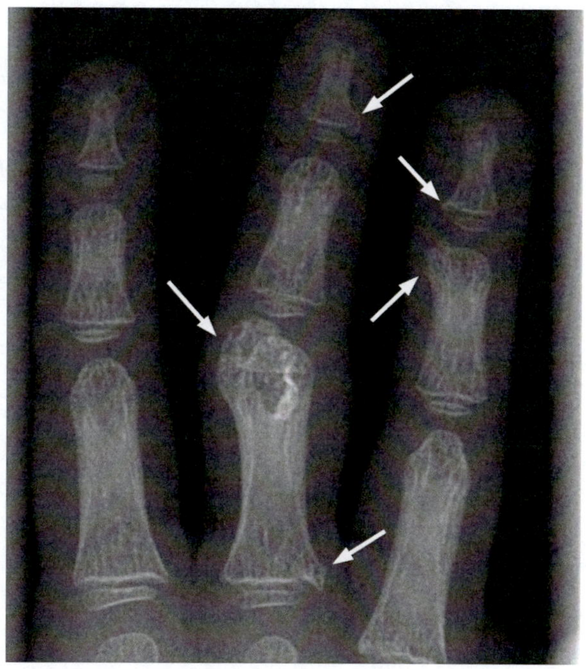

Fig. 32 Ollier's disease—multiple exostoses (*arrows*)

include trisomy 13, Meckel-Gruber syndrome, Bardet-Biedl syndrome, Smith–Lemli–Opitz syndrome, short rib-polydactyly syndromes and Ellis van Crevald syndrome (Lachman 2007).

Accessory digits may be well developed or rudimentary (Fig. 26) (Watson and Hennrikus 1997). Commonly the digit is rudimentary and held by a soft tissue bridge requiring only a simple excision

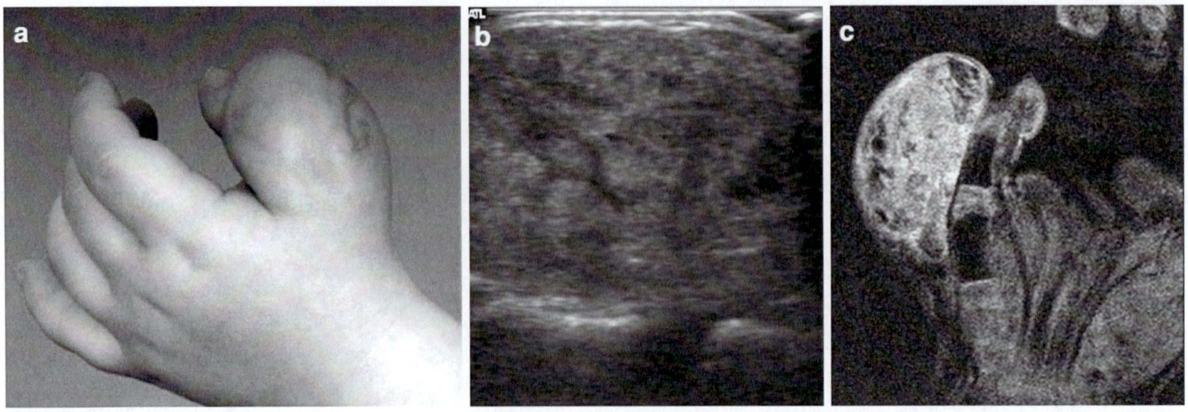

Fig. 33 **a** Large soft tissue mass on dorsum of thumb of 18 month old boy. Rapid growth raises possibility of malignant change, meriting initial urgent radiological investigation. Plain XR revealed no bony changes or calcification. This proved to be a benign lipoblastoma. **b** Ultrasound shows superficial heterogenous soft tissue mass. **c** Coronal T1 fat saturated sequence post contrast shows avid enhancement in the lipoblastoma adjacent to the thumb

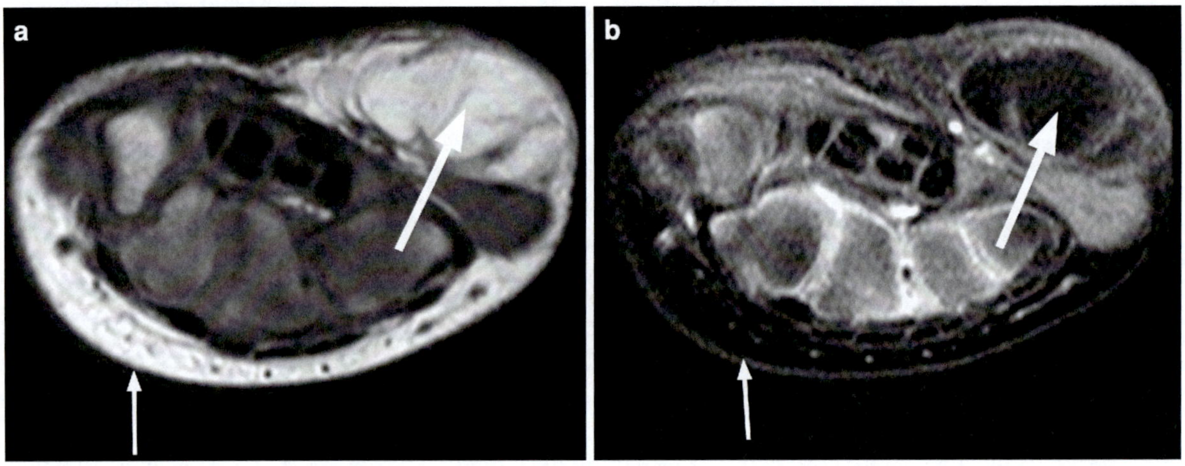

Fig. 34 MR of right hand shows. **a** on the T1 sequence the mass in the hypothenar eminence (*large arrow*) has the same signal as fat (*small arrow*). **b** on the T2 fat saturated sequence both fat and the mass saturate out, confirming the fatty nature of the mass

(Fig. 27a), though there can be bony attachments at proximal phalangeal or metacarpal level (Fig. 27b), requiring more involved surgery.

6.2 Pre-Axial Polydactyly

Although it is less common than post-axial polydactyly, it is more common in Caucasians and particularly in Orientals. The incidence is 1 in every 3,000 live births in the white population (Ress and Graham 1998). Duplication alone is usually unilateral and sporadic, however, if one of the duplicates is a triphalangeal thumb (Fig. 28a, b), a possible syndromic association should be considered (Rypens et al. 2006) and this can be inherited in an autosomal dominant pattern.

Thumb duplications are classified according to the level of duplication, and Wassel's classification is the most widely used and accepted (Fig. 29a, b, c, d). The most common type [Wassel type IV (Fig. 30a)] involves a duplicated proximal and distal phalanx sharing a common metacarpal articulation (Watt and Chung 2009).

Treatment usually involves creation of one good thumb out of the two duplicates, particularly if they

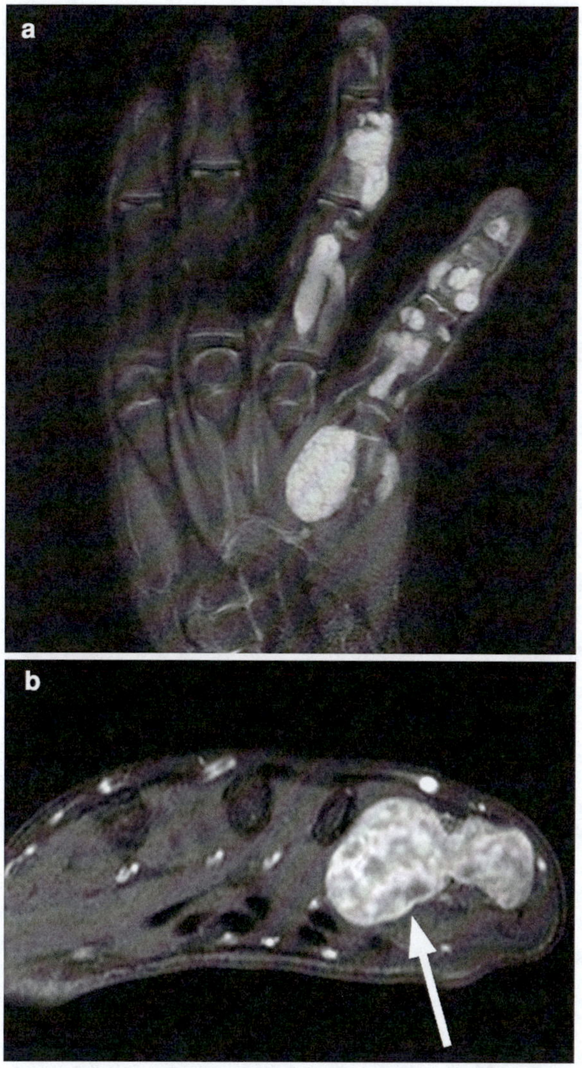

Fig. 35 Ollier's disease MRI. **a** T2 fat saturated coronal image shows the distribution of the high signal enchondromata **b** T1 fat saturated axial image post contrast shows a typical mottled chondroid type enhancement pattern in one lesion (*arrow*)

are of a fairly even size match, (i.e., amalgamation rather than excision) (Fig. 30b) and therefore plain radiographs are vital for surgical planning.

6.3 Central Polydactyly

This includes duplications that involve the index, middle or ring fingers and is often accompanied by syndactyly and cleft hand (Ress and Graham 1998; Tada et al. 1982).

6.4 Mirror-Hand and Mirror-Hand Spectrum

Duplication of the ulna, absence of the radius and thumb and duplication of the ring and small fingers about a common central finger characterize this exceedingly rare deformity. Only six cases of true mirror hand have been described in the literature (Watt and Chung 2009).

7 Overgrowth Conditions

These account for a small proportion of CHD and the region affected ranges from the entire limb, forearm, hand or digit. Overgrowth syndromes which may involve the hand include nerve territory orientated macrodactyly, lipomatous overgrowth, Proteus syndrome (Fig. 31), hemihypertrophy, Maffucci Syndrome, Ollier disease (Fig. 32), Parkes Weber Syndrome, Klippel-Trenaunay Syndrome and CLOVE syndrome (capillary malformations (C), lipomatous overgrowth of the trunk or extremities (LO), vascular malformations (V), epidermal naevi (E)) and generalized skeletal abnormalities) (Sapp et al. 2007).

In such cases, ultrasound and MRI can be very useful in clarifying the nature and soft tissue origin of the overgrowth (Figs. 33a, b, c; 34a, b; 35a, b). The typical MRI features of lipofibromatous hamartoma of the median nerve are illustrated (Fig. 36a, b, c).

7.1 Nerve Territory Oriented Macrodactyly and Lipomatous Macrodactyly

This is the most common overgrowth condition presenting to a hand surgeon. It is usually unilateral with a male predominance and no familial inheritance (Carty and Taghinia 2009). The lipomatous overgrowth may correspond with the ulnar or median nerve distribution within the hand (Fig. 37a, b). The affected nerves within the palm are characteristically grossly enlarged and compression neuropathies are common. The intrinsic muscles, joints, periarticular structures and skeletal parts are enlarged but blood vessels are of normal size. This latter fact is of great importance as the relative ischaemia in this condition can lead to difficulties in healing post surgery.

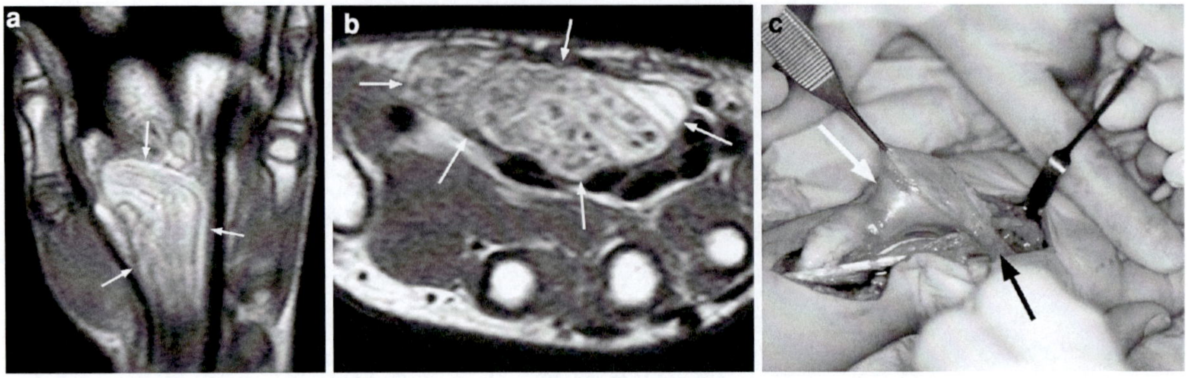

Fig. 36 Lipofibromatous hamartoma of the median nerve. **a** Coronal T1 shows high signal mass in the carpal tunnel (*arrows*) **b** Axial T1 sequence again shows the mass infiltrating the median nerve (*arrows*) **c** Operative photograph shows massive enlargement (*white arrow*) of the median nerve in the distal forearm and carpal tunnel caused by extensive and diffuse fatty infiltration, with relative sparing and more normal dimensions distally (*black arrow*)

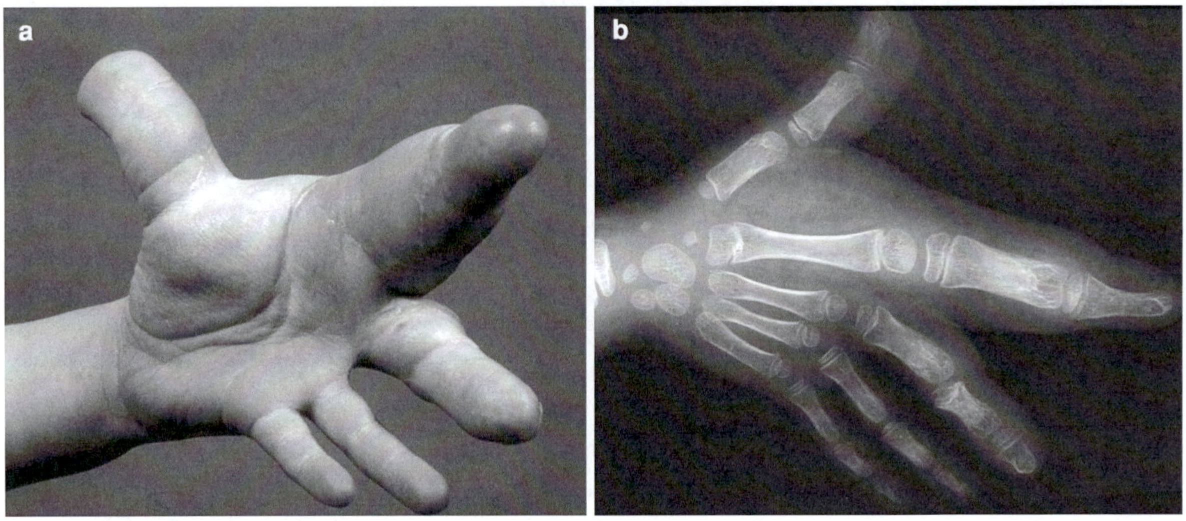

Fig. 37 **a** and **b** Nerve orientated macrodactyly following the median nerve distribution

8 Undergrowth Including Hypoplastic Thumb

This results from complete formation of the part during the embryonic period but incomplete growth and development during the fetal period (Van Heest et al 1996).

This group consists largely of the spectrum of hypoplasia of the thumb which can occur as an isolated entity, or more commonly in association with radial deficiencies. It is frequently bilateral and is often found in association with other hand differences including multiple other short digits, duplicated thumbs and a number of syndromes (Netscher and Baumholtz 2007).

The classification of thumb hypoplasia by (Blauth 1967) is useful in treatment planning, with less severe types requiring either no surgery or augmentation procedures (such as tendon transfers, ligament reconstruction and web-space deepening), whereas more severe forms (Fig. 38) require the creation of a new thumb by pollicisation of the adjacent index finger (Fig. 39a, b).

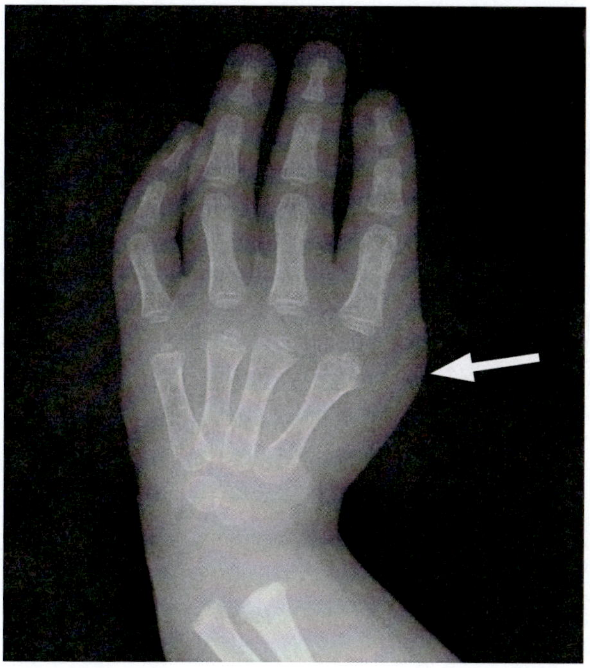

Fig. 38 Total aplasia of the thumb (Blauth grade 5)

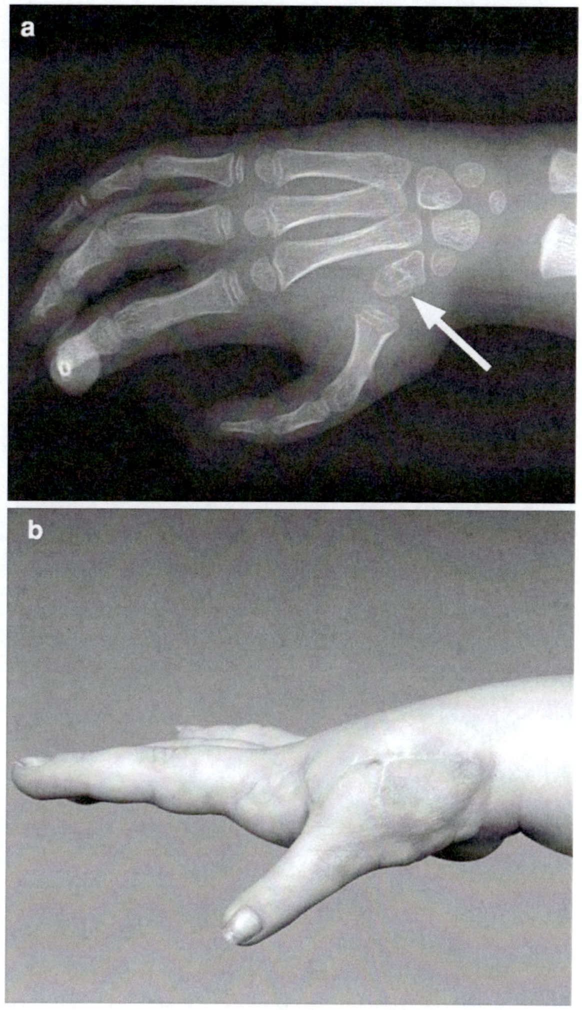

Fig. 39 Pollicisation of index finger for patient in Fig. 38 **a** Neo trapezium created by head of index metacarpal. **b** Pollicisation in such cases greatly upgrades the function of the hand

Plain radiographs are vital in the assessment of the hypoplastic thumb as the absence of a well-formed thumb basal joint (Fig. 40), indicates that augmentation procedures would be unlikely to produce a useful thumb, and requires a pollicisation of the index finger, with removal of the poorly-developed original thumb.

Hypoplasia of the fingers most commonly affects the index and little fingers with the middle phalanx being the most commonly affected bone (Fig. 41). This CHD is frequently inherited in an autosomal dominant pattern, and is associated with numerous congenital syndromes including Treacher Collins, Apert, Poland, Cornelia de Lange and Bloom syndromes (Flatt et al 1994).

9 Constriction Ring Syndrome

This is a rare condition where the fetus may become entangled in the amniotic membrane although the exact etiology remains controversial. It had been postulated that early amniotic rupture leads to the development of fibrous bands, which entangle the digits and limbs leading to intrauterine amputations and malformations (Torpin 1965). It has also been described as amniotic band syndrome. Prenatal risk factors include prematurity, low birth weight, maternal drug exposure, maternal illness or trauma during pregnancy (Kawamura and Chung 2009). The reported incidence is 1 in 15,000 live births. There is no sex predilection and 60% have an abnormal antenatal history (Foulkes and Reinker 1994).

The abnormalities are characteristically asymmetric and the most common findings include distal ring constrictions (Fig. 42a, b, c), intrauterine amputations (Fig. 43a, b, c, d) and acrosyndactyly (distal fusion of digits with a proximal fenestration that communicates the dorsal side with the volar side) (Fig. 44). The fingers may be truncated, a small cleft remains at the

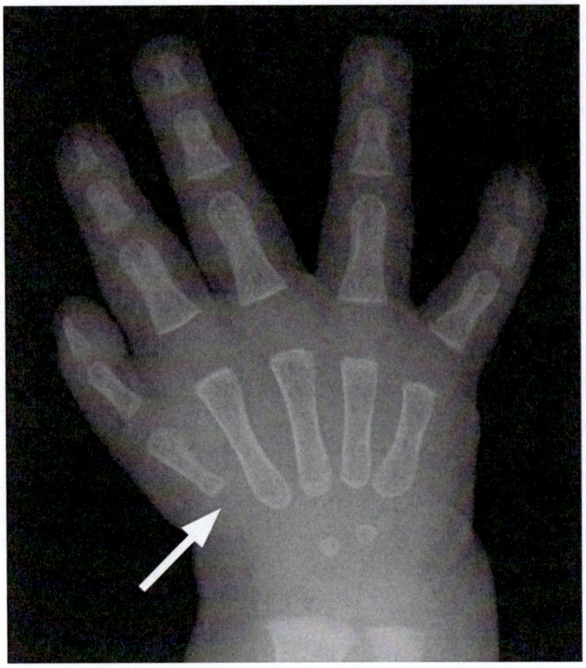

Fig. 40 A poorly developed basal joint in thumb hypoplasia (Blauth grade 3c) makes it very difficult to augment it into a useful thumb, though free metatarsophalangeal joint transfer from the foot has been used

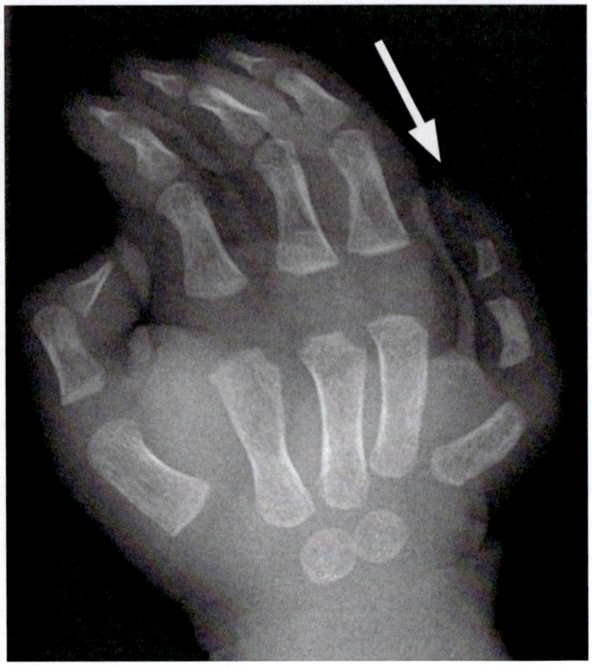

Fig. 41 Little finger hypoplasia. The marked attenuation of the fifth ray makes it difficult to augment, and was therefore treated in this case by ray amputation

site of the web space, and lower limb constriction bands and talipes deformities may be seen, (Kozin 2003; Wiedrich 1998; Foulkes and Reinker 1994). These features are not typically present with syndactyly resulting from inheritable and sporadic causes.

Interpretation of plain radiographs can be difficult in the more severe forms, in which the digits can be entwined and fused (Fig. 45a, b; 46a, b).

10 Generalized Skeletal Abnormalities

This includes conditions that do not fit into the other six categories described by Swanson, and includes skeletal hand deformities that are characteristic of a generalized bone and connective tissue disorder. The "tumour" like bone dysplasias including diaphyseal aclasia, and the fibrous disorders including neurofibromatosis and fibrous dysplasia are covered in separate chapters.

More than 250 skeletal dysplasias have been described with a complex classification system involving more than 30 groups organized by genetic and radiologic similarities. A comprehensive description of all the skeletal dysplasias involving the hand and wrist is therefore beyond the scope of this chapter, and reference should be made to a detailed text on this topic, (Lachman 2007; Spranger et al. 2002).

Antenatal ultrasound is able to diagnose many skeletal dysplasias (Dighe et al. 2008). In addition, low dose prenatal CT is starting to be used in large centers from the second trimester onward to provide further diagnostic information and aid antenatal counseling (Cassart 2010; Cassart et al. 2007). Post-delivery examination, plain film assessment, post mortem and genetic testing are, however, vital for determining a specific diagnosis for recurrence risk and counseling (Tretter et al. 1998).

A skeletal survey for the assessment of a skeletal dysplasia includes plain films of the skull, entire spine, chest, pelvis and extremities and there should be a systematic approach in the assessment of the bony skeleton.

It is important initially to determine the presence of any disproportionate shortening of the extremities and identify the presence of rhizomelia (proximal shortening of humerus or femur), mesomelia (middle segment shortening of tibia, fibula, radius and ulna) and/or acromelia (distal segment shortening of the hands and

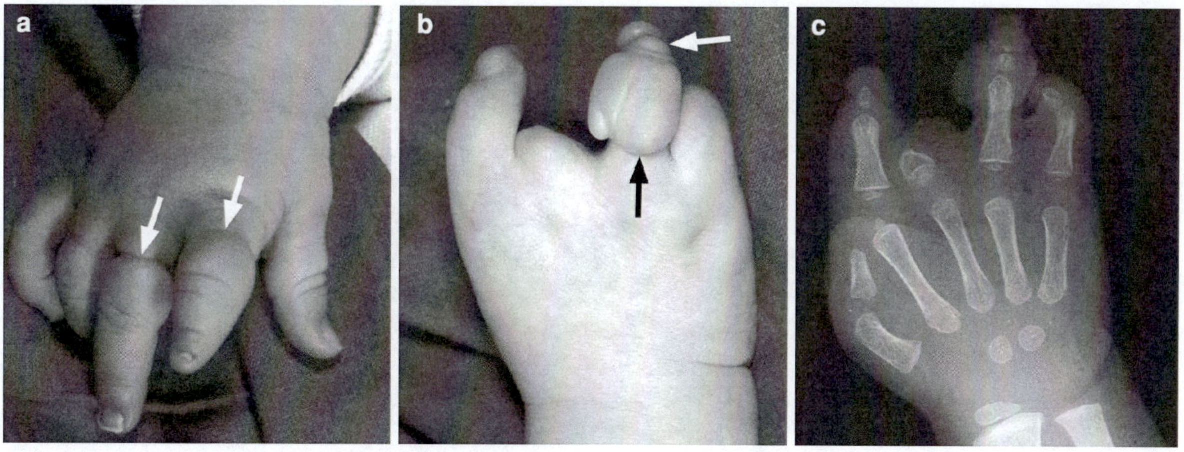

Fig. 42 Ring constriction syndrome. **a** Tight constrictions (*arrows*) with distal lymphoedema, needs relatively urgent release. **b** Marked distal lymphoedema, with rings at two levels on the same digit (*arrows*), plus autoamputations. **c** XR confirms involvement of all digits to varying degrees

feet). In reality, there is often a combination of shortening proximally and distally but the abnormality is categorized according to the predominant finding.

Disproportionate shortening may be present in isolation or as part of a more generalized skeletal dysplasia (Figs. 47, 48, 49, 50). The absence of hand and foot shortening in the presence of other abnormalities can suggest a diagnosis of a spondyloepiphyseal dysplasia congenita (Lachman 2008).

Secondly, assessment of the shape of the epiphyses, metaphyses and diaphyses and the appearance of epiphyseal ossification centers should be performed with particular attention to marginal irregularity, cortical thickness, flaring or flattening. Carpal bone ossification should be assessed for age and the presence of duplications, carpal fusions or accessory bones.

Findings should be organized and differential diagnosis and gamuts tables consulted in more specialist texts (Lachman 2007). Abnormalities should be differentiated from normal variants, always taking into consideration the clinical manifestations in conjunction with the radiologic findings.

This section will illustrate several more common examples with manifestations in the hand and wrist.

10.1 Achondroplasia Group

This includes three specific conditions, thanatophoric dysplasia, achondroplasia and hypochondroplasia. All have FGFR3 (fibroblast growth factor 3) mutations.

Thanatophoric dysplasia is also known as thanatophoric dwarfism and represents the second most common lethal bone dysplasia after osteogenesis type II. This condition is subdivided into types I and II, both of which are autosomal dominant mutations. In the extremities, there is generalized micromelia (shortening of all segments) and marked limb curvature (Fig. 51).

Achondroplasia is the most common, non-lethal skeletal dysplasia. It is an autosomal dominant condition with a spontaneous mutation rate of 80%. Most patients have a combination of rhizomelic, mesomelic and acromelic changes. In the hands, there is typically brachydactyly, metacarpal metaphyseal cupping and phalangeal metaphyseal widening (Lachman 2008) (Figs. 52, 53, 54).

Hypochondroplasia is also relatively very common, and shares many of same features of achondroplasia. The radiologic findings are milder and there is typically a later presentation, but there is always interpedicular widening in the lumbar spine.

10.2 Short Rib-Polydactyly Group

All conditions in this group are autosomal recessive and are similar radiologically.

Short rib-polydactyly dysplasias have the shortest ribs of all the dysplasias. In the hands, there is often severe brachydactyly with hypoplastic middle and distal phalanges. Polydactyly is commonly present.

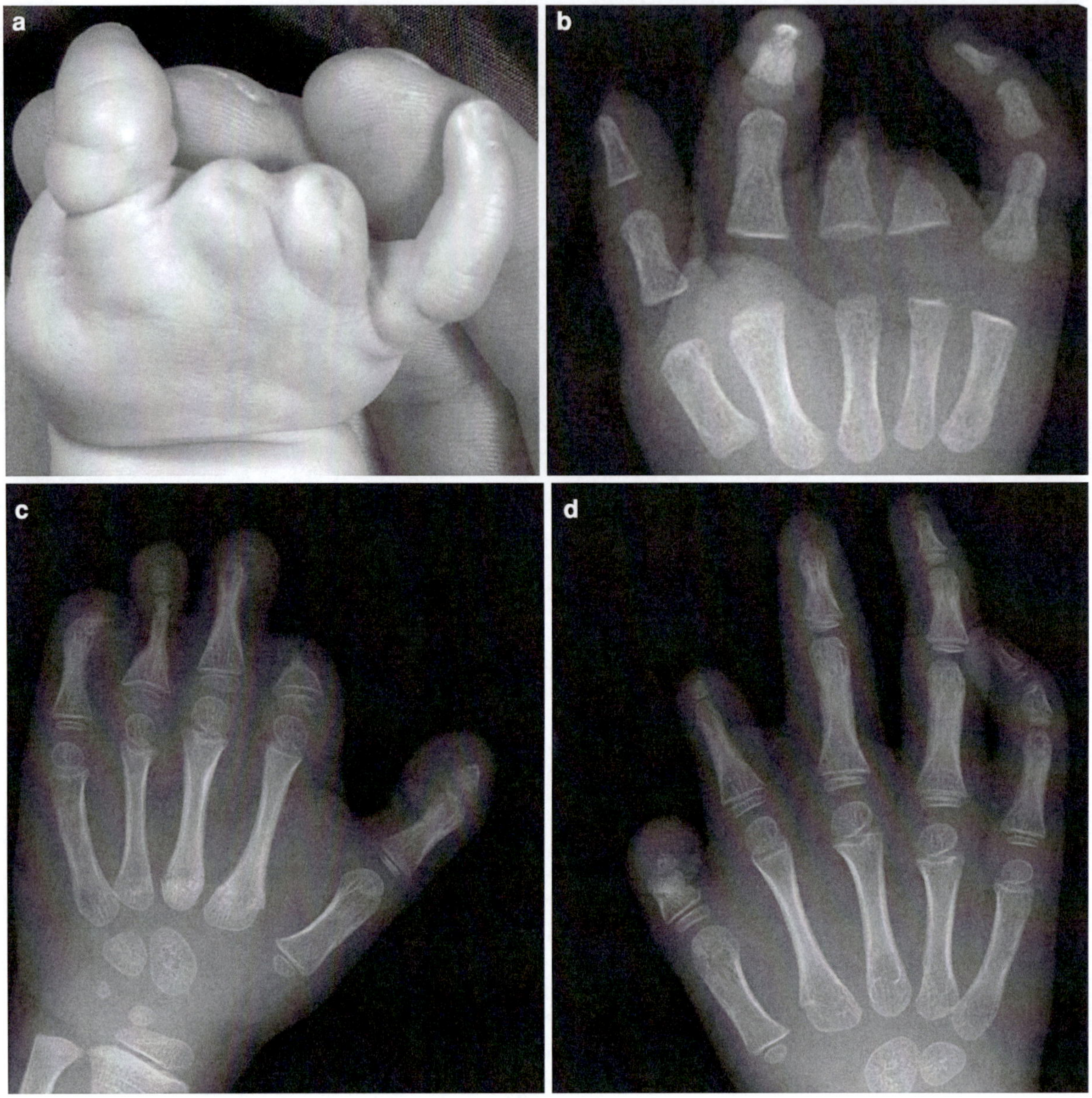

Fig. 43 **a** and **b** Autoamputations. **c** and **d** Bilateral asymmetrical involvement

Chondroectodermal dysplasia or Ellis van Crevald syndrome is a short-limbed dwarfism with dysplastic nails, hair and teeth accompanied by post-axial polydactyly and congenital heart disease. In the hands, as well as post-axial polydactyly, there are characteristic findings of carpal fusions, extra carpal bones and cone shaped epiphyses (Lachman 2008) (Fig. 55).

Asphyxiating Thoracic Dysplasia or Jeune Syndrome has similar radiologic appearances to Ellis-van Crevald syndrome with cone-shaped epiphyses in the hands. Uncommonly polydactyly is present.

10.3 Multiple Epiphyseal Dysplasia and Pseudoachondroplasia Group

In multiple epiphyseal dysplasia, the epiphyses of the hand are small, irregular and flattened and the carpal

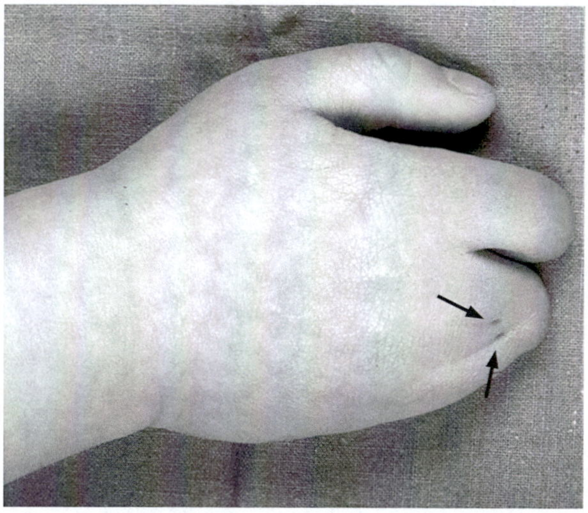

Fig. 44 Ring constriction syndrome with acrosyndactyly, and proximal fenestrations (*arrows*)

bones are small and irregular. There may be cone shaped epiphyses resulting in shortening of the short tubular bones of the hand.

Pseudoachondroplasia is a short limb, short trunk form of skeletal dysplasia. In the hands there is typically brachydactyly. The metacarpals are rounded proximally and there are mini-epiphyses in the hands with irregular carpal bones (Fig. 54).

10.4 Metaphyseal Disorders

Involvement of the hands occurs to varying degrees with the different metaphyseal dysplasias. Marked involvement of the hands is one of the main characteristics of metaphyseal chondrodysplasia McKusick Type. There is marked shortening of the hands, and flaring and cupping fragmentation of the metaphyses of the metacarpals and phalanges. The Jansen type metaphyseal chondrodysplasia demonstrates wide separation of epiphyses from metaphyses, with metaphyseal expansion and cupping. Schmid type metaphyseal chondrodysplasia, however, often has no hand involvement (Lachman 2008).

10.5 Dysostosis Multiplex Group

This group contains all the mucopolysaccharidoses, mucolipidoses and multiple storage diseases that produce a skeletal dysplasia.

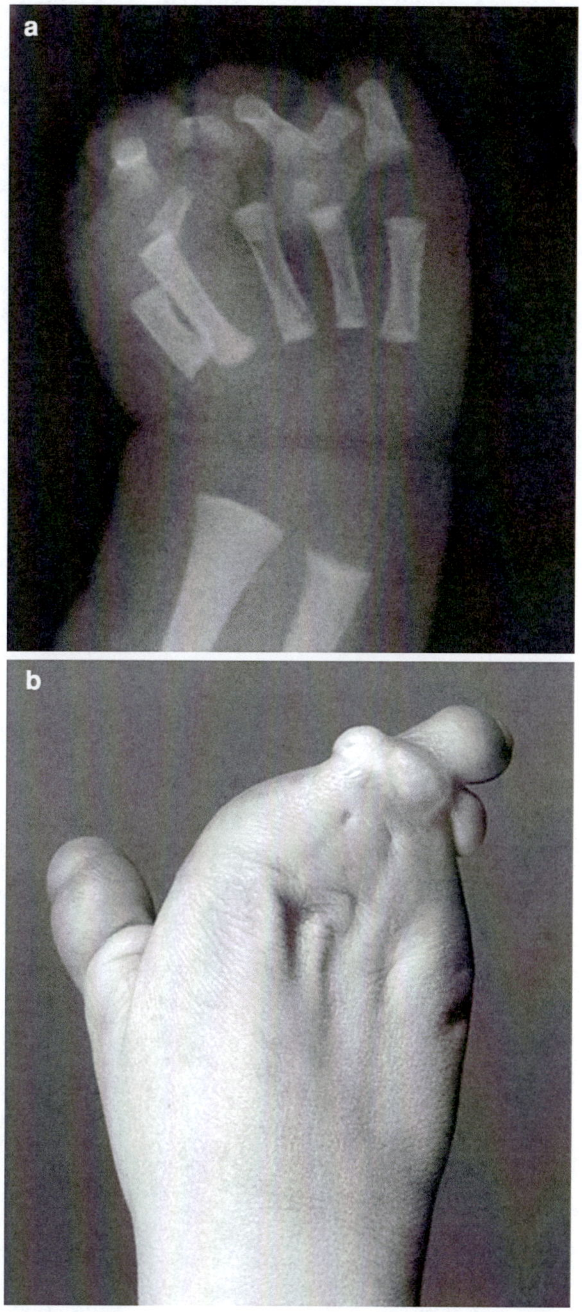

Fig. 45 **a** and **b** Ring constriction with complex arrangement of acrosyndactylies, necessitating very early release to prevent intractable bony deformities

Hurler syndrome (mucopolysaccharidosis type IH) has a recessive pattern of inheritance and most cases present in late infancy or early childhood. The hands characteristically exhibit brachydactyly, proximal

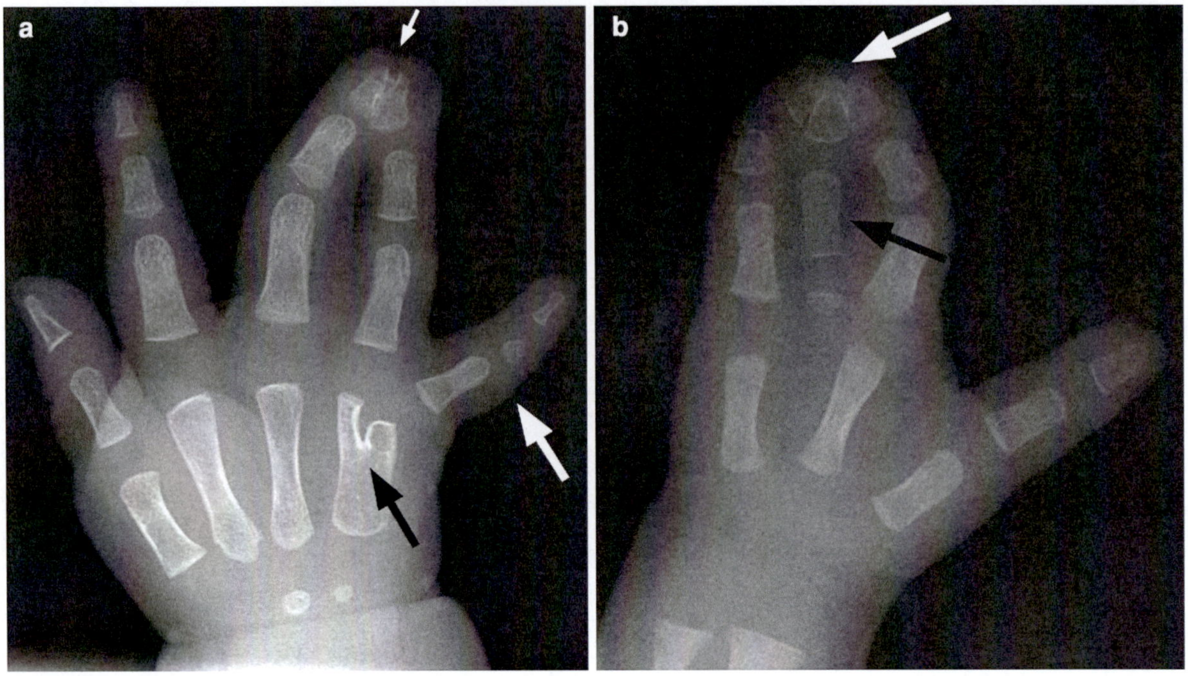

Fig. 46 Difficulties of classification. **a** Elements of syndactyly (*small white arrow*), hypoplasia (*large white arrow*) and bony synostosis (*black arrow*) in same hand. **b** Central duplication (*black arrow*), failure of formation (missing rays) and complex syndactylies (*white arrow*) in same hand

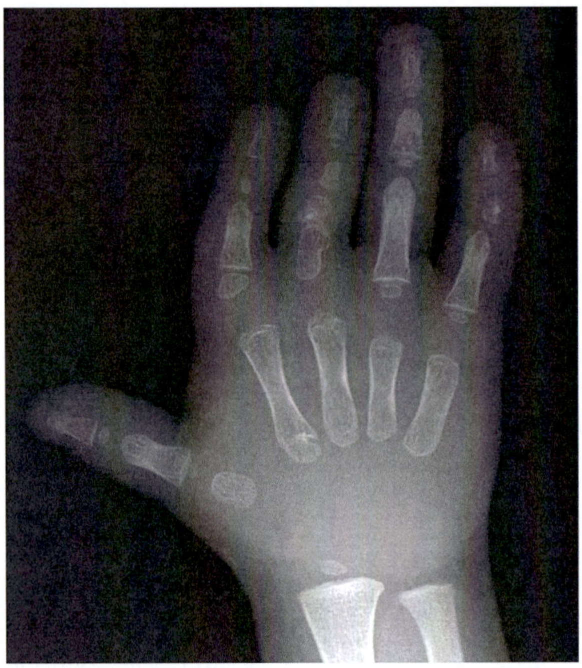

Fig. 47 Brachydactyly with absent carpal bone ossification, shortened metacarpals and shortened and dysplastic phalanges

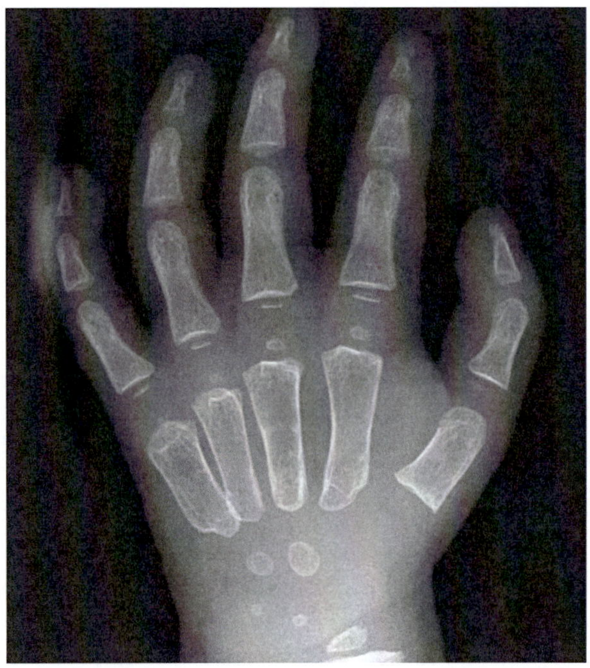

Fig. 48 Widened diaphyses of the metacarpals, proximal and middle phalanges with "pointing" of the proximal ends of the 2nd–5th metacarpals. The epiphyses are also dysplastic

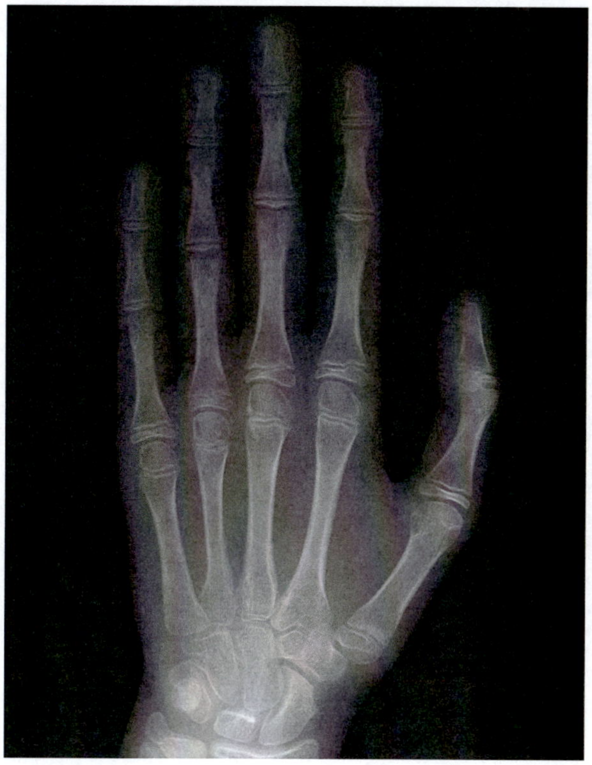

Fig. 49 Slender osteopenic bones with a metacarpal index of 10.4 in a patient with Marfans

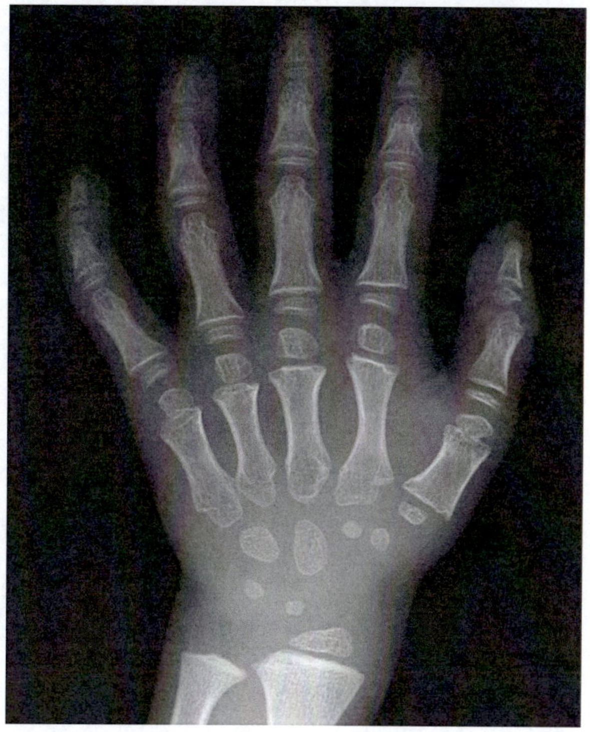

Fig. 50 Symmetrical shortening of the metacarpals with rounded, proximal metacarpals in a patient with Morquio syndrome. The carpal centers are small with delayed bone maturation

metacarpal "pointing", diaphyseal widening of metacarpals and proximal/middle phalanges and small irregular carpal bones with epiphyseal ossification delay (Lachman 2008) (Fig. 48).

Morquio syndrome (mucopolysaccharidosis type IVA and IVB) shows proximal metacarpal rounding, not "pointing" in the hands (Lachman 2008) (Fig. 50). The inheritance pattern is autosomal recessive (Hall 1997).

10.6 Dysplasias with Decreased Bone Density

These are represented primarily by osteogenesis imperfecta. Four main types have been described with osteogenesis imperfecta type II being the most common lethal skeletal dysplasia. In the extremities, in osteogenesis type II, there is generalized osteoporosis with or without fractures and shortened, widened long bones with thin cortices (Lachman 2008).

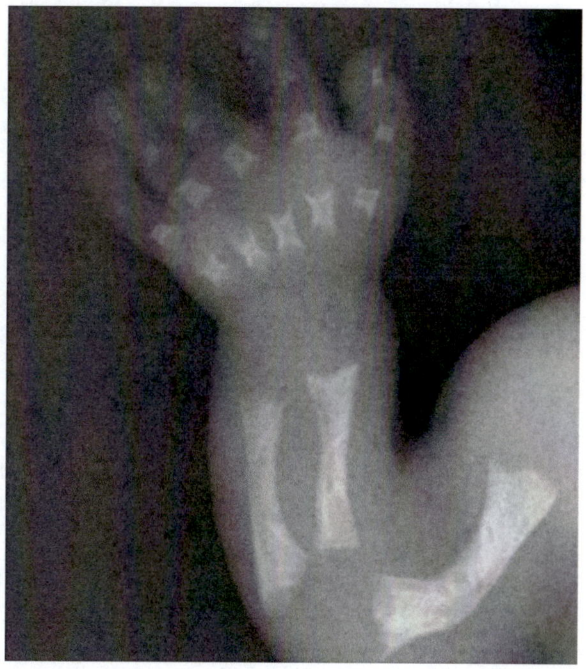

Fig. 51 Shortening and broadening of the tubular bones of the hand in a 20-week fetus with thanatophoric dysplasia type I

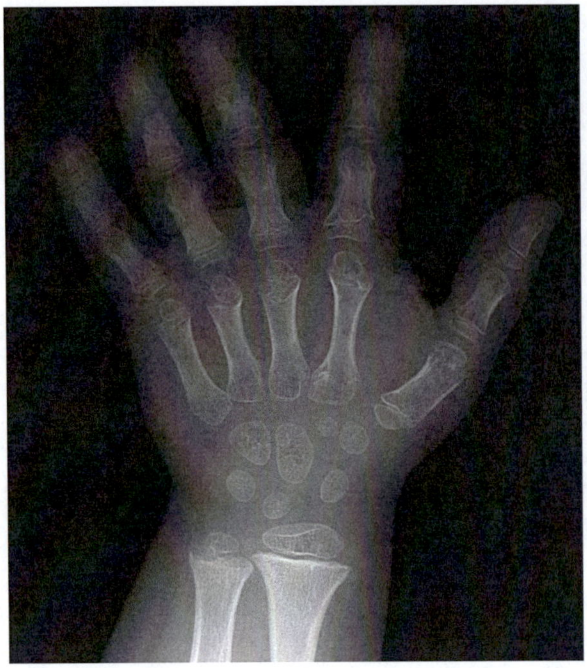

Fig. 52 Brachydactyly, metacarpal metaphyseal cupping and phalangeal metaphyseal widening in a patient with achondroplasia. In this patient, there is also flaring of the distal ulnar metaphysis

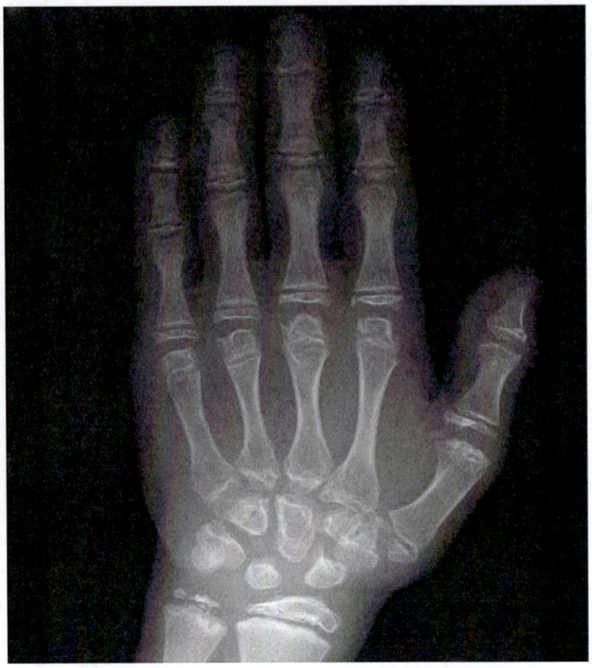

Fig. 54 Small carpals with irregular contours, shortened metacarpals and dysplastic, irregular epiphyses throughout the hand, some of which appear fragmented in a patient with pseudoachondroplasia

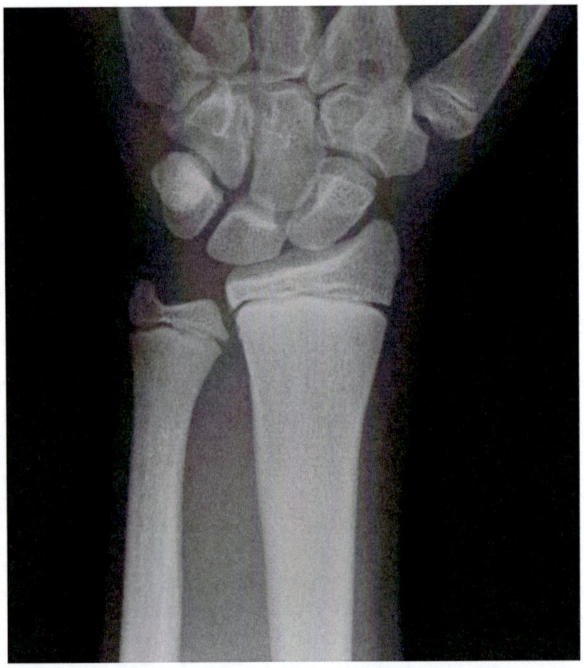

Fig. 53 Osteosclerosis of the bony skeleton and undertubulation of the distal radial diametaphysis in a patient with osteopetrosis

10.7 Sclerosing Bone Dysplasias

This can be divided into those conditions with increased bone density without alteration of bone shape (osteopetrosis and pyknodysostosis) and the craniotubular dysplasias (craniodiaphyseal dysplasia, craniometaphyseal dysplasia and Pyle dysplasia).

The long bones in osteopetrosis demonstrate metaphyseal expansion and osteosclerosis. There may be a "bone within a bone" appearance of the short tubular bones of the hand due to variation in disease activity (Lachman 2008) (Fig. 53).

Pyknodysostosis can be differentiated by the dysplastic or absent terminal phalanges, in combination with wide-open fontanelles and hypoplasia of the clavicles (Wynne-Davies et al. 1985).

10.8 Increased Limb Length

Marfans syndrome is a connective tissue disorder with autosomal dominant inheritance caused by mutations in the extracellular matrix protein fibrillin I. Typically, the

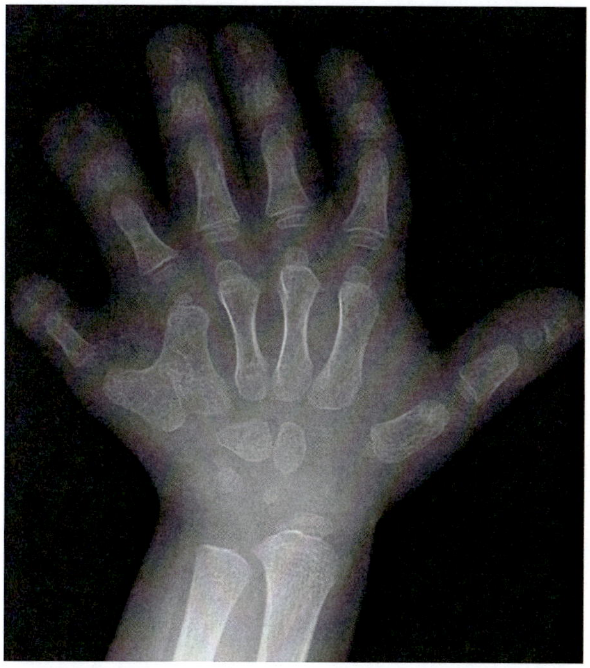

Fig. 55 Post-axial hexadactyly, middle and distal phalangeal hypoplasia, cone-shaped epiphyses of the middle phalanges, broadening of the hamate bone and early carpal coalition in a patient with Ellis van Crevald syndrome. The metacarpal of the duplicated digit is fused proximally to the metacarpal of the fifth finger. There is broadening of the fifth finger with duplicated distal phalanges articulating with a broadened middle phalanx

patient is tall with long, slender limbs and digits. Arachnodactyly can be determined by an abnormal metacarpal index above nine (sum of the lengths of the second to fifth metacarpals divided by the sum of the widths of the same bones) (McAlister et al. 2008) (Fig. 49).

11 Summary

While the classification of CHD presented is broadly and most commonly used in clinical practice it has many limitations, not least that some differences could comfortably be placed in several groups (e.g., Fig. 46a, b).

Radiology is vital for the assessment, treatment planning and follow up of all but the mildest cases of CHD, with plain films remaining the main imaging modality. Ultrasound and MRI are reserved for specific indications. Ultrasound can be extremely helpful in the assessment of tendons, and in the clarification of the nature of isolated swellings. MRI may provide additional information in selected cases, and is particularly important in the management of more complex overgrowth syndromes. Obstetric ultrasound now allows diagnosis of CHD earlier in fetal life, and advances in this modality will continue to raise the possibility of novel management opportunities and present new dilemmas.

Several CHD are associated with systemic syndromes and the reporting radiologist should be aware of these to highlight the need for further evaluation.

The management of CHD must be within a multidisciplinary environment with a team able to deal with all of the complex issues presented by this challenging group of patients.

References

Barsky AJ (1964) Cleft hand: classification, incidence and treatment. Review of the literature and report of nineteen cases. J Bone Joint Surg Am 46:1707–1720

Bayne LG, Klug MS (1987) Long term review of the surgical treatment of radial deficiencies. J Hand Surg (Am) 12:169–179

Benson LS, Kaplan EB (1994) Camptodactyly: classification and results of nonoperative treatment. J Pediatr Orthop 14(6):814–819

Blauth W (1967) Der hypoplastiche daumen. Arch Orthop Unfall Chir 62:225–246

Carty MJ, Taghinia A (2009) Overgrowth conditions: a diagnostic and therapeutic conundrum. Hand Clin 25:230

Cassart M (2010) Suspected fetal skeletal malformations or bone diseases: how to explore. Pediatr Radiol 40:1046–1051

Cassart M, Massez A, Cos T et al (2007) Contribution of three-dimensional computed tomography in the assessment of fetal skeletal dysplasia. Ultrasound Obstet Gynecol 29:537–543

De Smet L (2002) Classification for congenital anomalies of the hand: the IFSSH classification and the JSSH modification. Genet Couns 13(3):331–338

Dighe M, Fligner C, Cheung E et al (2008) Fetal skeletal dysplasia: an approach to diagnosis with illustrative cases. Radiographics 28:1061–1077

Ezaki M (1999) Angled digits. In: Green DP, Hotchkiss RN, Pederson WC (eds) Green's operative hand surgery, 4th edn. Churchill Livingstone, New York, pp 517–521

Flatt AE (1994) The care of congenital hand anomalies, 2nd edn. Quality Medical Publishing, St Louis, pp 99–117 pp228–248, pp366–410

Foulkes GD, Reinker K (1994) Congenital constriction band syndrome. A seventy year experience. J Pediatr Orthop 14(2):242–248

Frantz CH, O'Rahilly R (1961) Congenital limb deficiencies. J Bone Joint Surg Am 43:1202–1224

Giele H, Giele C, Bower C et al (2001) The incidence and epidemiology of congenital upper limb anomalies: a total population study. J Hand Surg Am 26(4):628–634

Goldfarb CA, Manske PR, Busa R et al (2005) Upper extremity phocomelia re-examined: a longitudinal dysplasia. J Bone Joint Surg Am 87(12):2639–2648

Hall JG (1997) Arthrogryposis multiplex congenital: etiology, genetics, classification, diagnostic approach and general aspects. J Pediatr Orthop B 6(3):159–166

Ireland DC, Takayama N, Flatt AE (1976) Poland's syndrome: a review of forty three cases. J Bone Joint Surg Am 58:52–58

James MA, McCarroll HR Jr, Manske PR (1999) The spectrum of radial longitudinal deficiency: a modified classification. J Hand Surg Am 24:1145–1155

James MA, Green HD, McCarroll HR Jr et al (2004) The association of radial deficiency with thumb hypoplasia. J Bone Joint Surg Am 86A(10):2196–2205

Jones GB (1964) Delta phalanx. J Bone Joint Surg Br 46:226–228

Kawamura K, Chung K (2009) Constriction band syndrome. Hand Clin 25:257–264

Koman LA, Toby EB, Poehling GG (1990) Congenital flexion deformities of the proximal interphalangeal joint in children: a subgroup of camptodactyly. J Hand Surg (Am) 15(4):582–586

Kozin SH (2001) Syndactyly. J Am Soc Surg Hand 1:1–13

Kozin SH (2003) Upper extremity congenital anomalies. J Bone Joint Surg 85A(8):1564–1576

Kozin SH (2004) Pediatric hand surgery. In: Beredjiklian PK, Bozentka DJ (eds) Review of hand surgery. Saunders, Philadelphia, pp 223–245

Lachman RS (2007) Taybi and lachman's radiology of syndromes, metabolic disorders and skeletal dysplasias, 5th edn. Mosby, St Louis

Lachman RS (2008) Skeletal dysplasias. In: Slovis TL (ed) Caffeys's paediatric diagnostic imaging, vol 2, 11th edn. Elsevier, Philadelphia, pp 2613–2670

Lourie GM, Lins RE (1998) Radial longitudinal deficiency. A review and update. Hand Clin 14:85–99

McAlister WH, Herman T, Kronemer KA (2008) Selected syndromes and chromosomal disorders. In: Thomas SL (ed) Caffeys's paediatric diagnostic imaging, vol 2, 11th edn. Mosby, Elsevier, pp 2687–2688

McCarroll HR (2000) Congenital anomalies: a 25 year overview. J Hand Surg (Am) 25(6):1007–1037

Mennen U, Van Heest A, Ezaki M et al (2005) Arthrogryposis multiplex congenital. J Hand Surg (Br) 30(5):468–474

Miller JK, Wenner SM, Kruger LM (1986) Ulnar deficiency. J Hand Surg Am 11(6):822–829

Miura T, Suzuki M (1984) Clinical differences between typical and atypical cleft hand. J Hand Surg (Br) 9:311–315

Netscher DT, Baumholtz MA (2007) Treatment of congenital upper extremity problems. Plast Reconstr Surg 119(5):101e–129e

Ogino T (1990a) Cleft hand. Hand Clin 6:661–671

Ogino T (1990b) Teratogenic relationship between polydactyly, syndactyly and cleft hand. J Hand Surg (Br) 15:201–209

Ploeckinger-Ulm B, Ulm MR, Lee A, Kratochwil A, Bernaschek G (1996) Antenatal depiction of fetal diagnosis with three-dimensional ultrasonography. Am J Obstet Gynaecol 175:571–574

Ress AM, Graham TJ (1998) Finger polydactyly. Hand Clin 14(1):49–64

Rypens F, Dubois J, Garel L, Fournet JC, Michaud JL, Grignon A (2006) Obstetric ultrasound: watch the fetal hands. Radiographics 26(3):811–829

Sapp JC, Turner JT, van de Kamp JM et al (2007) Newly delineated syndrome of congenital lipomatous overgrowth, vascular malformations and epidermal naevi (CLOVE syndrome) in seven patients. Am J Med Genet 143A:2944–2958

Schmidt CC, Neufield SK (1988) Ulnar ray deficiency. Hand Clin 14:65–76

Sells JM, Jaffer KM, Hall JG (1996) Amyoplasia, the most common type of arthrogryposis: the potential good outcome. Pediatrics 97(2):225–231

Sheldon W (1932) Amyoplasia congenital. Arch Dis Child 7:117–136

Smith RJ, Kaplan EB (1968) Camptodactyly and similar atraumatic flexion deformities of the proximal interphalangeal joints of the fingers: a study of thirty one cases. J Bone Joint Surg Am 50(6):1187–1203

Spranger JW, Brill PW, Poznanski A (2002) Bone dysplasias: an atlas of genetic disorders of skeletal development, 2nd edn. Oxford University Press Inc, NY

Swanson AB (1976) A classification for congenital limb malformations. J Hand Surg (Am) 1(1):8–22

Swanson AB, Swanson GD, Tada K (1983) A classification for congenital limb malformation. J Hand Surg (Am) 8:693–702

Tada K, Kurisaki E, Yonenobu K et al (1982) Central polydactyly- a review of 12 cases and their surgical treatment. J Hand Surg (Am) 7(5):460–465

Torpin R (1965) Amniochorionic mesoblastic fibrous strings and amniotic bands: associated constricting fetal malformations or fetal death. Am J Obstet Gynecol 91:61–75

Tretter AE, Saunders RC, Meyers CM, Dungan JS, Grumbach K, Sun C-CJ, Campbell AB, Wulfsberg EA (1998) Antenatal diagnosis of skeletal dysplasias. Am J Med Genet 75:518–522

Ty J, James M (2009) Failure of differentiation:part II (arthrogryposis, camptodactyly, clinodactyly, madelung deformity, trigger finger and trigger thumb). Hand Clin 25(2):200

Van Heest AE (1996) Congenital disorders of the hand and upper extremity. Paediatr Clin North Am 43(5):1113–1133

Watson BT, Hennrikus WL (1997) Postaxial type B polydactyly. Prevalence and treatment. J Bone Joint Surg Am 79:65–68

Watt AJ, Chung KC (2009) Duplication. Hand Clin 25(2):215–227

Wiedrich TA (1998) Congenital constriction band syndrome. Hand Clin 14:29–38

Wynne-Davies R, Hall CM, Graham AA (1985) Atlas of skeletal dysplasias. Churchill Livingstone, pp 454–464

Hand Trauma

Anand Kirwadi, Nikhil A. Kotnis, and Andrew Dunn

Contents

A. Kirwadi (✉) · N. A. Kotnis
Department of Radiology, Northern General Hospital, Sheffield Teaching Hospitals NHS Foundation Trust, Herries Road, Sheffield, S5 7AU, UK
e-mail: anandkirwadi@doctors.org.uk

A. Dunn
Department of Radiology, Royal Liverpool University Hospitals NHS trust, Prescot Street, Liverpool, L7 8XP, UK

Abstract

Hand injuries account for a large proportion of all injuries presenting to emergency departments. Avulsion injuries of the FDP tendons are a common sporting injury. Bowstringing of the flexor tendons are an important imaging sign of multiple annular pulley injuries. Mallet finger is the most common closed tendon injury in a sportsman. Rupture of the volar plate is a common complication of hyperextension injury. Imaging plays a crucial role in management of collateral ligament injuries. The extensor mechanism of the fingers is extremely intricate. Understanding relevant anatomy is quintessential for diagnosing and treating extensor mechanism injuries. Intra-articular metacarpal base fractures are commonly missed on initial presentation and pronated oblique radiographs help demonstrate the severity of this injury. Imaging evaluation of sports-related injuries of the hand should begin with radiographs. Ultrasound and magnetic resonance imaging play a vital role in diagnoses of soft tissue injuries. CT may be useful in understanding complex bony injuries.

1 Introduction

Traumatic hand injuries account for a large proportion of the workload of all emergency departments. Of a study of 50,272 patients, Angermann and Lohmann found that hand and wrist injuries made up 28.6 % of all injuries (Angermann and Lohmann 1993). Of these, 87 % involved the hand. Hill et al. found that the majority of isolated cases of hand and wrist

A. M. Davis et al. (eds.), *Imaging of the Hand and Wrist*, Medical Radiology. Diagnostic Imaging,
DOI: 10.1007/174_2012_768,

injuries arise from either a fall or sports-related injury (Hill et al. 1998).

In this chapter, we describe the most common traumatic soft tissue and bone injuries to the hand. We pay attention to the anatomy and mechanism of injury as this is fundamental to understanding and recognising patterns of injury on imaging. We also briefly mention some of the key management options that are important to be aware of whilst assessing the imaging of these injuries.

2 Volar Soft Tissue Injuries

2.1 Flexor Tendons

First described by Von Zander in 1891, avulsion injuries of the flexor tendon are common injuries in athletes. However, flexor tendon injuries are not as common as injuries to the extensor apparatus (Clavero et al. 2002).

The flexor mechanism of the digits comprises two tendons: the flexor digitorum superficialis (FDS) that inserts on the midportion of the middle phalanx, and the flexor digitorum profundus (FDP) which inserts on the volar aspect of the base of the distal phalanx. At the metacarpal head, the FDS splits and passes round the FDP tendon forming a ring aperture through which the FDP passes to become the more superficial tendon at the level of the proximal phalanx shaft (Clavero et al. 2002). These tendons run underneath the annular (A1–A5) and cruciform (C1–C3) pulleys lined by a synovial sheath that provides lubrication and nutrition. The vincula, which also provide blood supply to the tendons, connect the tendon to the synovial sheath (Hunter 1984).

Based on the mechanism of injury, these can be classified as open or closed injuries. For further discussion, we will concentrate on closed injuries. Open injuries are commonly due to lacerations. Closed injuries commonly occur when the finger is forcibly extended during maximum contraction of the profundus muscle—when a player is attempting to make a tackle and the ring finger slips off of the opposing player's shorts or jersey, hence the name "Jersey finger"(Aronovitz and Leddy 1998). Although it can occur in any finger, the ring finger is the most commonly involved finger accounting for 75 % cases (Hong 2005). McMaster in 1933 showed that the tendon was the strongest link in the musculotendinous chain and that rupture most commonly occurs at the bony insertion (McMaster 1933). When the tendon ruptures from its insertion, it may or may not avulse a bone fragment of variable size.

The most reliable finding is a complete loss of active flexion at the Distal Interphalangeal (DIP) joint (Buscemi and Page 1987). Because pain and swelling often mask the inability to flex the DIP joint (DIPJ), it is not uncommon for this injury to be missed initially and go untreated (Aronovitz and Leddy 1998).

Treatment and prognosis are influenced by several of the following factors: the level to which the tendon retracts, the remaining blood supply to the tendon, the length of time between injury and treatment and the presence and size of a bony avulsion fragment (Aronovitz and Leddy 1998). Based on the level of retraction and presence of bony fragment, Leddy and Packer have classified this injury into three main types (Table 1).

Buscemi et al., after describing four cases of FDP tendon injuries have suggested that avulsion of the FDP tendon with a separate intra-articular fracture of the base of the distal phalanx should be classified as a Type IV injury in the Leddy and Packer classification (Buscemi and Page 1987).

Radiographs may show an avulsed bone fragment from the distal phalanx. Severe comminution of the distal phalanx precludes accurate restoration of the articular surface and is important to note as it is a contra-indication to early FDP re-insertion (Jebson 1998).

At ultrasound, normal tendons are echogenic in the hand and wrist compared to muscle. They also show a typical fibrillar echotexture, which reflects their histological structure of longitudinally oriented bundles of collagen fibres (Jeyapalan et al. 2008). In cases of tendon rupture, discontinuity with a gap in the flexor tendon may be seen. The gap may be filled with disorganised, echogenic fibrinous material (Jeyapalan et al. 2008). In the presence of tendon rupture, discontinuity of the flexor tendon is seen with the gap at the rupture site (Figs. 1 and 2). In some patients, the tendon remains in continuity but is attenuated with subtle loss of fibrillar pattern due to partial division. These tendons may show less excursion than tendons in the neighbouring fingers on dynamic ultrasound assessment (Jeyapalan et al. 2008).

Table 1 Leddy and Packer classification of closed FDP injuries (Leddy and Packer 1977)

Type I	Retraction of the tendon into the palm with disruption of the vincular system resulting in loss of blood supply to the tendon
Type II	Most common type. Tendon retracts to the level of PIP joint, being held by the intact long vinculum preserving some blood supply
Type III	Large bony fragment that gets held in place by the A4 pulley
Type IV (Buscemi and Page 1987)	Tendon rupture with attached bony fragment and concomitant separate intra-articular fracture fragment

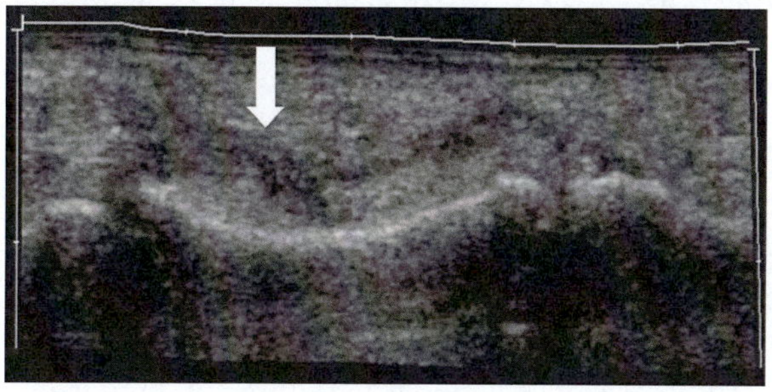

Fig. 1 Ultrasound of the finger using a linear probe in longitudinal plane showing empty FDP tendon sheath (*arrow*). DIPJ and PIPJ are on the *left* and *right* side of the image, respectively

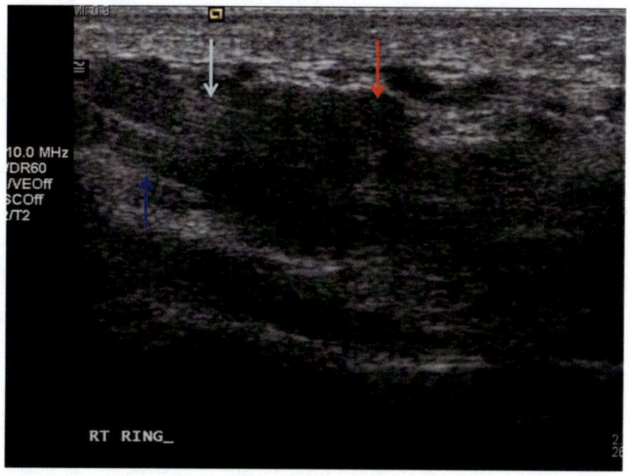

Fig. 2 Ultrasound of the ring finger using (different patient to Fig. 1) a high-frequency linear probe showing FDS rupture (*Red arrow* – at torn end), FDS (*Green arrow*) lying superficial to the FDS (*Blue arrow*)

On all magnetic resonance (MR) sequences, the flexor tendons appear as low-signal-intensity structures. In general, T1-W images provide good anatomical detail, while T2-W images are useful in assessment of inflammatory change that is associated with most pathological conditions (Clavero et al. 2002). Magnetic resonance imaging provides a non-invasive method to identify the site of tear, the degree of retraction of the torn fibres and other associated soft tissue injuries (Peterson and Bancroft 2006). In the presence of trauma, the associated oedema, haematoma and fibrosis compromise the tendon image quality and a tendon rupture is unlikely to be identified (Beltran et al. 1987).

Based on the current literature review, there is a general consensus that prompt reinsertion of an acute FDP avulsion injury is the preferred choice of treatment. In chronic injuries, the patient may be asymptomatic as they adapt by passively assisting DIPJ flexion, and do not require any further treatment (Aronovitz and Leddy 1998; Jebson 1998). If there is instability of the DIPJ with weakness of pinch or recurrent dorsal dislocations, joint arthrodesis or tenodesis should be considered (Aronovitz and Leddy 1998).

2.2 Annular Pulleys

Normal finger flexion is a complex fine motor action that requires the integrity and orchestration of a number of delicate structures that are centred around the flexor tendon system (Hauger et al. 2000). The flexor tendon sheath pulley system is of paramount biomechanical importance in flexion, not only for accurate tracking of the tendon but also to maintain the apposition of tendon and bone across the joint and provide a fulcrum to elicit flexion and extension (Lin et al. 1989). Doyle and Blythe in 1975 originally defined a pulley system of four annular and three cruciate pulleys. In 1981, Kleinhert and Broudy defined an additional fifth pulley arising distal to the fourth annular pulley.

In recent years, the number of people involved in climbing sports has increased exponentially as a result of easy and readily available access to artificial rock-climbing walls and indoor rock climbing facilities. The annular pulley injuries are caused by climbing techniques where the entire body weight is placed on one or two fingerholds, especially in overhung wall climbs. These techniques place high forces on the proximal interphalangeal (PIP) joint and the digital pulley system, resulting in finger injuries known as climber's finger (Klauser et al. 1999). The ring and middle fingers are most commonly affected, as they are most often used in climbing and are diagnosed in up to 30 % of climbers with finger injuries (Le Viet et al. 1996). Injury to the pulley system can result in loss of strength and decreased range of motion within the affected finger, bowstringing of the FDP tendon and fixed flexion contracture of the PIP joint (PIPJ). Pain and soft tissue swelling can make clinical evaluation a difficult and limited exercise. Many studies have claimed that bowstringing of the FDP tendon across the PIPJ with resisted flexion of the fingertips is diagnostic of A2 pulley rupture. However, in a laboratory study of 21 cadaveric fingers by Marco et al. (1998), isolated or even combined rupture of A2 and A4 pulley did not result in detectable bowstringing. Rupture of at least three pulleys was required to produce obvious bowstringing in this study. Early recognition of the injury and appropriate treatment are important in avoiding complications like fixed flexion contractures (Bollen 1990).

The A2 and A4 annular pulleys, located at the proximal third of the proximal phalanx and middle phalanges, respectively, are the broader and the most functionally important annular pulleys (Lin et al. 1989). Experimental studies performed by Marco et al. (1998) showed that the A4 pulley is predisposed to rupture first when the hand is in the crimp grip. The A2 pulley usually fails from its distal to its proximal edge, whereas the A4 pulley tears from its proximal to its distal edge (Marco et al. 1998). It is important to accurately differentiate the complete from incomplete tears, as decision for operative versus non-operative management depends on this vital finding.

Various studies have been published advocating the use of ultrasound (Klauser et al. 1999, 2002; Martinoli et al. 2000; Hauger et al. 2000); computed topography (CT) (Le Viet et al. 1996) and MR (Hauger et al. 2000, Klauser et al. 2002). An inability to directly delineate the pulleys along with the exposure to ionising radiation and relatively higher cost in comparison to ultrasound, make CT an unsuitable modality for diagnosing pulley injuries.

The magnetic resonance imaging (MRI) criteria for identifying pulley injuries include direct signs such as disrupted A2 and A4 pulleys (Hauger et al. 2000) or indirect signs like bowstringing (appreciated as increased tendon–phalangeal (TP) distance) or fluid in between the phalanx and tendon (Gabl et al. 1998). The MR has been the most accurate modality for imaging in the diagnosis of A4 lesions (Hauger et al. 2000). However, the expense, length of the examination and lack of real-time assessment are some of the drawbacks of MR examination.

Dynamic assessment gives ultrasound an advantage in the evaluation of pulley injuries. Ultrasound can demonstrate visualisation of fluid between the tendon and phalanx and allows assessment of the gliding ability of the tendons. Ultrasound demonstrated a sensitivity of 98 %, specificity of 100 %, a positive predictive value of 100 % and a negative predictive value of 97 % for the detection of finger pulley injuries (Klauser et al. 2002). Martinoli et al. (2000) demonstrated that examination in the longitudinal plane alone was sufficient as transverse sonograms added no significant information. Hauger et al. (2000) has suggested using TP distance measurements following a study performed using a cadaveric model (see Figs. 3a, b and c). A TP distance of greater than 1.0 mm was indicative of pulley system injury. An increase of the TP distance with forced flexion less than 3.0 mm was considered a sign of incomplete A2 pulley rupture, while a distance greater than 3.0 mm was considered a sign of complete rupture. Further increase in the TP distance to more than 5.0 mm was used as a sign for complete combined rupture of A2 and A3 pulley. An increase of TP distance equal to or greater than 2.5 mm was used as a sign for complete rupture of A4 pulley. Maximal active forced flexion during dynamic ultrasound examination is the most important factor for assessment of TP distance and detection of finger pulley injuries (Klauser et al. 2002).

Indications for non-operative or operative treatment are based on the clinical finding of bowstringing, functional disability, persistent pain, failure of

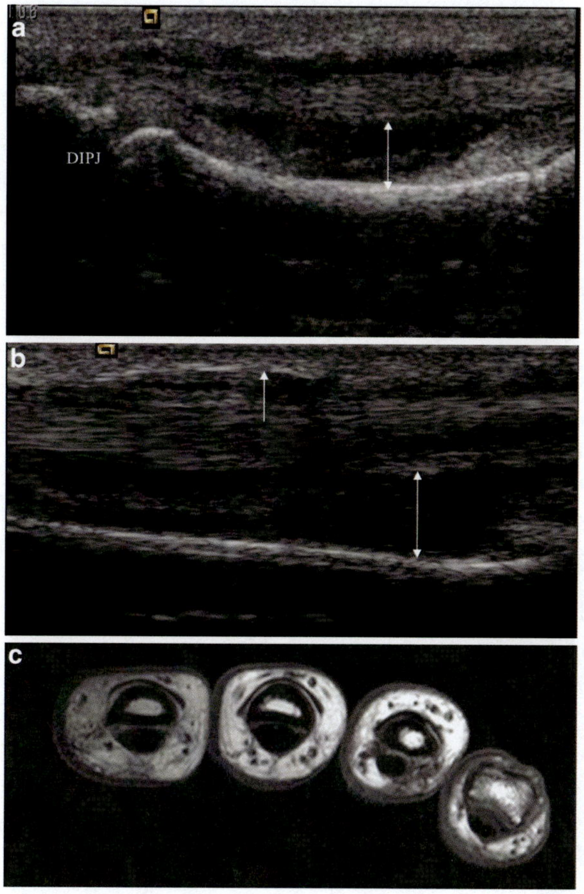

Fig. 3 **a**, **b** Both images taken in the same patient show increased tendo-phalangeal distance (*double arrow heads*) over the middle and proximal phalanges respectively, indicating rupture of the A2 and A4 pulleys. *Arrow* in **b** shows the ruptured A2 pulley. **c** Axial MR image shows increased tendo-phalangeal distance (*double arrow heads*) due to chronic rupture of the A2 pulley

non-operative treatment and on the amount of bowstringing of the involved flexor tendons (Gabl et al. 1998). Incomplete tears are normally treated conservatively, while complete tears are treated surgically. The treatment of complete tears with surgery has been controversial. In a study conducted by Gabl et al. (1998), complete ruptures were treated with surgery after non-operative treatment had failed. In the same study, functional outcome after non-operative and operative therapy was equal. Diagnosis and treatment at an early stage will prevent the progression of lesions and decrease the risk of long-term complications that are associated with fixed finger contracture (Hauger et al. 2000).

2.3 Volar Plate

Volar plate (VP) injury results as a consequence of hyperextension injury to the PIPJ. There may or may not be an associated intra-articular fracture (Yoong et al. 2010). Even when present, the fracture can be easily overlooked resulting in significant instability of the PIPJ (Nance Jr et al. 1979).

The VP is a multi-layered condensation of dense fibrocartilaginous tissue that lies between the flexor tendons and the PIPJ capsule. The VP attaches firmly only at the critical corner of the middle phalanx base, without strong insertion centrally. Proximally, the VP blends directly with the periosteum rather than direct insertion into the bone (Williams et al. 1998). Its important functions at the PIPJ level include providing stability against hyperextension, acting as a meniscus at the PIPJ, forming part of the intracavitary lining of the PIPJ and providing a smooth gliding surface for the flexor tendon (Williams et al. 1998).

The most common mechanism of injury is forced or sudden hyperextension at the PIPJ (Phair et al. 1989). The diagnosis of VP injury is usually made clinically, with tenderness over the volar aspect of the PIPJ, pain on passive hyperextension and instability with loss of pinch power (Nance Jr et al. 1979). The commonly used classifications are shown in Tables 2 and 3 below.

Along with AP and lateral views of the involved PIPJ, oblique views can also be helpful. In a study of 58 cases conducted by Nance Jr et al., 65 % of the fractures were best seen on the lateral view, while most of the others were best appreciated on the oblique projection (Nance Jr et al. 1979). Subtle dorsal subluxation can be identified by observing a V-shaped gap between the articular surfaces of the PIP joint—'V' sign. On ultrasound examination, the VP is seen as a wedge-shaped structure of intermediate echogenicity interposed between the flexor tendon and underlying PIPJ (Yoong et al. 2010). The complex three-layered collagen fibres running in different orientations (Williams et al. 1998) probably account for its mixed echogenic appearance on ultrasound. The VP is best seen in the sagittal plane and is of low signal on all MRI sequences (Fig. 4) (Yoong et al. 2010). To the best of our knowledge, there are currently no studies comparing the efficacy of ultrasound or MRI for diagnosing VP injuries.

Table 2 Eaton classification of VP injuries (Eaton 1971)

Type 1	No fracture or dislocation
Type 2	Dorsal dislocation without fracture
Type 3 stable	Fracture–dislocation with <40 % PIP joint surface
Type 3 unstable	Fracture–dislocation with >40 % PIP joint surface

Table 3 Stability-based classification (Keifhaber and Stern 1998)

Stable	<30 % articular surface
Tenuous	30–50 % articular surface
Unstable	>50 % articular surface

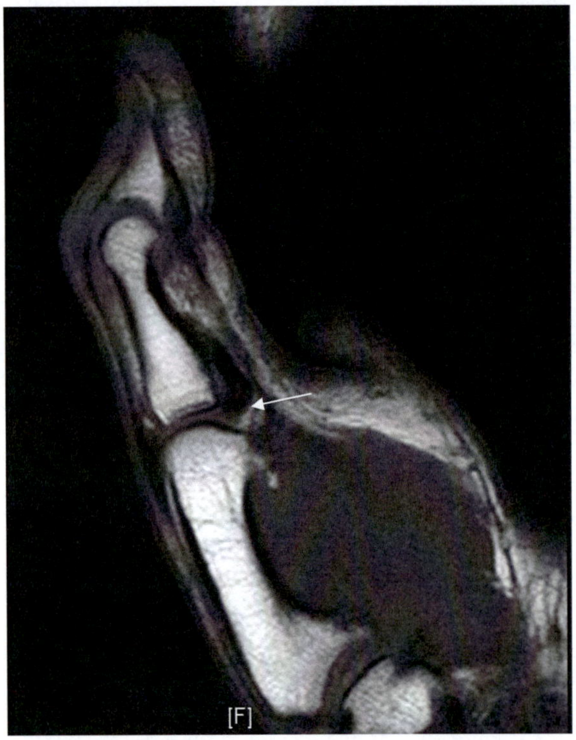

Fig. 4 Sagittal T1 W MR image of the thumb showing chronic type 1 volar plate injury (*White arrow*)

There is a consensus that the stable injuries involving less than 30 % of articular surface are treated conservatively either by splinting with extension-block or neighbour strapping. Various studies (Phair et al. 1989; Gaine et al. 1998) have shown favourable results with early active and passive mobilisation rather than splinting. Unstable injuries involving >50 % of articular surface are treated surgically with open reduction and internal fixation using various techniques or palmar plate arthroplasty, with later being preferred (Keifhaber and Stern 1998). The tenuous fractures involving 30–50 % of articular surface can be treated conservatively, if the articular surface congruity can be maintained with 30° flexion; if not they are best managed operatively (Keifhaber and Stern 1998).

3 Extensor Mechanism Injuries

3.1 Anatomy

The anatomy and function of the extensor mechanism of the hand comprise of a complex set of interlinked muscles, tendons and ligaments that are intricately coordinated to bring about the fine movements of the digits. The extensor mechanism of the hand can be divided into eight zones to aide in the evaluation and treatment of acute injuries (Kleinhert and Verdan 1983). The even-numbered zones are over bones, with the odd-numbered zones over the joints. Owing to the lesser number of the phalanges in the thumb, the numbering system is slightly different.

The extrinsic and intrinsic muscles of the hand make up the extensor mechanism. Zone VIII, containing the musculotendinous junctions of the extrinsic muscles is the most proximal zone. In zone VII, the extensor tendons are contained within the extensor retinaculum over the wrist joint. In zone VI, the tendons of the middle, ring and little finger are connected by juncturae tendinum. These interconnections must be considered when evaluating extensor tendon injuries (Newport 1997). In zone V, the extensor tendons are located centrally and are stabilised over the dorsum of the metacarpal head by the extensor hood. The sagittal bands (SB) are the main components of the extensor hood, which starts at the VP and has a dorsal tendinous point of insertion, gliding with the extensor system as the digit moves (Clavero et al. 2002). Distal to metacarpophalangeal (MCP) joint, the extensor mechanism becomes more complicated as the extrinsic and intrinsic muscles blend into the dorsal apparatus. The extrinsic extensor tendons divide into central and lateral slips with the central slip inserting into the dorsal aspect of the base of middle phalanx. The intrinsic muscles contribute to form the lateral slips to form conjoint tendons, which converge distally to form the terminal tendon that inserts on the base of the distal phalanx (Kleinhert and Verdan 1983). The intrinsic tendons are directed volar to the axis of MCP joint (MCPJ), flexing this joint and directing dorsal to the axis of PIPJ and DIPJs, extending these joints (Newport 1997).

On MR images, the normal extensor apparatus appear as low-signal structures at the expected locations, axial and sagittal planes being most useful (Clavero et al. 2002).

3.2 Mallet Injury (Zone 1)

Disruption of the terminal extensor tendon at the DIPJ, caused by sudden forced flexion of the extended finger results in extension lag deformity at the DIPJ called mallet finger. Other terms like ‘baseball finger’ and ‘drop finger’ have been used to describe this. This terminal extensor tendon can rupture at or near its insertion into the distal phalanx (soft tissue mallet injury) or can avulse a bony fragment from the base of distal phalanx (bony mallet injury) (Handoll and Vaghela 2004). As a result of this injury, the DIPJ cannot be actively extended. A mallet finger may be open, but is more often a closed injury (Rockwell et al. 2000). It is the most common closed tendon injury in sports persons (Posner 1977) and can occur either after a direct blow to the DIPJ or a relatively minor trauma to the fingertip. The middle finger is most often involved, followed by the little finger (Stark et al. 1962). Doyle has classified this injury into four types as follows (Table 4).

Table 4 Doyle classification of mallet injuries (Doyle 1999)

Type 1	Closed or blunt trauma, with or without avulsion fracture (most commonest type)
Type 2	Rupture of the tendon near or at the DIP joint
Type 3	Open, with deep abrasion of the tissues
Type 4	Trans-epiphyseal fracture in children, fractures involving a large part of the joint surface

The patient may present with swelling and bruising over the DIPJ. This being a rarely painful condition, patients frequently seek help late in the course of the event (Perron et al. 2001). Also, the extensor lag at the DIPJ may not appear for several days. Patients rarely complain of functional disability because there are relatively few activities which require full digital extension (Brzezienski and Schneider 1995). On clinical examination, apart from the fixed flexion deformity, the patient will be unable to actively extend the DIPJ. However, the deformity is correctable by passive extension.

Plain radiographs are routinely performed to exclude bony involvement (Fig. 5). Ultrasound may demonstrate: discontinuity of the extensor tendon with partial or complete tear; avulsion fracture; no real-time movements of the extensor tendon; and fluid in the region of the extensor tendon insertion (Kleinbaum et al. 2005). These findings can be used to differentiate traumatic mallet finger from others caused by fixed flexion deformity. In cases with no bone avulsion on plain film, sagittal MR images can be used to assess for terminal extensor tendon injuries and thus can be used to decide treatment (Clavero et al. 2002; Tabbal et al. 2009).

The most common type of mallet injury, closed type 1 injuries are generally managed conservatively with hyperextension splint for around 6–8 weeks. This is followed by further 4 weeks of splinting at night. Surgical treatment is usually reserved for open injuries, DIPJ instability/subluxation or a large (>30 %) displaced articular fracture fragment. A cadaveric study conducted by Hussain et al. concluded that palmar subluxation of a DIPJ without preexisting arthritic deformity is expected when more than one half of the dorsal articular surface is injured (Hussain et al. 2008).

3.3 Boutonniere Deformity (Zone III Injury)

A boutonniere deformity occurs as a result of an injury to the central slip at or near its insertion at the base of the middle phalanx. The term *boutonniere* is derived from the French for ‘buttonhole’, as the head of the proximal phalanx can pass through the defect in the extensor mechanism (Aronowitz and Leddy 1998). Most of these are caused by an unrecognised volar lateral dislocation of the PIPJ or less commonly by a blow to the dorsal aspect of the middle phalanx that forces the PIPJ into flexion while the finger is being actively extended (Aronowitz and Leddy 1998; Perron et al. 2001). This injury can either be open or

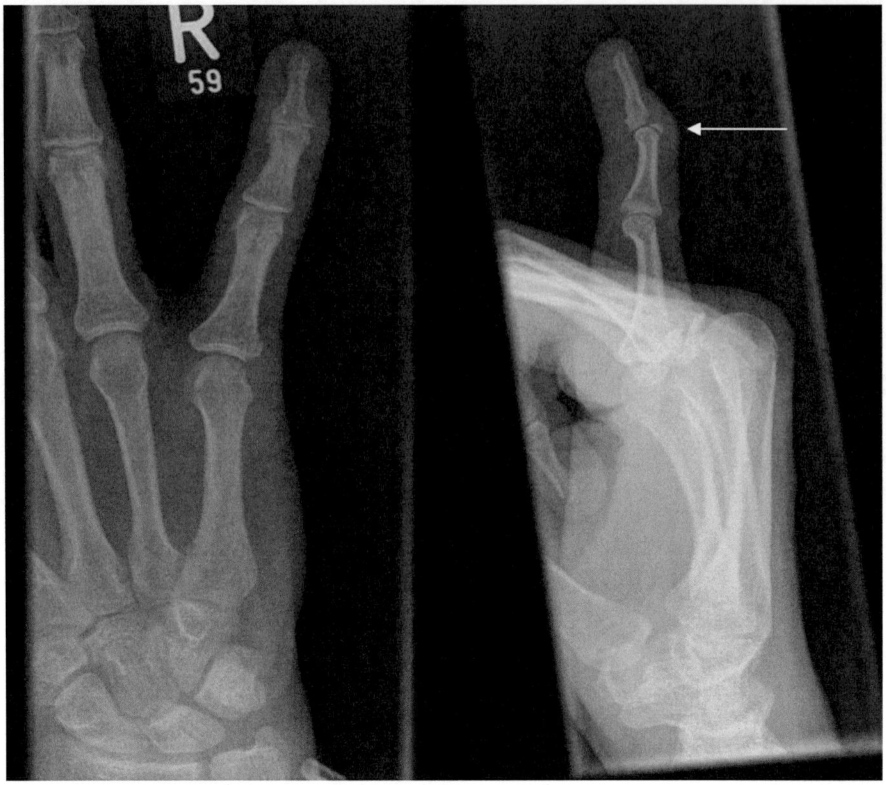

Fig. 5 AP and Lateral radiographs of right little finger. Lateral radiograph demonstrates avulsion fracture (*white arrow*) at the site of extensor tendon insertion into the base of the terminal phalanx, usually seen in closed traumatic extensor tendon disruption with avulsion fracture (type 1)

closed, and the central slip may avulse with or without a bony fragment.

The patient usually presents with pain and swelling with maximal tenderness at the PIPJ. The classic boutonniere deformity is rarely seen in the acute phase (Aronowitz and Leddy 1998). In the early acute phase, active extension is retained by the normally orientated lateral slips; but the head of the proximal phalanx eventually goes through the central slip resulting in migration of the lateral slips palmar to the PIPJ, which flexes the PIPJ and hyperextends the DIPJ resulting in the classic boutonniere deformity (Griffin et al. 2012). The above described deformity usually occurs 1–2 weeks after the initial injury (Hart et al. 1993).

Burton has described three stages of the boutonniere deformity (Table 5).

The Elson test, which demonstrates rigidity of the DIPJ during attempted PIP extension from a flexed position, has been shown to reliably diagnose an early central slip injury. However, the drawbacks of this test are it will not demonstrate partial rupture of the central slip and may be impeded by pain (Elson 1986). Initially, plain radiographs are obtained to evaluate for an avulsion fracture at the base of the middle phalanx (Fig. 6). In equivocal cases, where clinical evaluation is difficult owing to pain and swelling, MRI can be an effective method for detecting central slip lesions (Clavero et al. 2002). Magnetic resonance imaging can also provide valuable information about associated VP and ligamentous lesions of the PIPJ. To the best of our knowledge, there are no current studies available comparing the efficiency of clinical examination, ultrasound or MRI in diagnosing the central slip injuries.

Treatment of central slip injuries remains highly controversial. Generally these are treated closed with extension splinting of the PIPJs for 4–6 weeks followed by 2 weeks of night time splinting (Aronowitz and Leddy 1998). Surgical treatment is implemented when (1) displaced avulsion fracture, (2) axial and lateral instability of the PIPJ associated with loss of active or passive extension of the joint and (3) failed conservative treatment (Griffin et al. 2012). However, surgical reconstruction is the treatment of choice for a chronic symptomatic boutonniere deformity (Aronowitz and Leddy 1998).

Table 5 Stages of the boutonniere deformity (Burton 1982)

Stage 1	Dynamic imbalance, fully correctable passively
Stage 2	Extensor mechanism contracture, not passively correctable but does not involve the joint structure
Stage 3	Fixed contracture with joint changes involving collateral ligament, volar plate scarring and intra-articular adhesions

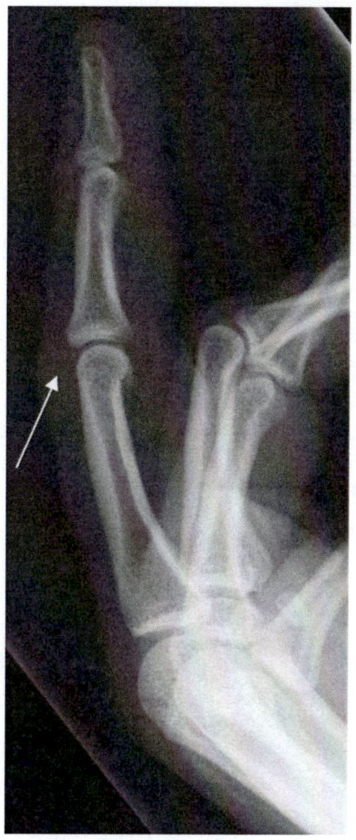

Fig. 6 Lateral radiograph showing a subtle avulsion fracture (*white arrow*) with associated soft tissue swelling at the base of the left middle finger intermediate phalanx

It is important to differentiate between a boutonniere and a pseudo-boutonniere deformity so that appropriate treatment plan can be implemented. Although, the appearances may be similar their aetiology is different. The pseudo-boutonniere deformity results from a PIPJ VP injury due to PIPJ hyperextension and resulting in PIPJ flexion contracture, rather than an injury to the central slip (Hong 2005). Typically, the flexion contracture of the PIPJ is fixed, and passive extension is not possible (Aronowitz and Leddy 1998). In a pseudo-boutonniere deformity, radiographs may slow calcification along the volar lateral aspect of the proximal phalanx. These injuries are managed conservatively by dynamic splinting, if the flexion contracture is less than 45° and surgical release may be needed to restore extension if the PIP flexion contracture is more than 45° (Aronowitz and Leddy 1998).

3.4 Boxer's Knuckle (Zone V Injury)

The extensor hood at the MCPJ is a retinacular system comprising the sagittal, oblique and transverse bands that stabilise the extensor tendon at the dorsal aspect of the MCPJ and keeps the tendon in place during flexion and extension. The SB is the most important structure of the extensor hood; this composes of a superficial and deep layer forming a tunnel through which the extensor tendon passes through (Kichouh et al. 2011). Sagittal band ruptures referred to as 'Boxer's Knuckle' can occur spontaneously, secondary to trauma or can be associated with synovial disorders like rheumatoid arthritis (Kichouh et al. 2011). Congenitally absent or lax SBs have been previously reported (Inoue and Tamura 1996). The most commonly injured finger is the middle finger, and the most frequently involved SB is the radial with ulnar instability (Rayan and Murray 1994). It has been thought that underlying normal ulnar inclination of the index and middle finger may predispose them to radial band disruption (Lopez-Ben et al. 2003). However, ruptures of the ulnar SB resulting in radial instability have also been reported in the literature. Patients commonly present with pain, swelling, loss of full extension and subluxation of the extensor tendon. Rayan and Murray classified SB injuries into three types as shown in Table 6.

However, the overlying soft tissue swelling and pain can make clinical assessment difficult to diagnose tendon subluxation (Lopez-Ben et al. 2003). As a result, accurate diagnosis of SB rupture may be difficult without imaging. Advantages of ultrasound over MRI include dynamic assessment, cost-effectiveness and easy availability.

Various studies have been published describing the use of ultrasound and MRI for diagnosing SB injuries. The SB is best seen in the axial plane with the MCP in slight flexion, appearing as a linear hypoechoic structure. Focal hyperechoic thickening of the SB or disappearance of the normal architecture of the SB can be demonstrated in patients with extensor hood injuries (Kichouh et al. 2011). Dynamic ultrasound

Table 6 Rayan and Murray classification of sagittal band injuries (Rayan and Murray 1994)

Type I	Mild injury with no instability
Type II	Moderate injury with extensor tendon subluxation
Type III	Severe injury with tendon dislocation

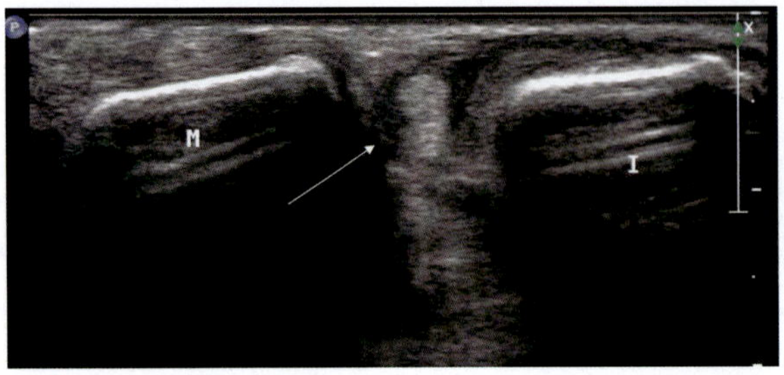

Fig. 7 Ultrasound image at MCPJ level shows subluxation of the index finger (I) extensor tendon (*white arrow*), secondary to extensor hood injury (not shown in this image)

with the fingers alternatively extended and then flexed in a clenched fist enables excellent visualisation of extensor tendon subluxation and dislocation at the MCPJ (Fig. 7) (Lopez-Ben et al. 2003).

On MRI, the SB is depicted as uniform low-signal intensity structure on all sequences. The T2W sequences are more accurate than T1W or post-contrast T1W sequences and post-contrast imaging does not improve the sensitivity in depicting the SB (Drape et al. 1994). The MR findings in acute injuries include morphologic and signal intensity changes, together with poor definition, focal discontinuity and focal thickening (Clavero et al. 2002). Magnetic resonance imaging of MCPJs in different kinematic positions has also been found useful in diagnosing SB injuries (Lopez-Ben et al. 2003). The role of oblique and transverse bands is not well known currently and these are also difficult to demonstrate on ultrasound and MRI (Kichouh et al. 2011).

Like other extensor mechanism injuries, the treatment of SB injuries also remains highly controversial. Ritts et al. advocate conservative treatment with splinting of the MCPJ in extension, while Hame and Melone Jr concluded that direct surgical repair with realignment of the central tendon is highly successful (Ritts et al. 1985; Hame and Melone Jr 2000). These will need to be treated as open infected injuries if the extensor mechanism or the SB injury is secondary to human bites with surgical debridement, intravenous antibiotics and splinting (Matzon and Bozentka 2010).

4 Collateral Ligament Injuries

4.1 Ulnar Collateral Ligament of the Thumb

The ulnar and radial collateral ligaments are primary stabilisers of the thumb MCPJ against radial and ulnar stress, respectively. Injury to these structures may result in joint instability, leading to significant disability and pain (Tang 2011). A correct early diagnosis influences management decisions and treatment outcomes (Sollerman et al. 1991). The thumb MCPJ is stabilised by static and dynamic stabilisers (Tsiouri et al. 2009). The static restraints include the VP, the dorsal capsule and the ulnar and radial collateral ligaments. The extrinsic and intrinsic muscles of the thumb make up the dynamic stabilisers. The ulnar collateral ligament (UCL) comprises a proper and an accessory ligament (Tsiouri et al. 2009). In flexion, the proper collateral ligament is taut, while the accessory collateral ligament is taut in extension.

Two acronyms are commonly used to describe UCL injuries, Gamekeeper's thumb and Skier's thumb. Gamekeeper's thumb was first reported by Campbell in 1955 to describe chronic attritional attenuation of the UCL in Scottish gamekeepers, secondary to strain induced on the first Web space (Campbell 1955). The Skier's thumb is used to describe acute injuries where the thumb is forced into abduction and hyperextension against the ski pole (Gerber et al. 1981). Thumb UCL injuries are the second most common skiing-related injury, after medial collateral ligament injury of the knee (Tsiouri et al. 2009).

Injury to the UCL is caused by sudden excessive valgus stress on the thumb MCPJ. Although this was attributed to the straps of the ski pole initially, later studies have showed that the incidence of the injury remained the same even with new pole designs without a strap (Derkash et al. 1987). In approximately 90 % of cases, the thumb UCL avulses from the base of the proximal phalanx (Coyle 2003). Although less frequent, it can avulse from proximal attachment or tear in the midsubstance. In 1962, Stener described a lesion in which the distal end of the avulsed UCL is displaced superficial to the adductor aponeurosis and is prevented from reapproximation to its anatomic insertion site (Stener 1962). Avulsion of UCL can be accompanied by more than one bony avulsion fragment with failure of the ligament bone complex at the site of the ligament–bone interface and also within the bone itself (Giele and Martin 2003).

Patients with acute injuries present with pain, swelling and reduced range of motion. Chronic presentations include deformity and loss of strength in particular pinching or grasping. On examination, tenderness to palpation will be present at the site of injury. A palpable mass on the medial side may represent the superficially displaced end of the UCL, suggestive of a Stener lesion. However, the absence of a palpable mass does not definitively rule out a Stener lesion (Heyman et al. 1993).

Evaluation of joint stability is the most important part of examination. The primary aim is to determine whether the injury is incomplete (Grade 1 or 2) or complete (Grade 3) (Tang 2011). Current consensus include testing the joint in zero degrees of extension and 30° flexion to evaluate accessory and proper collateral ligament components, respectively. Instability is defined as radial deviation of the proximal phalanx on the metacarpal head of >30–35° (Heyman et al. 1993). Stress examination demonstrating a firm end-point indicates an incomplete tear whilst opening of the MCPJ without a firm end-point indicates a complete tear (Patel et al. 2010).

Plain radiographs are routinely performed to rule out a fracture or subluxation (Fig. 8a). Previously, stress radiography, ultrasound and MR with or without arthrography have been used to assess thumb UCL injuries. In addition to the discrepancies concerning the performance and interpretation of stress radiographs, the most significant drawback is their inability to direct the treatment because they do not differentiate between a non-displaced tear and a Stener lesion (Green and Rowlan 1984). In a study conducted by Harper et al. comparing the efficacy of stress radiography versus MR examination with and without arthrography, the overall sensitivity of stress radiography was found to be only 64 % (Harper et al. 1996).

Ultrasound is useful in detecting partial and complete tears of the thumb UCL and has shown promising results in differentiating between complete tears and Stener lesions (Schnur et al. 2002). The normal thumb UCL appears as a hyperechoic structure spanning the ulnar side of the first MCPJ. Displaced UCL tears appear as a retracted, folded-on-itself structure which is displaced proximal and superficial to the adductor aponeurosis, creating the appearance of a 'yo–yo on a string' on coronal MRI scans (Ebrahim et al. 2006). The positive predictive value for ultrasound in identifying UCL tears is very high (87.5 % Schnur et al. and 94 % Jones et al.). However, the specificity varies between 83 % for displaced ruptures and 91 % for non-displaced ruptures (Hergan et al. 1995). Inexpensive and easy availability along with good overall comparable results with MR make ultrasound an attractive tool for evaluation of UCL tears. The primary disadvantage of ultrasound is that it is operator dependent. Ultrasound has been recommended to be used only in the 1st week after injury, as scarring may decrease accuracy of the method (Hergan et al. 1997).

Excellent soft tissue characterisation makes MR examination a very good modality to use in UCL injuries (Fig 8b). The sensitivity and specificity have been shown to be 100 % (Harper et al. 1996; Hergan et al. 1995). Thus, MR plays a vital role in making management plans for patients with UCL tears. Cost-effectiveness and availability remain the major deterrents for using MR as the primary modality in diagnosing UCL tears. Various pitfalls as described by Hergan et al. (1997) can cause misinterpretation between displaced and non-displaced UCL tears which can have serious implications on patient recovery. Hence, MR examination has been advocated when a non-displaced UCL tear is suspected by ultrasound (Hergan et al. 1997).

Conservative versus surgical management of UCL tears has been controversial and extensively debated over the last four to five decades. Grade 1 and 2 tears are managed conservatively. Surgery is indicated in the following instances: a Stener lesion is suspected; a displaced avulsion fracture exists, where there is an acute, grossly unstable joint; in symptomatic chronic injury; and in cases of volar subluxation seen on radiographs (Smith 1977). Surgical treatment has been widely accepted as treatment of choice for Grade 3 UCL tears.

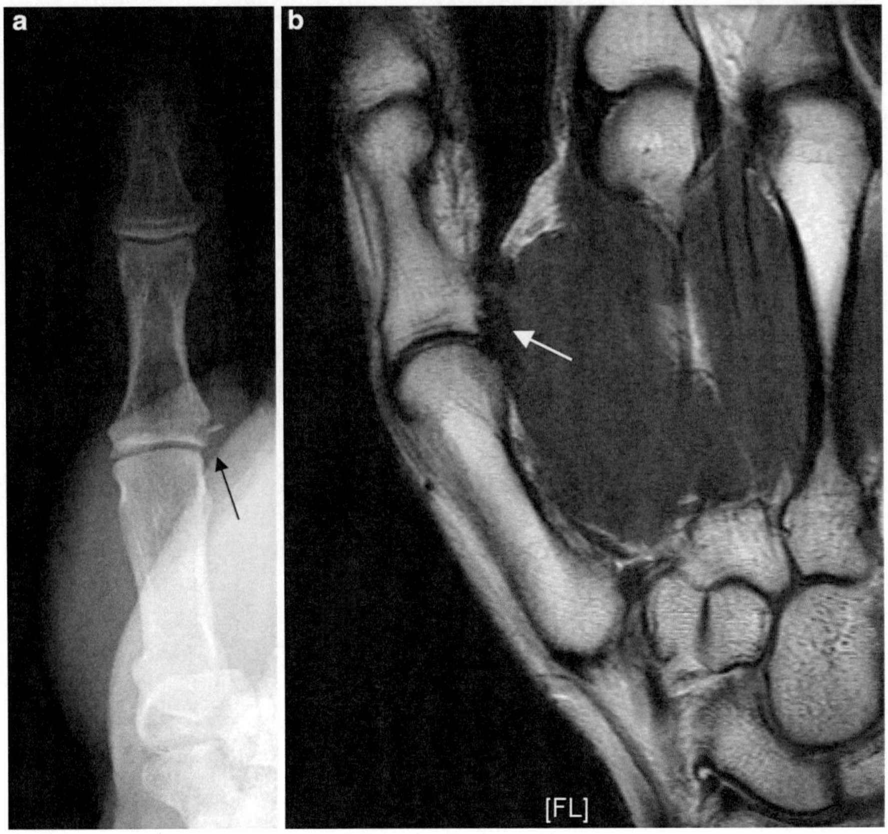

Fig. 8 **a, b** Plain radiograph AP view (**a**) and Coronal T1W MRI (**b**) showing bony avulsion fracture (*arrow*) at the site of UCL insertion

4.2 Radial Collateral Ligament

Injuries of radial collateral ligament (RCL) comprise 10–14 % of the collateral ligament injuries to the thumb MCPJ (Coyle Jr 2003). These have been referred to as "reverse gamekeeper's thumb" (Cooney et al. 1990).

The RCL originates dorsally on the lateral condyle of the metacarpal head and extends in a distal and palmar direction to insert into the lateral tubercle of the proximal phalanx. (Edelstein et al. 2008). Like UCL, the RCL also consists of proper and accessory collateral ligaments which act as static restraints when MCPJ is in flexion and extension, respectively.

Injuries of the RCL result from forced and sudden adduction of the MCPJ which can occur from a fall or during sports when a ball or player strikes the thumb. Acutely, the patient presents with pain, stiffness, swelling and deformity. In the chronic situation, once the swelling and pain has subsided, patients present with persistent pain with activities that require a radial-sided force such as closing a door (Edelstein et al. 2008).

It is important to identify partial from complete RCL tears as complete tears are treated surgically, while partial tears are treated conservatively. Radial stress test and drawer tests may be used to assess for RCL injury. A recent study by Coyle Jr found proximal tears (55 %) are commoner than distal (29 %) or midsubstance tears (16 %) (Coyle 2003). This can be explained by the fact that the distal width of the RCL insertion is equal to or wider than the RCL origin at the metacarpal (Lyons et al. 1998). Complete RCL tear can result in both static and dynamic instability (Edelstein et al. 2008). Although there are several classification systems for UCL injuries, there are no specific ones for the RCL injuries. A generalised classification is used instead. Grade 1: Small incomplete tear, Grade 2: larger but still incomplete tear and Grade 3: complete tear.

Conventional radiographs are obtained to assess for avulsion fractures and subluxation. Volar subluxation of the phalanx >3 mm is much more common with RCL injury than with the UCL injury (Tang 2011) as RCL is a primary support preventing volar subluxation. Stress dynamic fluoroscopy may also aid

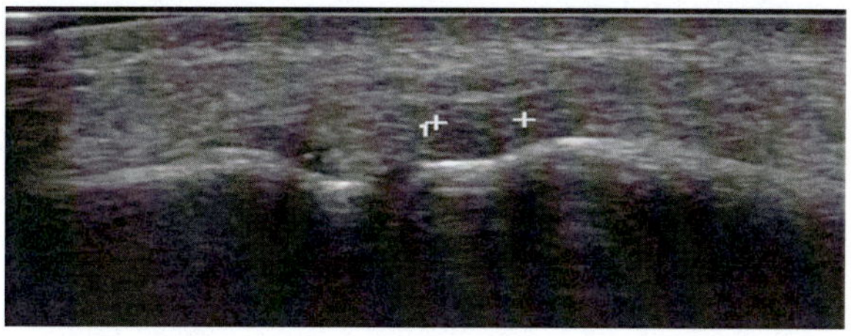

Fig. 9 Longitudinal ultrasound image showing rupture of radial collateral ligament

in evaluation of instability. Because of the high correlation between stress examination and operative findings, arthrography, ultrasonography (Fig. 9) or MRI are usually not needed (Edelstein et al. 2008).

On the basis of the current available literature, RCL and UCL injuries can be managed in a similar manner (Patel et al. 2010). Generally, Grade 1 and 2 injuries are treated conservatively, while treatment of Grade 3 injuries remains controversial. Various surgical methods have been described in the literature for Grade 3 injuries and no general agreement is present.

5 Fractures

Among the injuries sustained during sporting activities in the general population, it is fractures of the upper limb that predominate. The vast number of patients attending emergency department due to these injuries reflects this. In a retrospective study conducted by Aitken and Court-Brown looking at nearly 6000 fractures, 24 % of them occurred in hand and 22.4 % of these were sporting injuries. The thumb and the little fingers were most commonly involved fingers accounting for up to 57.3 % (Aitken and Court-Brown 2008). Metacarpal fractures of the thumb and little fingers are discussed below.

5.1 Thumb Fractures

The thumb provides up to 40 % of hand function (Carlsen and Moran 2009). Injuries to the thumb are predominantly fractures of the proximal phalanx or the metacarpal and ligamentous injuries around the MCPJ. Ligamentous injuries have been discussed in detail along with other soft tissue injuries of the hand. Thumb fractures are found to occur most commonly in children and the elderly (Stanton et al. 2007).

Thumb metacarpal base fractures form an important subset and will be discussed further.

5.1.1 Bennett Fracture

In 1882, Edward Hallaran Bennett first described the fracture involving the base of the thumb metacarpal. However, a Bennett fracture now refers to a two-part intra-articular fracture or dislocation involving the base of the thumb metacarpal (Rettig 2004). The mechanism of injury is classically an axial load to the flexed and adducted thumb (Hong 2005). The volar–ulnar fragment is held in place by its ligamentous attachment to the trapezium, known as the anterior oblique ligament, also described as the beak ligament (Bettinger et al. 1999). As a result of the injury, the remainder of the first metacarpal shaft subluxes in a dorsal, proximal and radial direction due to the pull of the abductor pollicis longus, extensor pollicis longus, extensor pollicis brevis and the adductor pollicis longus (Carlsen and Moran 2009). Gedda in 1954 has classified Bennett fractures as follows (Table 7).

Following clinical examination, a radiographic evaluation forms an integral part of the initial clinical assessment (Fig. 10). True antero–posterior and lateral views can be obtained with the Robert's and Bett's view, respectively, to look for fracture displacement and joint congruency (Carlsen and Moran 2009). These fractures are unstable and should be promptly referred to a hand surgeon for appropriate management. Closed reduction with percutaneous pin fixation is recommended if the fragment is less than 25 % of the articular surface and if the fragment is larger than 25 % of articular surface, and those irreducible by closed techniques should be opened, reduced and internally fixed (Weinstein and Hanel 2002).

5.1.2 Rolando Fracture

This was first described by Silvio Rolando in 1910, a Y-pattern fracture of the thumb metacarpal base (Fig. 11). Currently, this eponym is used widely for any comminuted intra-articular fracture of the thumb metacarpal base (Hong 2005). These are similar in location and etiology to Bennett fracture (Hong 2005). This fracture pattern is considerably more difficult to treat and has a worse prognosis than that of the Bennett fracture (Carlsen and Moran 2009). When there are two large fragments without considerable comminution, open reduction and internal fixation can

Table 7 Gedda classification of Bennett fractures (Gedda 1954, cited by (Carlsen and Moran 2009)

Type 1	Large single ulnar fragment and metacarpal base subluxation
Type 2	Impaction fracture without metacarpal base subluxation
Type 3	Small ulnar avulsion fragment with metacarpal dislocation

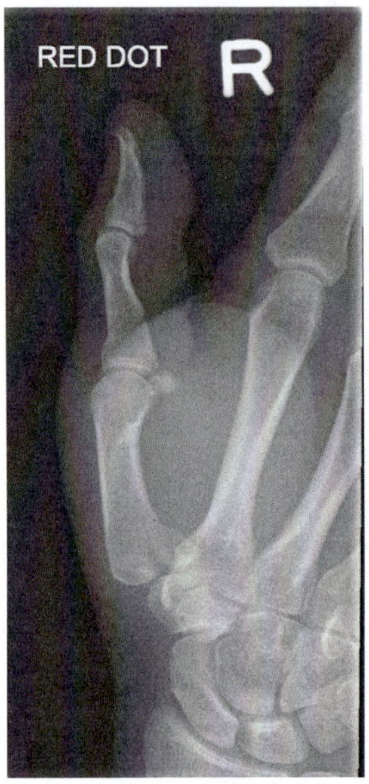

Fig. 10 Lateral radiograph of thumb showing fractures of the metacarpal base (Bennett fracture type 1) and proximal phalanx shaft

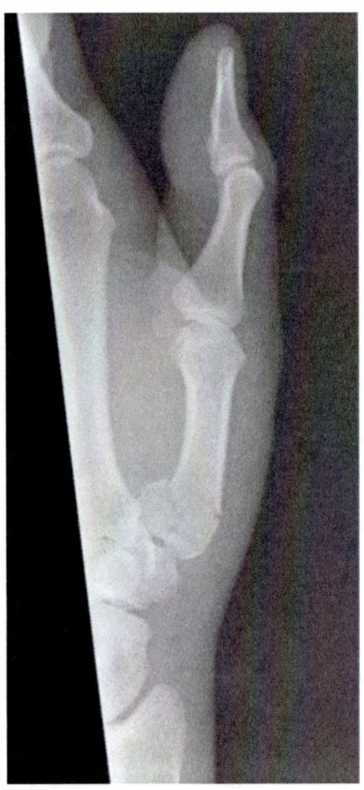

Fig. 11 Rolando fracture of the metacarpal base on a lateral radiograph of the thumb

be successful. For markedly comminuted fractures, distraction and reliance on ligamentous reduction of the fragments may be necessary (Carlsen and Moran 2009).

5.2 Boxer's Fracture

The most common fracture of the hand is fracture of the little finger metacarpal, accounting for up to 50 % of all metacarpal fractures and 20 % of all fractures of the hand (Lee and Jupiter 2000). A fracture to the little finger metacarpal neck is referred to as boxer's fracture. These result from incorrect technique in swinging a fist, that puts an oblique force applied to the smallest, weakest metacarpal (Walsh 2004). The fracture occurs just below the metacarpal head and is normally displaced in a volar direction (Fig. 12). It is important to assess for malrotation by examining the direction of the fingers in flexion (Hong 2005). Apex volar angulation of up to 40° is acceptable and can be treated conservatively with immobilisation in a gutter splint with ring and little finger MCPJs in a 90° flexed position (Hong 2005). Fractures that are markedly comminuted or angulated may need open reduction and internal fixation (Peterson and Bancroft 2006).

5.3 Intra-articular Fractures and Dislocations of the Carpometacarpal Joints

Intra-articular metacarpal base fractures are high-energy injuries that are often missed on initial presentation (Liaw et al. 1995). These are associated with carpometacarpal (CMC) dislocations and most commonly occur in the ring and little fingers.

The mechanism of injury involves axial load transmission through the fourth metacarpal onto the carpal bones (Cain et al. 1987). The ring and little finger CMC joints being modified saddle joints, allow considerable movement in the antero–posterior plane that predisposes these joints to dislocation (Liaw et al. 1995). At a certain stage when the ring finger metacarpal is unable to dissipate the force, a fracture occurs resulting in shortening of the ring finger metacarpal. The axial load is then transferred to the little finger metacarpal causing the little finger CMC joint injury (Liaw et al. 1995). The degree of the little finger metacarpal flexion determines the type and degree of hamate injury (Cain et al. 1987). Flexion of

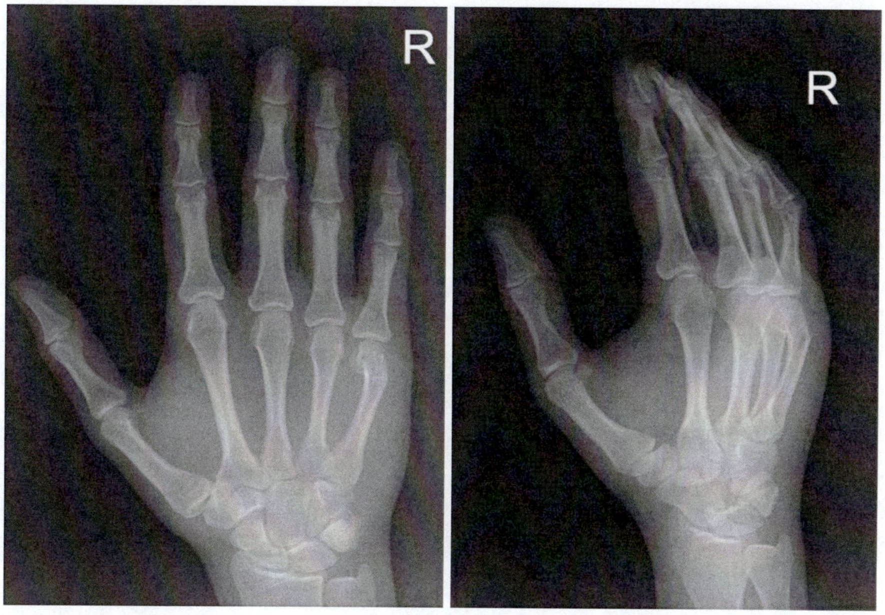

Fig. 12 AP and oblique radiographs showing little finger metacarpal neck fracture (Boxer's fracture) with volar angulation

the metacarpal during impact may cause dorsal dislocation of the little finger metacarpal base, dorsal CMC ligament disruption and hamate fracture. In the little finger, the ECU, FCU and abductor digiti minimi tendon exert deforming forces on the fracture fragments (Weinstein and Hanel 2002). Cain et al. in 1987 have classified the combined ring and little finger metacarpal fracture and little finger CMC joint injury into three categories as follows (see Table 8).

Table 8 Cain et al. classification of intra-articular fractures and dislocations of carpometacarpal joints (Cain et al. 1987)

Type	Characteristic features
1A	Subluxation or dislocation of the little finger metacarpal base without hamate fracture
1B	Type 1A + small dorsal rim hamate avulsion fracture
2	Dorsal hamate comminution is present
3	Coronal splitting of the hamate

The routine AP and lateral radiographs of the hand may not reveal the full extent of the ring and little finger CMC joints (Fig. 13) and a CT scan may be needed to demonstrate the full extent of the injury (Fig. 14). The 45° pronated oblique and 15° pronated oblique views are helpful in assessing the severity of this injury (Liaw et al. 1995).

The treatments of these injuries depend on the severity and stability of the CMC joints. Type 1 stable injuries treated conservatively. Closed reduction and percutaneous pinning can be used to treat unstable type 1 injuries (Cain et al. 1987). Type 2 and 3 injuries are potentially unstable and will require open reduction and internal fixation (Liaw et al. 1995).

5.4 Phalangeal Fractures

Phalangeal fractures can occur at head, neck, shaft or base of the phalanges. There are many variations of these involving various locations. Shaft fractures can be transverse, oblique, spiral or comminuted (Hong 2005). Displacement and angulation of phalangeal fractures result from a combination of two main factors: the mechanism of injury and the deforming nature of the fracture (Peterson and Bancroft 2006). A direct blow can result in transverse or comminuted fracture, while a twisting injury often results in an oblique or spiral fracture (Lee and Jupiter 2000).

Condylar fractures of the head of proximal phalanx are typically the result of axial loading. London described three types of Condylar fractures that influence prognosis and management: a type I stable, undisplaced unicondylar fracture; a type II unstable, displaced, unicondylar and type III comminuted bicondylar fracture (London 1971).

Along with standard AP and lateral radiographs, CT can provide further information that may assist the surgeons in management.

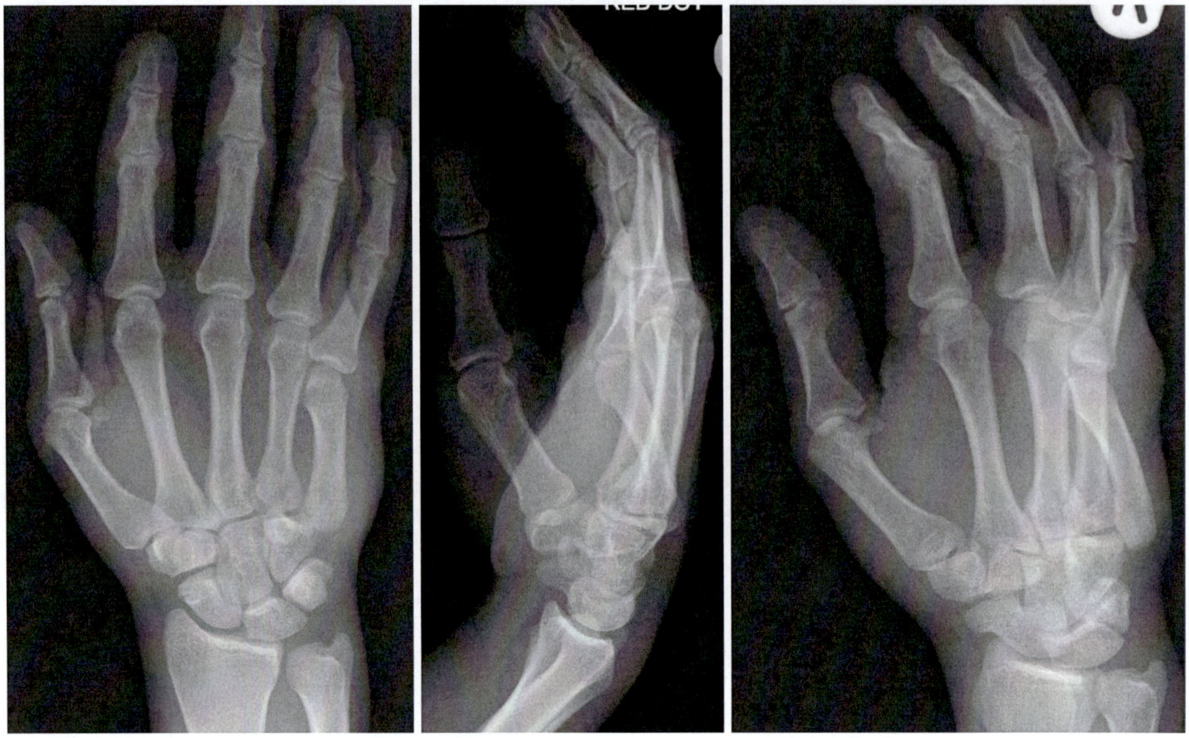

Fig. 13 AP, lateral and oblique radiographs of the right hand showing little finger CMC joint dislocation. Note hamate fracture (seen on CT—Fig. 14) is not visible on these plain films

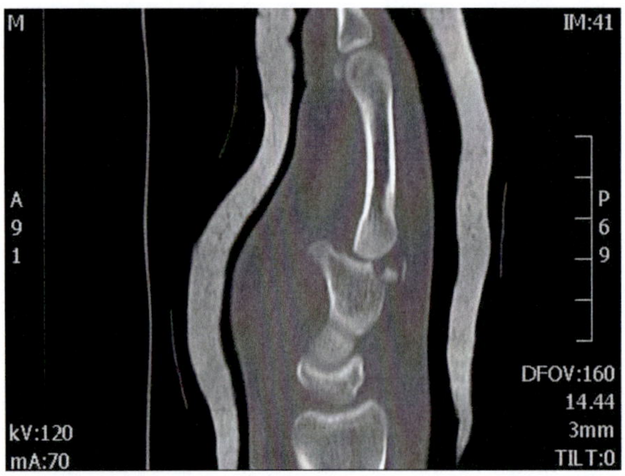

Fig. 14 Sagittal CT image shows little finger CMC joint subluxation with rim fracture of the hamate (Cain et al. type 1B CMC joint injury)

Oblique or spiral fractures may be associated with malrotation. No malrotation is acceptable for phalangeal fractures, because this leads to overlap and malalignment of the digit (Peterson and Bancroft 2006). Acceptable reduction is less than 6 mm of shortening, less than 15° of angulation and with no rotational deformity (Lee and Jupiter 2000).

Non-displaced fractures are treated conservatively, while displaced and malrotated fractures should be reduced; closed at first, but then surgically if needed (Hong 2005). For condylar fractures, London types II and III are treated surgically and stable type I injuries are managed conservatively (Stern 2005).

5.5 Interphalangeal Joint Dislocations

Interphalangeal (IP) dislocations are common injuries in athletes. These injuries usually result from significant force and may result in ligamentous injury or tear. Most IP joint dislocations involve the PIPJ (Morgan et al. 2001). The PIPJ is susceptible especially to forced abnormal motion produced in ball sports and in sports resulting in axial loading of the digit (Morgan et al. 2001). Most IP joint dislocations are dorsal, with dorsal dislocation of the middle phalanx and disruption of the VP (Fig. 15) (Hong 2005).

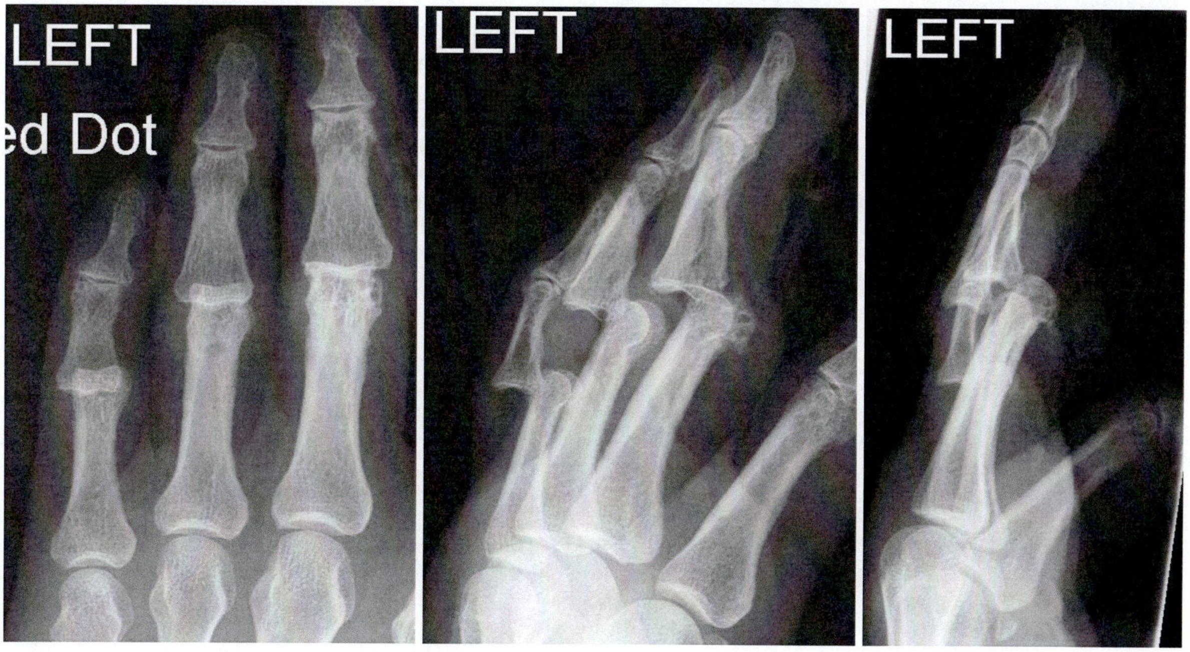

Fig. 15 AP, oblique and lateral radiographs of the middle, ring and little fingers showing dorsal dislocation of the proximal interphalangeal joints

6 Conclusion

This chapter has described the most common soft tissue and bone injuries to the hand. We have related the anatomy and mechanism of these injuries to the imaging assessment. We have also discussed factors that influence management decisions which enable a more thorough imaging assessment.

Acknowledgments The authors wish to sincerely thank Dr. David Moore, Dr. Steven L. J. James and Dr. Andrew J. Grainger for providing some of the images used in this chapter.

References

Aitken S, Court-Brown CM (2008) The epidemiology of sports-related fractures of the hand. Injury 39:1377–1383

Angermann P, Lohmann M (1993) Injuries to the hand and wrist. A study of 50,272 injuries. J Hand Surg Br 18(5):642–644

Aronowitz ER, Leddy JP (1998) Closed tendon injuries of the hand and wrist in athletes. Clin Sports Med 17:449–467

Beltran J, Noto AM, Herman LJ, Lubbers LM (1987) Tendons: High field strength surface coil MR imaging. Radiology 162:735–740

Bettinger PC, Linscheid RL, Berger RA, Cooney WP III, An KN (1999) An anatomic study of the stabilizing ligaments of the trapezium and trapeziometacarpal joint. J Hand Surg 24(4):786–798

Bollen (1990) Injury to the A2 pulley in rock climbers. J Hand Surg Br. May 15(2):268–70

Brzezienski MA, Schneider LH (1995) Extensor tendons injuries at the distal interphalangeal joint. Hand Clin 11:373–386

Burotn RI (1982) Extensor tendon-late reconstruction. In Green DP (ed): Operative HandSurgey. New York, Churchill Livinstone p. 2073

Buscemi MJ, Page BJ (1987) Flexor digitorum profundus avulsions with associated distal phalanx fractures: A report of four cases and review of the literature. Am J Sports Med 15:366–370

Cain JE, Shepler TR and Wilson MR (1987) Hamatometacarpal fracture-dislocation: classification and treatment. J Hand Surg. 12A:5(1):762–767

Campbell CS (1955) Gamekeeper's thumb. J Bone Joint Surg Br 37:148–149

Carlsen BT, Moran SL (2009) Thumb trauma: Bennett fractures, rolando fractures, and ulnar collateral ligament injuries. J Hand Surg Am 34(5):945–952

Clavero JA, Alomar X, Monill JM, Esplugas M, Golano P, Mendoza M, Salvador A (2002) MR imaging of ligament and tendon injuries of the fingers. RadioGraphics 22: 237–256

Cooney WP, Arnold D, Grace J (1990) Collateral ligament injury of the thumb. Adv Orthop Surg 13:235–248

Coyle MP Jr (2003) Grade III Radial collateral ligament injuries of the thumb metacarpophalangeal joint: Treatment

by soft tissue advancement and bony reattachment. J Hand Surg Am 28(1):14–20
Derkash RS, Matyas JR, Weaver JK et al (1987) Acute surgical repair of the skier's thumb. Clin Orthop Relat Res 216:29–33
Doyle JR (1999) Extensor tendons—acute injuries. In: Geen DP, Hotchkiss RN, Pederson WC (eds) Green's operative hand surgery, 4th edn. Churchill Livingstone, Edinburgh, pp 1950–1986
Drape JL, Dubert T, Silbermann O, Thelen P, Thivet A, Benacerraf R (1994) Acute trauma of the extensor hood of the metacarpophalangeal joint: MR imaging evaluation. Radiology 192:469–476
Eaton RG (1971) Joint injuries of hand. Charles C. Thomas, Springfield
Ebrahim SF, De Maeseneer M, Jager T, Marcelis S, Jamadar DA, Jacobson JA (2006) US diagnosis of UCL tears of the thumb and stener lesions: technique, pattern-based approach, and differential diagnosis. Radiographics 26: 1007–1020
Edelstein DM, Kardashian G, Lee SK (2008) Radial collateral ligament injuries of the thumb. J Hand Surg 33A:760–770
Elson RA (1986) Rupture of the central slip of the extensor hood of the finger. A test for early diagnosis. J Bone Joint Surg Br 68(2):229–231
Gabl M, Rangger C, Lutz M, Fink C, Rudisch A, Pechlaner S (1998) Disruption of the finger flexor pulley system in elite rock climbers. Am J Sports Med 26:651–655
Gaine WJ, Beardsmore J, Fahmy N (1998) Early active mobilisation of volar plate avulsion fractures. Injury 29:589–591
Gerber C, Senn E, Matter P (1981) Skier's thumb: Surgical treatment of recent injuries to the ulnar collateral ligament of the thumb's metacarpophalangeal joint. Am J Sports Med 9:171–177
Giele H, Martin J (2003) The two-level ulnar collateral ligament injury of the metacarpophalangeal joint of the thumb. J Hand Surg 28B:92–93
Green DP, Rowlan SA (1984) Fractures and dislocations in the hand. In: Rockwood CA Jr, Green DP (eds) Fractures in adults, 2nd edn. JB Lippincott, Philadelphia, pp 388–394
Griffin M, Hindocha S, Jordan D, Saleh M, Khan W (2012) Management of extensor tendon injuries. Open Orthop J 6(Suppl 1:M4):36–42
Hame SL, Melone CP Jr (2000) Boxer's knuckle in the professional athlete. Am J Sports Med 28:879882
Handoll HHG, Vaghela M (2004) Interventions for treating mallet finger injuries. Cochran Database Syst Rev (1)
Harper MT, Chandnani VP, Spaeth J, Santangelo JR, Providence BC, Bagg MA (1996) Gamekeeper thumb: Diagnosis of ulnar collateral ligament injury using magnetic resonance imaging, magnetic resonance arthrography and stress radiography. J Magn Reson Imaging 6(2):322–328
Hart RG, Uehara DT, Kutz JE (1993) Extensor tendon injuries of the hand. Emerg Med Clin North Am 11(3): 637–649
Hauger O, Chung CB et al (2000) Pulley System in the fingers: normal anatomy and simulated Lesions in cadavers at MR Imaging, CT and US with and without contrast material distention of the tendon sheath. Radiology 217:201–212
Hergan K, Mittler C, Oser W (1995) Ulnar collateral ligament: differentiation of displaced and nondisplaced tears with US and MR imaging. Radiology 194:65–71
Hergan K, Mittler C, Oser W (1997) Pitfalls in sonography of the gamekeeper's thumb. Eur Radiol 7:65–69
Heyman P, Gelberman RH, Duncan K, Hipp JA (1993) Injuries of the ulnar collateral ligament of the thumb metacarpophalangeal joint: Biomechanical and prospective clinical studies on the usefulness of valgus stress testing. Clin Orthop Relat Res 292:165–171
Hill C, Riaz M, Mozzam A, Brennen ND (1998) A regional audit of hand and wrist injuries. J Hand Surg (Br Eur) 23B(2):196–200
Hong E (2005) Hand injuries in sports medicine. Prim Care 32:91–103
Hunter JM (1984) Anatomy of the flexor tendons: pulley, vincular, synovial, and vascular structures. In: Spinner M (ed) Kaplan's functional and surgical anatomy of the hand, 3rd edn. Lippincott, Philadelphia, pp 65–92
Hussain SN, Dietz JF, Kalainov DM, Lautenschlager EP (2008) A biomechanical study of distal interphalangeal joint subluxation after mallet fracture injury. J Hand surg 33A:26–30
Inoue G and Tamura Y (1996). Dislocation of the extensor tendons over themetacarpophalangeal joints. J Hand Surg(Am) 21:464–469
Jebson PJL (1998) Flexor digitorum profundus tendon avulsions. Oper Tech Orthop 8:63–66
Jeyapalan K, Bisson MA, Dias JJ, Griffin Y, Bhatt R (2008) The role of ultrasound in the management of flexor tendon injuries. J Hand Surg (Eur) 33E(4):430–434
Keifhaber TR, Stern PJ (1998) Fracture dislocations of the proximal interphalangeal joint. J Hand Surg Am 23:368–380
Kichouh M, De Maesenner M, Jager T, Marcelis S, Van Hedent E, Van Roy P, De Mey J (2011) Ultrasound findings in injuries of dorsal extensor hood: Correlation with MR and follow-up findings. Eur J Radiol 77:249–253
Klauser A, Bodner G, Frauscher F, Gabl M, Xur Nedden D (1999) Finger injuries in extreme rock climbers assessment of high-resolution ultrasonography. Am J Sports Med 27:733–737
Klauser A, Frauscher F, Bodner G, Halpern E, Schoke MF, Springer P, Gable M, Judamaier W, Nedden D (2002) Finger pulley injuries in extreme rock climbers: depiction with dynamic US. Radiology 222:755–761
Kleinbaum Y, Heyman Z, Ganel A, Blankstein A (2005) Sonographic imaging of mallet finger. Ultraschall Med 26(3):223–226
Kleinhert HE, Verdan C (1983) Report of the committee on tendon injuries. J Hand Surg (Am) 8(5 pt 2):794–798
Le Viet D, Rousselin B, Roulot E, Lantieri L, Godefroy D (1996) Diagnosis of digital pulley rupture by computed tomography. Hand Surg 21A:245–248
Leddy JP, Packer JW (1977) Avulsion of the profundus tendon insertion in athletes. J Hand Surg (Am) 2:66–69
Lee SG, Jupiter JB (2000) Phalangeal and metacarpal fractures of the hand. Hand Clin 16:323–332
Liaw Y, Kalnins G, Kirsh G, Meakin I (1995) Combined fourth and fifth metacarpal fracture and fifth carpometacarpal joint dislocation. J Hand surg (Br Eur) 20B(2):249–252

Lin GT, Amadio PC, An KN, Cooney WP (1989) Functional anatomy of the human digital flexor pulley system. J Hand Surg Am 14:949–956
London PS (1971) Sprains and fractures involving the interphalangeal joints. Hand 3:155–158
Lopez-Ben R, Lee DH, Nicolodi DJ (2003) Boxer knuckle (injury of the extensor hood with extensor tendon subluxation: diagnosis with dynamic us—report of three cases. Radiology 228:642–646
Lyons RP, Kozin SH, Failla JM (1998) The anatomy of the radial side of the thumb: static restraints in preventing subluxation and rotation after injury. Am J Orthop 27:759–763
Marco RA, Sharkey NA, Smith TS, Zissimos AG (1998) Pathomechanics of closed rupture of the flexor tendon pulleys in rock climbers. J Bone Joint Surg Am 80:1012–1019
Martinoli C, Bianchi S, Nebiolo M, Dechi LE, Garcia JF (2000) Sonographic evaluation of digital annular pulley tears. Skeletal Radiol 29:387–391
Matzon JL, Bozentka DJ (2010) Extensor tendon injuries. J Hand surg 35A:854–861
McMaster PE (1933) Tendon and muscle ruptures: clinical and experimental studies on the causes and location of subcutaneous ruptures. J Bone Joint Surg 15:705
Morgan WJ, Slowman LS (2001) Acute hand and wrist injuries in athletes: evaluation and management. J Am Acad Orthop Surg 9:389–400
Nance EP Jr, Kaye JJ, Milek MA (1979) Volar plate fractures. Radiology 133:61–64
Newport ML (1997) Extensor tendon injuries in the hand. J Am Acad Orthop Surg 5:59–66
Patel S, Potty A, Taylor EJ, Sorene ED (2010) Collateral ligament injuries of the metacarpophalangeal joint of the thumb: a treatment algorithm. Strat Trauma Limb Reconstr 5:1–10
Perron AD, Brady WJ, Keats TE, Hersh RE (2001) Orthopaedic pitfalls in the emergency department: closed tendon injuries of the hand. Am J Emerg Med 19:76–80
Peterson JJ, Bancroft LW (2006) Injuries of the fingers and thumb in the athlete. Clin Sports Med 25:527–542
Phair IC, Quinton DN, Allen MJ (1989) The conservative management of volar avulsion fractures of the PIP joint. J Hand Surg Br 14:168–170
Posner MA (1977) Injuries to the hand and wrist in athletes. Orthop Clin North Am 8:593–618
Rayan GM, Murray D (1994) Classification and treatment of closed sagittal band injuries. J Hand Surg 19A:590–594
Rettig AC (2004) Athletic injuries of the wrist and hand. Part II: overuse injuries of the wrist and traumatic injuries to the hand. Am J Sports Med 32:262–273
Ritts GD, Wood MB, Engber WD (1985) Nonoperative treatment of traumatic dislocations of the extensor digitorum tendons in patients without rheumatoid disorders. J Hand Surg 10A:714–716
Rockwell WB, Butler PN and Byrne BA (2000) ExtensorTendon: Anatomy, Injury, and Reconstruction. Plastic and Reconstructive surgery 106: 1592-1603
Schnur DP, DeLone FX, McClellan MR, Bonavita J, Witham RS (2002) Ultrasound: A powerful tool in the diagnosis of ulnar collateral ligament injuries of the thumb. Ann Plast Surg 49:19–23
Smith RJ (1977) Post-traumatic instability of the metacarpophalangeal joint of the thumb. J Bone Joint Surg (Am) 59-A:14–21
Sollerman C, Abrahamso SO, Lundborg G, Adalbert K (1991) Functional splinting versus plaster cast for ruptures of the ulnar collateral ligament of the thumb. Acta Orthop Scand 62:524–526
Stanton JS, Dias JJ, Burke FD (2007) Fractures of the tubular bones of the hand. J Hand Surg 32E:626–636
Stark HH, Boyes JH, Wilson JN (1962) Mallet finger. J Bone Joint Surg Am 44(6):1061–1068
Stener B (1962) Displacement of the ruptured ulnar collateral ligament of the metacarpo-phalangeal joint of the thumb. J Bone Joint Surg (Br) 44-B:869–879
Stern PJ (2005) Fractures of the metacarpals and phalanges. In: Green DP (ed) Green's operative hand surgery, 5th edn. Elsevier Churchill Livingstone, Philadelphia
Tabbal GN, Bastidas N, Sharma S (2009) Closed mallet thumb injury: a review of the literature and case study of the use of magnetic resonance imaging in deciding treatment. Plast Reconstr Surg 124(1):222–226
Tang P (2011) Collateral ligament injuries of the thumb metacarpophalangeal joint. J Am Acad Orthop Surg 19:287–296
Tsiouri C, Hayton MJ, Baratz M (2009) Injury to the ulnar collateral ligament of the thumb. Hand 4:12–18
Walsh JJ (2004) Fractures of the hand and carpal navicular bone in athletes. South Med J 97:762–765
Weinstein LP, Hanel DP (2002) Metacarpal fractures. J Am Soc Surg Hand 2:168–180
Williams EH, McCarthy E, Bickel KD (1998) J Hand Surg Am 23A:805–810
Yoong P, Goodwin RW, Chojnowski A (2010) Phalangeal fractures of the hand. Clin Radiol 65:773–780

Imaging of Wrist Trauma

Nigel Raby

Contents

N. Raby (✉)
Department of Radiology, Westen Infirmary,
Glasgow, G11 6NT, UK
e-mail: N.Raby@clinmed.gla.ac.uk;
nigel.raby@ggc.scot.nhs.uk

Abstract

This chapter will principally describe and illustrate acute bony injuries of the distal radius and carpus occurring as a result of trauma. Plain films form the bulk of investigations, but where indicated use of CT and MR imaging is also included. Chronic traumatic injuries principally overuse, or stress injuries will also be considered but in less detail.

1 Introduction

1.1 Radiographic Anatomy and Projections

Standard radiographic views for the evaluation of wrist are a postero-antererior (PA) and lateral. These projections are described with the relevant anatomy in Radiography and Arthrography and will not be repeated here. These 2 views will allow evaluation of injuries of the distal radius and ulna, an assessment of the carpal bones, and the carpo-metacarpal junction. Additional views may be obtained in special specific circumstance most commonly when there is clinical suspicion of a scaphoid fracture.

1.2 Analysis of Radiographs

On the PA view, inspect each bone in turn looking for cortical disruption that would indicate a fracture. It is important to consider in turn the distal radius and ulna, then the eight carpal bones and finally the bases of the metacarpals. Next, undertake scrutiny of the normal uniform spacing of 1–2 mm around each carpal bone.

A. M. Davis et al. (eds.), *Imaging of the Hand and Wrist*, Medical Radiology. Diagnostic Imaging,
DOI: 10.1007/174_2010_110,

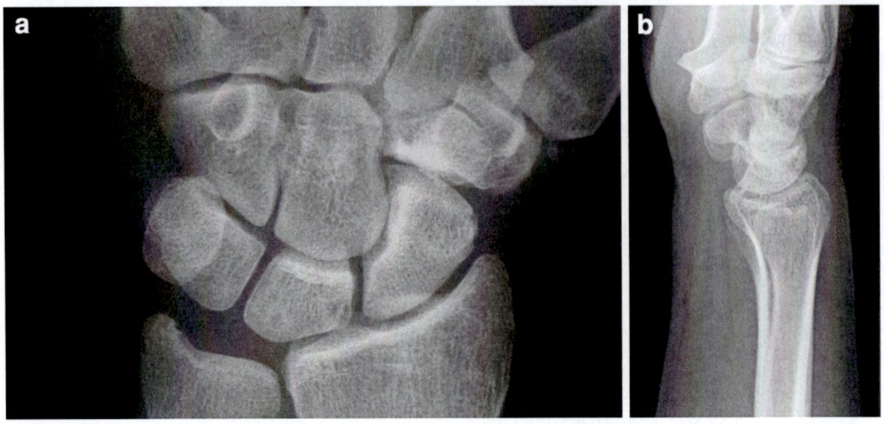

Fig. 1 **a** Normal AP radiograph. Note the uniform spacing between the carpal bones including the carpo-metacarpal junction. The 3 carpal arcs are smooth. The ulnar side of the 3rd metacarpal aligns with the space between the capitate and hamate. **b** Normal lateral radiograph. Observe the normal volar tilt of the distal radius. The dorsal cortex of the radius should be smooth with no steps or crinkles. Observe the normal alignment of the radius lunate and capitate

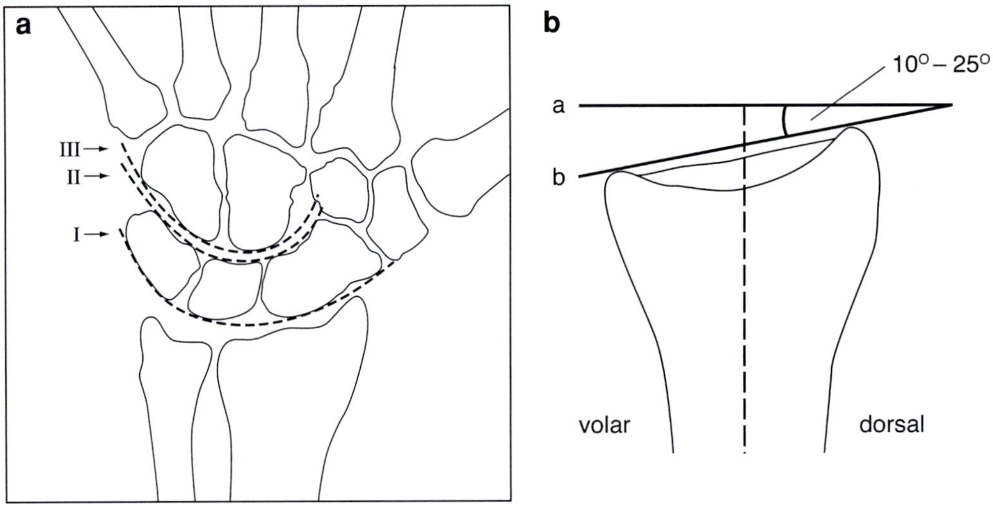

Fig. 2 **a** Line drawing indicating the position of the three carpal arcs. **b** The normal volar tilt of the distal radius

This spacing also occurs at the carpo-metcarpal junction. Loss of this spacing should lead to very careful inspection of the abnormal area, as often this will indicate significant carpal or carpo-metacarpal disruption (Fig. 1). One should also observe the arrangement of the carpal bones into smooth arcs. Three arcs have been described (Gilula 1979). The first delineates the proximal surface of the proximal row of carpal bones (scaphoid, lunate, triquetral). The second is formed by the distal articular surface of the same bones. The third is along the proximal curvature of the capitate and hamate (Fig. 2).

These arcs should normally be smooth with no steps or disruption. Interruption of any of these smooth arcs indicates a disruption of the normal arrangement of bony structures at the point of the step in the arc. Note should also be taken of the normal alignment of the metacarpals with the distal row of carpal bones, in particular, the relationship of the 3rd metacarpal with the distal capitate. A line drawn down the ulnar side of the metacarpal should pass through the joint between the capitate and hamate (Fig. 1). Loss of this normal alignment indicates a carpo-metacarpal disruption most commonly a dislocation. This sign is akin to the alignment of the tarsometatarsal joint in the foot.

Much important information is to be found on the lateral film. A key observation is that of the distal radial angle. The normal distal radius has a volar tilt of approx 10°. This represents the angle between a line drawn along the long axis of the radius and a line drawn from the dorsal to the volar rim of the radius and has a normal range of 2°–20° (Figs. 1b, 2b). Alteration of this angle occurs when there is a subtle fracture of the distal radius. Normal relationship of the distal radius and carpal bones is best assessed on the lateral view, and this is discussed further in the Sect. 3.3. Displacement of the distal radial epiphysis and disruption of carpal alignment are often only evident on this view. Fractures of the triquetral bone will only be seen on the lateral radiograph.

CT is rarely used to confirm or refute the presence of a fracture. A fracture is usually evident on the plain films, but CT is helpful to define the exact anatomy in complex fractures and dislocations to aid surgical planning. This is particularly true when there is involvement of the articular surface of the radius such a Bartons fracture dislocation and die punch injuries. The exception is when an injury of isolated carpal bones is suspected. Fractures of these, particularly hamate and capitate, may be seen only on CT. CT is of value in some carpal dislocations but is particularly of value in cases of metacarpal dislocations which can be difficult to identify on plain films. In the current era of multislice scanners, there is no longer any need to be overly prescriptive about scan planes and slice thickness. Modern scanners allow very rapid multiplanar and 3D reconstruction with isotropic voxels, so that the injured wrist can be scanned in any position and reviewed in the best plane for the injury under investigation without any loss of information or degradation of the image.

MR is not generally utilised to evaluate acute wrist trauma, but it is the investigation of choice when an occult scaphoid fracture is suspected clinically.

1.3 Ligamentous Anatomy of Wrist

The ligamentous anatomy of the wrist is extremely complex. There is disagreement between authors with considerable variation in the description of the ligament anatomy. This anatomy has been dealt with in detail elsewhere in this book and will not be reiterated here. This level of understanding is important when evaluation of the ligaments by imaging is being undertaken. However, for the purposes of this chapter, such detail is not required. What is required is knowledge of important ligaments and their attachments. This information allows a better understanding of the patterns of bony injury and associated findings. Here, I will outline the key ligaments and indicate where in the later text this ligamentous knowledge applies. Of necessity, this is a much simplified account of the ligaments.

Ligaments are divided into extrinsic and intrinsic both dorsal and volar. The volar ligaments are stronger and more functionally significant. Extrinsic ligaments link the distal radius and ulna to the carpal bones. The intrinsic or intercarpal ligaments link carpal bones to one another.

On the dorsal aspect two ligaments are of importance in this chapter. They are the dorsal radiotriquetral (extrinsic) and the dorsal intercarpal ligament. Both attach to the triquetral bone. It is the attachment of these ligaments that account for the avulsion fracture of the triquetral (see below) (Fig. 3a).

On the volar aspect, there are 2 key ligaments. The radio scapho-capitate (RSC) and the radio lunate triquetral (RLT), both extrinsic ligaments (Fig. 3b). The position of the RSC helps understand the propensity of the scaphoid to fracture (see Sect. 3.1).

When the wrist is dorsiflexed, these two ligaments separate resulting in what is termed the space of Poirier. This space between the ligaments is an area of weakness which accounts for the carpal dislocations that occur around the lunate (see Sect. 3.3).

The attachments of the RSC and RLT to the radius account for the isolated fracture of the radial styloid which is essentially an avulsion injury. (See isolated fracture of radial styloid.)

In addition to the RSC and RLT, there are other ligaments that arise from the volar aspect of the radius to attach to carpal bones. Their names and arrangement are not important in this setting, but the multiple ligaments account for the bone fragments seen on the volar aspect of the wrist in patients with dorsal radio carpal dislocations (see Sect. 3.3).

On the ulnar aspect of the wrist lies the triangular fibrocartilage complex (TFCC). Again this has very complex anatomy, but for our purposes it is sufficient know that there are paired ligaments on dorsal and volar aspects of the wrist. The radio-ulnar ligaments pass horizontally between the radius and the ulna styloid process. There are also two ligaments running

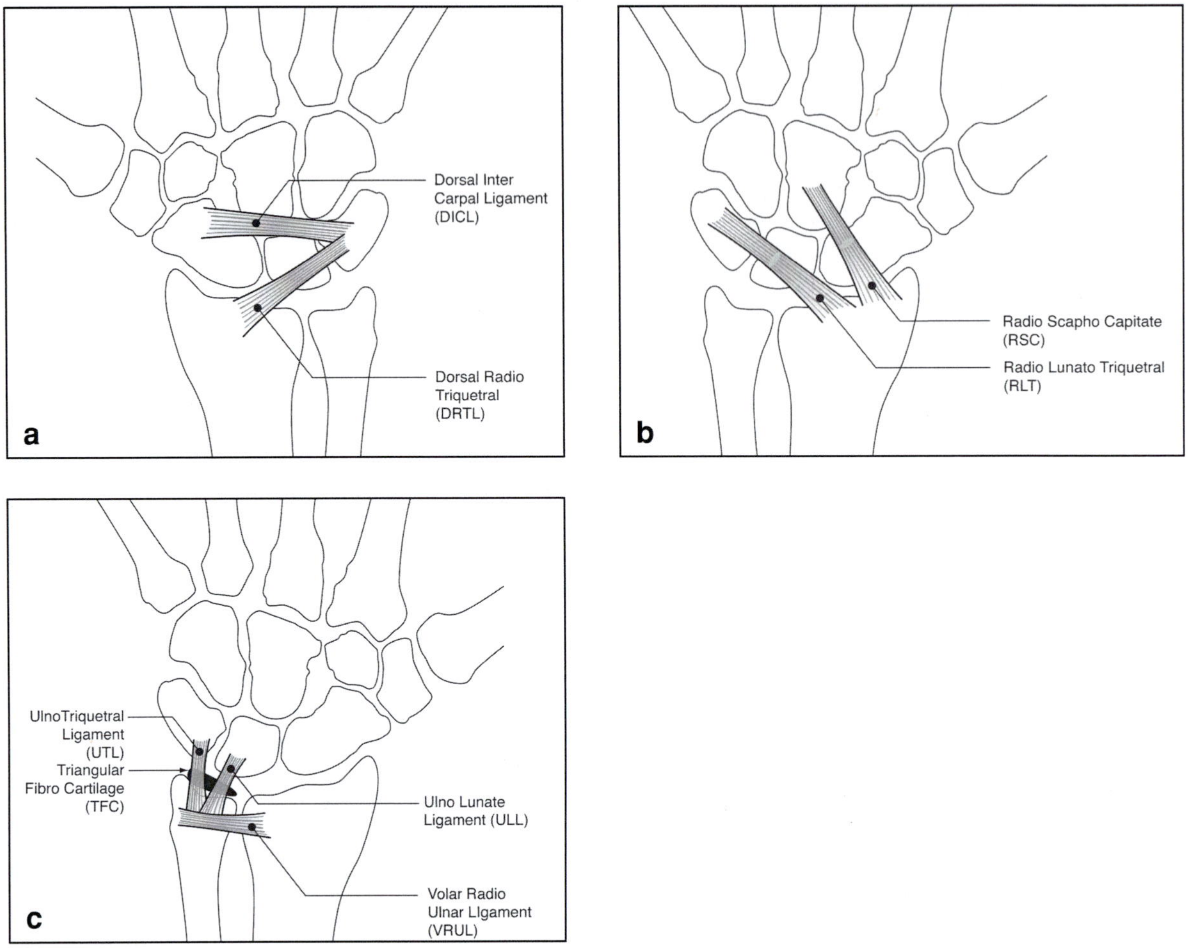

Fig. 3 **a** Important dorsal ligaments. **b** Volar ligaments radial aspect. **c** Volar ligaments and TFC

from the base of ulna styloid to the lunate and triquetral bone. These four ligaments account for the fractures of the ulna styloid seen in several injuries including Colles fractures and distal radio ulna joint disruption (Fig. 3c).

Of the very many intrinsic ligaments, only those connecting scaphoid, lunate and triquetral bones are of significance with respect to acute bony injuries. Thus, the scapho-lunate ligament is disrupted with scaphoid rotatory subluxation.

2 Injuries of Radius and Ulna

Most commonly injuries result from fall on the outstretched wrist. The type of injury sustained is age related.

2.1 Children

In young children, fractures of the radius proximal to the epipyhseal plate predominate in age group 6–10. These fractures often involve both radius and ulna and may be grossly displaced (Fig. 4). After this, until epipyhseal fusion injuries most commonly involve the epipyhseal plate and are thus Salter Harris fractures. Typically, there is dorsal displacement of the epiphysis with or without an associated fracture fragment from the adjacent metaphysis resulting in either a Salter-Harris type one or two injury (Fig. 5). The degree of displacement is often gross, but on occasion the anteroposterior radiograph can appear quite normal. As with adults, it is careful inspection of the lateral film which will reveal the abnormal alignment

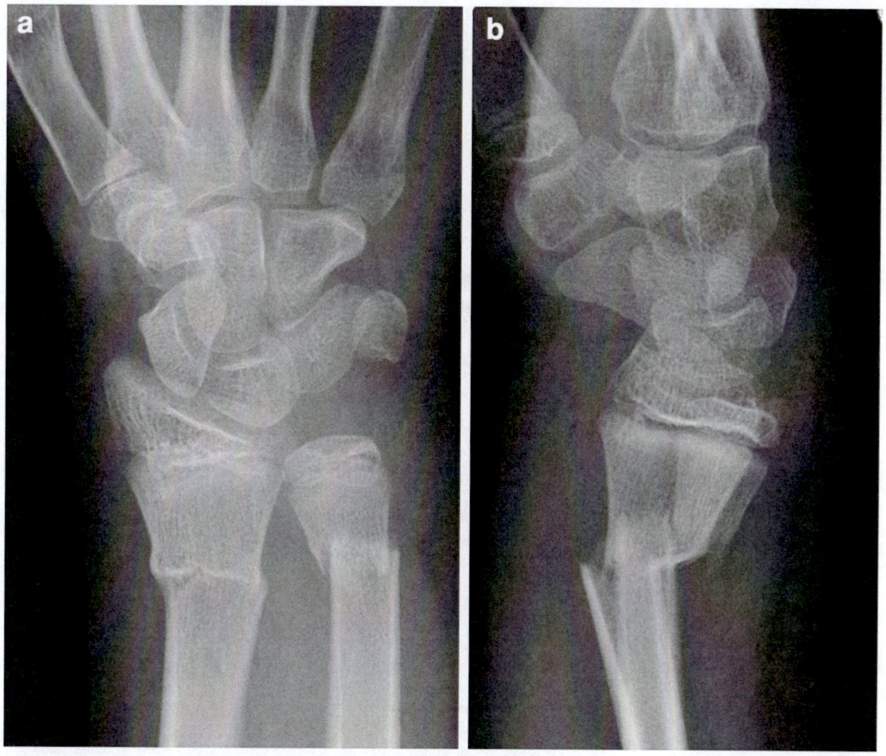

Fig. 4 **a** and **b** AP and lateral radiographs demonstrate fracture of radius and ulna in a child. There is considerable angulation and overlap at the fracture site. The fracture is proximal to the epiphysis which is not involved. This is the typical site and appearance of wrist injuries in children under the age of 10

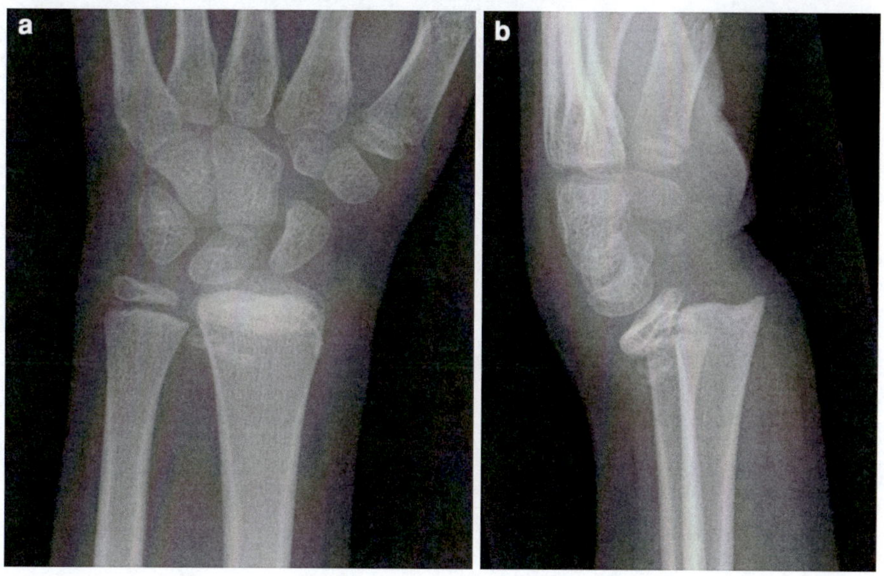

Fig. 5 **a** AP radiograph with no obvious abnormality. Observe however the loss of clarity of the radial epipyhseal plate with increased sclerosis. **b** Lateral radiograph shows that the epiphysis is displaced dorsally. There is a small fragment of bone from the metaphysis in addition which means this is a Salter Harris type 2 injury. This is the commonest type of injury seen at the epipyhseal plate

of the distal radial epiphysis. Colles type fractures do not occur in this age group. Greenstick and buckle or Torus fractures of the radius occur only in children. Torus fractures are a compression failure of bone usually at the junction of diaphysis and metaphysis. The term comes from Latin meaning a "protuberance" or "rounded swelling". The injury is due to compression forces resulting in a circumferential buckling of the cortex. Thus, the abnormality can be seen on both views although it may be more evident on the lateral projection (Fig. 6). It is a relatively minor injury that will heal well with only minimal immobilisation required (Davidson et al. 2001). Scaphoid fractures do not occur in children

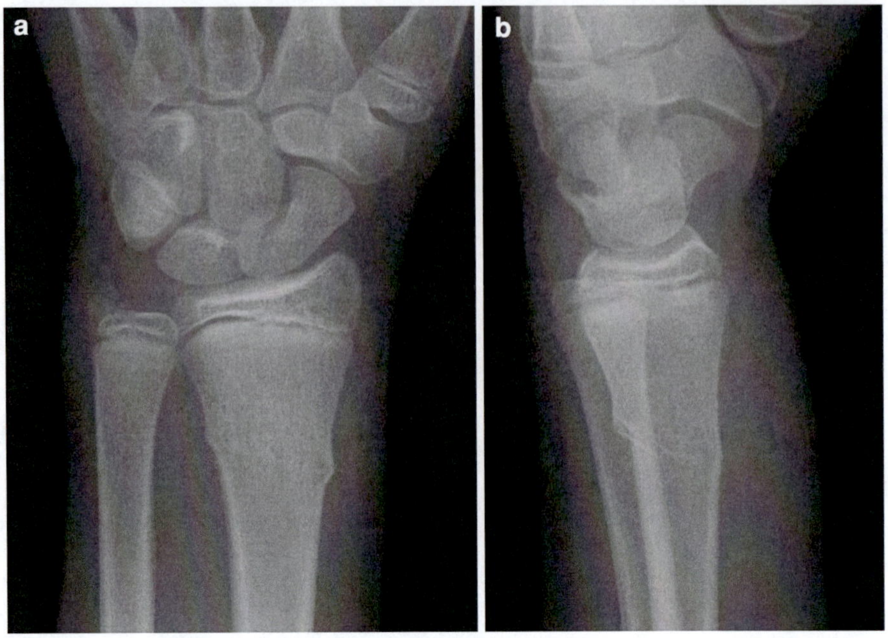

Fig. 6 **a** and **b** There is buckling of the cortex of the radius. This is a circumferential injury and thus seen on both AP and lateral views. It is referred to as a Torus fracture and is seen exclusively in children

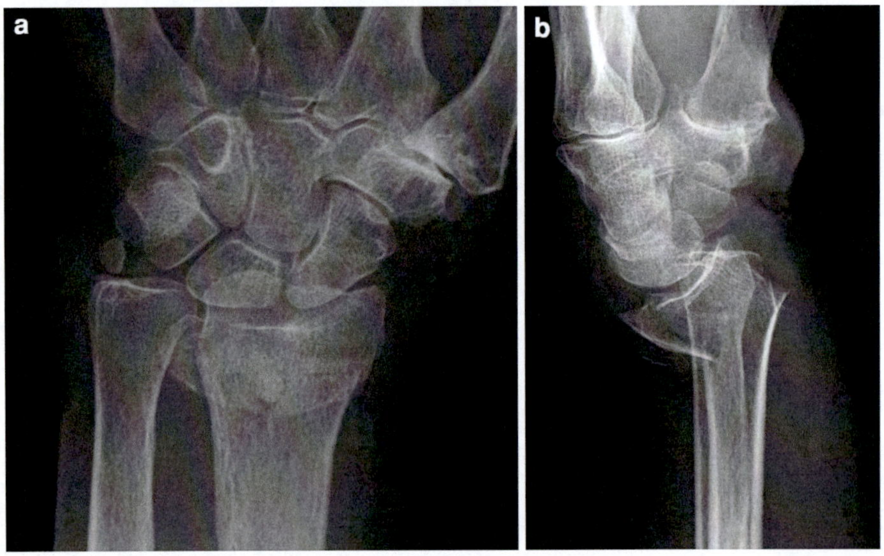

Fig. 7 **a** and **b** Colles fracture. There is fracture of the distal radius with dorsal angulation. The articular surface is not involved. There is some radial displacement, and there is an associated fracture of the ulnar styloid process. All of the above need to be present to fulfil the original description of a Colles fracture

under 10 and are rare in older children (Thornton and Gyll 1999).

2.2 Adults

Colles fracture is the commonest wrist injury in patients over age of 40. Increasing frequency with age suggests a relationship to osteoporosis. It was first defined by Abraham Colles professor of surgery in Dublin in his 1814 paper "On the Fracture of the Carpal Extremity of the radius". His definition includes the following: (1) fracture of radius within 2 cm of distal radial articular surface but not involving it, (2) dorsal angulation of distal fragment, (3) dorsal displacement of the fragment, and (4) associated fracture of ulnar styloid process. In addition, there is also often some lateral (radial) displacement of the distal radial fragment (Fig. 7). The mechanism of injury with resultant forces applied to

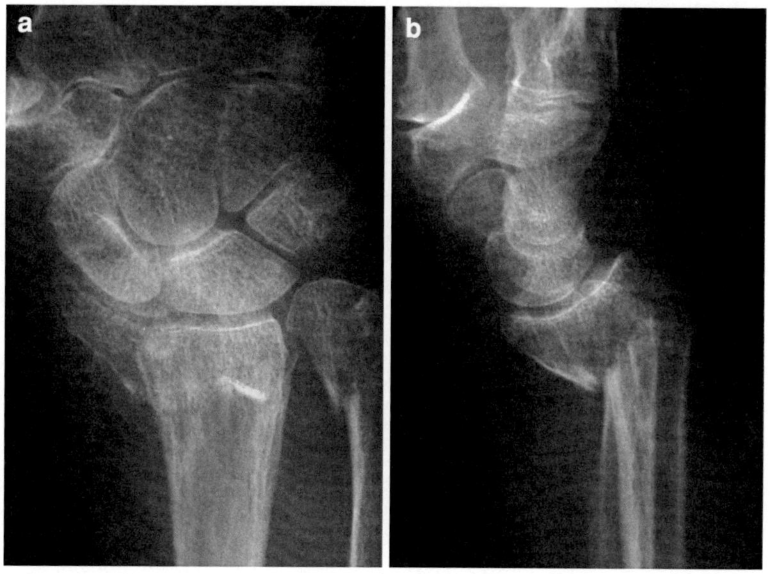

Fig. 8 **a** and **b** Smiths fracture. The distal radial fracture fragment is angulated and displaced in a volar direction. The articular surface not involved. There is an associated distal ulna fracture

the distal forearm bones explains these findings. With fall onto the outstretched hand in extension, impact occurs on the thenar eminence. There are compression forces transmitted along the dorsal cortex of the radius with traction forces along the volar aspect. This results in the fracture with displacement described above. The ulnar styloid fracture occurs due to radial shortening with traction on the ulnar styloid process via the triangular fibrocartilage complex principally the ligaments which attach to the process.

Smith (1847) described a variation of the above where the distal radial fragment is displaced and angled volarly and medially. This is typically caused by falling onto the wrist whilst it is flexed. Again a key feature is that the articular surface remains intact (Fig. 8). Subsequently, this fracture has been subclassified by some to include volarly displaced fractures with an intra-articular component. This injury is indistinguishable from the reversed Bartons fracture discussed below.

Barton described an injury of the distal radius (Barton 1838) as follows: "a subluxation of the wrist consequent to a fracture through the articular surface of the carpal extremity of the radius… The fragment… usually is quite small, and is broken from the end of the radius on the dorsal side" (Fig. 9). This fracture differs from Colles and Smiths fractures due to involvement of the articular surface of the radius. It is a shearing injury through the articular surface. The term is now often incorrectly ascribed to any intra-articular fracture. Barton's description also includes the presence of dislocation or subluxation of the radiocarpal joint. A similar injury but with the bone fragment from the volar margin is known by some as a reversed Bartons fracture. It is in fact the volar fracture with volar displacement which occurs more commonly. The fracture fragment varies in size but may involve up to 50% of the articular surface (Fig. 10). The key feature is that the articular surface of the lunate remains in contact with the displaced rim fragment of the distal radius (Fig. 9), and it is this finding that distinguishes this injury from a radio carpal dislocation.

Subtle radial fractures can be easily overlooked. The signs to look for are a subtle crinkle in the cortex of the radius usually on the dorsal aspect and seen only on the lateral film (Fig. 11). Alteration in the radial angle from the usual 10° volar angulation will provide confirmatory evidence but is not present in every case. It has been suggested that soft issue signs around the wrist such as loss of the pronator fat stripe which is normally seen as a lucent area on the volar aspect of the distal radius is a useful adjunct to identifying subtle radial fractures (MacEwan 1964) However, a recent review of the utility of this observation has shown it to be of limited value with a sensitivity of only 26% (Annamalai and Raby 2003).

Isolated fracture of the radial styloid process (Fig. 12) is also known as Hutchinsons or Chauffeurs Fracture. This refers to an intra-articular fracture that

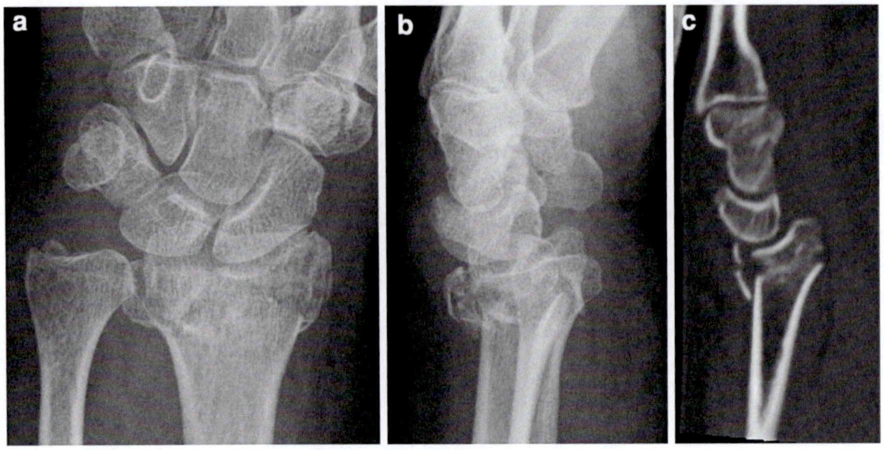

Fig. 9 **a** There is a fracture of the distal radius with extension into the radial articular surface. **b** The distal fracture fragment is angled dorsally, the carpus is subluxed posteriorly. **c** Sagittal CT confirms the intra-articular component of the fracture and the dorsal subluxation of the carpus

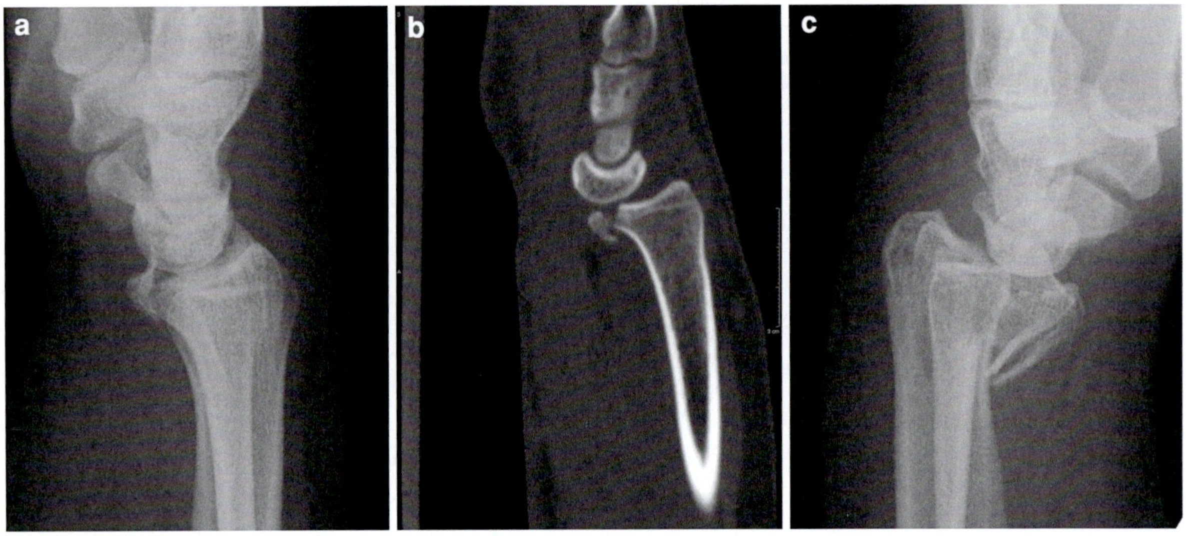

Fig. 10 **a** Lateral radiograph with a small fracture fragment of the distal radius on volar aspect. **b** Sagittal CT demonstrates the degree to which the carpus has subluxed volarly. **c** A second case where the volar fracture and carpal displacement is clearly evident on the radiograph. It involves nearly 50% of the articular surface

runs obliquely across the distal radius from the radial cortex into the joint separating the radial styloid from the parent bone. The injury is explained by the ligamentous attachments. The strong RSL and RLT ligaments attach to the radius on the styloid side and result in this avulsion injury.

Die punch injuries occur due to impaction of the lunate on the lunate fossa of the radius which results in a depressed comminuted intra-articular fracture of the radial articular surface which may have both sagittal and coronal components (Fig. 13). The full fracture extent may be difficult to see on plain films, but CT will demonstrate the disrupted articular surface which has both sagittal and coronal components. Depression of the fracture fragments arising in or near the lunate fossa is a key finding. There may be up to four fracture fragments. Commonly, this type of injury is seen as part of a more complex injury of the radius.

The use of eponymous names is prone to misuse. Unless all fully understand precisely what it describes, clinical confusion can result. Many

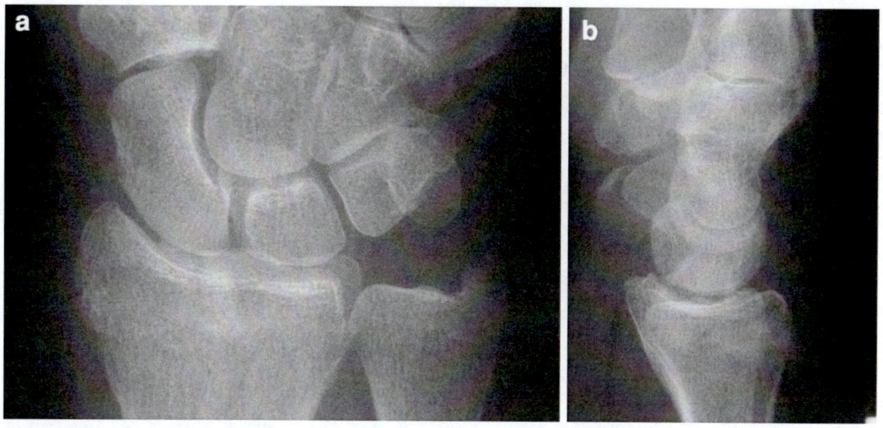

Fig. 11 **a** AP view there is some disruption of the normal trabecular pattern in the distal radius, and there is a slight step of the cortex. **b** On the lateral, there is a subtle buckling of the dorsal cortex. Note that the normal volar tilt of the distal radial articular surface has been reversed

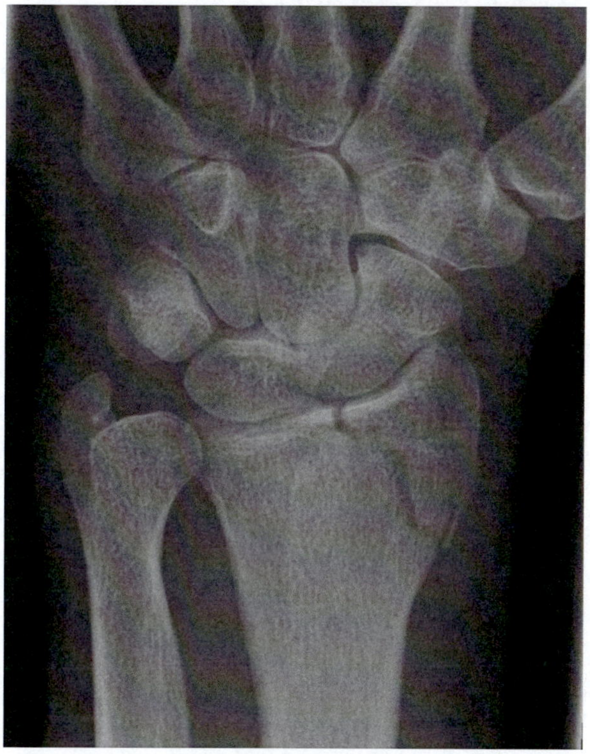

Fig. 12 There is an isolated fracture of the distal radius running obliquely through the distal radius to reach the articular surface. This separates the radial styloid from the rest of the bone

fractures do not fall precisely into any of the exact original descriptions. It must be appreciated that descriptions of injures that now have eponymous names attached were derived from clinical examination and cadaveric studies in the pre radiology era. The variations that can occur with all these injuries were not appreciated at that time. For this reason, it is probably better to give a full description of the fracture lines, fragments displacement and angulation and extent of articular involvement if any. To try and improve on this situation, several classification systems have been proposed (Frykman 1967; Fernández 1993; Melone 1986; Jupiter and Fernandez 1997). These are based variously on the mechanism of injury or the anatomy of the fracture. These systems attempt to provide a framework for treatment options by the orthopaedic surgeon, but none have been universally adopted. Unless locally agreed practice is to use one of the classifications to communicate findings to your orthopaedic surgeons, they are of little practical value to the reporting radiologist on a day-to-day basis. For this reason, they have not been included in this chapter.

2.3 Distal Radio-Ulnar joint

In the acute setting, disruption of the distal radio-ulnar joint (DRUJ) is seen in association with 3 types of fracture.

By far the most common is in association with fracture of the distal radius. Any significant radial shortening may result in disruption of the distal radio ulnar joint. The incidence of this is between 11 and 19% of distal radial fractures (May et al. 2002).

A different circumstance exists with the so-called Galeazzi fracture dislocation. In this event, a fracture of the shaft of the radius occurs with angulation and/or overlap of bone at the fracture site. Unless there is a fracture of the ulna as well, there will be dislocation

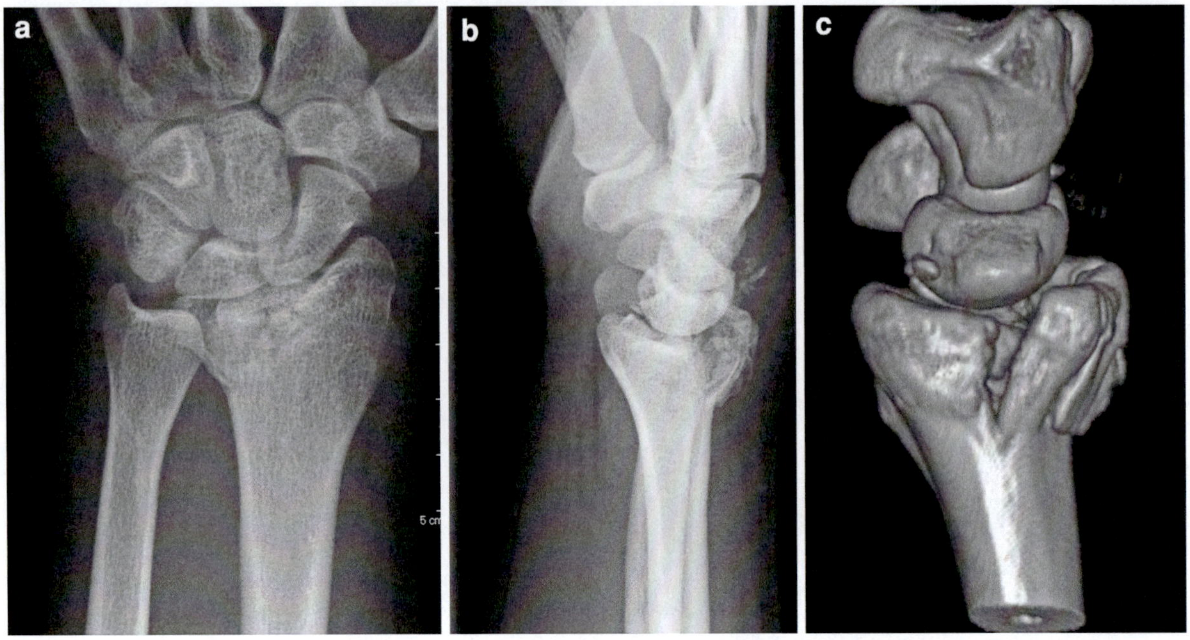

Fig. 13 **a** AP radiograph shows abnormality of the distal radius with comminution of the articular surface of the radius on the ulnar side. This is the lunate fossa of the radius. **b** The lateral view demonstrates disruption of the dorsal cortex. The lunate has been driven down onto the radius causing this injury pattern. **c** This 3D volume reconstructed CT is looking from the ulnar side of the wrist (the ulna has been removed). The lunate is seen disrupting the lunate fossa of the radial articular surface

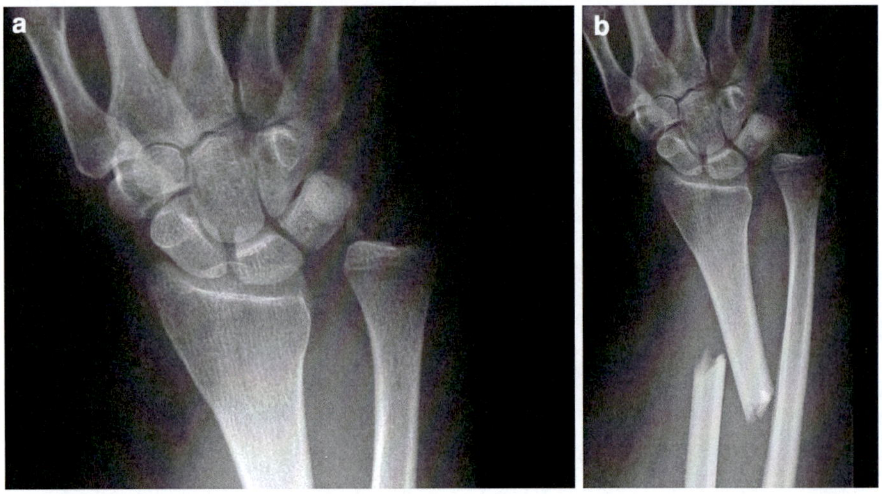

Fig. 14 **a** AP of wrist demonstrates a wide separation and displacement of the distal radio-ulnar joint, It is impossible for this to occur in isolation. There must be a more proximal fracture of the radius with angulation or overlap at the fracture site. **b** Radiograph of forearm demonstrates such a fracture

of the DRUJ. Conversely, if a DRUJ dislocation is evident on a wrist radiograph, then a more proximal radial fracture is likely to have occurred and radiographs of the whole forearm must be obtained (Fig. 14).

The third fracture associated with distal radio ulna joint disruption is the Essex-Lopresti fracture dislocation. This occurs when a fall on the outstretched hand results in an axial force driving the radius proximally with disruption of the DRUJ and the distal interosseous membrane finally resulting in fracture and or dislocation of the radial head. The injury is generally only sustained by a severe force.

Isolated disruption of the DRUJ is much less common and can be difficult to diagnose (Nicolaidis et al. 2000; Tsai and Paksima 2009). It is thought to

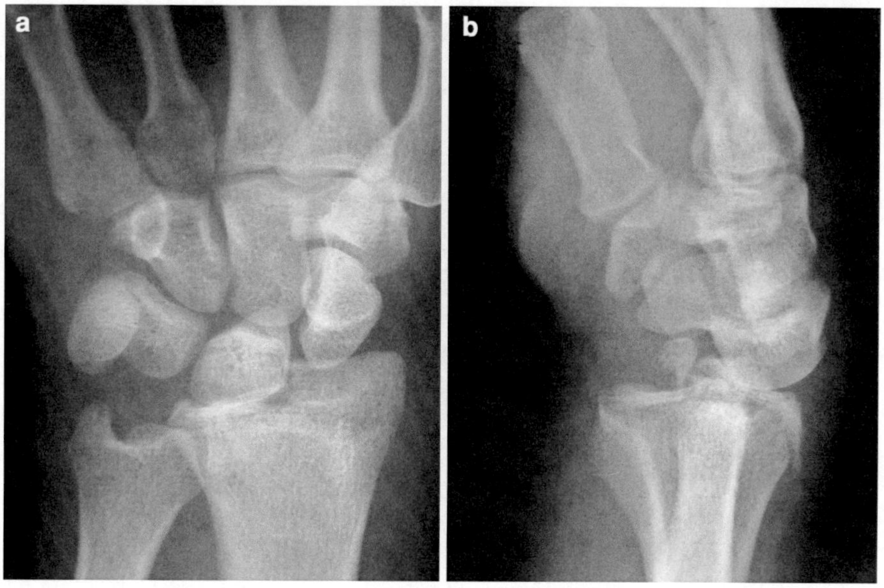

Fig. 15 **a** AP view of wrist with evidence of disruption of the carpal arcs. **b** On the lateral view, the whole carpus is displaced dorsally. The bony fragments on the volar aspect are due to avulsion by the volar ligaments attached to the volar aspect of the radius

occur with hyperpronation with fall on the outstretched hand. A fracture of the ulnar styloid process may be present, but this seen more commonly in association with a radial fracture. DRUJ disruption in turn is associated with injury of the TFCC and the associated stabilising ligaments. Thus, this tends to present more often as chronic wrist pain often with no definite acute incident.

Plain radiographs (Nakamura et al. 1995; Lo et al. 2001) and CT (Nakamura et al. 1996) have been utilised to evaluate the DRUJ, but can be difficult to assess with considerable overlap between normal and abnormal. There is an association between DRUJ disruption, ulna styloid process fracture and damage of the underlying TFCC.

Radiocarpal fracture dislocations (RCFD) are rare and occur due to high-energy injuries with both shearing and rotational components (Ilyas and Chaitanya 2008). They can occur in isolation but more commonly are associated with fracture of the distal radius. Dorsal displacement is more common than volar (Fig. 15). These injuries need to be differentiated from the Bartons fracture where a rim fracture of the radius is also present. In the Bartons fracture, the radial articular surface remains in contact with the proximal carpal row. With RCFD, the radial articular surface is no longer in alignment with the carpal row. This is best appreciated on the lateral radiograph by observing the position of the lunate relative to the radius. The dislocation may occur in isolation, but often a dorsal dislocation is associated with a volar rim fracture of the radius. This apparent paradox is explained by the ligamentous attachments. When the carpus dislocates dorsally, the volar extrinsic ligaments attached to the volar rim of the radius may avulse a bone fragment from this site (Lozano-Calderón et al. 2006). RCFD are also associated with intra-carpal fractures and fracture dislocations (see below).

There are two classifications for these injuries. Moneim et al. (1985) classified these injuries into 2 groups depending on whether there was associated intercarpal injury or not. An alternative classification is based on the size of the radial fracture fragment (Dumontier et al. 2001). In those with no or only a small radial fragment, there is likely to be major ligamentous disruption resulting in multidirectional instability. In those with a large radial styloid fragment separated from the underlying bone, the radiocarpal ligaments are likely to be intact. Reduction of the dislocation with fixation of the fracture is likely then to restore wrist stability.

3 Carpal Injuries

3.1 Scaphoid

The scaphoid is by far the most common of the carpal bones to sustain an injury and accounts for at least

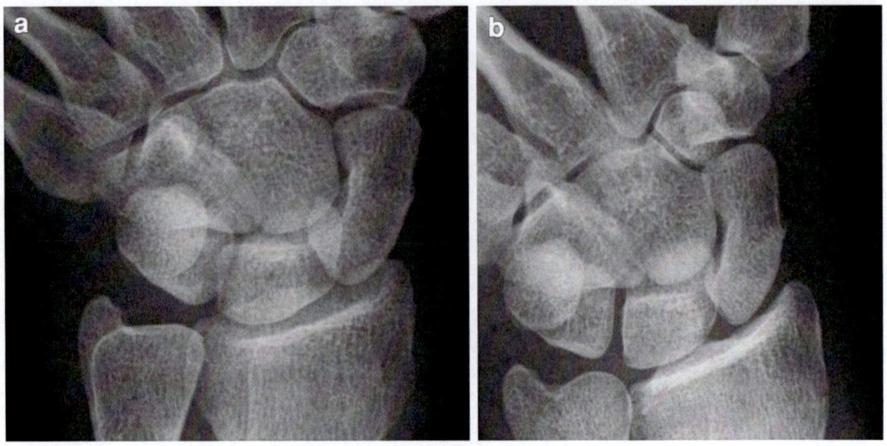

Fig. 16 In addition to the conventional AP and lateral views of wrist, if a scaphoid fracture is suspected, then additional view must be obtained. These are with **a** ulnar deviation of the wrist and **b** deviation and angulation of the tube towards the elbow

Table 1 Relative incidence of carpal bone fractures

Scaphoid	68.2%
Triquetrum	18.3%
Trapezium	4.3%
Lunate	3.9%
Capitate	1.9%
Hamate	1.7%
Pisiform	1.3%
Trapezoid	0.4%

60% of all carpal fractures (Gaebler 2006; Table 1). The propensity for this bone to fracture more often than all the other carpal bones combined is explained by its anatomy. Unique among the carpal bones the scaphoid bridges the proximal and distal carpal rows. As these two rows move to different degrees during wrist dorsiflexion, this places increased stress on the bridging scaphoid. This is compounded by the presence of the radiocapitate ligament that lies across the waist of the scaphoid. Both of these forces act to maximise the stress forces at the waist of the scaphoid thus accounting for the high incidence of injuries at this site. Furthermore, in extreme dorsiflexion, the scaphoid waist may impact upon the dorsal rim of the radius providing an additional mechanism of injury.

Radiography The scaphoid lies at about the angle of about 45° relative to the radial shaft in the sagittal plane. It is overlapped by the lunate, capitate and pisiform on the lateral view. Hence, the two conventional views of the wrist may fail to demonstrate some scaphoid fractures. With the PA view in particular, the X-ray beam passes obliquely through the scaphoid rather than at right angles to it, so a fracture line through the waist of the scaphoid will be traversed obliquely by the beam. Therefore, unless the fracture is widely separated, it is often not detected on this view. To overcome these problems, it is essential when a scaphoid injury is suspected clinically that additional dedicated views are obtained. Typically, 2 more radiographic projections are employed with the intention of elongating the scaphoid, projecting it clear of other carpal bones and allowing the X-ray beam to pass through the scaphoid perpendicular to its long axis. The projections used vary, but in the authors department a second PA view with ulnar deviation plus one with the tube angled at 45° towards the elbow is obtained (Figs. 16, 17).

This small bone causes more diagnostic and management difficulties than almost any other due to the nature of its blood supply. Its blood supply is unusual with the blood entering the distal pole first then passing into the proximal pole. The result is that when fracture occurs through the waist of the scaphoid which is the commonest site (80% of cases) and the proximal pole (10%) the blood supply to the proximal pole is interrupted (Fig. 18). This brings with it the danger that the proximal pole loses its vascular supply and develops avascular necrosis. Fractures of the waist are associated with 30% incidence of AVN, and disruption of the proximal pole almost always leads to this complication (Fig. 19). Alternatively, the lack of blood supply hinders healing at the fracture site and non-union of the fracture occurs (Fig. 20).

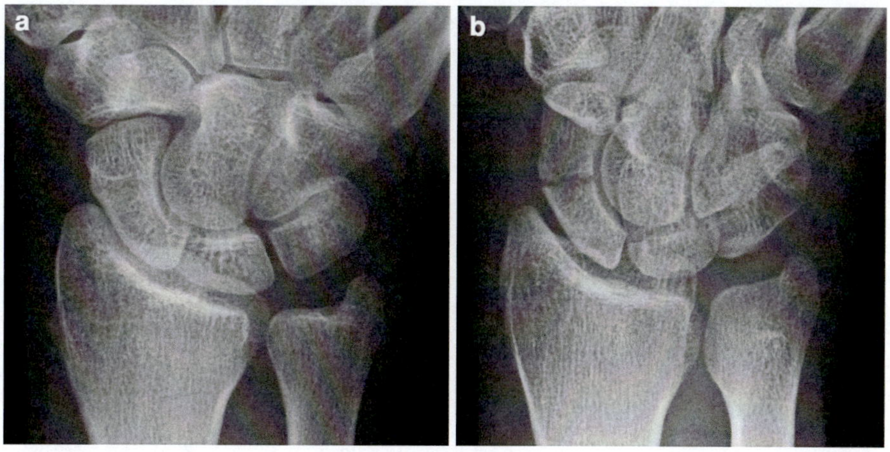

Fig. 17 Effect of scaphoid views. **a** Conventional AP view does not show any definite abnormality. **b** Angled view clearly demonstrates a now obvious fracture

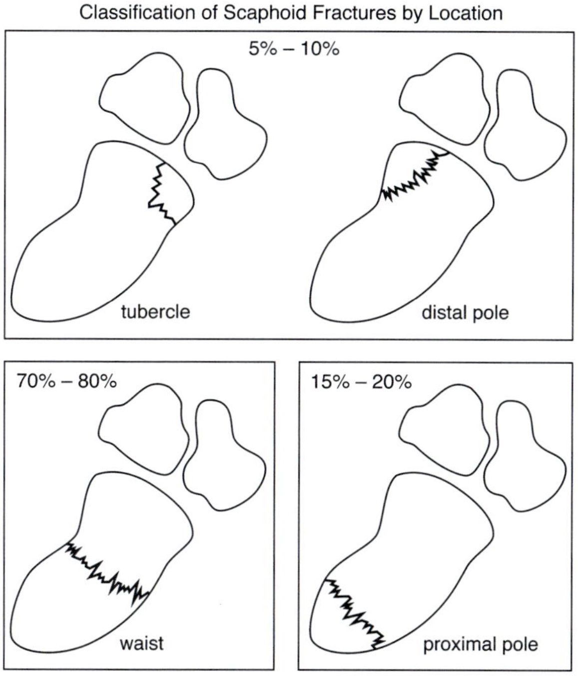

Fig. 18 The sites of scaphoid fracture with frequency of occurrence. Fractures of the waist account for the great majority

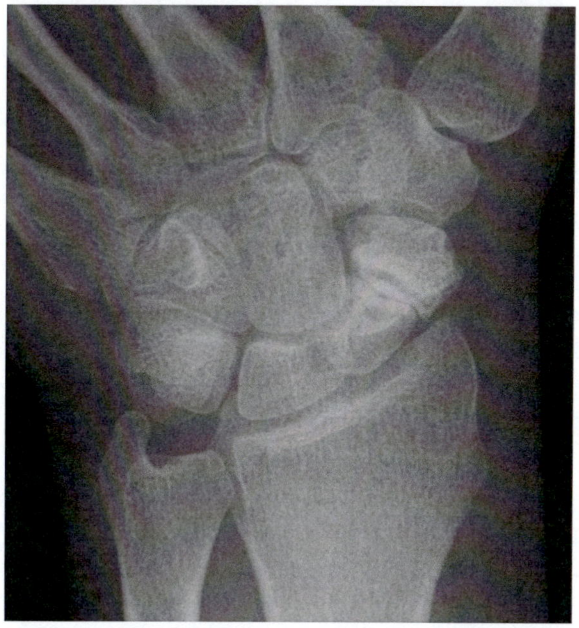

Fig. 19 Initial radiograph taken at time of injury demonstrated a fracture of the waist of the scaphoid. This radiograph taken 18 months later shows that the fracture line remains well demarcated with sclerotic edges. This represents established non-union of the fracture

Historically, extreme care has been taken in managing patients with suspected scaphoid injuries. Because of the difficulties that may occur in identifying scaphoid fractures on radiographs, a combined clinical and radiological approach has been adopted to minimise the possibility that a fracture has been over looked. In patients with an appropriate history and clinical findings suggestive of scaphoid fracture, an initial scaphoid series of radiographs is obtained. If a fracture is identified, the wrist is immobilised and managed accordingly. If no fracture identified, it is recognised that this does not completely exclude a fracture due to the difficulties described above. Accordingly, because of the possible long-term complications that may arise after suboptimal treatment of a fracture the patient is managed as if a fracture is present and the wrist is immobilised. The patient is then reviewed at about 10 days when further radiographs are obtained. It is stated that resorption

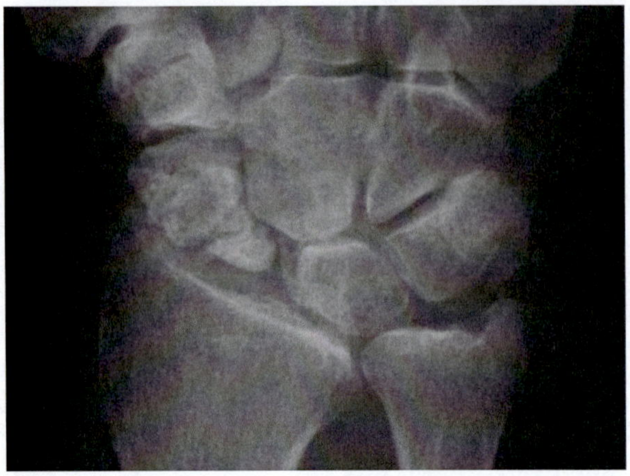

Fig. 20 The proximal pole of the scaphoid is sclerotic and shrunken. This is the appearance of established avascular necrosis some 5 years after initial injury

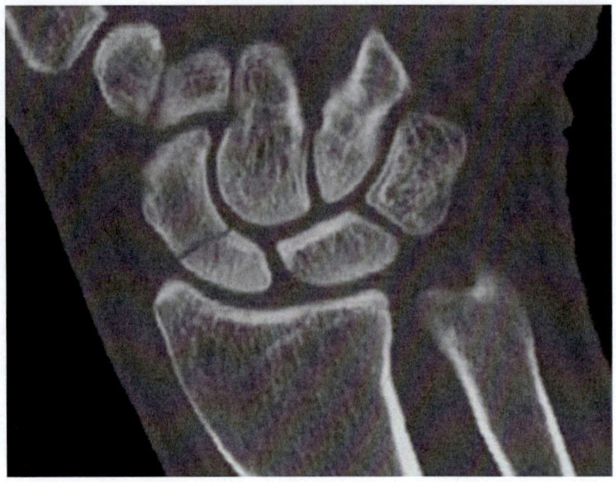

Fig. 21 Multislice CT with coronal reconstruction demonstrates a fracture of the scaphoid. No abnormality was evident on the plain radiographs

will occur around a fracture site rendering it visible on delayed radiographs. This process may need to be repeated on several occasions until either a fracture is clearly identified or the patient's symptoms resolve. "We overtreat a lot of patient to avoid undertreating a few" (Barton 1992).

This practice or similar modifications remain in common use (Brookes-Fazakerley et al. 2009); however, it has been questioned in the era of more sophisticated imaging options. To understand the validity of the management rationale, some basic back ground information is required.

How many fractures are present but not visible at the time of the initial radiographs?

Most studies have shown that in fact a great majority of fractures (85% or more) are visible on the initial films (Leslie and Dickson 1981; Brøndum et al. 1992). Some even consider that all fractures can be identified (Duncan and Thurston 1985).

How many patients develop non-union or avascular necrosis?

The same authors independently found that these complications occurred in 5% of patients with a scaphoid fracture.

How often are fractures identified on follow-up films?

In a recent study using MR as the gold standard, it was found that detection of occult fractures on follow-up films was extremely inaccurate, with sensitivity as low as 9% and very poor interobserver reliability (Low and Raby 2005). This confirmed observations by others (Tiel-Van Buul et al. 1992a, b). It is apparent that clinicians rely on clinical findings rather than radiographs to guide management.

To improve on this situation, for many years other imaging modalities have been utilised including isotope bone scan CT and MRI. A recent international survey (Groves et al. 2006) however has shown that despite the extensive evidence base the majority of departments still undertake repeat radiographs when no fracture is seen. Alternative imaging modalities are employed only as a secondary investigation and in order of frequency these are MR CT and isotope scan.

Isotope bone scans are sensitive but non-specific. Whilst almost all fractures will show evidence of increased isotope uptake if scanned 3 or more days after the acute event, approximately 35% of increased isotope up take in the carpus is due to abnormality other than a scaphoid fracture, and additional imaging may be needed to resolve this issue (Tiel-Van Buul et al. 1992a, b; Tiel-Van Buul et al. 1993; Waizenegger et al. 1994; Beeres et al. 2007).

CT is utilised more than isotope scans (Groves et al. 2006). Whilst CT can undoubtedly identify some occult fractures (Fig. 21), there is still an error rate (Adey et al. 2007), and it has been shown that trabecular bone injury will not be detected although the relevance of this is debatable (Memarsadeghi et al. 2006; La Hei et al. 2007).

MRI Is now the investigation of choice (Foex et al. 2005), but use remains limited due to perceptions that

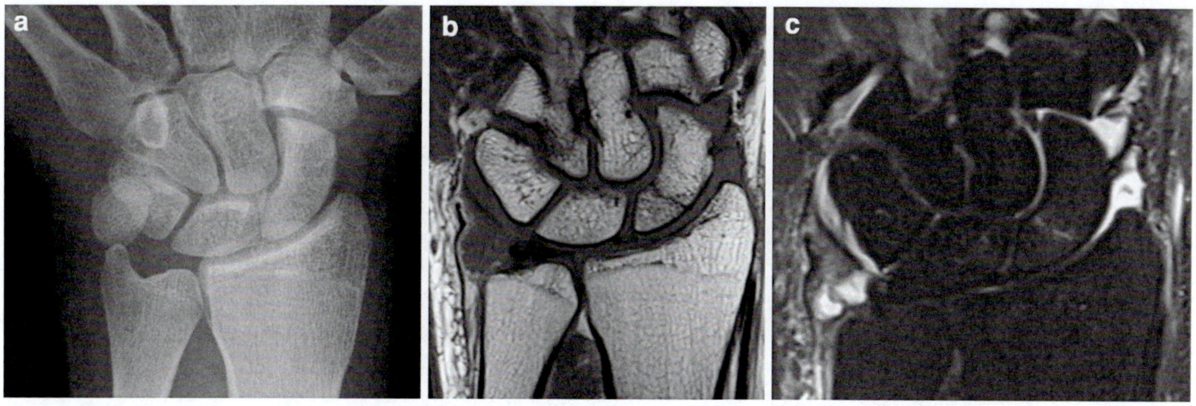

Fig. 22 **a** Radiographs are normal. No scaphoid fracture identified on any view. **b** and **c** Coronal T1-weighted and STIR MR demonstrates a fracture across the scaphoid waist seen as a low signal linear line on the T1-weighted and high signal line on the STIR sequence

its availability is restricted. There is extensive literature regarding the use of MR in patients with suspected scaphoid fracture not evident on plain film (Fig. 22) (Raby 2001; Brydie and Raby 2003). This consistently indicates that MR accurately identifies scaphoid fractures, and other carpal or radial fractures that may be responsible for the patient's symptoms. Just as importantly a normal MR will exclude bony injury allowing early discharge of the patient from hospital care, and it is this fact that renders it cost effective (Kumar et al. 2005). Several studies have confirmed this to be the case. The ability to be able to reliably discharge patients without need for immobilisation, further hospital attendance or repeat radiographs is the most important benefit of this strategy (Dorsay et al. 2001).

Despite the best efforts of all concerned in the management of patients with scaphoid fractures, non-union or AVN still occurs in a small proportion of patients. Attention has thus been directed to imaging techniques that may indicate that a recognised fracture is either failing to unite or developing AVN in the hope that early detection of these complications would allow early intervention (Figs 23, 24). To date, evidence of ability to reliably detect these complications is limited. The major focus has been on the use of MRI with contrast enhancement. The theory is that as fracture of the scaphoid waist may interrupt the blood supply to the proximal pole, then on contrast enhanced scans lack of enhancement of the proximal pole will indicate lack of blood supply and thus poor prognosis with non-union or avascular necrosis as a long-term result (Dawson et al. 2001). Studies have had conflicting results, and the numbers in the studies have been small (Singh et al. 2004; Cerezal et al. 2000) There is no good evidence that contrast-enhanced MR can accurately predict either of these complications. However, whether or not these complications are detectable earlier by imaging is of little consequence if the final outcome remains unaltered. To date, there is no robust evidence that there is any improvement in outcome as a result of contrast-enhanced MR, and one study has shown no outcome benefit in a group of patients who underwent MR prior to surgery (Singh et al. 2004). Further studies with accumulation of large data sets are required to confirm or refute its value.

CT also has its advocates (Smith et al. 2009) with a recent paper suggesting benefit in the detection of AVN and non-union with improved outcome after surgery. Confirmatory evidence from other sources is awaited. CT however is undoubtedly of value in detecting certain other complications of scaphoid fracture. Some scaphoid fractures unite satisfactorily but may develop the so-called hump back deformity (Fig. 25). This occurs when the distal fracture fragment flexes in a palmer direction with the distal carpal row whilst the proximal fragment rotates dorsally with the proximal carpal row. This results in angulation occurring at the fracture site with a prominent dorsal bony protrusion and is best appreciated on CT. It is associated with persisting pain, restriction of movement and development of arthritic changes. CT can also assist in confirming that a fracture has united

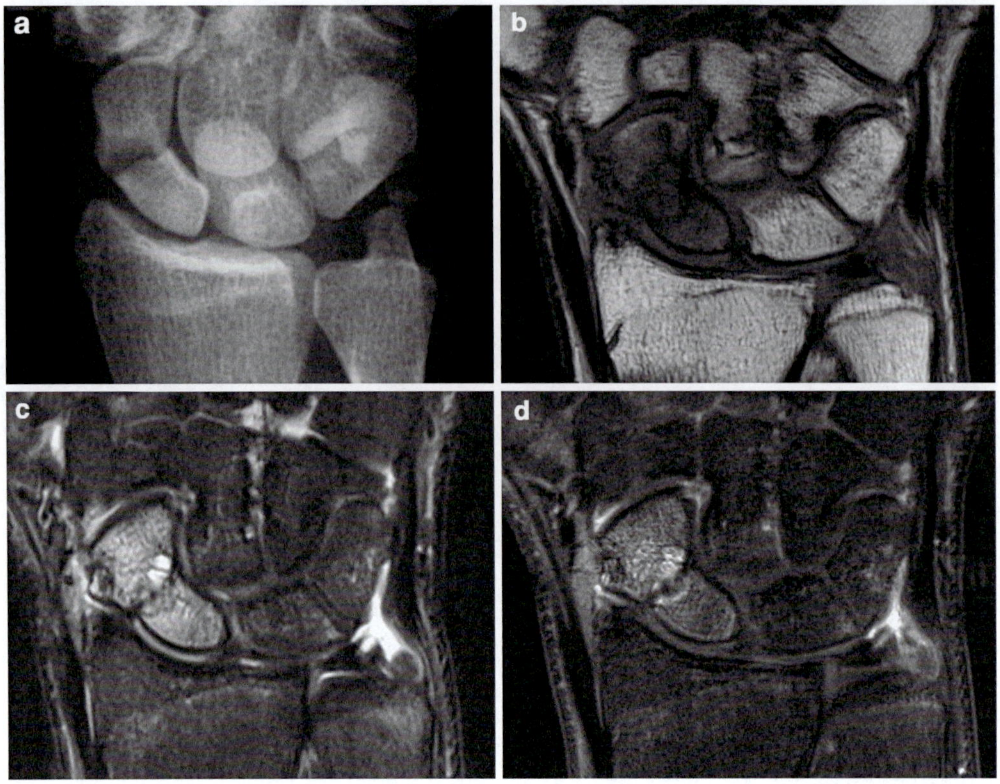

Fig. 23 **a** Radiograph shows scaphoid waist fracture with cystic bone resorption 5 months after initial injury. **b** Coronal T1-weighted image. There is loss of normal marrow signal in the proximal pole. **c** STIR sequence shows diffuse high signal indicating marrow oedema. **d** Post-contrast T1 weighting with fat saturation shows enhancement of the proximal pole suggesting it retains a vascular supply

when plain films suggest that a fracture line persists (Fig. 26).

3.2 Other Carpal Fractures

After the scaphoid, the triquetral bone is most commonly injured accounting for 18–20% of injuries (Table 1). This injury is usually due to a bony avulsion of the insertion of the radio and ulno triquetral ligaments. Typically, the fracture is not evident on the PA view but can be seen on the lateral as a bone fragment seen on the dorsal aspect of the wrist (Fig. 27). Transverse fracture can also occur due to extreme dorsiflexion with compression of the triquetrum between the ulna and hamate. These fractures may be seen in association with Perilunate dislocation (see below).

Other carpal bone injuries are all relatively rare, each of the other carpal bone accounting each for only 2–3% of injuries. CT or MR may have a useful role to play in these injuries that are often difficult to detect on plain films.

Fractures of the hamate can involve the hook in isolation or the body. Hook fractures are often associated with sporting activities since the handle of a bat or racquet abuts the hook. Conventional radiographs will often fail to demonstrate such injuries that may therefore be diagnosed as soft tissue injuries or "wrist sprain" only (De Schrijver and De Smet 2001). Additional views have been shown to demonstrate these fractures such as the so-called carpal tunnel view. However, if such a fracture is strongly suspected clinically, then CT will demonstrate them most clearly (Fig. 28) (Kato et al. 2000). Fracture of the body can occur in isolation but more often are associated with other carpal fractures or with fracture dislocation of the 5th metacarpal base. These injuries are usually evident on conventional radiographs (Fig. 29).

Capitate fractures in isolation are uncommon. Typically, fractures occur through the waist of the

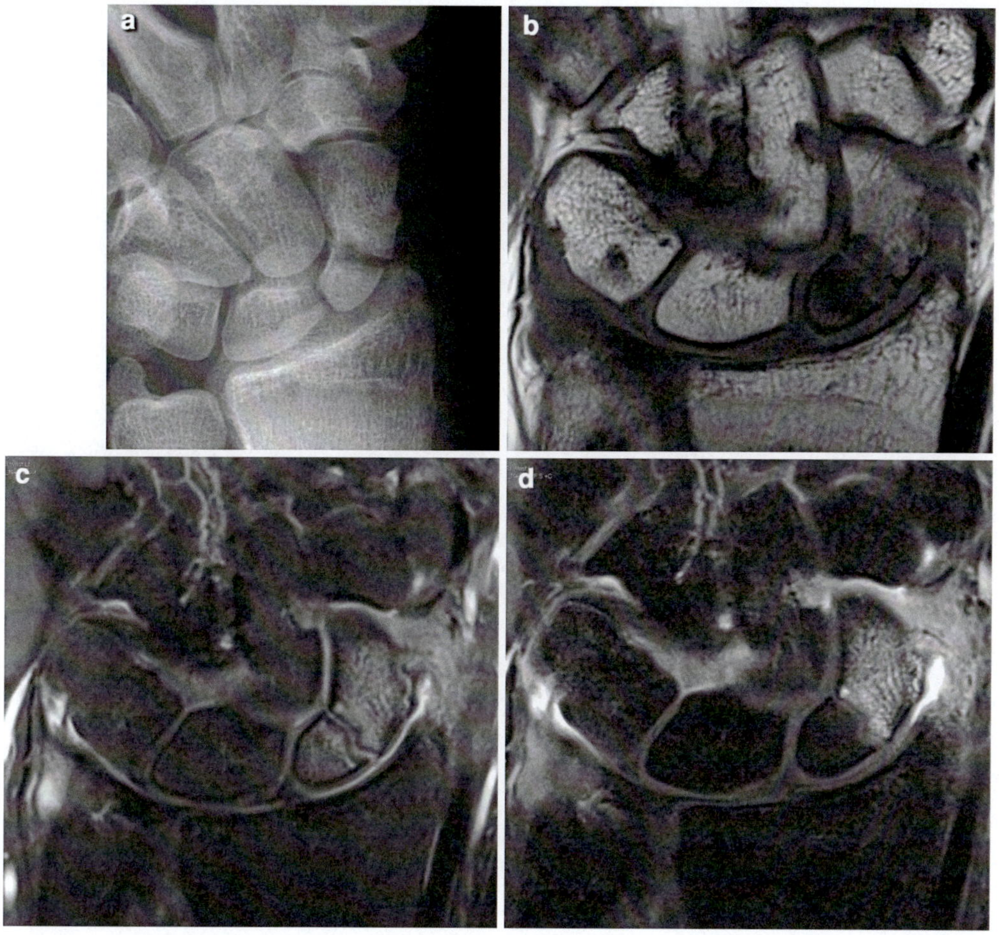

Fig. 24 **a** Fracture of scaphoid proximal pole now 6 months old. **b** There is complete loss of normal marrow signal in the proximal pole on T1-weighted image. **c** PD fat-saturated image shows diffuse marrow oedema. **d** Post-contrast T1-weighed with fat saturation. There is no enhancement of proximal pole suggesting loss of blood supply

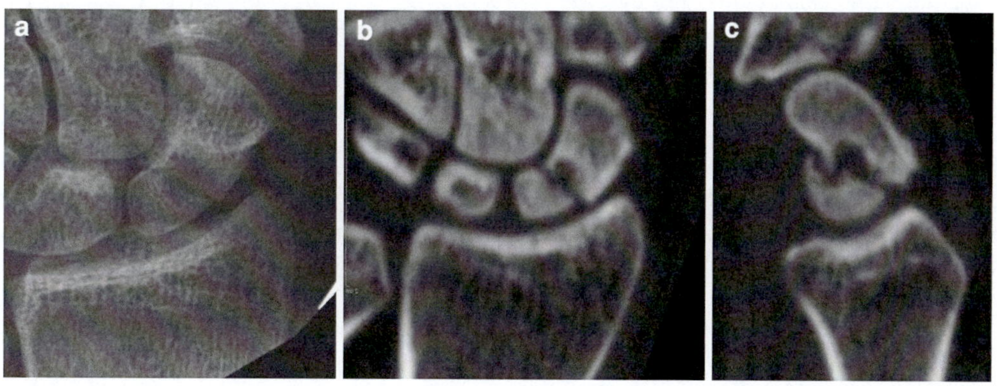

Fig. 25 **a** Radiograph shows a fracture across the proximal third of the scaphoid. Resorption at fracture site has resulted in cystic change at the fracture line. **b** CT undertaken to confirm non-union. There is no evidence of any bony continuity at the fracture site. **c** Sagittal reconstruction demonstrates displacement at the fracture site resulting in the so-called hump back deformity

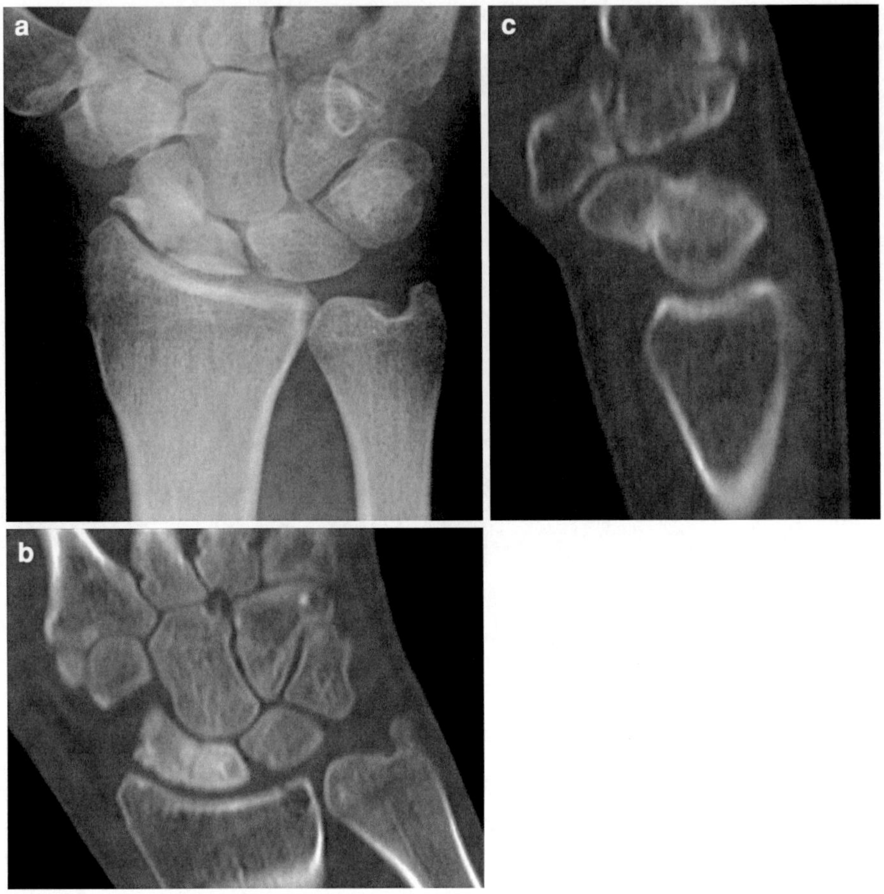

Fig. 26 **a** Radiograph of scaphoid fracture after 6 months. The fracture line persists suggesting possible non-union. **b** Coronal reformatted CT. The scaphoid is sclerotic with a linear lucency across the waist suggesting non-union. **c** Sagittal reformatted CT shows that in fact there is bony union across the majority of the fracture site. A step in the cortex is the cause of the linear lucency seen on the previous images mimicking a persistent fracture line

capitate. These can be seen on the AP view of the wrist (Fig. 30). More commonly capitate fractures occur in association with perilunate dislocation. Fractures occur as a result of wrist dorsiflexion. With more severe injury, the proximal pole of the capitate can be displaced and rotated through either 90° or 180° (Fig. 31). These findings are seen along with other fractures of the greater arc or zone of vulnerability.

Lunate fractures are uncommon and typically are small chip or avulsion fractures. Only occasionally do the fractures extend through the bone. The principal complication is that of avascular necrosis (Keinbock's disease). Pisiform and trapezoid fractures are rare and are not considered further.

3.3 Carpal Dislocations

The proximal carpal row (scaphoid, lunate and triquetral) act as a functional unit and is referred to as an intercalated (inserted in between) segment. That is a functional row of bone inserted between the distal radius and the distal carpal row. These three bones act as a keystone coordinating wrist motion and transmitting force between wrist and hand. The proximal row of carpal bone has no tendons attached and relies on complex ligamentous attachments as well as bony configuration for stability. The pisiform although it lies proximally is not functionally associated with these bones. It is a sesamoid bone within the tendon of flexor carpi ulnaris.

The distal row of trapezium, trapezoid, capitate and hamate is more stable and forms a transverse arch supporting the metacarpal bones. The distal row of carpal bones are rarely disrupted unless associated with other injuries (see below). The scaphoid that lies at an angle bridges the proximal and distal carpal row and normally contributes to stability of the carpus. Fractures of the waist of the scaphoid break this bony linkage between the two rows. Most carpal fractures and dislocations occur due to falling on the

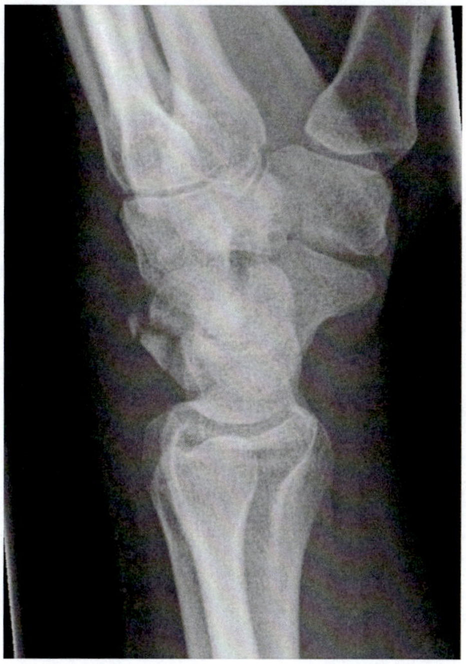

Fig. 27 This lateral radiograph shows several bone fragments on the dorsal aspect at mid-carpal level. This finding almost invariably indicates a triquetral fracture although the AP view will usually be normal. Further investigation by cross-sectional imaging to prove the origin of the bone fragments is generally not required or indicated

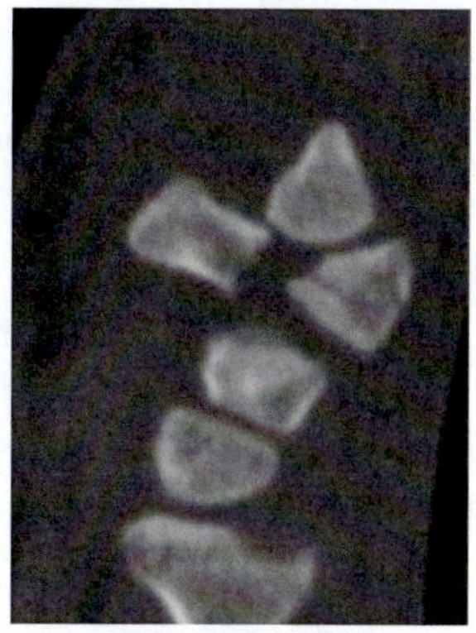

Fig. 28 Sagittal CT demonstrating a fracture of the hook of the hamate. This was not visible on conventional radiographs

outstretched wrist with the wrist forced into a hyperextended position. Evaluation of these injuries is aided by the evaluation of lines or arcs drawn through the carpus. Somewhat confusingly this nomenclature does not relate to the same arcs used to describe normal carpal alignment (Yeager and Dalinka 1985). In this terminology, the lesser arc separates the lunate from the adjacent carpal bones (Fig. 32). The greater arc passes through the scaphoid, capitate, hamate, triquetral (and in some modifications the distal radius and ulna). Injury through the lesser arc represents a lunate dislocation. Injuries of the greater arc indicate a perilunate injury. This may be an isolated perilunate dislocation or with associated fracture(s) of bones along this arc. Virtually, all combinations of fracture can occur along this zone. This is best referred to as the "Zone of Vulnerability" (Johnson 1980). An abnormality anywhere along this arc should prompt a thorough search of all points to identify associated fractures. Injuries of the greater arc are twice as common as those of the lesser arc.

Carpal dislocations thus most commonly involve the proximal row of bones, and the lunate is most often involved. Understanding the lateral radiograph

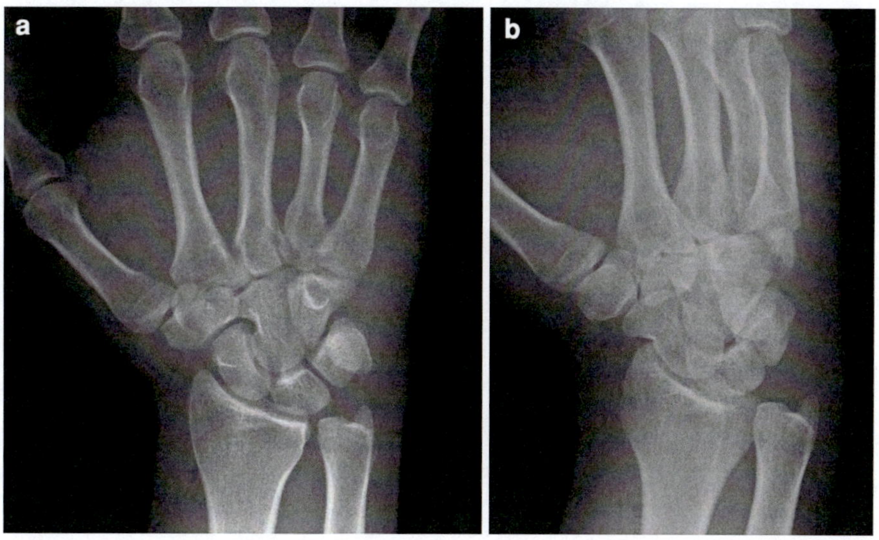

Fig. 29 **a** AP radiograph of wrist is normal. **b** Oblique view demonstrates a vertical fracture of the hamate

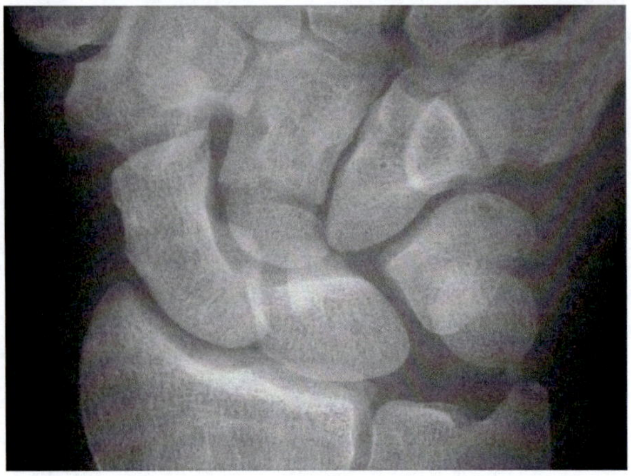

Fig. 30 There is fracture through the proximal third of the capitate. This is unusual in isolation

is key to detect these injuries although valuable information is also available on the PA view. On a normal lateral view of the wrist, there should be alignment of the lunate with the distal radius and the capitate. That is to say that a line drawn through the centre of the lunate should inferiorly pass through the radial articular surface and superiorly should pass through the centre of the capitate (Fig. 33). If this rule is broken, a carpal dislocation is certain. We (Raby et al. 2005) have likened this to a saucer (the radial articular surface) with a cup (the lunate) sitting on it. Within the cup, there should sit an apple (the capitate). Lunate dislocation occurs with hyperextension injuries. On a PA radiograph, the normal intercarpal

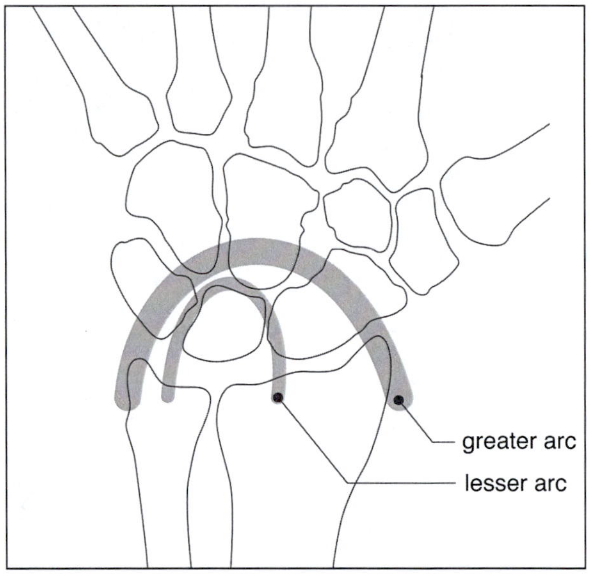

Fig. 32 Carpal fracture dislocations occur along the greater arc or zone of vulnerability

distances are disrupted with bony overlap evident. The lunate appears to have a triangular shape where normally it has a trapezoid appearance. It is on the lateral film however where the diagnosis is most easily detected. Here, a dislocated lunate will be seen displaced to the volar aspect. It is rotated so that is has the appearance of a new moon (Fig. 34). The alignment of the radius and capitate is preserved, but the lunate (the cup) lies palmer to the line drawn through the radius and capitate. Lunate dislocation is most

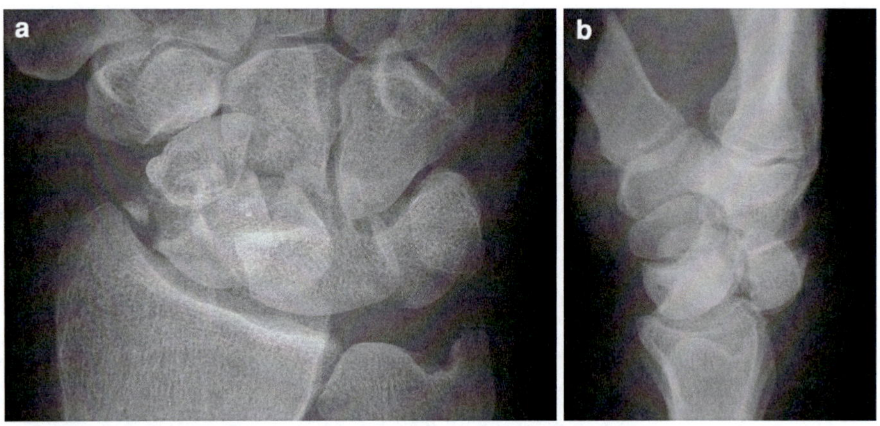

Fig. 31 **a** Complex mid carpal fracture dislocation. There are fractures of the scaphoid and proximal third of the capitate. **b** On the lateral view, the proximal capitate articular surface can be seen rotated through 90° lying dorsal to the lunate. There is perilunate dislocation of the carpus. Capitate fracture are more commonly seen in association with these mid-carpal injuries

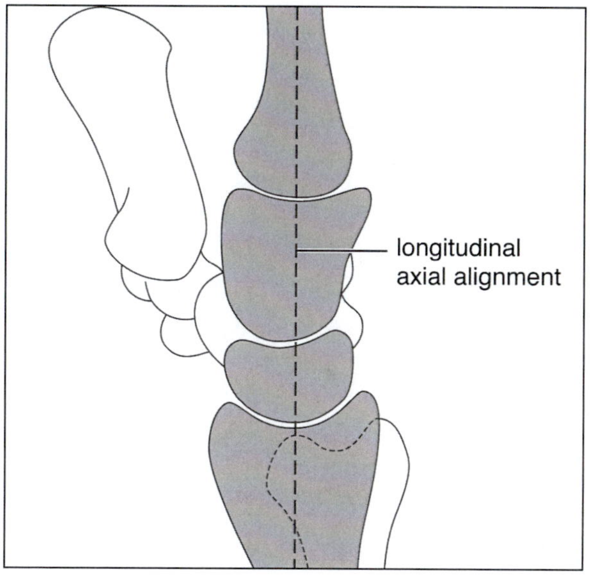

Fig. 33 The normal alignment of the three key bones on the lateral view. The capitate sits on the lunate which sits on the radius. A line drawn through the capitate should pass through the approximate centre of the lunate and distal radial articular surface

commonly an isolated finding with additional fractures found only uncommonly. The maxim "the cup should never be empty" is a simplistic but effective way of detecting these injuries.

Perilunate dislocation is also a hyperextension injury and is often associated with other carpal injuries (see above) most commonly a fracture of the scaphoid. It is more common than lunate dislocation. In this injury, the lunate remains aligned with the radius, but the capitate and the rest of the distal carpal row are displaced in a volar direction (Fig. 35). For this to occur, there must be disruption of some of the intra-carpal ligaments. The injury is often not apparent on the PA views, but on the lateral film the lunate (cup) remains on the saucer (distal radius). The capitate (apple) does not sit in the cup but lies posterior (volarly). As already seen perilunate dislocation is typically associated with other fractures along the greater arc zone of vulnerability (Fig. 36). When there are both fractures and perilunate dislocation present, the convention is to describe first the fractures then the dislocation. In this case, the description should be of a trans-scaphoid, trans–triquetral and perilunate dislocation.

Scapho-lunate disassociation is also known as rotatory subluxation of the scaphoid. It is a ligamentous injury occurring with forced wrist extension. Several ligaments are disrupted in this injury. In sequence, the radioscaphoid, the volar radiocapitate and finally the scapho-lunate ligament fail. This allows the distal scaphoid pole to rotate in a volar direction. On plain radiographs, the injury can be identified by noting a widening of the intercarpal distance between scaphoid and lunate. This is the so-called Terry Thomas sign. The rotation of the

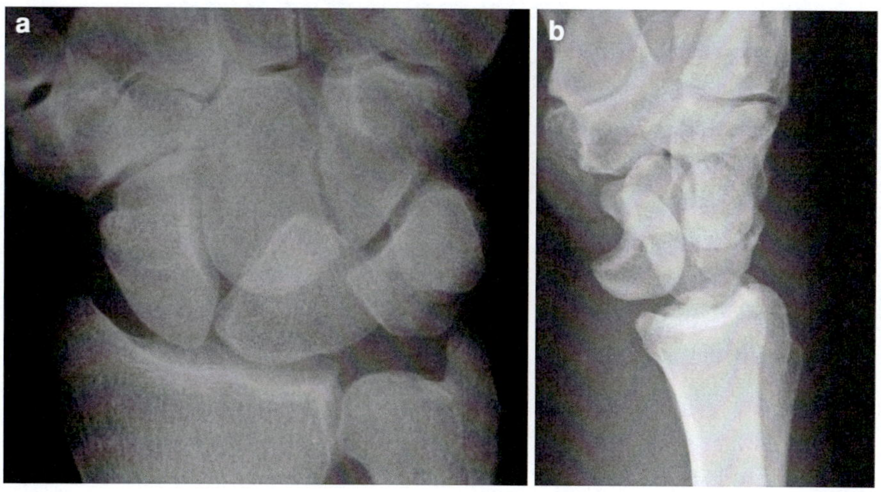

Fig. 34 **a** There is disruption of the proximal carpal arc with interruptions at the junctions of lunate with the scaphoid and triquetral. The lunate has a triangular configuration compared with the normal quadrilateral shape. **b** Lateral view demonstrates loss of the normal alignment of the radius, lunate and capitate with the lunate rotated and displaced volarly. These are all signs of lunate dislocation

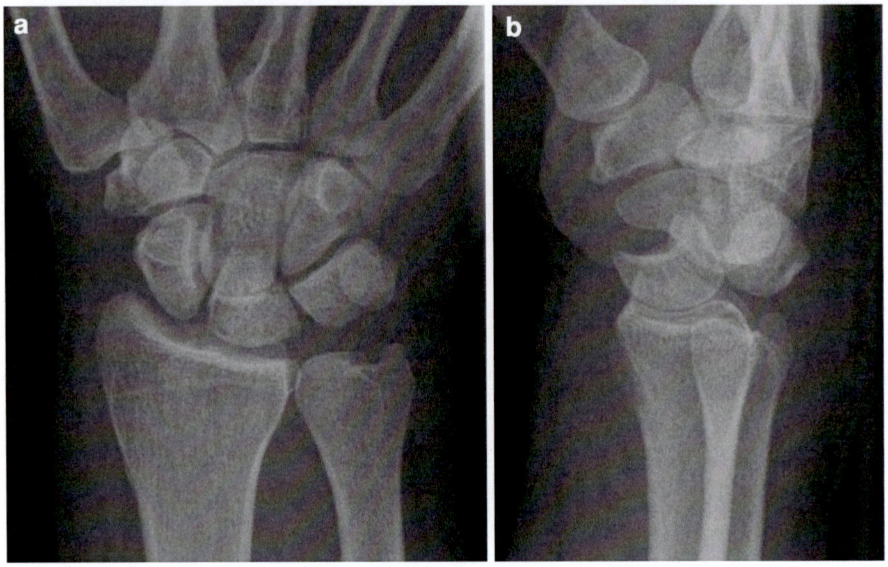

Fig. 35 **a** There is little to see on the AP view of the wrist apart from the triangular configuration of the lunate. The arcs are maintained. **b** On the lateral view, however, there is loss of the normal carpal alignment. The lunate sits normally on the radius, but the capitate now lies dorsal to the lunate indicating a perilunate dislocation. The cup of the lunate is empty

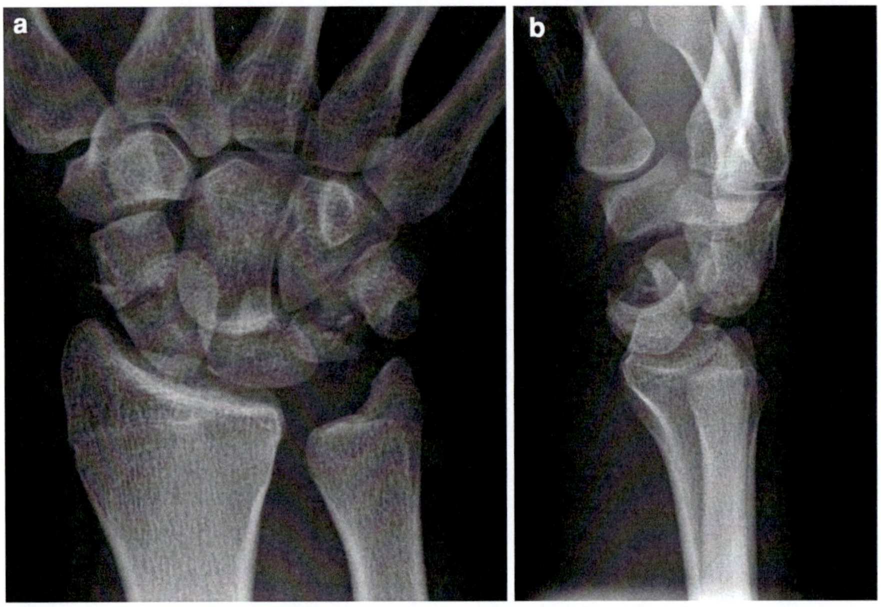

Fig. 36 **a** AP radiograph demonstrates fractures of the waist of the scaphoid and triquetral bones. There is disruption of the second carpal arc with loss of the normal intercarpal spacing. There is marked overlap of both scaphoid and lunate with the capitate. The lunate has an abnormal triangular appearance. **b** The lateral view demonstrates the capitate does not sit on the lunate but lies dorsal to it. This is a trans-scaphoid trans-triquetral perilunate dislocation

scaphoid causes it to be foreshortened, and the distal pole seen end on has a ring-like appearance (Fig. 37) (Hudson et al. 1976). On occasion, the radioscaphoid ligament avulses a bone fragment from the radial styloid attachment, but more often there is no fracture evident so that this is injury that can be easily overlooked.

4 Carpo-Metacarpal Injuries

There is normally little movement at the carpo-metacarpal joints. Strong ligaments bind the distal carpal row to the base of the metacarpals, and there is little movement possible either on palmer or

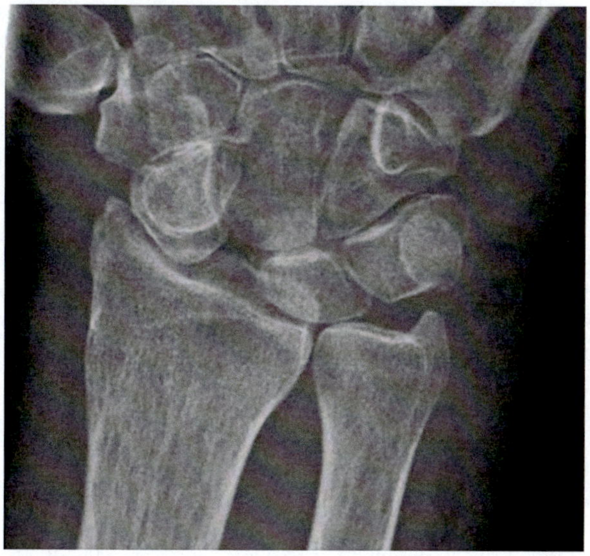

Fig. 37 There is widening of the gap between lunate and scaphoid. The scaphoid has rotated and appears foreshortened. There is a ring-like appearance of the distal pole due to the pole now being seen end on. This indicates disruption of the scapholunate ligament. Known correctly as rotatory subluxation of the scaphoid, it has been known as the "Terry Thomas sign" in the UK after an actor who had a large gap between his front teeth

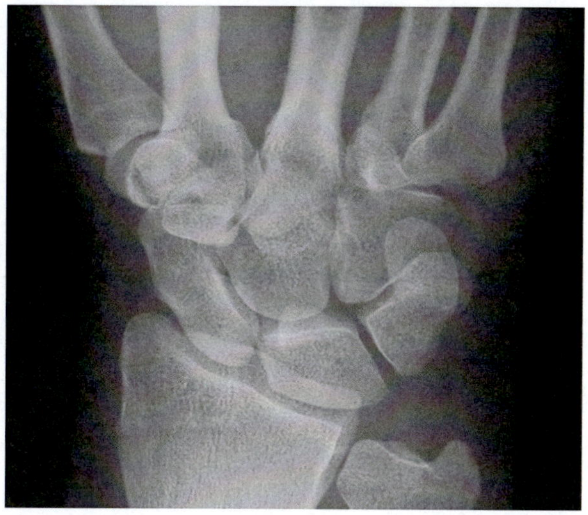

Fig. 38 AP radiograph of wrist. There is loss of the carpometacarpal spaces with increased bone density at the base of the 2nd and 3rd metacarpals due to bone overlap indicating dislocation at this site

dorsiflexion. Dislocations at this site only rarely occur in isolation and are more commonly associated with fractures of the metacarpal bases or the adjacent carpal bones, most commonly the hamate and capitate. These injuries are rare and result from high-energy axial loading of the metacarpals such as occurs when delivering a punch. The site of injury often leads to request from the referring clinician for radiographs of the hand rather than the wrist. An AP and oblique view will be obtained.

Disruption of the carpo-metacarpal joint may occur in isolation or may be associated with fracture of either the proximal metacarpal or the adjacent carpal bone. Isolated dislocations without associated fracture are difficult to identify. These injuries can be detected by observation of the loss of the normal gaps between the distal carpal row and the base of the metacarpals and/or by identifying areas of increased bone density due to the resultant bone overlap (Fig. 38). Fisher et al. (1983) described the appearance of the carpo-metacarpal joint from the second to fifth metacarpal as having an elongated M shape. The articular surfaces of the metacarpals and adjacent carpal bones form two parallel lines with this M shape. Loss of this normal configuration should alert the viewer to a possible metacarpal dislocation. All of these findings are best seen on the AP view. Where there is suspicion on the standard radiograph series, a lateral of the hand may add further useful information. The displaced metacarpal will then be visible as almost all are dislocated dorsally (Fig. 39). Metacarpal fractures when present aid identification of the injury. Carpal fractures may be impossible to see on plain films and may only be evident on subsequent CT (Fig. 40) (Kaewlai et al. 2008; You et al. 2007). A common injury is that of fracture dislocation of the 5th metacarpal, and this accounts for 50% of single ray dislocations. It is likely that this is due to the attachment of the extensor and flexor carpi ulnaris tendons to the 5th metacarpal base which draw the dislocated bone proximally resulting in bony overlap. The second metacarpal accounts for 25% of solitary dislocations. Multiple dislocations are more common. Dislocation of the 5th metacarpal plus one or more of the other metacarpals accounts for 80% of injuries at this level (Rodgers 2001).

5 Acute Soft Tissue Injuries

In acute trauma, soft tissue injuries are common but are usually overshadowed by the presence of bony fractures and dislocations. Thus, injuries of the

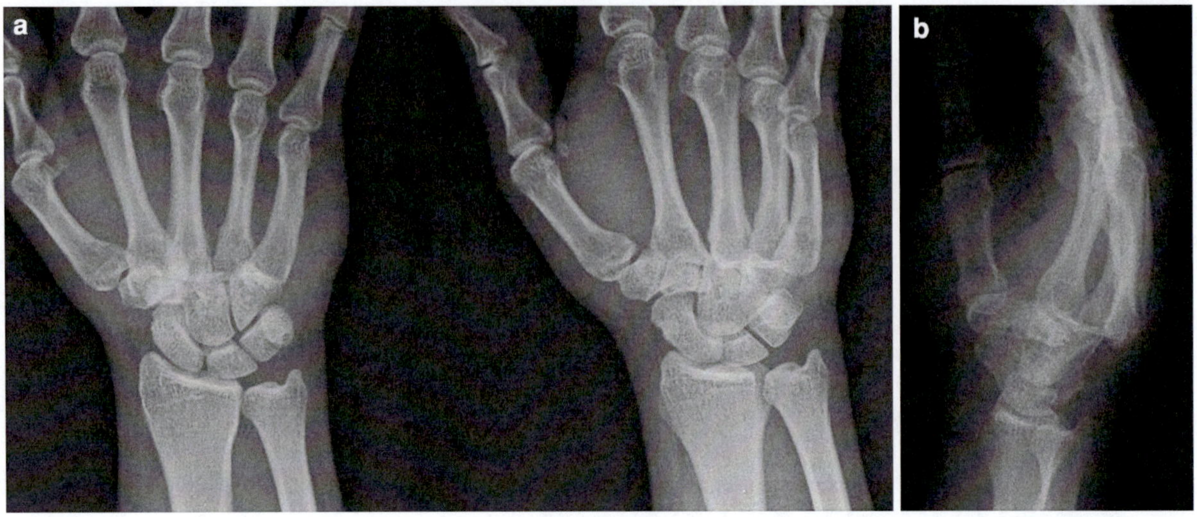

Fig. 39 **a** AP and oblique radiographs of wrist and hand. There is loss of the normal carpal-metacarpal spacing at the base of the 3rd to 5th metacarpals. Increased sclerosis is also evident, meaning there must either be bone impaction or overlap. **b** An additional lateral view demonstrates dorsal dislocation of the metacarpals

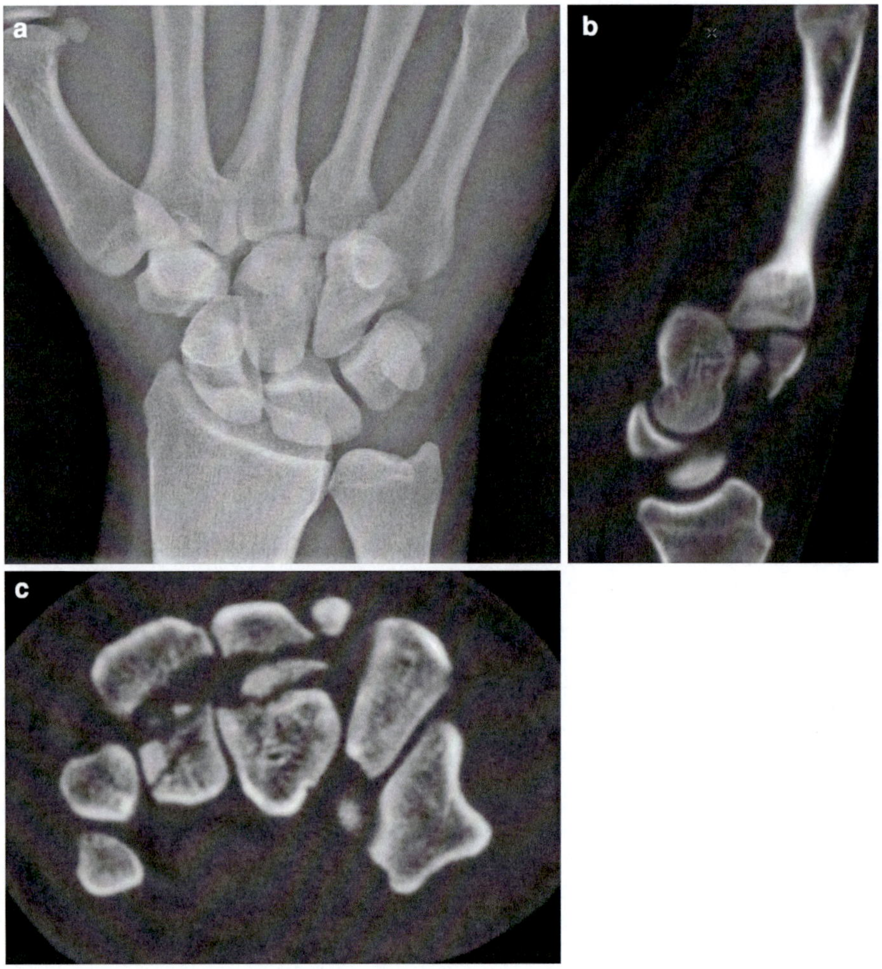

Fig. 40 **a** Loss of carpo-metacarpal space at 5th metacarpal. Note also there is loss of alignment of the third metacarpal with the capitate. **b** Sagittal CT image demonstrates dorsal dislocation of a metacarpal with fractures of the capitate. **c** Axial CT image shows fractures of capitate and hamate. CT will often identify additional fractures in this type of injury

Table 2 Palmer classification of TFCC tear

Traumatic injury	Comments
A. Central perforation	
B. Ulnar avulsion	May have avulsion of ulna styloid Associated with injury to palmar and dorsal radio-ulnar ligaments. May result in instability
C. Distal avulsion	Distal avulsion of ulna lunate or ulna triquetral ligaments
D. Radial avulsion	Avulsion of insertion into radius, may be associated with a fracture

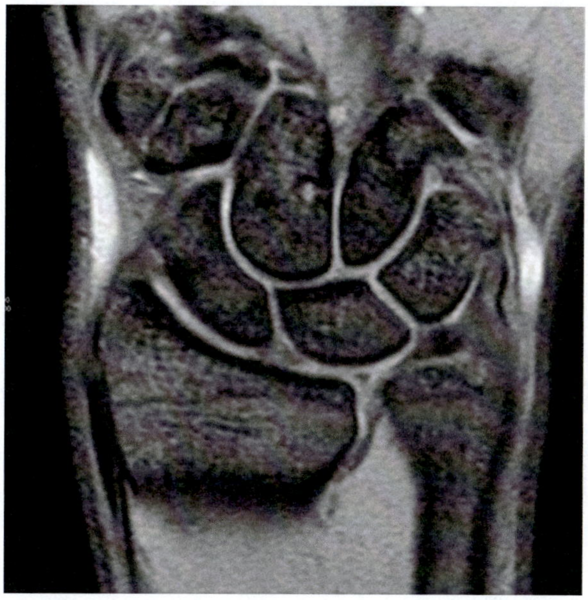

Fig. 41 Twenty-one-year male with pain persisting after a fall on the wrist some 6 weeks previously. Coronal T2* GE MR of wrist. There is a central perforation of the articular disc of the TFCC

intercarpal ligaments which occur in most carpal dislocations are not specifically identified and treated. Isolated soft tissue injuries do occur as a result of trauma. Rupture of the scapho-lunate ligament with rotary subluxation of the scaphoid has already been considered. The triangular fibrocartilage complex is another soft tissue structure which can be injured acutely. Bony injuries may be present, but in many cases it is an isolated soft tissue injury. Palmer (1989) classified injuries of the TFCC into acute traumatic (Palmer class 1) and chronic degenerative (Palmer class 2). It is only the former that will be considered here. Palmer further subclassified these acute TFCC injuries into 4 groups depending on the site of perforation (Table 2). MR has proven to be accurate in the assessment of TFCC injuries (Fig. 41) (Oneson et al. 1996), but MR arthrography may be required to detect these injuries (Zanetti et al. 2007). Imaging at higher field strength (3T) has been shown recently to improve identification of the injuries without the use of intra-articular contrast (Magee 2009).

6 Chronic/Overuse Injuries

Chronic stress injuries of the upper limb are far less common than in the lower limb. This is self-evident as in normal circumstances the upper limb is not weight bearing rending it much less likely to come under repetitive stress during normal daily activities. Stress injuries of the upper limb are thus almost exclusively found in those who undertake activities outwith the norm. Principally, this involves athletes' or those with unusual jobs that require use of the upper limb in an unusual activity.

In a review of 44 cases of upper limb stress injuries in athletes, SINHA et al. (1999) found only 17 occurred in the wrist. The only stress fractures reported involve the distal radius, the distal ulna and the scaphoid. Stress injuries in athletes may occur as a result of repetitive stresses applied at the site of muscular attachments to bone such as may occur with weight lifters. Alternatively, repeated weight bearing especially if there is impact loading can also result in a bony stress response. This has been described most often in gymnasts usually females as their routines include many activities (Webb and Rettig 2008), which involve weight bearing on the upper limb often with impact forces in addition. The radiology findings on plain films have been described (Carter et al. 1988). In a series of 8 gymnasts aged 14–16, radiographs of the wrist demonstrated irregularity and widening of the radial epipyhseal growth plate bilaterally but asymmetrically. The irregularity of the growth plate was largely marked on the metaphyseal side (Fig. 42). Some of the cases also showed an ill-defined cystic appearance. In 5 cases, the ulna growth plate was also affected but to a lesser extent. The findings have likened to the appearances seen in rickets (Liebling et al. 1995). The MR appearances have been described (Shih et al. 1995). In an

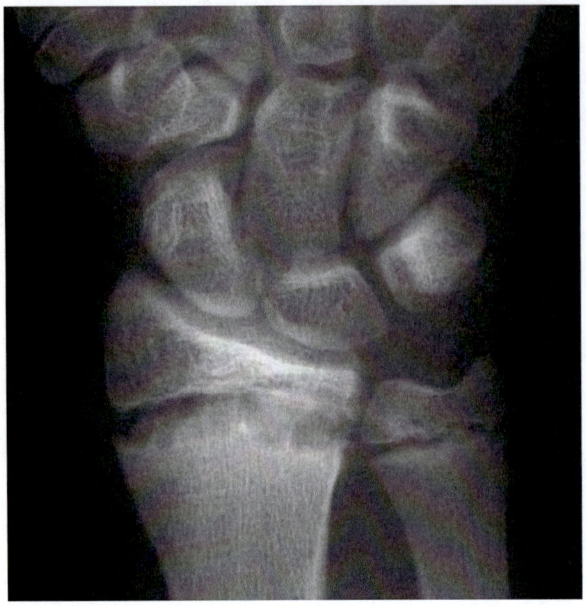

Fig. 42 AP radiograph of wrist of a young gymnast. There is widening of the epipyhseal plate with irregularity on the metaphyseal side

examination of 93 wrists in 47 gymnasts. The authors described several findings including widening of the growth plate, extension of the physeal cartilage into the metaphysis and or epiphysis. Also noted in some cases were vertical or horizontal fractures of the metaphysis. MR was more sensitive than plain films in the detection of most of these abnormalities. This has been confirmed in a recent paper (Dwek et al. 2009).

In addition to the metaphyseal stress injuries described above, the scaphoid has been reported to undergo stress fracture. Seven of Sinha's 44 cases had scaphoid stress fractures. These are seen in gymnasts but also in weight lifters. Weight bearing with the wrist in extension is the mechanism of injury which places repeated stress across the scaphoid waist. Stress fractures of the other carpal bones are exceptionally rare (Anderson 2006).

There are two further areas worth brief consideration. The first is the bone changes that may be seen within the wrist and carpus as a result of chronic vibration. Use of vibrating power tools such as pneumatic drills and chain saws may result in a spectrum of clinical disorders including white finger syndrome and carpal tunnel syndrome representing respectively vascular and neural changes as a result of exposure to repeated vibration over a long period of time. Furthermore, cystic changes visible on radiographs within the carpal bones particularly have been reported to occur in these workers. These changes in cysts measuring between 2 and 5 mm occur most commonly in the lunate and scaphoid. The association of these findings with occupational exposure is however inconsistent with some finding these changes almost as frequently within age-matched controls (Malchaire et al. 1986). There seems little evidence that those at risk should have regular screening radiographs of the wrists and in those with symptoms radiographic findings need to be treated with caution as cause and effect have not been proven (Gemne and Saraste 1987).

Finally, there are a few reports of instances of cysts developing at the site of healing fractures (Fig. 43). This is seen particularly in children with greenstick fractures, and the distal radius is the commonest site. The cystic change is seen initially at or close to the fracture site but persists and appears to migrate proximally into the diaphysis with time. On cross sectional imaging, the lesion is seen to lie not within the medullary cavity but in a juxtacortical or subperiosteal position (Roach et al. 2002). The pathogenesis is debated (Phillips and Keats 1986) with subperiosteal fat (Papadimitriou et al. 2005) subperiosteal (Durr et al. 1997) and intra-osseous haemorrhage all mooted as possible causes. The presence of a lucent lesion of bone away from the fracture site some time after the injury which may have healed can lead to diagnostic confusion with a tumour (Houshian et al. 2007) being considered as a possible cause. Thus, recognition of this entity with the typical cross-sectional appearance will prevent this erroneous diagnosis being entertained for too long.

7 Summary/Key Points

Careful evaluation of both AP and lateral radiographs is essential to avoid overlooking significant injury of the wrist and carpus. Understanding of ligamentous anatomy aids understanding of the injury patterns that occur.

Identification of one injury should alert one to the possibility of other associated injuries. Knowledge of the pattern of these injuries allows a systematic directed search to be undertaken.

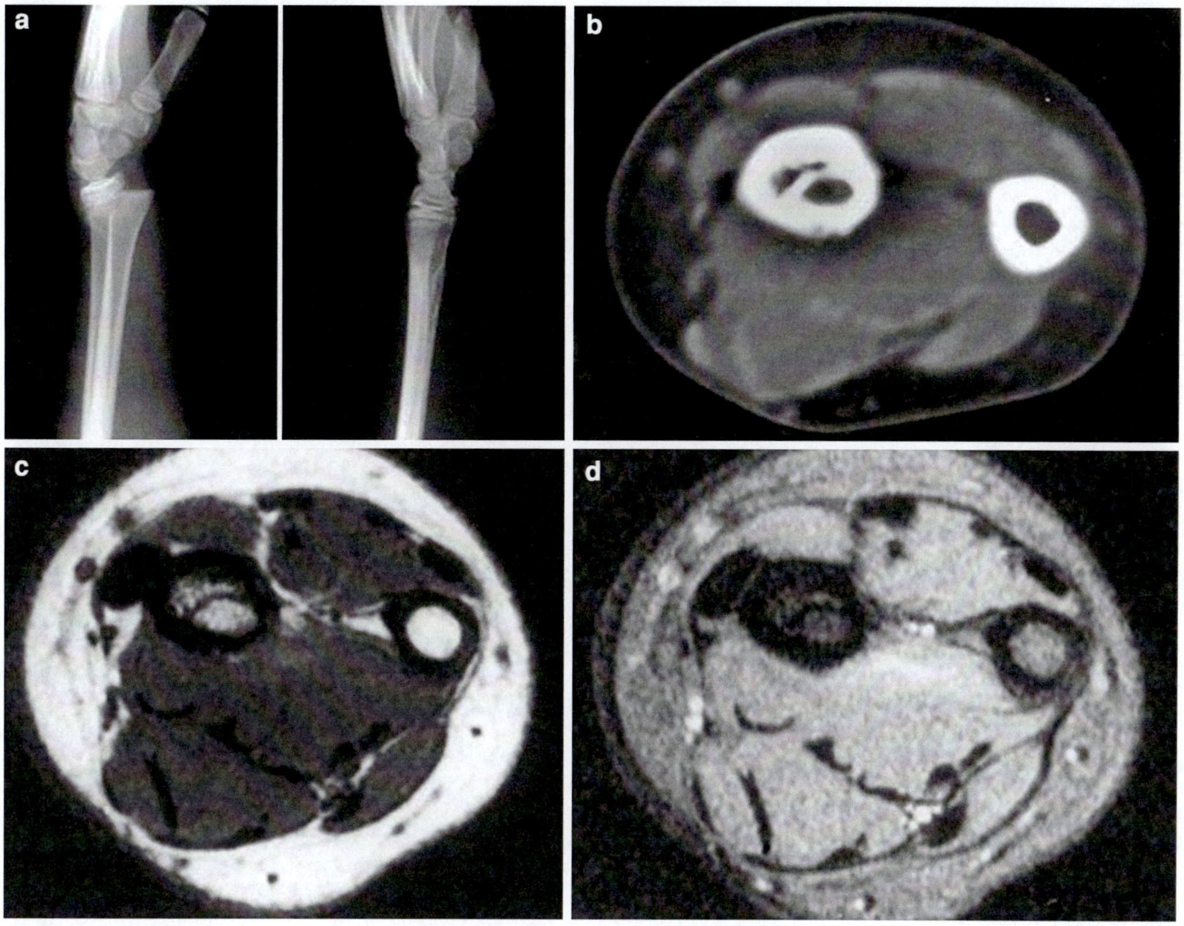

Fig. 43 **a** Lateral radiograph at time of injury demonstrating a Salter-Harris type 2 injury (left image) Later radiograph with fracture healed but cystic change evident on volar cortex (right image). **b** CT of lesion shows cystic area lies within cortex. **c** Axial T1- and **d** T2-weighted MR confirms fatty marrow content of lesion. Case reproduced with permission from reference 71

Lateral radiograph contains much vital information. It is essential to become familiar with its appearances and understand the normal anatomical relationships.

MR is a technique of choice for detecting occult scaphoid fractures.

Describe fractures and dislocations systematically rather than using eponymous names.

References

Adey L, Souer JS, Lozano-Calderon S, Palmer W, Lee SG, Ring D (2007) Computed tomography of suspected scaphoid fractures. J Hand Surg Am 32(1):61–66

Anderson MW (2006) Imaging of upper extremity stress fractures in the athlete. Clin Sports Med 25(3):489–504

Annamalai G, Raby N (2003) Scaphoid and pronator fat stripes are unreliable soft tissue signs in the detection of radiographically occult fractures. Clin Radiol 58(10):798–800

Barton JR (1838) Views and treatment of an important injury of the wrist. Med Exam 1:365–368

Barton NJ (1992) Twenty questions about scaphoid fractures. J Hand Surg[Br] 17B:289–310

Beeres FJ, Hogervorst M, Rhemrev SJ, den Hollander P, Jukema GN (2007) A prospective comparison for suspected scaphoid fractures: bone scintigraphy versus clinical outcome. Injury 38(7):769–774

Brøndum V, Larsen CF, Skov O (1992) Fracture of the carpal scaphoid: frequency and distribution in a well-defined population. Eur J Radiol 15(2):118–122

Brookes-Fazakerley SD, Kumar AJ, Oakley J (2009) Survey of the initial management and imaging protocols for occult scaphoid fractures in UK hospitals. Skeletal Radiol 38(11):1045–1048

Brydie A, Raby N (2003) Early MRI in the management of clinical scaphoid fracture. Br J Radiol 76(905):296–300

Carter SR, Aldridge MJ, Fitzgerald R, Davies AM (1988) Stress changes of the wrist in adolescent gymnasts. Br J Radiol 61(722):109–112

Cerezal L, Abascal F, Canga A, García-Valtuille R, Bustamante M, del Piñal F (2000) Usefulness of gadolinium-enhanced MR imaging in the evaluation of the vascularity of scaphoid nonunions. AJR Am J Roentgenol 174(1):141–149

Davidson JS, Brown DJ, Barnes SN, Bruce CE (2001) Simple treatment for torus fractures of the distal radius. J Bone Joint Surg (Br) 83-B:1173–1175

Dawson JS, Martel AL, Davis TR (2001) Scaphoid blood flow and acute fracture healing a dynamic MRI study with enhancement with gadolinium. J Bone Joint Surg [Br] 83-B:809–814

De Schrijver F, De Smet L (2001) Fracture of the hook of the hamate, often misdiagnosed as "wrist sprain". J Emerg Med 20(1):47–51

Dorsay TA, Major NM, Helms CA (2001) Cost-effectiveness of immediate MR imaging versus traditional follow-up for revealing radiographically occult scaphoid fractures. AJR 177:1257–1263

Dumontier C, Meyer zu Reckendorf G, Sautet A, Lenoble E, Saffar P, Allieu Y (2001) Radiocarpal dislocations: classification and proposal for treatment. A review of twenty-seven cases. J Bone Joint Surg Am 83-A(2):212–218

Duncan DS, Thurston AJ (1985) Clinical fracture of the scaphoid–an illusionary diagnosis. J Hand Surg 10B(3):375–376

Durr HR, Lienemann A, Stabler A, Kuehne J-H, Refior HJ (1997) MRI of posttraumatic cyst-like lesions of bone after a greenstick fracture. Eur Radiol 7:1218–1220

Dwek JR, Cardoso F, Chung CB (2009) MR imaging of overuse injuries in the skeletally immature gymnast: spectrum of soft-tissue and osseous lesions in the hand and wrist. Pediatr Radiol 39(12):1310–1316

Fernández DL (1993) Fractures of the distal radius: operative treatment. In: Heckman JD (ed) Instructional Course Lectures, vol 42. American Academy of Orthopaedic Surgeons, Park Ridge, pp 73–88

Fisher MR, Rogers LF, Hendrix RW (1983) Systematic approach to identifying fourth and fifth carpometacarpal joint dislocations. Am J Roentgenol 140(2):319–324

Foex B, Speake P, Body R (2005) Best evidence topic report. Magnetic resonance imaging or bone scintigraphy in the diagnosis of plain X-ray occult scaphoid fractures. Emerg Med J 22(6):434–435

Frykman G (1967) Fracture of the distal radius including sequelae-shoulder-hand-finger syndrome, disturbance in the distal radio-ulnar joint and impairment of nerve function. A clinical and experimental study. Acta Orthop Scand Suppl 108:3

Gaebler C (2006) Fractures and dislocations of the carpus. In: Buchholz RW, Heckmen JD, Court-Brown C (eds) Rockwood and green's fractures in adults, 6th edn. Lippincott Williams & Wilkins, Philadelphia, pp 857–908

Gemne G, Saraste H (1987) Bone and joint pathology in workers using hand-held vibrating tools. An overview. Scand J Work Environ Health 13(4):290–300

Gilula LA (1979) Carpal injuries: analytic approach and case exercises. Am J Roentgenol 133(3):503–517

Groves AM, Kayani I, Syed R, Hutton BF, Bearcroft PP, Dixon AK, Ell PJ (2006) An international survey of hospital practice in the imaging of acute scaphoid trauma. Am J Roentgenol 187(6):1453–1456

Houshian S, Pedersen NW, Torfing T, Venkatram N (2007) Post-traumatic cortical cysts in paediatric fractures: is it a concern for emergency doctors? A report of three cases. Eur J Emerg Med 14(6):365–367

Hudson TM, Caragol WJ, Kaye JJ (1976) Isolated rotatory subluxation of the carpal navicular. Am J Roentgenol 126(3):601–611

Ilyas A, Chaitanya C (2008) Radiocarpal fracture dislocations. J Am Acad Orthop Surg 16:647–655

Johnson RP (1980) The acutely injured wrist and its residuals. Clin Orthop 149:33–44

Jupiter JB, Fernandez DL (1997) Comparative classification for fractures of the distal end of the radius. J Hand Surg Am 22(4):563–571

Kaewlai R, Avery LL, Asrani AV, Abujudeh HH, Sacknoff R, Novelline RA (2008) Multidetector CT of carpal injuries: anatomy, fractures, and fracture-dislocations. Radiographics 28(6):1771–1784

Kato H, Nakamura R, Horii E, Nakao E, Yajima H (2000) Diagnostic imaging for fracture of the hook of the hamate. Hand Surg 5(1):19–24

Kumar S, O'Connor A, Despois M, Galloway H (2005) Use of early magnetic resonance imaging in the diagnosis of occult scaphoid fractures: the CAST Study. NZ Med J 118:1209

La Hei N, McFadyen I, Brock M, Field J (2007) Scaphoid bone bruising–probably not the precursor of asymptomatic non-union of the scaphoid. J Hand Surg Eur Vol 32(3):337–340

Leslie IJ, Dickson RA (1981) The fractured carpal scaphoid: natural history and factors influencing outcome. J Bone Joint Surg 63-B(2):225–230

Liebling MS, Berdon WE, Ruzal-Shapiro C, Levin TL, Roye D Jr, Wilkinson R (1995) Gymnast's wrist (pseudorickets growth plate abnormality) in adolescent athletes: findings on plain films and MR imaging. Am J Roentgenol 164(1):157–159

Lo IK, MacDermid JC, Bennett JD, Bogoch E, King GJ (2001) The radioulnar ratio: a new method of quantifying distal radioulnar joint subluxation. J Hand Surg Am 26(2):236–243

Low G, Raby N (2005) Can follow-up radiography for acute scaphoid fracture still be considered a valid investigation? Clin Radiol 60(10):1106–1110

Lozano-Calderón SA, Doornberg J, Ring D (2006) Fractures of the dorsal articular margin of the distal part of the radius with dorsal radiocarpal subluxation. J Bone Joint Surg Am 88:1486–1493

MacEwan DW (1964) Changes due to trauma in the fat plane overlying the pronator quadratus muscle: a radiologic sign. Radiology 82:879–881

Magee T (2009) Comparison of 3-T MRI and arthroscopy of intrinsic wrist ligament and TFCC tears. Am J Roentgenol 192(1):80–85

Malchaire J, Maldague B, Huberlant JM, Croquet F (1986) Bone and joint changes in the wrists and elbows and their association with hand and arm vibration exposure. Ann Occup Hyg 30(4):461–468

May MM, Lawton JN, Blazar PE (2002) Ulnar styloid fractures associated with distal radial fractures: incidence and implications for distal radioulnar joint instability. J Hand Surg [Am] 27(6):965–971

Melone CP (1986) Open treatment for displaced articular fractures of the distal radius. Clin Orthop 202:101–111

Memarsadeghi M, Breitenseher MJ, Schaefer-Prokop C, Weber M, Aldrian S, Gäbler C, Prokop M (2006) Occult scaphoid fractures: comparison of multidetector CT and MR imaging–initial experience. Radiology 240(1):169–176

Moneim MS, Bolger JT, Omer GE (1985) Radiocarpal dislocation–classification and rationale for management. Clin Orthop Relat Res 192:199–209

Nakamura R, Horii E, Imaeda T, Tsunoda K, Nakao E (1995) Distal radioulnar joint subluxation and dislocation diagnosed by standard roentgenography. Skeletal Radiol 24(2):91–94

Nakamura R, Horii E, Imaeda T, Nakao E (1996) Criteria for diagnosing distal radioulnar joint subluxation by computed tomography. Skeletal Radiol 25(7):649–653

Nicolaidis SC, Hildreth DH, Lichtman DM (2000) Acute injuries of the distal radioulnar joint. Hand Clin 16(3):449–459

Oneson SR, Scales LM, Timins ME, Erickson SJ, Chamoy L (1996) MR imaging interpretation of the Palmer classification of triangular fibrocartilage complex lesions. Radiographics 16(1):97–106

Palmer AK (1989) Triangular fibrocartilage complex lesions: a classification. J Hand Surg 14A:594–606

Papadimitriou NG, Christophorides J, Beslikas TA, Doulianaki EG, Papadimitriou AG (2005) Post-traumatic cystic lesion following fracture of the radius. Skeletal Radiol 34(7):411–414

Phillips CD, Keats TE (1986) The development of post-traumatic cyst-like lesions in bone. Skeletal Radiol 15:631–634

Raby N (2001) Magnetic resonance imaging of suspected scaphoid fractures using a low field dedicated extremity MR system. Clin Radiol 56(4):316–320

Raby N, Berman L, de Lacey G (2005) Accident and emergency radiology a survival guide, 2nd edn. Elsevier, Amsterdam

Roach RT, Cassar-Pullicino V, Summers BN (2002) Paediatric post-traumatic cortical defects of the distal radius. Pediatr Radiol 32(5):333–339

Rodgers LF (2001) Radiology of skeletal trauma, 3rd edn, Chap. 17. Churchill Livingstone, London

Shih C, Chang CY, Penn IW, Tiu CM, Chang T, Wu JJ (1995) Chronically stressed wrists in adolescent gymnasts: MR imaging appearance. Radiology 195:855–859

Singh AK, Davis TR, Dawson JS, Oni JA, Downing ND (2004) Gadolinium enhanced MR assessment of proximal fragment vascularity in nonunions after scaphoid fracture: does it predict the outcome of reconstructive surgery? J Hand Surg Br 29(5):444–448

Sinha AK, Kaeding CC, Wadley GM (1999) Upper extremity stress fractures in athletes: clinical features of 44 cases. Clin J Sport Med 9(4):199–202

Smith ML, Bain GI, Chabrel N, Turner P, Carter C, Field J (2009) Using computed tomography to assist with diagnosis of avascular necrosis complicating chronic scaphoid nonunion. J Hand Surg Am 34(6):1037–1043

Thornton A, Gyll C (1999) Children's fractures. WB Saunders, London

Tiel-Van Buul MM, Van Beek EJ, Van Dongen A, Van Royen EA (1992a) The reliability of the 3 phase bone scan in suspected scaphoid fracture: an inter- and intra-observer variability analysis. Eur J Nucl Med 19:848–852

Tiel-Van Buul MMC, Van Beek EJR, Broekhuizen AH, Nooitgedacht EA, Davids PHP, Bakker AJ (1992b) Diagnosing scaphoid fractures: radiographs cannot be used as a gold standard. Injury 23(2):77–79

Tiel-Van Buul MN, Van Beek EJ, Born JJ, Gobler FN, Broekhuizen AH, Van Royen EA (1993) The value of radiographs and bone scintigraphy in suspected scaphoid fracture: a statistical analysis. J Hand Surg [Br] 18:403–406

Tsai P, Paksima N (2009) The distal radio ulnar joint. Bull NYU Hosp Jt Dis 67(1):90–96

Waizenegger M, Wastie ML, Barton NJ, Davis TRC (1994) Scintigraphy in the evaluation of the "clinical" scaphoid fracture. J Hand Surg [Br] 19B(6):750–753

Webb BG, Rettig LA (2008) Gymnastic wrist injuries. Curr Sports Med Rep 7(5):289–295

Yeager BA, Dalinka MK (1985) Radiology of trauma to the wrist: dislocations, fracture dislocations, and instability patterns. Skeletal Radiol 13(2):120–130

You JS, Chung SP, Chung HS, Park IC, Lee HS, Kim SH (2007) The usefulness of CT for patients with carpal bone fractures in the emergency department. Emerg Med J 24(4):248–250

Zanetti M, Saupe N, Nagy L (2007) Role of MR imaging in chronic wrist pain. Eur Radiol 17:927–938

Wrist Instability

Milko C. de Jonge, G. J. Streekstra, S. D. Strackee, R. Jonges, and M. Maas

Contents

M. C. de Jonge · M. Maas (✉)
Department of Radiology, Academic Medical Center, Amsterdam, The Netherlands
e-mail: m.maas@amc.uva.nl

M. C. de Jonge
Department of Radiology, Zuwe Hofpoort Ziekenhuis, Woerden, The Netherlands

G. J. Streekstra · R. Jonges
Department of Biomedical Engineering and Physics, Academic Medical Center, Amsterdam, The Netherlands

S. D. Strackee
Department of Plastic, Reconstructive and Hand Surgery, Academic Medical Center, Amsterdam, The Netherlands

M. Maas
Radiology Room C1-120, Meibergdreef 9, 1105A2 Amsterdam, The Netherlands

Abstract

The painful clunking, unstable wrist has been an area of specific interest for clinicians and radiologists for many years. This chapter aims to focus on the unstable wrist, reviewing the clinical problem, exploring current hypotheses, critically evaluating radiological tools in aiding the clinician, and illustrating the integrative views of the authors based on their fundamental research and clinical practice. This chapter cannot provide a complete overview as this is a controversial area with an extremely extensive literature.

1 Introduction

Carpal instability is a problem of unknown extent, of which sparse literature suggests an incidence of 2.6 % in adults (Mink van der Molen 1997). The lack of reliable data relating to incidence is partly due to the lack of consensus relating to diagnosis and terminology and also the result of differences between ways in which carpal instability is classified (Kobayashi et al. 1997). The wrist has a complex anatomy involving 15 bones comprising the radius and ulna, carpal bones, and metacarpal bases. However the biomechanical principles governing carpal kinematics and instability remain poorly understood.

2 Anatomy

With the exception of flexor carpi ulnaris on the pisiform, none of the tendons that move the wrist insert onto carpal bones. This means stabilization of

A. M. Davis et al. (eds.), *Imaging of the Hand and Wrist*, Medical Radiology. Diagnostic Imaging, DOI: 10.1007/174_2012_699,

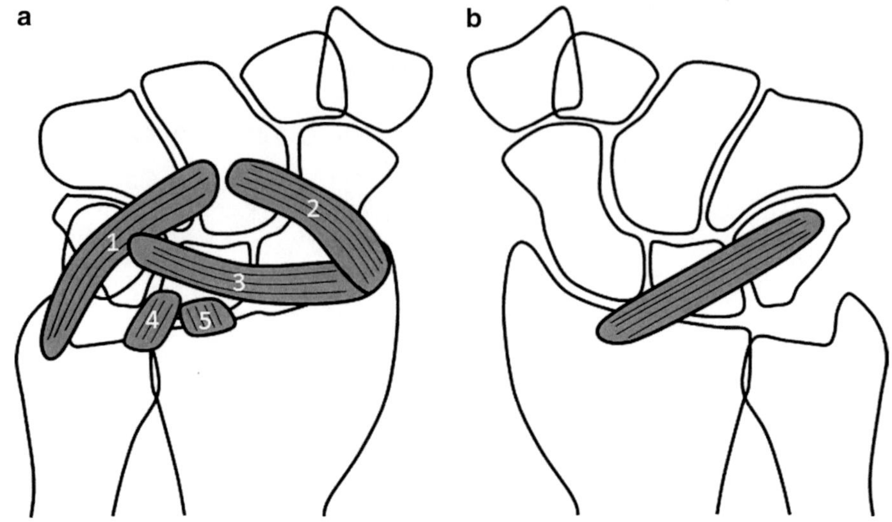

Fig. 1 Diagram showing the major extrinsic ligaments of the wrist. **a** Volar showing 1 = ulnotriquetralcapitate, 2 = radioscaphoidcapitate, 3 = radiolunatetriquetral, 4 = ulnolunate, 5 = radiolunate. **b** Dorsal showing the radiotriquetral ligament which also has an attachment to the lunate

the carpal bones is almost entirely passive, movements being dependent on the shapes of the articulations between bones and their passive stabilization by a complicated series of intrinsic ligaments.

Wrist ligaments fall into two groups: the extrinsic ligaments linking the radius or ulna to the carpal bones and the intrinsic ligaments running between carpal bones. The two most important intrinsic ligaments lie in the proximal carpal row, between the scaphoid and lunate (scapholunate) and between the lunate and triquetral (lunatetriquetral) bones.

The scapholunate (SL) and lunatetriquetral (LT) ligaments have a complex structure with strong fibrous volar and dorsal components and a thinner membranous central portion. The membranous portion has no stabilizing function and only the volar and dorsal components act as true ligaments. Small perforations in the membranous portion of the ligaments may exist in the normal population. The dorsal component of the SL and the volar component of the LT ligaments are the thickest and most important components for stabilization (Cerezal et al. 2012). The lunate attachments of the two ligaments are stronger than the scaphoid and triquetral attachments which means injury will tend to occur at the scaphoid attachment of the SL ligament and at the triquetral attachment of the LT ligament.

The extrinsic ligaments lie on the volar and dorsal aspects of the wrist. On the volar aspect of the wrist the ligaments tend to course from the radius and ulna toward the capitate (radioscaphocapitate and ulnotriquetralcapitate ligaments) or toward the lunate (radiolunate and ulnolunate ligaments). On the dorsal aspect of the wrist the most important extrinsic ligament is the dorsal radiotriquetral ligament which also sometimes has attachments to the lunate which it stabilizes against volar flexion (Viegas et al. 1999) (Fig. 1).

3 The Clinical Problem

The classical presentation of carpal instability is a patient presenting with reduced range of motion and wrist pain and mechanical symptoms, usually a clunk. Such a presentation requires the clinician to establish the cause of the mechanical symptoms by identifying the site of instability.

A clunk is described as a low-pitched dull sound, caused by sudden subluxation or reduction of a partially dislocated carpal bone (Gilula et al. 2002). Various types are described (Garcia-Elias 2008). The origin may be from a particular carpal row with disruption of the SL ligament within the proximal carpal row the most frequently described entity (Amadio 1991). LT instability is a less frequently encountered pattern of proximal carpal row instability. In the authors' experience midcarpal laxity or instability (MCI) is the most frequently encountered cause of the clunking wrist in daily practice.

The most frequently used and widely recognized system for the classification of carpal instability is the MAYO classification. This system identifies four categories of instability (Dobyns 1998).

Type I: Carpal instability dissociative (CID), representing instability occurring within a carpal row with S-L or L-T intercarpal ligament disruption as examples.

Type II: Carpal instability non-dissociative (CIND), described as carpal instability between rows. This falls into three broad groups: instability between the radius and proximal carpal row, instability between the proximal and distal carpal rows, or a combination of the two.

Type III: Carpal instability complex (CIC), a combination of types I and II.

Type IV: Adaptive carpal instability (CIA), in which abnormal carpal kinematics result from trauma such as a distal radial malunion, or congenital dysplasia.

The reality is frequently more complex than this apparently simple classification suggests and the clinical situation is rarely clear. Because of this imaging assessment is commonly required.

4 Imaging

4.1 Conventional Radiography

The primary imaging modality for wrist problems in general and specifically for patients with an unstable wrist is conventional radiography. It is recommended that both wrists are imaged enabling comparison; this can only be done if standardized techniques are used. Although this standardized technique is well described in the literature (Gilula et al. 2002; Peh and Gilula 1994; Weiss et al. 2007), awareness of such standardization among radiographers and clinicians is often lacking. Training of radiology technicians and radiographers in how to achieve optimal and reproducible images should be part of the clinical responsibility of the supervising radiologist. The measurement of specific angles that are extensively described in the literature with respect to carpal instabilities can only be done reliably on these standardized images (Gilula et al. 2002). Ideally, the technician should be part of the team dealing with wrist pathologies.

Although the use of conventional PA and lateral radiographs is widely adopted, the value of additional views is questionable and debated in the literature and among clinicians. Several additional views (instability series and/or stress views) are described; PA views with maximal ulnar and maximal radial deviation, and AP clenched fist views are among the ones most commonly used (Gilula et al. 2002; Peh and Gilula 1994; Weiss et al. 2007; De Filippo et al 2006; Metz et al. 1997; Pliefke et al. 2008). In some cases up to 15 different additional views to analyze the wrist of a single patient are described (Metz et al. 1997). However, the literature on standardization of technique and reproducibility of these additional views is very limited. Although these views are described as being advantageous for analyzing wrist instability in the authors' opinion they hold significant limitations. Too many variables are introduced, for instance the maximum ulnar or radial deviation differs enormously between patients and within the same patient at different time points. Furthermore, these views have not been tested in a healthy population with no established normal parameters (Toms et al. 2011). An additional problem is that views with maximal ulnar and radial deviation only provide information on the end points of deviation and lack information on the whole pathway of the movement (see section on 4D imaging). One also has to be aware of the normal movement patterns of the carpals and their projection on the radiographs in normal situations. In maximal radial deviation the projection of the scaphoid and lunate is completely different compared to views in maximal ulnar deviation. If the radiologist is unaware of this phenomenon, adequate interpretation of these views is difficult.

4.2 Signs and Angles

The classic signs described on PA and lateral radiographs of the wrist are the dorsal intercalated segmental instability (DISI) and volar intercalated segmental instability (VISI) pattern (Gilula et al. 2002). It must be remembered that these are not diagnoses as such; they are merely signs reflecting underlying pathology although they are also seen in healthy individuals (then sometimes referred to as DISI or VISI configuration (Metz et al 1997)).

A DISI deformity is characterized by dorsal tilting of the lunate compared to the scaphoid. This will result in an increased scapho-lunate (SL) angle, generally above 60–80 degrees (there is some variation in the normal values given in the literature). A DISI pattern is

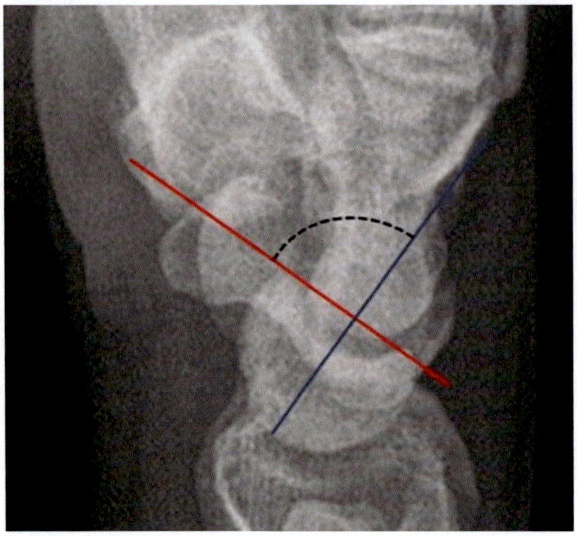

Fig. 2 DISI deformity on lateral wrist radiograph. There is an increase in the scapholunate angle (see "Radiography and Arthrography") (*dotted line*) between the axis of the scaphoid (*red line*) and the axis of the lunate (*blue line*)

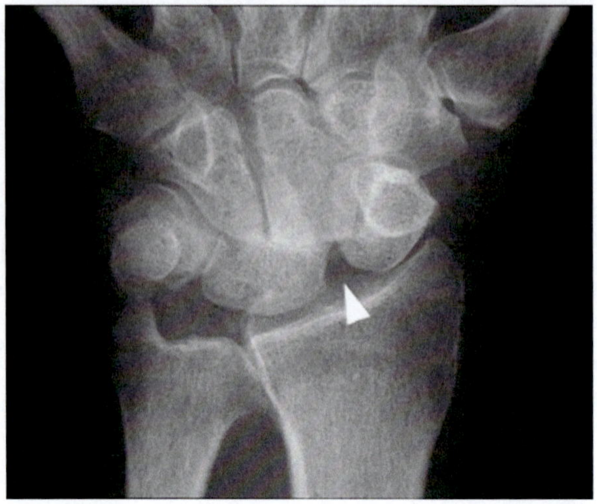

Fig. 3 Scapholunate dissociation. There is widening of the scapholunate interval (*arrowhead*) and the resulting flexion of the scaphoid results in overlapping of the body and distal pole of the scaphoid giving the signet-ring sign

classically described in patients with lesions of the SL ligament (Fig. 2) while a VISI pattern is classically described in patients with lesions of the LT ligament however this is actually infrequently seen in LT ligament lesions. A VISI stance is much more frequently encountered in midcarpal instability or a general lax wrist. However, it is important to realize that both are also seen in patients with intact SL and LT ligaments who have other injured ligaments (Dobyns 1998). A VISI deformity is identified when there is volar tilting of the lunate compared to the scaphoid resulting in a decreased scapho-lunate angle. Generally, this is described as below 30 degrees although again numbers vary in the literature. For details of methods of measuring these angles see "Radiography and Arthrography" in the chapter by Davies, this volume.

4.3 Type I Instabilities

Lesions of the scapholunate ligament are the most common lesions encountered in daily clinical practice. They usually present after a fall on an outstretched hand. Initial radiographs are frequently normal. Although the natural course of an undetected SL ligament injury is unknown, the DISI pattern will usually take some time to develop. Initially carpal stabilization is maintained, predominantly by other intrinsic ligaments (for example the STT ligaments. Extrinsic ligaments play no role in maintaining carpal stability in a neutral position, but come under tension in extreme flexion, extension and deviation. It is in the later stages, when other ligaments begin to fail that the DISI deformity starts to develop (Theumann et al. 2006). Other classic signs of a lesion of the SL ligament are widening of the SL distance (traditionally called "Terry Thomas" sign) (Fig. 3). An increase in distance between the scaphoid and lunate bone on a PA wrist radiograph of more than 2 mm can be regarded as suspicious for injury to the ligament, while a gap of greater than 4 mm is considered abnormal. Because of intra-observer differences in measurements it is helpful to recognize that the distance between the individual carpal bones is approximately equal given the cartilage thickness over the carpal bones shows little variation. It may be helpful to image the contralateral wrist as not infrequently the patient has the same SL configuration on each side which may be indicative of a preexisting condition such as congenital laxity of the SL ligament (Vitello and Gordon 2005). Dissociation of the scaphoid and lunate bones as a result of SL ligament disruption results in the scaphoid tending to move into volar flexion. When the normal constraints are removed, the lunotriquetral block has the tendency to move into dorsiflexion. This will result in the DISI pattern and consequently increased SL angle. Another sign on the PA wrist view will be foreshortening of the

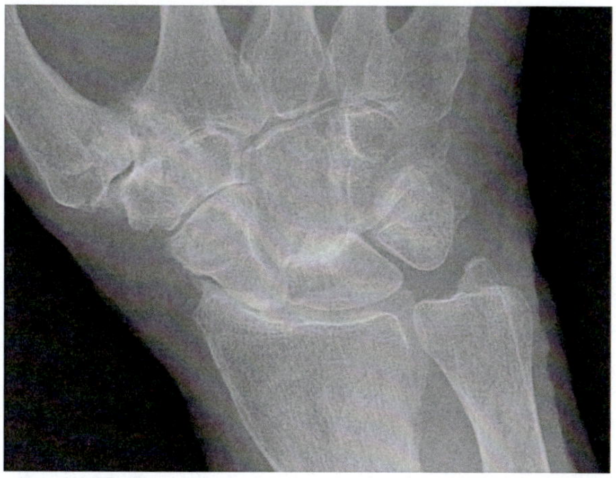

Fig. 4 Scapoholunate advanced collapse (SLAC). Long-standing scapholunate dissociation has resulted in osteoarthritis with joint space loss and sclerosis at the midcarpal and radioscaphoid joints

scaphoid leading to overlapping of the distal pole of the scaphoid and the body of the scaphoid resulting in the so-called signet-ring sign (Weiss et al. 2007) (Fig. 3). However, this is also seen in a substantial number of normal wrists and will also be seen on inadequate PA views in which there is (even mild) radial deviation (Pliefke et al. 2008). It has to be noted that the flexed position of the scaphoid and the extended position of the lunate is much more easily recognized on the lateral view. In long-standing, often missed, SL lesions a Scapho-Lunate-Advanced-Collapse (SLAC) wrist will develop, although it is unknown how fast this may occur. Depending on the stage of the disease the radiograph will show the SL dissociation combined with osteoarthritis typically at the radioscaphoid and/or the midcarpal joints (Fig. 4). Radiologists need to detect and recognize early SL ligament lesions, in order to prevent this often devastating condition.

If an SL lesion is obvious on a plain radiograph together with the appropriate clinical picture, the diagnosis of a static instability is made (Taleisnik 1984). If the patient is clinically suspected of an SL instability pattern with a normal radiograph then additional imaging has to be performed to rule out a dynamic instability pattern. Several imaging modalities can be used for this purpose although in the authors' opinion cineradiogradiophy is extremely valuable (see Other Imaging Modalities/Cineradiography).

Lesions of the Luno-Triquetral (LT) ligament are, in our opinion, probably under diagnosed, but there is no data about the incidence or prevalence. The pattern of instability is the opposite to that seen in a SL lesion. Since the lunate is separated from the triquetrum but still firmly attached to the scaphoid, it will follow the scaphoid into volar flexion while the triquetrum will dorsiflex which can result in a VISI deformity. The distance between the lunate and triquetrum may be increased.

4.4 Type II Instabilities

Type II instability is instability occurring between carpal rows and/or the distal radius/ulna, at the level of the radiocarpal or midcarpal joint. It is often found in patients with increased laxity of the ligaments resulting in hypermobility. In these patients, there is no history of trauma present and the patient is completely asymptomatic. Nevertheless, extrinsic ligament injury can lead to painful instability. There is an ongoing confusing debate about the terminology, etiology, classification, treatment, and imaging of these conditions in the literature. The most common distinction is between palmar (Lichtman et al. 1993) and dorsal midcarpal instability (Louis et al 1984). The former is more commonly recognized as a clinical entity. The radiographic findings are diverse. All the abnormalities described earlier in SL or LT dissociations are found, although the VISI pattern is described as being the most common abnormality especially in the palmar instability subtype (Toms et al. 2011; Lichtman and Wroten 2006). Again several additional views are described as being helpful. Garcia-Elias describes the forced ulnar and radial deviation and the anterior and posterior drawing views to determine ligament laxity (Garcia-Elias 2008). The absence of normal values for these views and the degrees of laxity in healthy subjects without wrist pain make the use of these views in general practice debatable.

Although no scapholunate ligament tear is identified in mid carpal instability, scapholunate widening may be seen as a sign of general ligament laxity (Garcia-Elias 2008).

4.5 Other Imaging Modalities

4.5.1 MR Imaging and CT

The aim with cross-sectional imaging modalities is to identify the nature and extent of ligamentous

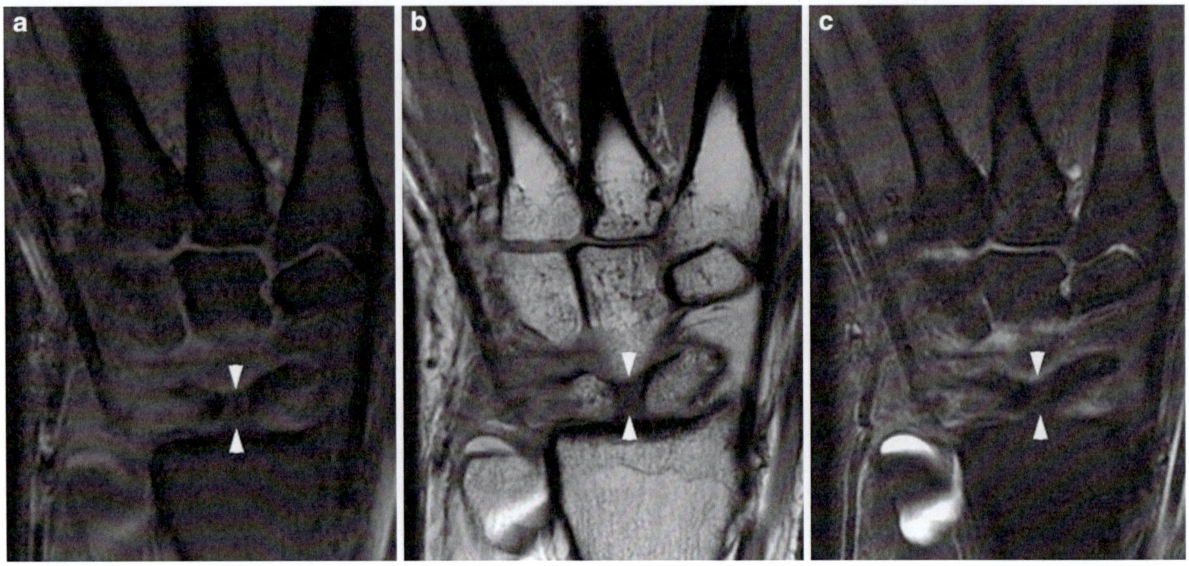

Fig. 5 Coronal 3T images (2mm, dedicated wrist coil) On T1 FS (**a**), PD (**b**) and T2 FS (**c**) the dorsal,functionally most important, component of the scapho-lunate intrinsic ligament (SLIL) is seen.The separate fibers are well delineated (*arrowheads*)

disruption and to identify any associated abnormality such as articular cartilage damage. As discussed above, the conventional radiographic signs only develop later after injury and direct visualization of the ligaments is required to diagnose their disruption. If primary ligament repair is planned this has to be undertaken early or there is a high risk of nonhealing (Garcia-Elias and Geissler 2005; Lindau 2010).

The sensitivity of MRI for SL ligament tear detection is reported as between 37 and 95 % (Johnstone et al. 1997; Manton et al 2001; Zlatkin et al. 1989). Using non-arthrographic 3T MRI the sensitivity is better for complete tears than for partial tears and the sensitivity and specificity for SL lesions is higher than for LT lesions. Sensitivity is considerably improved by the use of MR arthrography but this turns a non-invasive investigation into one with intra-articular injections in at least 1 or 2 compartments (radiocarpal and midcarpal joints). Sensitivity is reported as between 62 and 100 % (Braun et al. 2003; Meier et al 2002; Schmitt et al. 2003). It is not uncommon to have normal degenerative perforations in the membranous component of the intrinsic ligaments which means that the passage of contrast on MR arthrography between the radiocarpal and midcarpal joints is not in itself evidence of a symptomatic or significant ligament injury. Although 3T conventional MRI shows good sensitivity to intrinsic ligament disruption, arthrographic contrast still seems to improve sensitivity (Magee 2009). There are no comparative studies between 1.5 and 3T regarding lesions of the SL and/or LT ligament (Saupe 2009; Schmid et al. 2005; Stehling et al 2009). In the authors' experience 3T non-arthrographic studies provide adequate demonstration of the morphology of the important intrinsic wrist ligaments (Figs. 5, 6). When this is combined with functional assessment using videofluoroscopy MR arthrography is rarely needed.

Coronal and axial imaging provides the best means of assessing the intrinsic wrist ligaments. Full-thickness ligament disruption is seen as nonvisualization, or a full-thickness defect in the ligament (Figs. 7, 8). Partial ligament disruption may be appreciated as a focal discontinuity in a component of the ligament (Fig. 9). High signal intensity can be seen in the ligament of fat-saturated images. However, it should be noted that discontinuities in the membranous portion of the ligament may not be significant if the volar and dorsal components of the ligament are intact (Fig. 10).

MRI is the imaging modality of choice for the evaluation of the extrinsic ligaments of the wrist. The palmar scapho-capitate and triquetro-hamo-capitate ligaments, together often called the arcuate ligament are the most important ones to identify in patients with palmar midcarpal instability. The visualization of the arcuate ligament is described in cadavers using

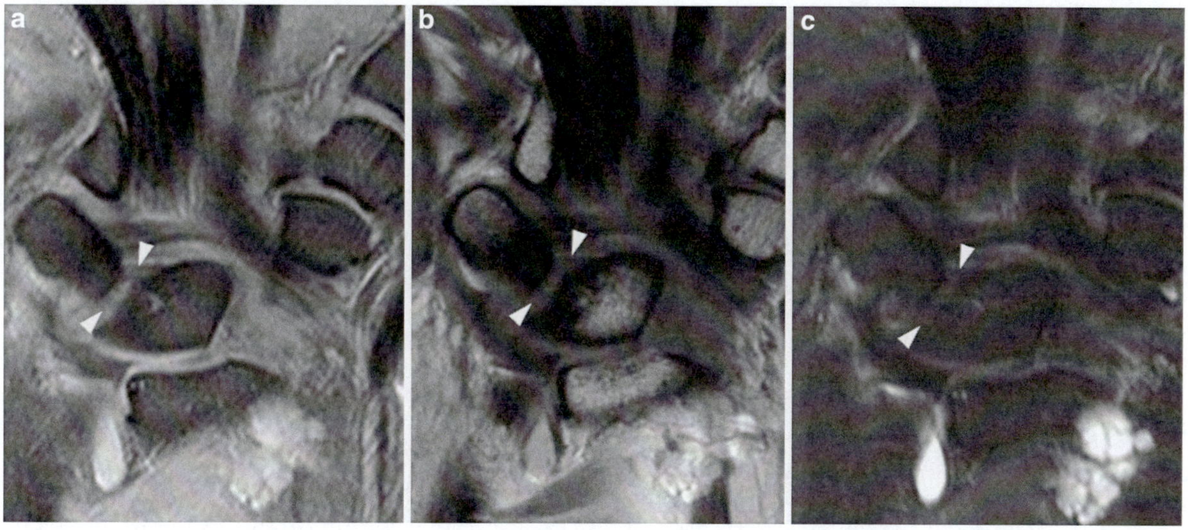

Fig. 6 Coronal 3T images (2mm, dedicated wrist coil) On T1 FS (**a**), PD (**b**) and T2 FS (**c**) thefunctionally most important volar component of the luno-triquetral intrinsic ligament (LTIL)is seen and separate fibers are well delineated (*arrowheads*)

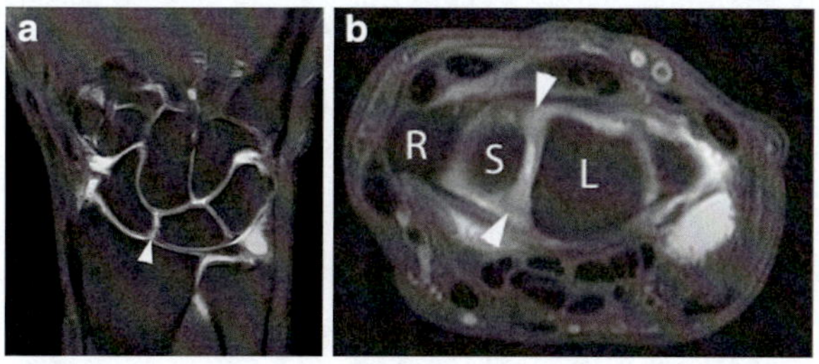

Fig. 7 Full-thickness tear of scapholunate ligament. **a** Coronal T1 fat suppressed image from MR arthrogram. Only the radial carpal joint was injected with gadolinium, but contrast passes freely through the scapholunate interval into the midcarpal joint as a result of a scapholunate ligament tear (*arrowhead*). Note also contrast is seen in the distal radioulnar joint as a result of a triangular fibrocartilage complex tear. This coronal section only shows the tear in the membranous portion of the ligament. **b** Axial T1 image from MR arthrogram. The proximal scaphoid (S) and lunate (L) are demonstrated with complete disruption of the volar and dorsal components of the scapholunate ligament arrowheads. R = radial styloid. Figure supplied by Dr AJ Grainger, Leeds, UK

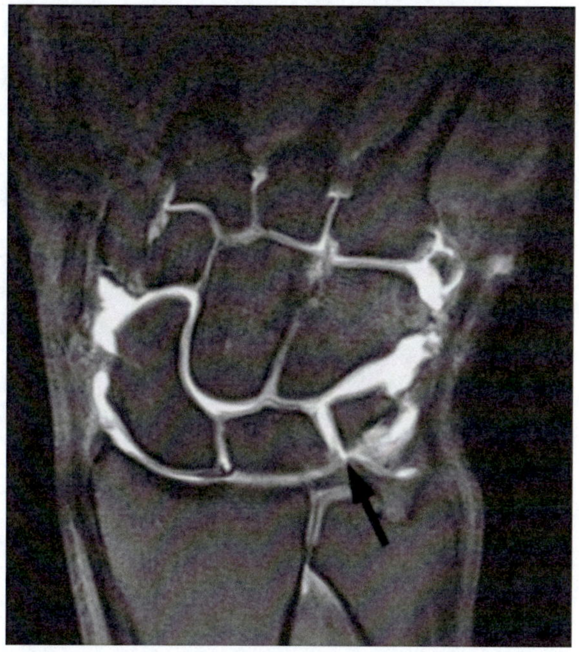

Fig. 8 Tear of lunate-triquetral ligament. Coronal T1 fat suppressed MR arthrographic image. There is diastasis of the lunate-triquetral joint with disruption of the lunate-triquetral ligament (*arrow*)

conventional MR imaging as well as with MR arthrography (Theumann et al. 2003, 2006; Chang et al. 2007); however clinical descriptions of its use are rare (Toms et al. 2011; Theumann et al. 2006).

CT on its own is of less value in the diagnosis of carpal instability. However, combined with an arthrographic injection demonstration of the intrinsic ligaments can be achieved and there is literature comparing MR imaging and MR arthrography versus CT arthrography in which the latter is more sensitive especially for partial injuries to the intrinsic ligaments (Schmid et al. 2005; Moser et al. 2007). CT can be useful to assess the later stages of the disease (SLAC wrist), especially to determine the amount of cartilage

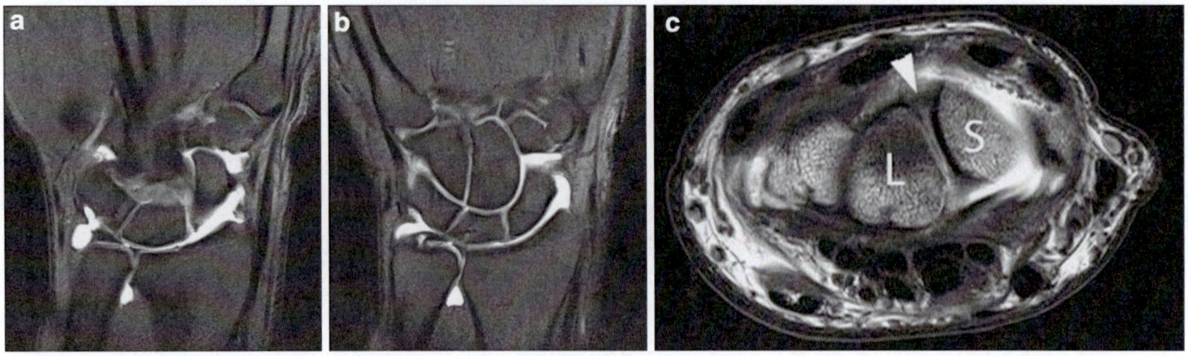

Fig. 9 Incomplete tear of scapholunate ligament. **a** Coronal T1 fat suppressed MR arthrographic image through the volar aspect of the scapholunate joint shows disruption of the scapholunate ligament. **b** An adjacent coronal section from the same series showing the scapholunate ligament is intact more dorsally. **c** Axial T1MR arthrographic image through the proximal scapholunate joint (S = Scaphoid, L = Lunate) confirms the volar scapholunate ligament disruption with an intact dorsal component (*arrowhead*). Note A and B also show a full-thickness perforation of the triangular fibrocartilage with passage of contrast into the distal radioulnar joint. Figure supplied by Dr AJ Grainger, Leeds, UK

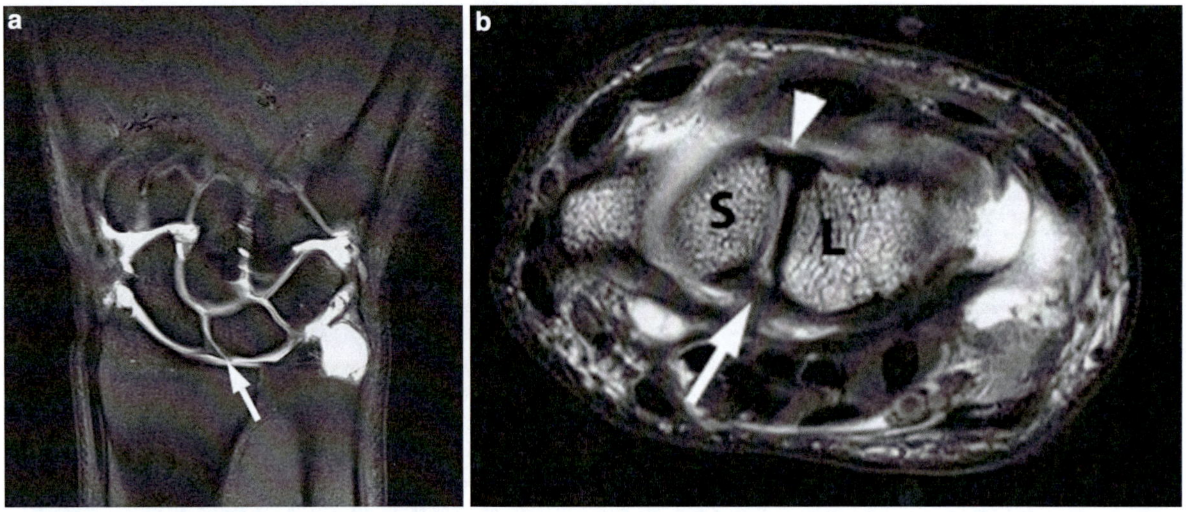

Fig. 10 Perforation of membranous component of scapholunate ligament. **a** Coronal T1 fat suppressed MR arthrographic image through the scapholunate joint shows a perforation in the ligament with contrast communicating through the ligament into the midcarpal joint (*arrow*). **b** Axial T1 MR arthrographic image through the proximal scapholunate joint shows the important fibrous components of the ligament on the volar (*arrow*) and dorsal (*arrowhead*) aspects of the joint are intact. S = Scaphoid, L = Lunate

damage. In the preoperative planning of salvage procedures, such as proximal row carpectomy or four corner fusion, Lunate-Capitate-Triquetrum-Hamate (LCTH) arthrodesis, CT scanning provides essential additional information for the hand surgeon.

4.5.2 Cineradiography

The drawback of cross-sectional imaging (as with radiographs) is the static nature of these modalities. Since instability is essentially a dynamic problem, dynamic imaging modalities such as cineradiography and fluoroscopy are particularly suited for its investigation (Protas and Jackson 1980). Both wrists can easily be examined, at relatively little cost and in a minimum amount of time compared to an MRI study. Examining both wrists offers the advantage that the examiner has a good idea of the movement pattern of the non-injured wrist and this can be compared with the injured wrist. The images obtained can be easily stored in PACS for reviewing and for demonstration

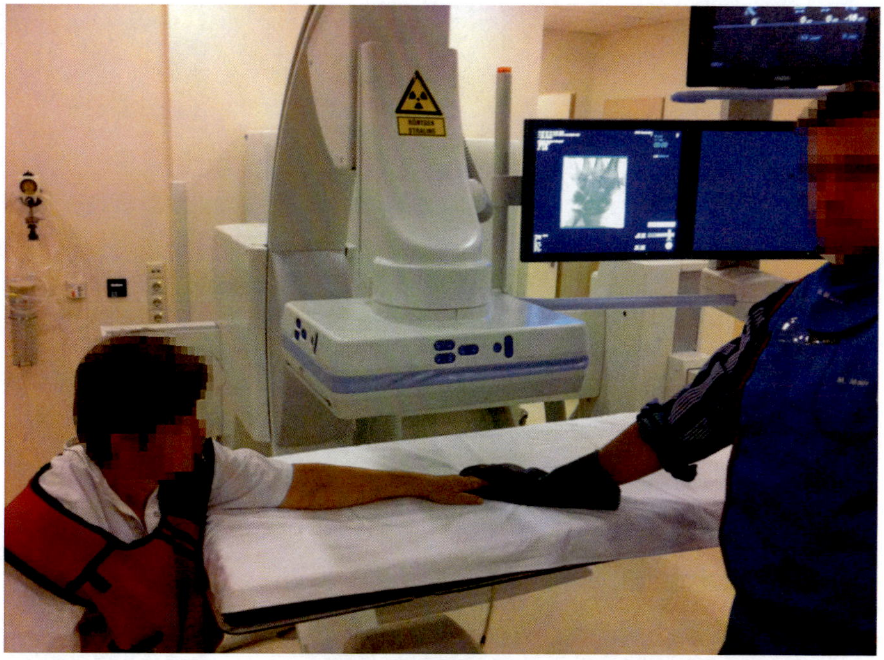

Fig. 11 Undertaking a cineradiographic examination of the wrist. The patient is seated at the end of the fluoroscopy table at the left side of the examiner. Both wear lead protection. The examiner wears protective lead gloves. The monitors are right in front of the examiner to evaluate the movement patterns in close detail

to the clinician. A standardized protocol has to be performed which should be developed after discussion with the hand surgeon. Different stress tests can be performed, although the Watson test (clinical test for scapho-lunate instability) is difficult to perform due to technical reasons (lead gloves worn by the examiner). In order to perform a fluoroscopic examination one has to understand the normal kinematic movements of the wrist. Normal kinematics are extensively described in several (experimental) studies (Arimitsu et al. 2008; Kaufmann et al. 2006). A routine assessment of the non-injured wrist also helps understanding these normal kinematic patterns.

It is important to position the patient well during fluoroscopy (Fig. 11). The arm rests with the elbow on the fluoroscopy table to eliminate as much muscle action of the upper and lower arm on the hand (Fig. 12). Our protocol consists of: PA and lateral view with radial and ulnar deviation (Fig. 13), lateral view with palmar and dorsal flexion (Fig. 14), lateral view with anterior and posterior drawer test (Fig. 15), and finally the Lichtman test (Fig. 16).

There are surprisingly few studies that deal with the diagnostic accuracy of cineradiography for SL lesions. A study by Pliefke et al. (2008) mentioned a sensitivity of 86 % with a specificity of 95 %. A study by Kwon and Baek 2008, using a cutoff point of a 2 mm scapho-lunate gap at fluoroscopy, mentioned a maximum sensitivity of 95 % (Kwon and Baek 2008). In an unpublished study by the authors a sensitivity of 95 % was found. In the authors opinion the most appropriate imaging modality after plain films in cases of SL instability should be a fluoroscopic examination of the wrist because of the aforementioned advantages.

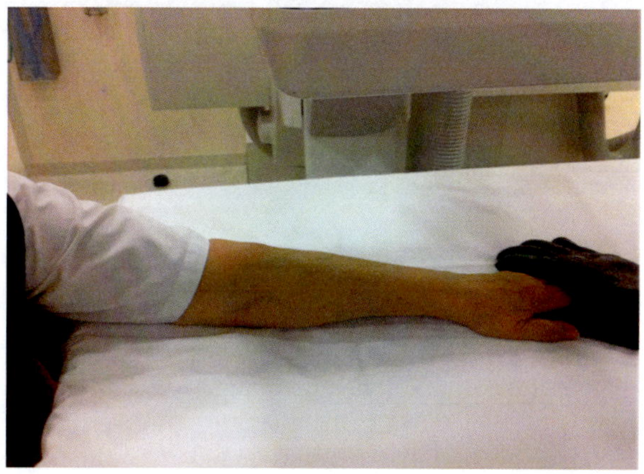

Fig. 12 Arm positioning. The elbow of the patient rests on the fluoroscopy table to eliminate forces exerted on the hand

In midcarpal instability the Lichtman test is, in our opinion the most important stress test to perform, both clinically as well as using cineradiography (Lichtman et al. 1981, 1993). In this test the thumb of the investigator is placed over the distal carpal row. With

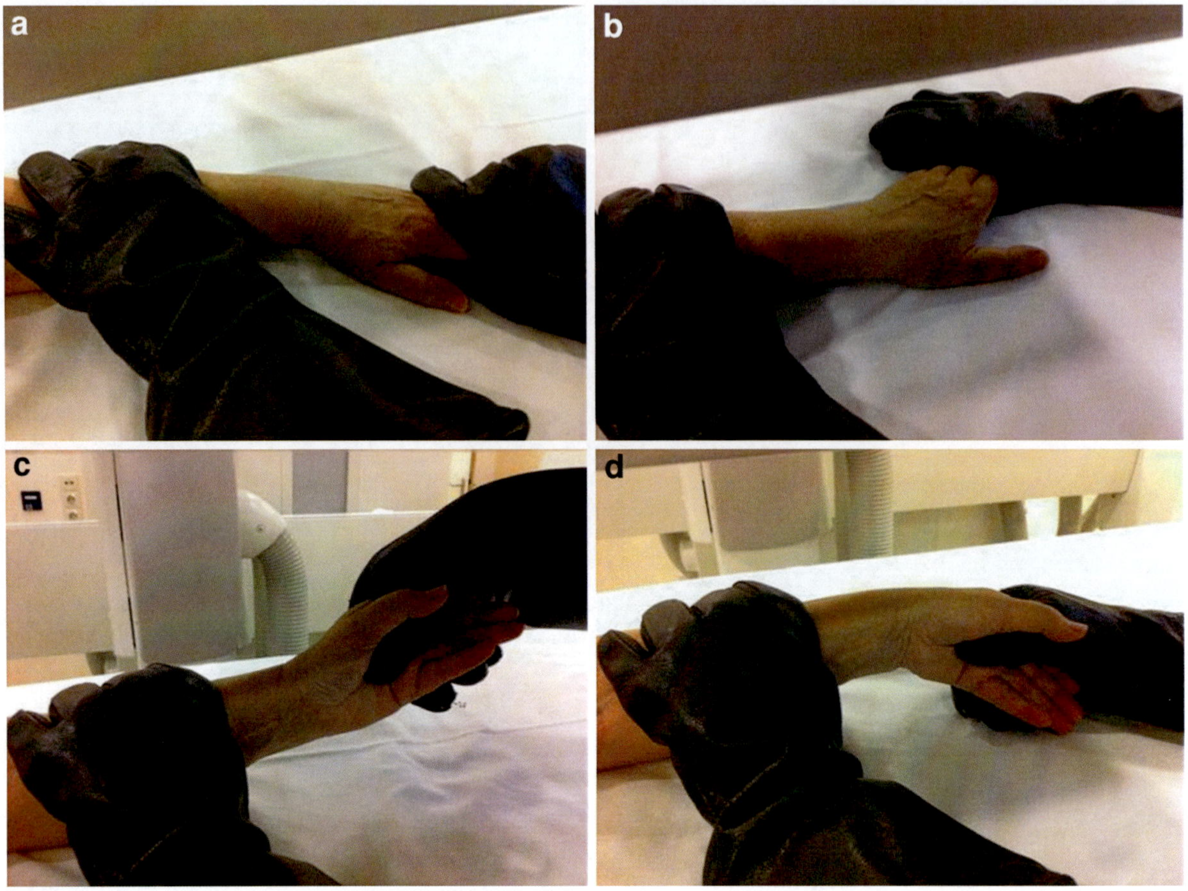

Fig. 13 The movements of the hand during the beginning of the examination. **a** PA view with radial deviation; **b** PA view with ulnar deviation; **c** lateral view with radial deviation; **d** lateral view with ulnar deviation

palmar translation of the carpus the proximal carpal row will move in flexion and with axial loading the wrist is moved from radial to ulnar deviation (Fig. 16). In midcarpal instability the proximal row will initially fail to translocate radially and extend but will then suddenly snap into position, the so-called "catch-up clunk". If this is painful the test is called positive and is considered a diagnostic indicator of a symptomatic midcarpal instability. The anterior and posterior drawer tests as described by Garcia-Elias (2008) are also important. The anterior drawing test is aimed at demonstrating laxity of the palmar ligaments especially the scaphotrapezial ligament; the posterior drawer test, in which the hand is translated dorsally compared to the wrist stresses the dorsal ligaments, especially the dorsal scaphotriquetral ligament. It is this test which is felt to be the most important test to demonstrate dorsal midcarpal instability.

5 Understanding of Wrist Biomechanics by 4D Imaging

As discussed above, analysis of motion patterns of the carpal bones is often useful in diagnosis of instability patterns. Analysis of the complete motion trajectory of the carpal bones has been shown to be particular beneficial when no diagnostic signs are found in radiographs and stress views at maximal radial or ulnar deviation also show no abnormalities (Protas and Jackson 1980; Braunstein et al. 1985; Obermann 1996; Schmitt et al. 2006).

For the past 30 years cineradiography has been the instrument to image these instability patterns. New developments in detecting motion patterns of carpal bones are devoted to 4D imaging of carpal kinematics. Four-dimensional imaging provides for visualization

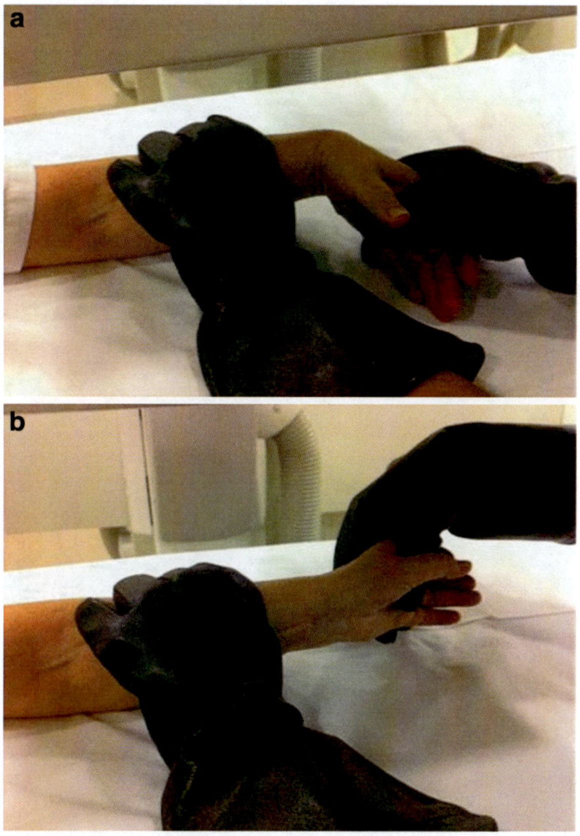

Fig. 14 Additional movements. **a** Lateral view with palmar flexion; **b** lateral view with dorsal flexion (extension)

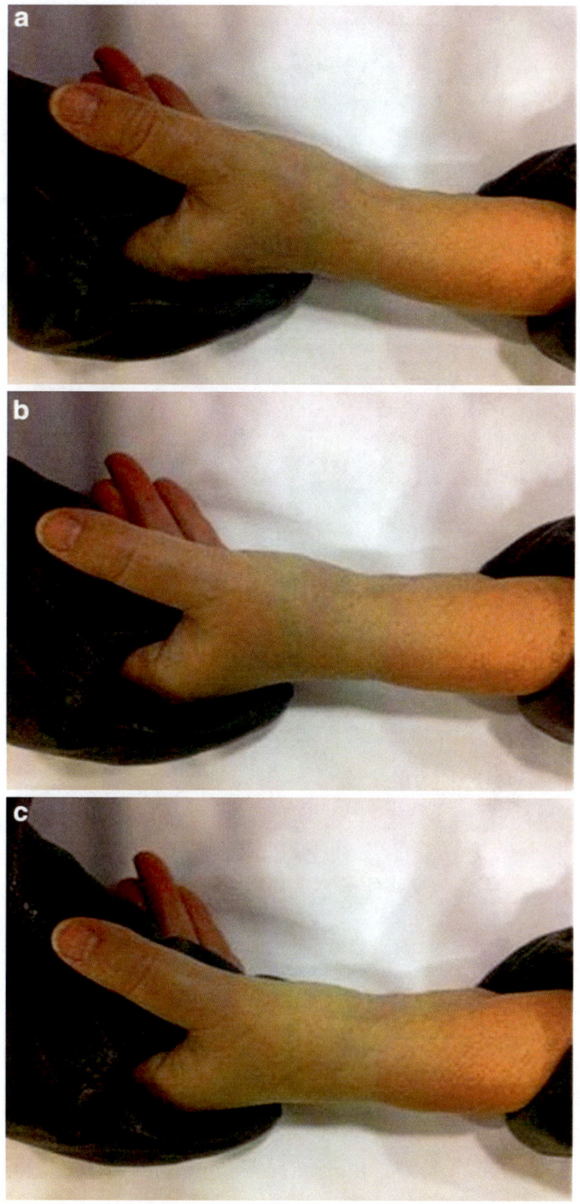

Fig. 15 Additional movements-drawer test. **a** Anterior drawer test is performed by applying pressure at the dorsal side of the hand. **b** The hand is then brought back into neutral. **c** The posterior drawer test is performed by applying pressure on the palmar side of the hand

and quantification of motion patterns of each individual carpal bone in 3D space (Carelsen et al. 2009; Crisco et al. 1999; Snel et al. 2000). Four-dimensional imaging methods are divided into quasi dynamic CT-imaging of the wrist using multiple static poses of the hand (Crisco et al. 1999; Snel et al. 2000) and also true dynamic 4D imaging of carpal bones during movement of the hand (Carelsen et al. 2009). These methods have advantage that they are potentially easier to interpret than cineradiography that uses 2D projections of the bone anatomy for each time frame. In 4D imaging the full 3D geometry of each carpal bone is available in each time frame. This also allows quantitative analysis of motion patterns in terms of translations and rotations of each individual bone as a function of time.

Currently, 4D imaging of the wrist joint is primarily used for basic research on joint biomechanics (Foumani et al. 2010a, b; Moojen et al. 2002, 2003; Moore et al. 2007; Streekstra et al. 2010) but has the potential to be used for clinical evaluation true 3D carpal instability patterns. An example of this potential is the detection of 3D motion pattern in a patient with SL dissociation. The motion pattern demonstrated reveals that widening of the bone gap between the scaphoid and lunate is not observed at maximal radial or ulnar deviation but at an intermediate of the

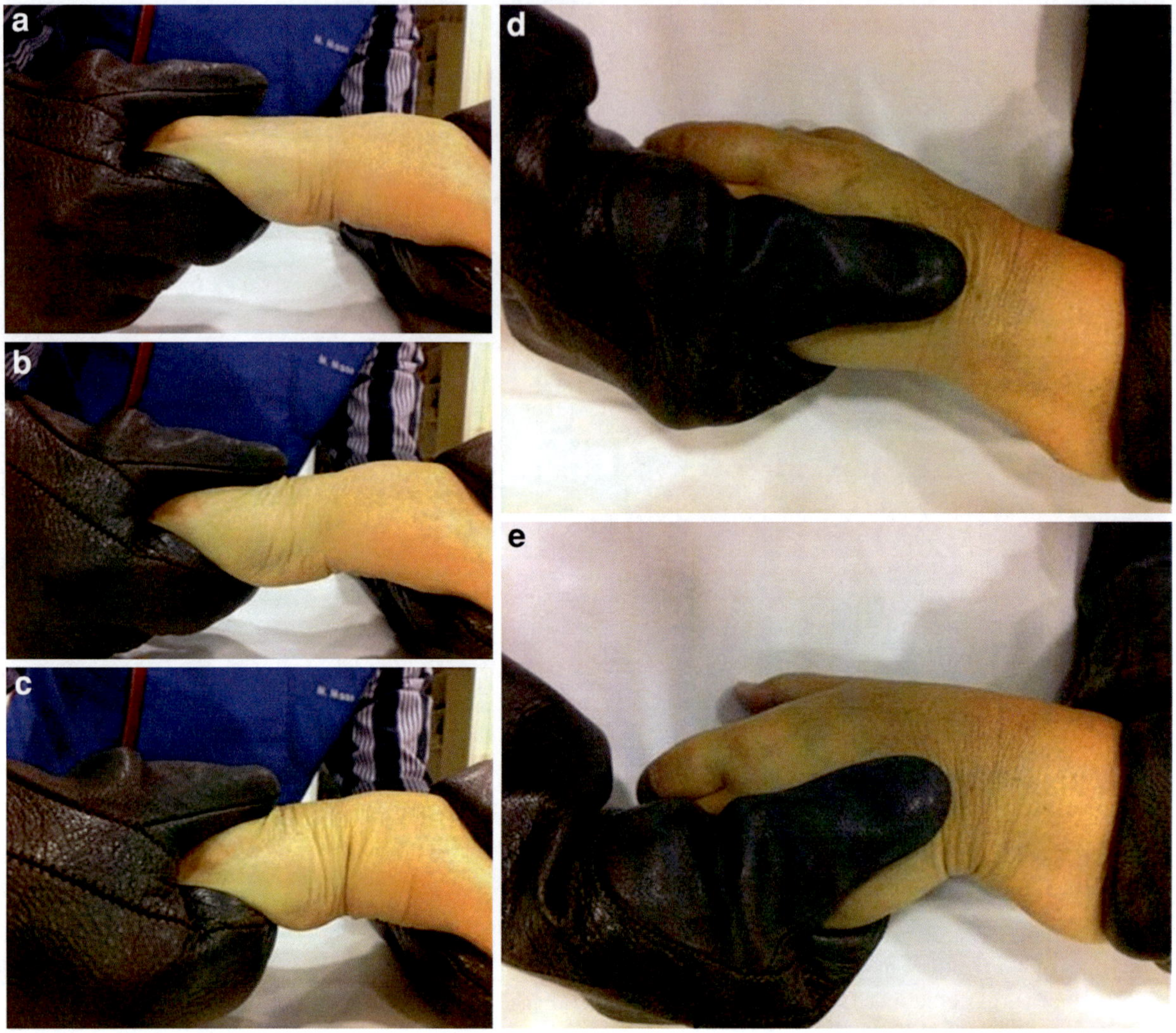

Fig. 16 The Lichtman or midcarpal shift test. **a** Initially the hand is in neutral position. **b** Dorsal pressure is applied. **c–e** Axial loading is then given and the hand is moved from radial to ulnar deviation

hand during the range of motion (Fig. 9). This is in agreement with qualitative cineradiographic observations of carpal motion through radial-ulnar deviation (Snel et al. 2000). The added value of 4D imaging is the quantitative nature of the observation in terms of translations and rotations of carpal bones that may help to develop more objective parameters to diagnose instability patterns of joints (Fig. 17).

Another example of the possible usefulness of the 4D approach in diagnosing wrist problems is the detection of joint space width as a representation of cartilage thickness over the entire joint surface area as a function of hand position (Fig. 18). In patients with SL-dissociation the joint space seems to be reduced over the entire joint surface compared to healthy volunteers (Foumani et al. 2010a, b).

6 Treatment and Clinical Perspective

One of the key purposes of non-invasive diagnostics is the triage between a conservative or invasive (arthroscopy or arthrotomy) therapeutic approach. In our setting cineradiography aids in tailoring the appropriate treatment for the specific patient with chronic undiagnosed wrist pain (CUWP), making the choice between surgical and physical therapy easier.

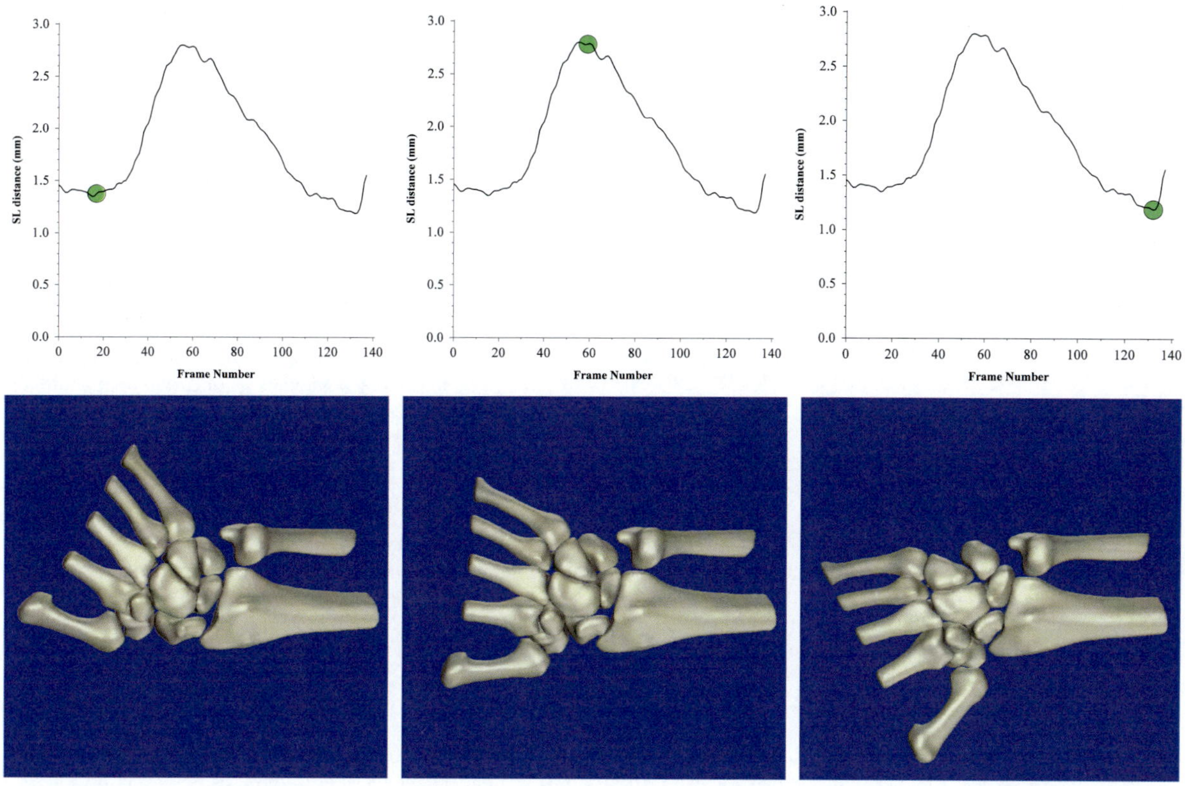

Fig. 17 Three time frames of a 4D image sequence of moving wrist bones in a patient with SL-dissociation. The image sequence shows widening and narrowing of the gap between the scaphoid and lunate (SL-distance) as a function of the hand position

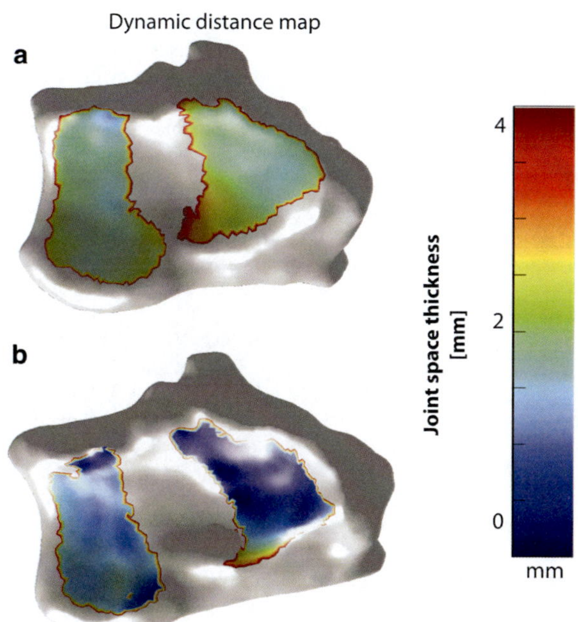

Fig. 18 Dynamic distance maps showing reduced minimal distance between adjacent joint surfaces in a follow up acquisition of patients and healthy volunteers. **a** Healthy Volunteers. **b** Patients with scapholunate dissociation

Fundamental research has shown that chronic wrist pain, without any morphological anatomical substrate detected by state-of-the-art diagnostic tools, could be controlled by non-surgical therapeutic strategies, such as adaptations in motor control (Smeulders et al. 2001). In a comparative study, Smeulders et al. 2001 found a significant difference in fluency of motion between patients and controls. They concluded that disturbance of fine motor control in CUWP may be a contributing factor to chronic wrist pain. A second case control study in patients with CUWP compared to healthy volunteers described a significant difference in fluency of movement between the two groups (Smeulders et al. 2002). This difference was strikingly found in the unaffected wrist, in which the authors hypothesized that chronic wrist pain is maintained by persistent abnormal cerebral motor function.

Since instability of the wrist is a possible cause for unilateral wrist pain, undiagnosed with standard radiography, MRI or CT, the cause of this may also be due to persistent abnormal motor function. This has led to the development of a specialized training regime for this CUWP patient group (Videler et al.

1998). This exercise program tackles unstable wrists combining central cerebral focused motor re-education and muscle strengthen coordination. The use of cine radiography as a triage modality may be a beneficial, cost-effective manner of managing patients with pain in the chronic unstable wrist. In excluding other causes of wrist pain, and a positive finding of midcarpal instability, cineradiography can play a pivotal role.

Acknowledgments We would like to thank M. Foumani MD and Mrs. M.R.W. Evers-van Bavel for their help in preparing the manuscript.

References

Amadio PC (1991) Carpal kinematics and instability: a clinical and anatomic primer. Clin Anat 4(1):1–12

Arimitsu S et al (2008) Analysis of radiocarpal and midcarpal motion in stable and unstable rheumatoid wrists using 3-dimensional computed tomography. J Hand Surg 33(2): 189–197

Braun H et al (2003) Direct MR arthrography of the wrist-value in detecting complete and partial defects of intrinsic ligaments and the TFCC in comparison with arthroscopy. RoFo: Fortschritte auf dem Gebiete der Rontgenstrahlen und der Nuklearmedizin 175(11):1515–1524

Braunstein EM et al (1985) Fluoroscopic and arthrographic evaluation of carpal instability. AJR Am J Roentgenol 144(6):1259–1262

Carelsen B et al (2009) Detection of in vivo dynamic 3-D motion patterns in the wrist joint. IEEE Trans Biomed Eng 56(4):1236–1244

Cerezal L et al (2012) MR and CT arthrography of the wrist. Semin Musculoskeletal Radiol 16(1):27–41

Chang W et al (2007) Arcuate ligament of the wrist: normal MR appearance and its relationship to palmar midcarpal instability: a cadaveric study. Skeletal Radiol 36(7): 641–645

Crisco JJ, McGovern RD, Wolfe SW (1999) Noninvasive technique for measuring in vivo three-dimensional carpal bone kinematics. J Orthop Res Off Publ Orthop Res Soc 17(1):96–100

De Filippo M et al (2006) Pathogenesis and evolution of carpal instability: imaging and topography. Acta Biomed Atenei Parmensis 77(3):168–180

Dobyns JH (1998) Classification of carpal instability. In: Cooney WP, Linscheid RL (eds) The wrist: diagnosis and operative treatment. Mosby, St. Louis, pp 490–500

Foumani M et al (2010a) In vivo dynamic and static three-dimensional joint space distance maps in the radiocarpal joint. In: 11th triennial congress of the international federation of societies for surgery of the hand, Seoul, Korea

Foumani M et al (2010b) The effect of tendon loading on in vitro carpal kinematics of the wrist joint. J Biomech 43(9):1799–1805

Garcia-Elias M (2008) The non-dissociative clunking wrist: a personal view. J Hand Surg Eur 33(6):698–711

Garcia-Elias M, Geissler WB (2005) Carpal instability. In: Green DP et al (eds). Green's operative hand surgery. Elsevier Churchill Livingstone, Philadelphia, pp 535–604

Gilula LA et al (2002) Wrist: terminology and definitions. J Bone Joint Surg Am 84-A(Suppl 1):1–73

Johnstone DJ et al (1997) A comparison of magnetic resonance imaging and arthroscopy in the investigation of chronic wrist pain. J Hand Surg 22(6):714–718

Kaufmann RA et al (2006) Kinematics of the midcarpal and radiocarpal joint in flexion and extension: an in vitro study. J Hand Surg 31(7):1142–1148

Kobayashi M et al (1997) Normal kinematics of carpal bones: a three-dimensional analysis of carpal bone motion relative to the radius. J Biomech 30(8):787–793

Kwon BC, Baek GH (2008) Fluoroscopic diagnosis of scapholunate interosseous ligament injuries in distal radius fractures. Clin Orthop Relat Res 466(4):969–976

Lichtman DM, Wroten ES (2006) Understanding midcarpal instability. J Hand Surg 31(3):491–498

Lichtman DM et al (1981) Ulnar midcarpal instability-clinical and laboratory analysis. J Hand Surg 6(5):515–523

Lichtman DM et al (1993) Palmar midcarpal instability: results of surgical reconstruction. J Hand Surg 18(2):307–315

Lindau T (2010) Arthroscopic management of scapholunate dissociation. In: Del Pinal F, Mathoulin C (eds) Arthroscopic management of distal radius fractures. Springer, Berlin, pp 99–108

Louis DS et al (1984) Central carpal instability—capitate lunate instability pattern: diagnosis by dynamic displacement. Orthopedics 7:1693–1696

Magee T (2009) Comparison of 3-T MRI and arthroscopy of intrinsic wrist ligament and TFCC tears. AJR Am J Roentgenol 192(1):80–85

Manton GL et al (2001) Partial interosseous ligament tears of the wrist: difficulty in utilizing either primary or secondary MRI signs. J Comput Assist Tomogr 25(5):671–676

Meier R et al (2002) [Scapholunate ligament tears in MR arthrography compared with wrist arthroscopy]. Handchirurgie, Mikrochirurgie, plastische Chirurgie : Organ der Deutschsprachigen Arbeitsgemeinschaft fur Handchirurgie : Organ der Deutschsprachigen Arbeitsgemeinschaft fur Mikrochirurgie der Peripheren Nerven und Gefasse : Organ der Vereinigung der Deutschen Plastischen Chirurgen 34(6):381–385

Metz VM, Metz-Schimmerl SM, Yin Y (1997) Ligamentous instabilities of the wrist. Eur J Radiol 25(2):104–111

Mink van der Molen AB (1997) Carpale letsels, onderzoek naar de verzuimaspecten ten gevolge van carpale letsels in Nederland 1990–1993—(Carpal injuries, research of work-related absence due to carpal injuries in the Netherlands 1990–1993) Thesis, Rijksuniversity Groningen

Moojen TM et al (2002) Scaphoid kinematics in vivo. J Hand Surg 27(6):1003–1010

Moojen TM et al (2003) In vivo analysis of carpal kinematics and comparative review of the literature. J Hand Surg 28(1):81–87

Moore DC et al (2007) A digital database of wrist bone anatomy and carpal kinematics. J Biomech 40(11): 2537–2542

Moser T et al (2007) Wrist ligament tears: evaluation of MRI and combined MDCT and MR arthrography. AJR Am J Roentgenol 188(5):1278–1286
Obermann WR (1996) Wrist injuries: pitfalls in conventional imaging. Eur J Radiol 22(1):11–21
Peh W, Gilula LA (1994) Imaging of the wrist—a customized approach. Curr Orthop 8:23–31
Pliefke J et al (2008) Diagnostic accuracy of plain radiographs and cineradiography in diagnosing traumatic scapholunate dissociation. Skeletal Radiol 37(2):139–145
Protas JM, Jackson WT (1980) Evaluating carpal instabilities with fluoroscopy. AJR Am J Roentgenol 135(1):137–140
Saupe N (2009) 3-Tesla high-resolution MR imaging of the wrist. Semin Musculoskelet Radiol 13(1):29–38
Schmid MR et al (2005) Interosseous ligament tears of the wrist: comparison of multi-detector row CT arthrography and MR imaging. Radiology 237(3):1008–1013
Schmitt R et al (2003) Direct MR arthrography of the wrist in comparison with arthroscopy: a prospective study on 125 patients. RoFo : Fortschritte auf dem Gebiete der Rontgenstrahlen und der Nuklearmedizin 175(7):911–919
Schmitt R et al (2006) Carpal instability. Eur Radiol 16(10): 2161–2178
Smeulders MJ, Kreulen M, Bos KE (2001) Fine motor assessment in chronic wrist pain: the role of adapted motor control. Clin Rehabil 15(2):133–141
Smeulders MJ et al (2002) Motor control impairment of the contralateral wrist in patients with unilateral chronic wrist pain. Am J Phys Med Rehabil/Assoc Acad Physiatrists 81(3): 177–181
Snel JG et al (2000) Quantitative in vivo analysis of the kinematics of carpal bones from three-dimensional CT images using a deformable surface model and a three-dimensional matching technique. Med Phys 27(9):2037–2047
Stehling C et al (2009) Three-tesla magnetic resonance imaging of the wrist: diagnostic performance compared to 1.5-T. J Comput Assist Tomogr 33(6):934–939
Streekstra GJ et al (2010) 4D-Imaging of voluntary joint motion from biplane fluoroscopy images. In: 96th annual meeting of the radiological society of North America (RSNA), Chicago
Taleisnik J (1984) Classification of carpal instability. Bull Hosp Jt Dis Orthop Inst 44(2):511–531
Theumann NH et al (2003) Extrinsic carpal ligaments: normal MR arthrographic appearance in cadavers. Radiology 226(1):171–179
Theumann NH et al (2006) Association between extrinsic and intrinsic carpal ligament injuries at MR arthrography and carpal instability at radiography: initial observations. Radiology 238(3):950–957
Toms AP, Chojnowski A, Cahir JG (2011) Midcarpal instability: a radiological perspective. Skeletal Radiol 40(5): 533–541
Videler AJ, Kreulen M, Brandsma W (1998) An exercise program for patients with chronic, undiagnosed wrist pain. Physiopraxis 7(11):10–13
Viegas SF et al (1999) The dorsal ligaments of the wrist: anatomy, mechanical properties, and function. J Hand Surg 24(3):456–468
Vitello W, Gordon DA (2005) Obvious radiographic scapholunate dissociation: X-ray the other wrist. Am J Orthop 34(7):347–351
Weiss S, Schwartz DA, Anderson SC (2007) Radiography: a review for the rehabilitation professional, quiz 179. J Hand Ther Off J Am Soc Hand Ther 20(2):152–178
Zlatkin MB et al (1989) Chronic wrist pain: evaluation with high-resolution MR imaging. Radiology 173(3):723–729

Nerve Entrapment Syndromes

Stefano Bianchi, Lucio Molini, Marie Claude Schenkel, and Thierry Glauser

Contents

S. Bianchi (✉)
CIM SA, Cabinet Imagerie Medicale, Route de Malagnou 40, 1208 Geneva, Switzerland
e-mail: stefanobianchi@bluewin.ch

L. Molini
Struttura Complessa di Radiodiagnostica, Ospedale Galliera, Via Volta, 16128 Genoa, Italy

M. C. Schenkel
Cabinet de Rhumatologie, Rue de la Faïencerie 6, 1227 Carouge-Geneva, Switzerland

T. Glauser
CH8, Cabinet de Chirurgie de la Main, Rue Charles Humbert 8, Geneva, Switzerland

S. Bianchi
Clinique des Grangettes, Chemin de Grangettes 7, 1224 Geneva, Switzerland

Abstract

Compressive neuropathies (CN) occur when peripheral nerves (PN) are exposed to long-standing excessive pressure (Bard and Lioté 2007; Blancher and Kubis 2007; Graif et al. 1991; Hobson-Webb et al. 2008; Silvestri et al. 1995; Stewart 1993). The chronic compression is responsible for local internal changes in the nerve leading to impaired nerve function and clinical findings reflecting on the nerve affected as well as the duration of compression.

1 Introduction

Compressive neuropathies (CN) occur when peripheral nerves (PN) are exposed to long-standing excessive pressure (Bard and Lioté 2007; Blancher and Kubis 2007; Graif et al. 1991; Hobson-Webb et al. 2008; Silvestri et al. 1995; Stewart 1993). The chronic compression is responsible for local internal changes in the nerve leading to impaired nerve function and clinical findings reflecting on the nerve affected as well as the duration of compression.

The recent increasing interest on CN of the wrist can be explained by their growing frequency, often related to sport or occupational activities, financial consequences due to work absence and increased diagnostic possibilities related to new development in imaging techniques (Aagaard et al. 1998; Beekman and Visser 2004; Spratt et al. 2002). CN are quite common in the routine outpatient practice and can mimic, especially in the early stages, other musculoskeletal disorders. A carefully taken patient history and a well-performed accurate clinical examination

A. M. Davis et al. (eds.), *Imaging of the Hand and Wrist*, Medical Radiology. Diagnostic Imaging,
DOI: 10.1007/174_2010_111,

are the mainstays of a correct diagnosis (El Miedany et al. 2008). Nevertheless, instrumental examinations allow the confirmation of the clinical findings, identification of the level and degree of nerve compression and in most cases permit the assessment of the cause of the compression. There are two main types of clinical examinations obtained in PN assessment: electrodiagnostic and imaging studies. The first excel in the exquisite assessment of nerve function while imaging modalities such as magnetic resonance imaging (MRI) and ultrasound (US) permits a superb evaluation of the morphology of the affected nerves and of most compressive causes (Beekman and Visser 2002; Graif et al. 1991; Martinoli et al. 1996, 2000a, b; 2005; 2008; Padua et al. 2008; Valle and Zamorani 2007). MRI allows an optimal tissue contrast and an accurate assessment of all anatomic structures surrounding the nerves. Because of its multiplanar capability and large field of view, it is the most used imaging technique in local neoplastic disorders. Nevertheless, accurate assessment of thin nerves of the distal arm requires high field equipments and collaborative patients to avoid arm movements even in uncomfortable positions. Patients' claustrophobia limits the possibility of MRI. Presence of a cardiac pacemaker is well-known absolute contraindications to the examination. The advances in US technology have lead to an improvement in the assessment of the musculoskeletal system (Bianchi and Martinoli 2007; van Holsbeeck and Introcaso 2001). Nowadays, US is considered an optimal imaging technique to evaluate the normal anatomy and disorders of PN (Fornage 1988; Peer and Bodner 2008). Examination of the hand and wrist nerves is accurately performed by using high-frequency transducers with exquisite superficial focusing capability and very high definition (Bianchi et al. 1999, 2001). Advantages of US include the ability to assess long segments of nerve quickly and perform dynamic examinations. US is inexpensive, well tolerated by patients, has no contraindications and is currently considered by several authors to be the primary technique for imaging PN pathology.

Because of the high ability of US in assessing PN of the hand and wrist as well as of it low cost, we will focus this chapter on US. First, a review of the normal anatomy of the PN and of the basic pathologic physiology of CN is presented and then follows a description of the normal anatomy of the carpal and Guyon's tunnels, together with a description of the technique of US examination and US anatomy. Finally, we will present the US appearance of the main conditions causing wrist CN.

2 Normal Anatomy and US Anatomy of PN

Nerve axons, invested by a thin layer of connective tissue (endoneurium), packed together compose the nerve fascicles that are surrounded by the perineurium. The size and number of fascicles that form a nerve depend on the individual nerve, distance from site of origin and amount of pressure the nerve is subjected to. Fascicles are separated by connective tissue (interfascicular epineurium) housing vessels. The nerve trunk is finally surrounded by the superficial epineurium, a thick sheath containing loose connective with elastic fibers and vessels (Kaymak et al. 2008).

High-resolution US can accurately assess the echo texture of normal PN both in vitro and in vivo (Martinoli et al. 2000a, b; Silvestri et al. 1995) (Fig. 1). Longitudinal sonograms image them as composed of multiple hypoechoic parallel but discontinuous linear areas separated by hyperechoic bands. On transverse scans, the hypoechoic areas correspond to oval or rounded images, encircled by a hyperechoic background. Histological correlation demonstrated that the hypoechoic bands correspond to the fascicles that run longitudinally within the body of the nerve, while the hyperechoic background reflects the interfascicular epineurium. The overall number of fascicles detected by US is smaller than their actual number and their number diminishes with the frequency of the US transducers utilized (Silvestri et al. 1995).

3 Pathological Physiology of CN

PN are elastic structures that can adapt and deform secondary to external forces. They run in the extremities surrounded by fat and connective tissue that lessen frictions against adjacent rigid anatomic structures. When crossing joints, PN are usually contained in osteofibrous tunnels that prevent their dislocation during articular movements. A variety of

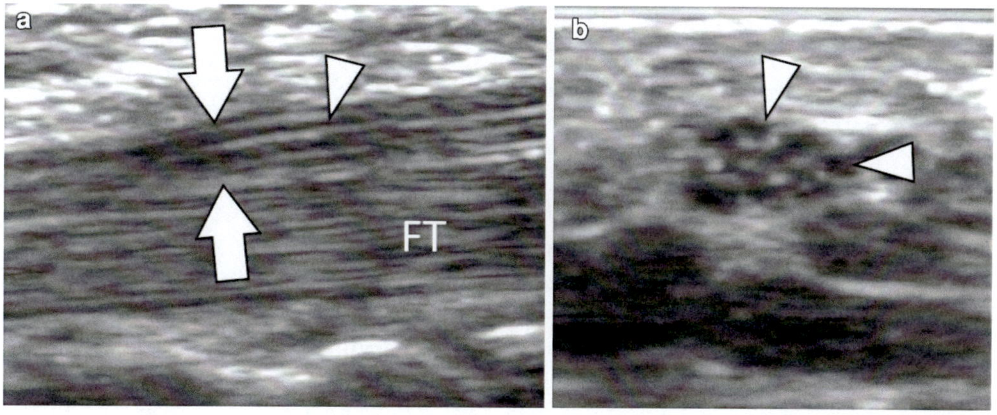

Fig. 1 Normal ultrasound anatomy of a peripheral nerve. Longitudinal and transverse sonograms. Longitudinal (**a**) and transverse (**b**) sonograms obtained on the median nerve at the carpal tunnel show the nerve (*arrows*) as a well-delimited structure made by multiple anechocoic nerve fascicles (*arrowheads*). The fascicles are surrounded by the hyperechoic perineurium. In (**a**), note the different appearance (fibrillar pattern) of the flexor tendons (FT) compared to the median nerve

pathomechanism can be involved in the development of CN. The most common mechanism is a direct extrinsic compression of nerves in anatomic locations in which they are retained in a relatively fixed position and cannot displace on the action of the compressive cause. A typical example is that of a nerve running inside an inextensible osteofibrous tunnel subject to extrinsic compression by a mass. Another mechanism is hypermobility of nerve. In these cases, the nerves are too mobile and are subject to compression or stretching against bony protuberance or fibrous ligaments during displacements.

In EN, nerve changes and clinical symptoms are dependent both on the degree of compression and on its duration. Low pressure applied for short time is relatively well tolerated, and complete recovery can be expected after withdrawal of external compression. On the other side, high pressure for long periods of time can severely alter the morphology and function of nerves and eventually can result in its irreversible damage. Long-standing external compression on a PN results in internal structural changes. First, impaired vein flow leads to increased intraneural interstitial pressure that results in reversible intraneural edema, mainly found at the level of connective tissue. In more prolonged compressions, ischemia due to damage of the vasa nervorum, the small vessels that are responsible for the vascularization of the nerve trunk, leads to irreversible internal fibrosis. This results lastly in myelin sheath and axonal degeneration. Such morphological changes alter nerve conduction with subsequent sensitive or motor impairment depending on the type of nerve affected.

Wrist CN are mainly observed as a consequence of nerve compression inside inextensible fibroosseous tunnels. The most frequent is the carpal tunnel syndrome (CTS), which follows the entrapment of the median nerve (MN) inside the carpal tunnel (CT) (Ashraf et al. 2009; Bianchi et al. 2007; Boutte et al. 2009; Buchberger et al. 1991, 1992; Duncan et al. 1999; Pinilla et al. 2008; Sernik et al. 2008). Entrapment of the ulnar nerve (UN) at the Guyon's tunnel (GT) is less frequent (Ashraf et al. 2009; Bianchi et al. 2004; Patel et al.).

4 Anatomy of the Nerves of the Wrist and Hand

The main nerves found in the wrist region are the MN, radial nerve (RN) and UN. The MN descends inside the anterior compartment of the forearm in a median position to enter the hand through the CT, a fibroosseous canal located at the volar aspect of the wrist (Bianchi et al. 2007). The CT is an inextensible structure delimited posteriorly by the carpal bones and anteriorly by the transverse carpal ligament (TCL). The TCL is a thick fibrous structure that is continuous with the anterior superficial fascia of the forearm proximally and blends distally with the palmar aponeurosis of the hand. From an anatomic point of view, two layers compose the TCL. The superficial layer is formed by the distal expansion of the palmaris gracilis tendon that prolongs into the palmar aponeurosis. The deep layer is made by thick transverse fibers forming a rectangular ligament of nearly 3–4 cm of craniocaudal size. The radial aspect of the TCL inserts into the tuberosity of the scaphoid and into the tubercle of the trapezium, while the ulnar attachments are into the pisiform and the hook of the hamate. A vertical septum origins from the inferior radial aspect of the TCL and delimitates a small lateral fibrous tunnel that houses the flexor carpi radialis tendon. The CT is larger proximally at the level of the pisiform and smaller distally at the level of the hook of the hamate. The TCL is thicker and more rigid distally. The CT contains nine tendons, four tendons of the flexor digitorum superficialis and four tendons of the flexor digitorum profundus for the 2nd–5th fingers and the tendon of the flexor pollicis longus. To facilitate tendons gliding inside the tunnel during flexion and extension of the fingers, synovial sheaths, formed by a visceral and a parietal layer, surround them. The visceral layer attaches firmly to the tendons, while the parietal layer adheres to the peritendineous structures. A small amount of synovial fluid retained between the two layers allows their gliding during tendon movements and their smooth gliding. Although a great variability exists in the arrangement of synovial tendon sheaths, they are usually two in number. The lateral surrounds the flexor pollicis longus tendon, while the larger medial one envelops the remaining tendons. Several anatomic variant of the CT can be encountered and can predispose to CTS. A variety of anomalous muscles can be found inside the CT (Touborg-Jensen 1970). They are mainly the result of cranial extension of lubricates muscles or distal extension of a flexor digitorum anomalous bellies. Other variants are less common.

At approximately 5 cm from the proximal wrist crease, the MN leaves the palmar cutaneous branch that supplies the proximal portion of the palm of the hand (Taleisnik 1973). The branch initially runs close to the main nerve trunk. Then, it leaves it to direct laterally and run between the palmaris and flexor carpi radialis tendon. The small sensitive branch then reaches the hand region either running superficially to the TCL or between its two layers. Knowledge of the anatomy and course of the superficial branch is important since it can be inadvertently injured during TCL section in CT release.

After having released the sensitive branch, the MN enters the tunnel along with the flexor tendons. Inside the CT, it lies just inferior to the TCL, superficial and parallel to the flexor tendons of the index and middle fingers and medial to the flexor pollicis longus tendon. The second branch of the nerve at this level is a thenar motor branch. The branch can detach from the trunk either proximal, inside or distal by rapport to the CT. The different types must be recognized by the surgeon to avoid their inadvertent surgical section. It supplies the thenar muscles. More distally, the MN splits into several sensory branches to the first, second and third digits and the radial half of the fourth digit. Some anatomic variations in the MN must be known since they can facilitate CTS. The most frequent is the so-called bifid MN (Iannicelli et al. 2000, 2001; Propeck et al. 2000). It is due to proximal division of the nerve into two separate nerves that run close one to the other inside the CT. A bifid NM can be seldom associated with persistence of the median artery, another common anatomic variant (Gassner et al. 2002; Kele et al. 2002). In these cases, the artery lies in between the two nerves and runs with them inside the CT. Thrombosis of this anomalous artery can be associated with CTS either because of its enlargement or because of secondary ischemia of the vasa nervorum (Kele et al. 2002). These variations can be easily detected by US. The bifid median nerve appears as a split of the nerve in two trunks that usually have a different size. The nerve can be separated by a variable distance, and usually, they are more easily detected at the level of the pronator quadratus on transverse sonograms. When they run inside the CT, they run closer and are more difficult to be distinguished. The persistent median artery can be easily followed by US since it originates from the ulnar artery at the level of the proximal forearm to descend close to the MN along the anterior aspect of the forearm. Since the artery has approximately the same diameter of the MN fascicles, an accurate technique of examination must be deployed to detect it. In case of doubt, gentle pressure with the transducer results in augmentation of its pulsatility. Color Doppler can be also used to assess the internal blood flow.

The small GT is located palmar and medial to the CT. It is formed by the palmar carpal ligament, which forms the roof, and by the TCL, the pisiform and the hook of the hamate that constitute the remaining walls. The tunnel houses the UN, and the ulnar artery and veins surrounded by loose connective tissue and fat. As for the CT, accessory muscles can be found running inside the GT (Patel et al.). The most common is the accessory abductor digiti minimi. This muscle takes origin from the antebrachial fascia of palmaris longus tendon at the distal aspect of the forearm. It then directs distally to enter the Guyon's tunnel. Inside the tunnel, it is mostly found running superficially to the UN and UA. Nevertheless, some muscles run in between the two. It then enters the palm of the hand to insert into the base of the proximal phalanx of the small fingers together with the abductor digiti minimi muscles.

5 Technique of US Examination and Normal US Anatomy

US can easily detect the MN and UN at the level of the distal forearm (Aleman et al. 2008; Bianchi et al. 2004, 2007; Jamadar et al. 2001). As for every anatomic district, knowledge of the normal anatomy and of the peculiar nerve echo texture is a definite prerequisite for the detection of PN and differentiation from other surrounding structures such as tendons. The MN can be easily detected since it runs between the tendons of the flexor digitorum superficialis and profundus muscles. The UN runs close to the UA that is readily detected at US because of its pulsatility. The nerve lies just medial to the artery. Detection of the smaller nerves such as the superficial branch of the RN is also possible but necessitates the use of high-frequency transducers and a good experience in PN evaluation.

US accurately depicts both tunnels and their contents (Bianchi and Martinoli 2007; Buchberger et al. 1991, 1992; Peer and Bodner 2008; van Holsbeeck and Introcaso 2001) (Fig. 2). The CT is visualized by transverse and sagittal sonograms. Transverse images are obtained first since they are more panoramic. If obtained with adequate transducers, i.e., larger then 4–5 cm, transverse sonograms allow the simultaneous visualization of all intracanal structures. They are obtained first proximal to the CT, at the level of the pronator quadratus muscle, to localize the different anatomic structures before they enter the canal. Moreover, it is important to explore the cranial portion of the MN since in CTS the MN is larger at this level. More distally, identification of different bone landmarks of the CT is essential in order to perform a correct US examination. At the proximal tunnel, the landmarks are the rounded appearances of the pisiform medially and of the scaphoid laterally. Both bones are covered by a flexor tendon: the flexor carpi radialis lies on the scaphoid, while the flexor carpi ulnaris inserts into the pisiform and, by its more superficial fibers, continues distally as the pisohamate ligament. The TCL appears as a curved linear hyperechoic band connecting the lower face of the pisiform to the scaphoid. Beneath the ligament are imaged the flexor tendons and the MN. Since these run obliquely, the transducer must be tilted toward cranial to correctly depict them and avoid anisotropy. Each tendon can be localized by its anatomic position and behavior at dynamic scan during the

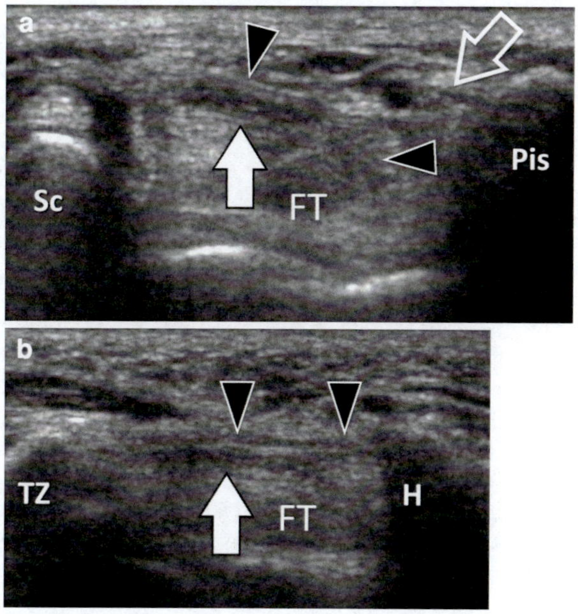

Fig. 2 In vivo normal ultrasound appearance of the carpal tunnel. Transverse images obtained from cranial (**a**) to distal (**b**). At the level of the proximal CT (**a**), the median nerve (*arrow*) lies inside the tunnel in a superficial location, between the transverse carpal ligament (*arrowheads*) and the flexor tendons (FT). *Sc* scaphoid; *Pis* pisiform. The Guyon's tunnel (*void arrow*) houses the ulnar artery and nerve. At the distal tunnel (**b**), the transverse carpal ligament appears rectilinear and the median nerve more flattened. *TZ* trapezium; *H* hamate hook

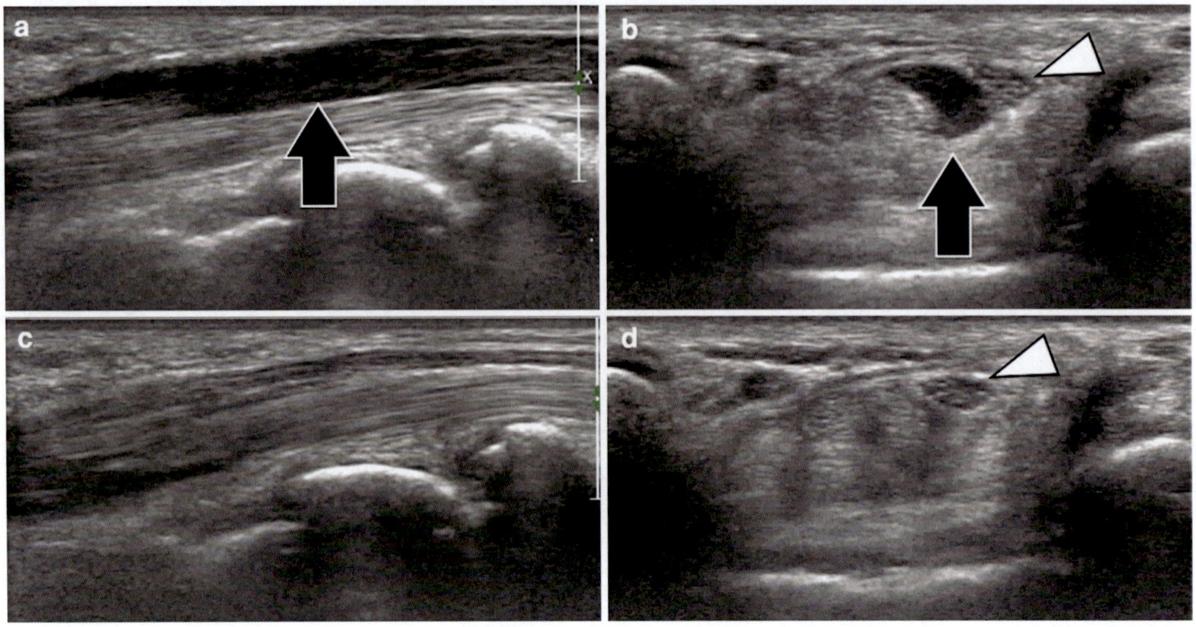

Fig. 3 Carpal tunnel. Anatomic variations: anomalous muscle. Longitudinal and transverse sonograms obtained with fingers in extension (**a**, **b**) and flexion (**c**, **d**). Images obtained in extension show a low-lying accessory bundle (*arrows*) of the flexor digitorum superficialis muscle. Transverse image shows the displacement of the median nerve (*arrowhead*) by the muscle. Note how the accessory muscle moves cranially to the carpal tunnel in fingers' flexion and is no more evident

movement of the fingers (Chen et al. 1997). No muscles can be found in normal condition inside the CT. In cases of accessory muscles, realization of dynamic examination during flexion and extension of the fingers is mandatory to detect them (Fig. 3). The MN appears as an oval hyperechoic structure containing several rounded hypoechoic fascicles. It lies just deep to the TCL. Bone landmarks of the distal tunnel are the pointed hook of the hamate medially and the flat volar surface of the trapezium laterally. Compared to the proximal tunnel, the distal tunnel is smaller. As a consequence, the flexor tendons appear crowded and hardly distinguishable and the MN more flattened. The distal TCL is ticker and more rectilinear. Sagittal images are then obtained over the flexor tendons and the MN that presents the characteristic fascicular internal appearance (Bianchi et al. 2007; Bianchi and Martinoli 2007). The occurrence of a bifid MN, found in as many as 2.8% of normal subjects, appears at US as a splitting of the nerve at the proximal level (Fig. 4). In the distal canal, the two nerves are found closer and are difficult to distinguish. Bifid MN can be also involved in CTS (Bayrak et al. 2008). The occurrence of an accessory median artery located close to a normal or bifid MN inside the CT is a well-known anatomic variation (Fig. 4). Its internal flow is readily assessed by color Doppler imaging. US findings of the anomalous artery correlate well with MRI appearance (Fig. 5).

As for the carpal tunnel, transverse images of the Guyon's tunnel are obtained at a proximal and distal level (Fig. 6) (Bianchi et al. 1999, 2004). Proximal sonograms, acquired at the pisiform level, show the thin palmar carpal ligament overlying the pulsatile UA. Once detected the artery, inclination of the transducer helps in depicting the UN that is located between it and the medial aspect of the pisiform. Distal sonograms show the superficial branches of the UA and UN overlying the tip of the hook of the hamate. Tilting the transducer in a way to study the medial aspect of the hypothenar muscles allows the visualization of the medial aspect of the hamate bone and detection of the deep ulnar artery branch and of the deep (motor) branch of the UN surrounded by the hypothenar muscles. Longitudinal sonograms of the branches of the UN are technically

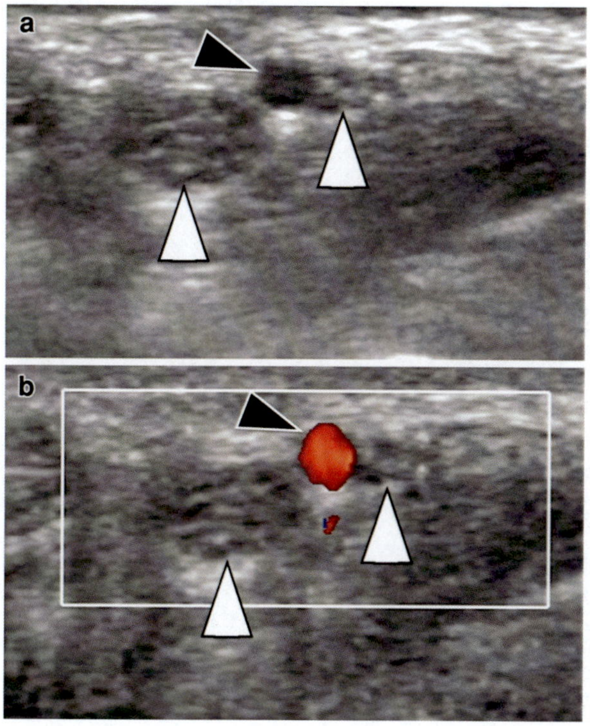

Fig. 4 Carpal tunnel. Anatomic variations: bifid median nerve with persistent median artery. Transverse (**a**) and transverse color Doppler (**b**) sonograms. Images show a median nerve made by two separate trunk of different size (*white arrowheads*). A persistent median artery runs between the two nerves (*black arrowheads*). The *artery* shows normal internal flow signal at color Doppler

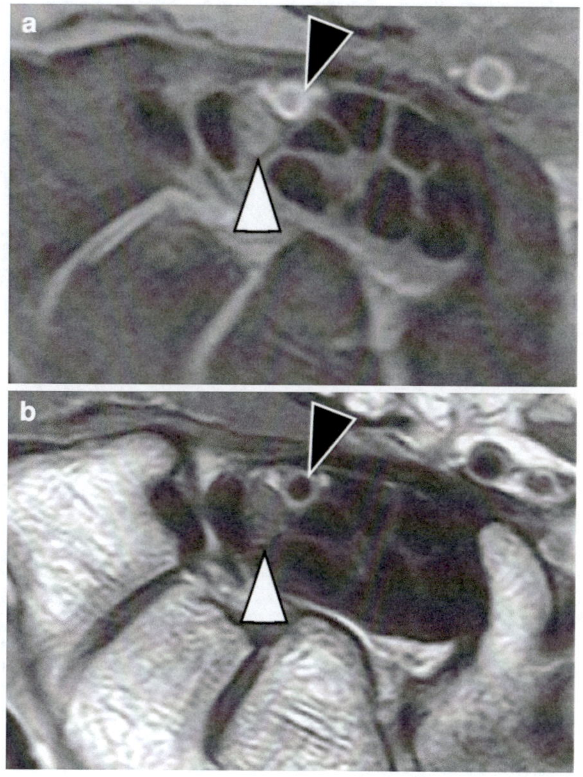

Fig. 5 Carpal tunnel. Anatomic variations: MRI appearance of persistent median artery. Transverse PD fat sat (**a**) and PD (**b**) MR images show the anomalous artery (*black arrowheads*) located close to the normal MN (*white arrowheads*)

more difficult to be obtained and are of limited help in the assessment of the GT.

Although injections of steroid inside the carpal tunnel are realized by clinical guidance in the vast majority of patients, US can seldom be used to avoid inadvertent MN injury (Smith et al. 2008).

6 CTS

Several articles have demonstrated a good correlation between US data and electrophysiologic measurements in CTS (Kaymak et al. 2008; Kwon et al. 2008; Mondelli et al. 2008). US findings have been extensively described (Bard and Lioté 2007; Bianchi et al. 2007; Buchberger et al. 1992; Hobson-Webb et al. 2008; Klauser et al. 2009; Padua et al. 2008). They can be arbitrary divided into alterations in MN and CT appearance and findings related to the compressive causes.

6.1 Changes in MN Appearance

In long-standing compression inside the CT, the MN shows the alteration in its size as well as morphologic changes. Regardless of the cause of local compression, the nerve presents typically a swollen appearance at the proximal tunnel and decrease in the size in the distal tunnel (Fig. 7). To objective these morphologic changes, two measures have been proposed. The first is the nerve cross-sectional area that is obtained at the proximal level. Two techniques of measurements have been proposed: the ellipse formula and direct tracing of the axial surface of the nerve that has been shown to be more accurate. A surface greater than 0.10 cm^2 has been reported to be a valuable criterion for the diagnosis. Different authors have defined different values with threshold suggested for MN abnormality between 9 and 14 mm^2. Klauser reported better results by comparing

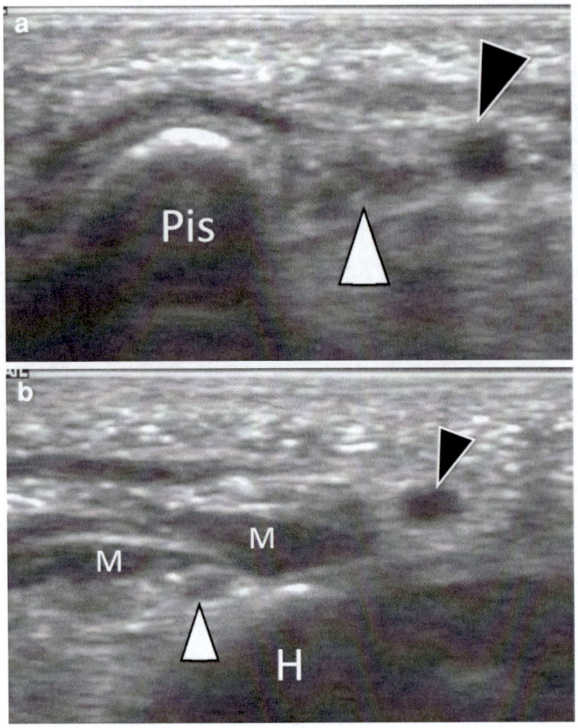

Fig. 6 In vivo normal ultrasound appearance of the Guyon's tunnel. Transverse images obtained from cranial (**a**) to distal (**b**). At the proximal level (**a**), the ulnar nerve (*white arrowhead*) lies inside the tunnel between the ulnar artery (*black arrowhead*) and the pisiform (Pis). At the distal tunnel (**b**), note the deep branch of the UN (*small white arrowhead*) located close to the hook of the hamate (H) and surrounded by muscles (M). The superficial branch of the UA runs in a more superficial location (*small black arrowhead*)

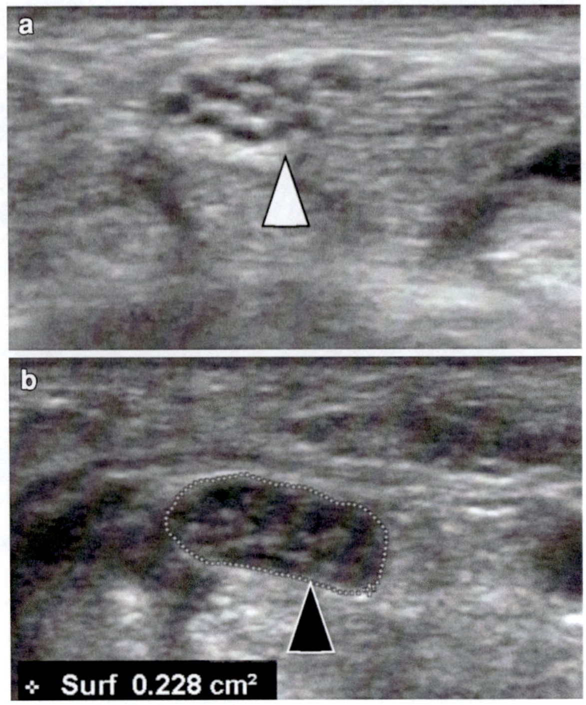

Fig. 7 Carpal tunnel syndrome. Morphologic changes in the median nerve. Transverse sonograms obtained in a patient with carpal tunnel syndrome proximal (**a**) and at the level of the tunnel (**b**). In (**a**), the nerve (*white arrowhead*) presents a regular internal aspect with the hypoechoic nerves fascicules well differentiated from the internal connective tissue. In (**b**), the nerve (*black arrowhead*) is swollen with a surface area evaluated at 22.8 mm^2. It presents a homogenous hypoechoic appearance due to internal edema or fibrosis

cross-sectional area measurements of the MN obtained at the level of the carpal tunnel with those obtained at the level of the pronator quadratus muscle (Klauser et al. 2009). The authors found that the difference between the two measurements (Delta CSA) allowed more specific and sensitive results. Use of a Delta CSA threshold of 2 mm^2 yielded the greatest sensitivity (99%) and specificity (100%) for the diagnosis of CTS (Klauser et al. 2009). The second measure is the so-called fattening ratio that is obtained at the distal level and is calculated by dividing the latero-lateral diameter of the nerve for its thickness. A value greater of 4 is associated with CTS.

High-resolution transducers can also show intraneural changes, i.e., reduced echogenicity and a disorganized internal fascicular pattern due to edema and fibrosis. Color Doppler techniques can show increased flow signals in the perineural plexus and among the nerve fascicles due to acute neuritis (Fig. 8).

6.2 Changes in CT Appearance

In the wide majority of patients, because of the increased intracanal pressure, the TCL presents a more pronounced convex appearance. This sign, the so-called bulging of TCL, is found either at proximal or at distal tunnel (Buchberger et al. 1991, 1992). Objective assessment of bulging has been reported at the distal tunnel and can be obtained by measuring the distance from the most superficial point of the TCL to a line connecting the tips of the hook of the hamate and the tubercle of the trapezium. A distance equal or greater then 4 mm is considered abnormal and

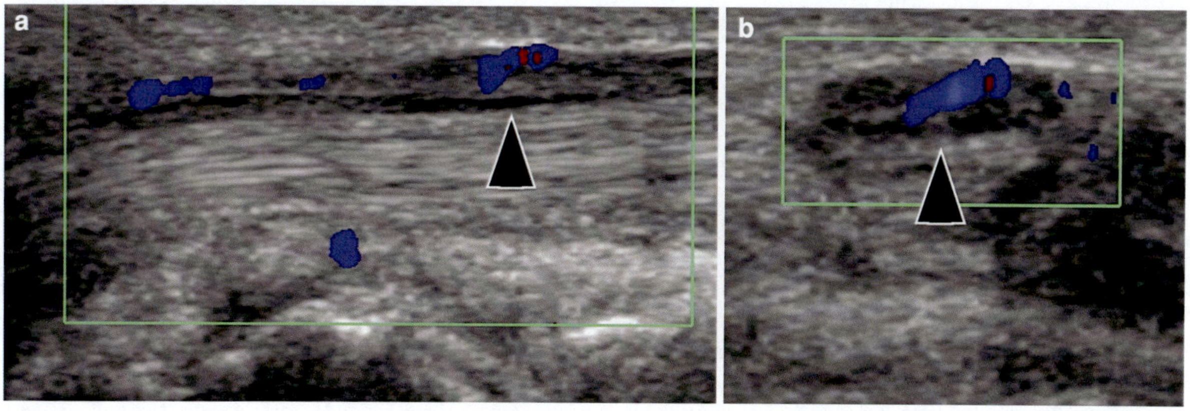

Fig. 8 Carpal tunnel syndrome. Color Doppler changes in the median nerve. Longitudinal (**a**) and transverse (**b**) sonograms obtained in a patient with carpal tunnel syndrome. In both images vascular signals inside the nerve (*arrowheads*) are evident due to hyperemia secondary to nerve compression

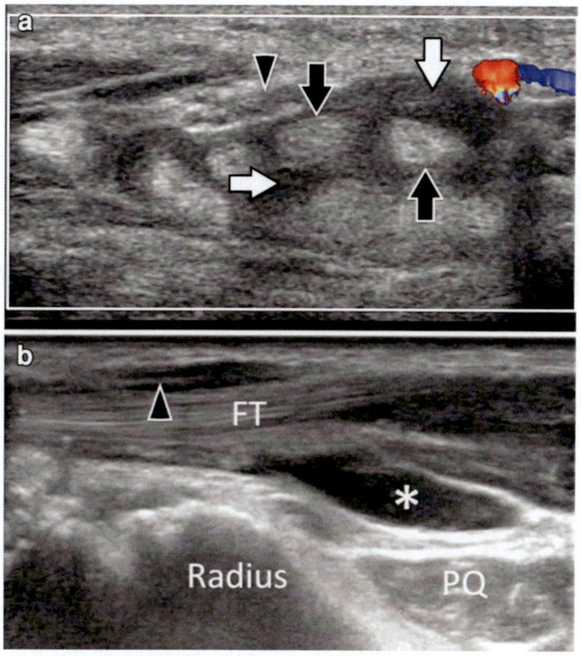

Fig. 9 Carpal tunnel syndrome. Causes of nerve compression. Tenosynovitis. **a** transverse color Doppler sonogram in a patient with carpal tunnel syndrome due to aspecific tenosynovitis. Images show the tendons (*black arrows*) surrounded by hypoechoic thickened synovium (*white arrow*). Note displacement of the median nerve (*arrowhead*). No hypervascular changes are noted inside the synovium. **b** serous tenosynovitis of the flexor tendons revealed by an anechoic effusion (*asterisk*) located inside the tendon sheath

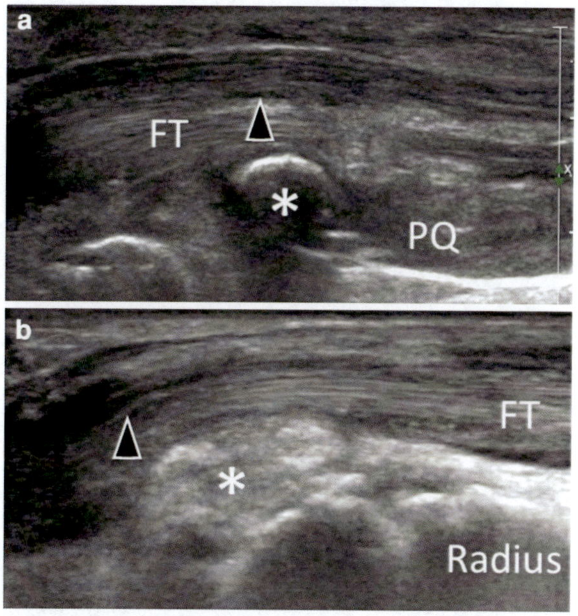

Fig. 10 Carpal tunnel syndrome. Causes of nerve compression. Longitudinal sonograms (**a**) volar displacement of an osseous fragment (*asterisk*) in fracture of the distal epyphisis of the radius (**b**) capsular thickening and calcification (*asterisk*) in chondrocalcinosis. *PQ* pronator quadratus muscle; *FT* flexor tendons, *arrowheads* median nerve

significantly associated with CTS. Sometimes increased thickness of the TCL can be noted together with focal calcifications.

6.3 Demonstration of Compressive Causes

The vast majority of CTS is due to aspecific tenosynovitis of the flexor tendons. US demonstrates tenosynovitis as a hypoechoic halo surrounding the

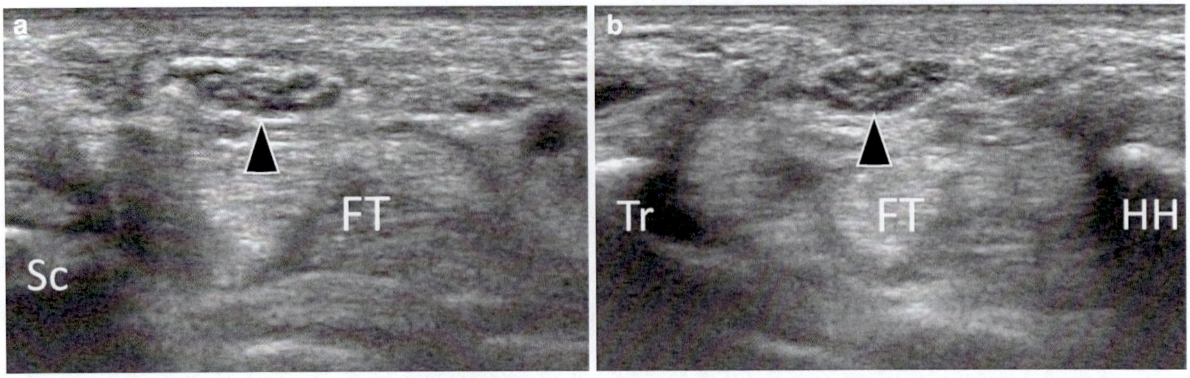

Fig. 11 Carpal tunnel syndrome. Post-surgical appearance. Normal findings at transverse sonograms obtained at the proximal (**a**) and distal (**b**) tunnel. Both images show a palmar displacement of the median nerve because of correct release of the transverse carpal ligament. *FT* flexor tendons; *Sc* scaphoid; *Tr* trapezium; *HH* hook of the hamate; *arrowheads* median nerve

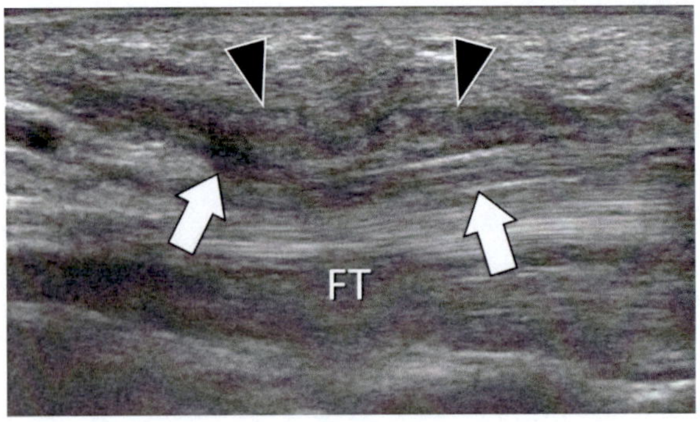

Fig. 12 Carpal tunnel syndrome. Post-surgical complications. Thickening of the transverse carpal ligament. Longitudinal sonogram. Image shows an irregular hypoechoic thickening of the transverse carpal ligament (*black arrowheads*) compressing the median nerve (*white arrows*). *FT* flexor tendons

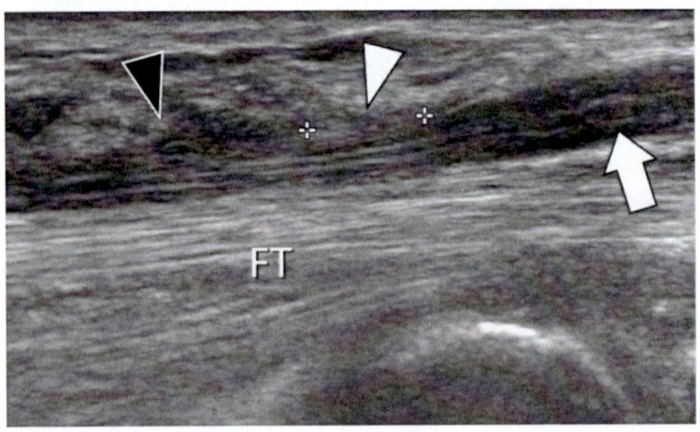

Fig. 13 Carpal tunnel syndrome. Post-surgical complications. Partial release of the transverse carpal ligament. Longitudinal sonogram. Image shows the release of the distal transverse carpal ligament that appears hypoechoic (*black arrowhead*). The proximal ligament was not sectioned at surgery and still compresses the median nerve. Note swelling and hypoechogenicity of the proximal to the compression site (*white arrow*). *FT* flexor tendons

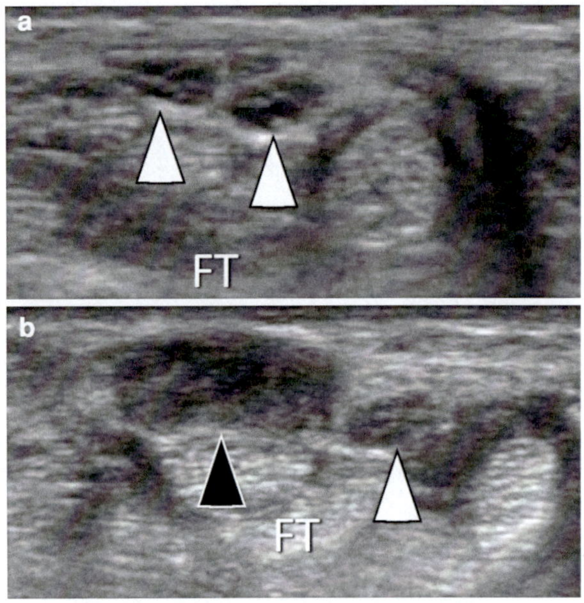

Fig. 14 Carpal tunnel syndrome. Post-surgical complications. Trauma of a bifid median nerve at transverse sonograms. Images obtained proximal to (**a**) and inside (**b**) the tunnel shows a hypoechoic traumatic neuroma of a trunk of the bifid median nerve secondary to local trauma during arthroscopy. *FT* flexor tendons; *arrowheads* bifid median nerve

tendons due to fluid effusion and thickening of the tendon synovial sheaths (Fig. 9). Typically, tenosynovitis facilitates the visualization and differentiation of the tendons running within the tunnel because of the increased contrast between the hypoechoic synovium and the hyperechoic tendons. Color Doppler can detect hyperemic changes within the inflamed synovium or more rarely inside the tendons. Sometimes a definite fluid effusion can be detected inside the tendons sheath as a hypoechoic collection located at the proximal cul-de-sac of the tendon sheath (Fig. 9). Unfortunately, the US appearance of tenosynovitis is aspecific, and US does not allow the differentiation among inflammation secondary to systemic arthropathies such as rheumatoid arthritis or infections and other possible etiologies.

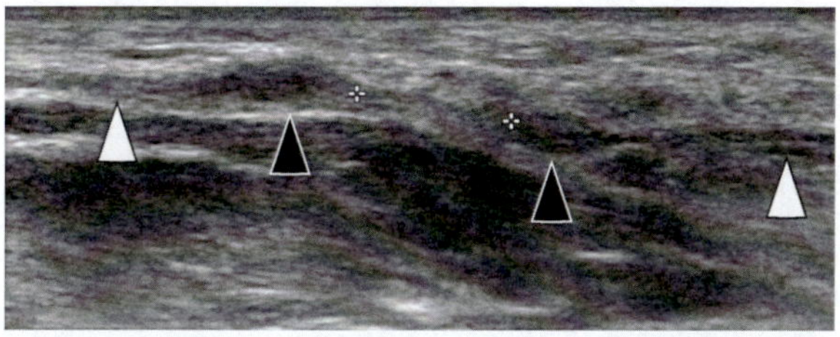

Fig. 15 Carpal tunnel syndrome. Post-surgical complications. Section of a branch of the median nerve. Longitudinal sonogram. Image obtained at the palm of the hand shows complete interruption of one of the distal branch of the median nerve (callipers) secondary to local trauma during arthroscopy. *Black arrowheads* proximal and distal stump neuroma; *white arrowheads* normal nerve portions

Focal masses inside the tunnel are easily detected by US. US can detect accessory muscles as well-delimited hypoechoic masses that exhibit the same internal echo texture of normal peripheral muscles (Fig. 3). Dynamic examination is particularly useful in their detection since it shows the muscle entering/leaving the CT during flexion/extension of the fingers. Transverse images are best suited to show the displacement and compression of the nerve during movements of the fingers. Ganglia are the most common masses found inside the CT. They are cystic lesions with fibrous wall, filled by tick mucinous fluid, that are depicted by US as polilobulated, hypoanechoic structures with well-defined borders and internal septa. Older ganglia show thickening of the peripheral wall and of the internal septa. No internal flow signals are depicted by color Doppler in uncomplicated ganglia, while discrete hyperemia can be detected in recent rupture. Amyloid deposits are rare causes of CTS and can be seen in long-standing renal failure. US images them as solid hypoechoic ill-defined lesions. Knowledge of the underlying systemic disorder is obviously a prerequisite for the US diagnosis. A hypertrophied callus secondary to a

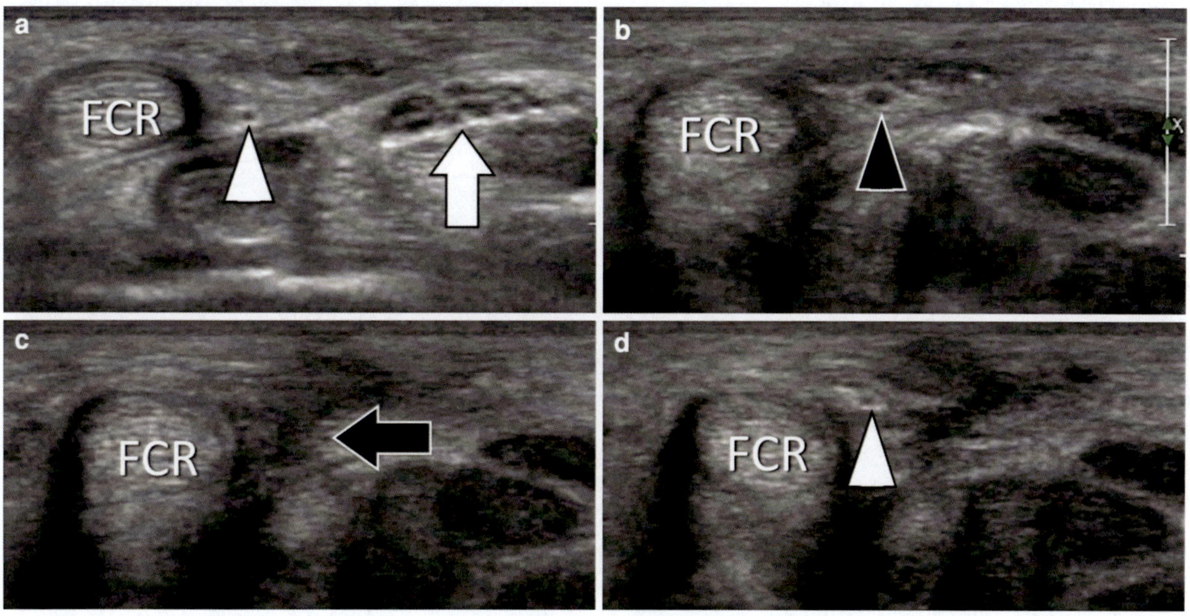

Fig. 16 Carpal tunnel syndrome. Post-surgical complications. Section of the sensitive superficial branch of the median nerve. Transverse sonograms obtained from proximal to distal (**a–d**). **a** In the more proximal image, the branch is normal (*white arrowhead*). *Arrow* median nerve. **b** More distally, the branch is swollen and hypoechoic due to traumatic neuroma (**c**) at the level of the section of the transverse carpal ligament, US shows an irregular area of fibrosis (*arrow*). The branch is not visible. **d** More distally, the branch presents a normal appearance. *FCR* flexor carpi radialis tendon

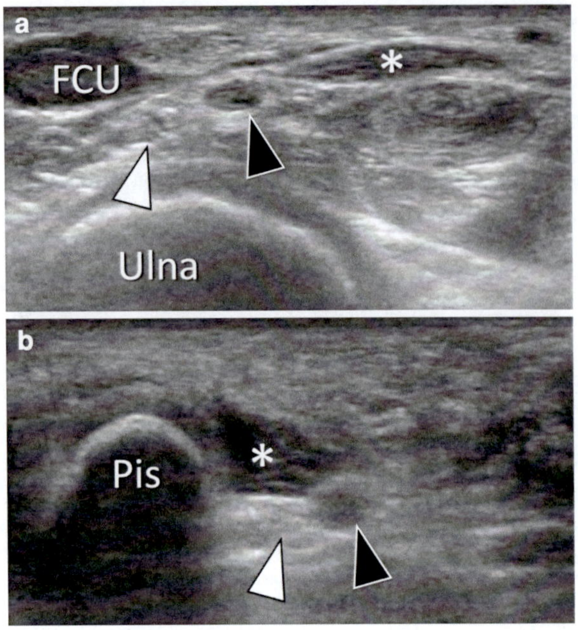

Fig. 17 Guyon's tunnel. Anatomic variations: anomalous muscle. Transverse sonograms obtained on the distal forearm (**a**) and at the level of the Guyon's tunnel (**b**). Proximal image (**a**) shows an accessory abductor digiti minimi muscle (*asterisk*) originating from the antebrachial fascia. In (**b**), the muscle run within the Guyon's tunnel. It displaces anteriorly the ulnar artery (*black arrowhead*) and nerve (*white arrowhead*). *FCU* flexor carpi ulnaris; *Pis* pisiform

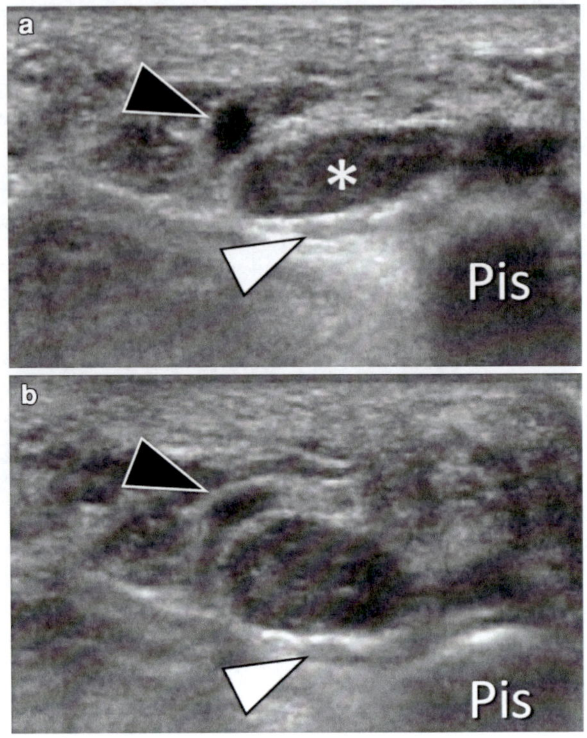

Fig. 18 Guyon's tunnel. Anatomic variations: anomalous muscle. Transverse sonograms obtained at the level of the Guyon's tunnel at rest (**a**) and during active abduction of the little finger (**b**).Images show an accessory abductor digiti minimi muscle (*asterisk*) located between the ulnar artery (*black arrowhead*) and nerve (*white arrowhead*). In (**b**), note the increase in the size of the accessory muscle (*asterisk*) during contraction and secondary displacement of the ulnar artery and nerve. *Pis* pisiform

fracture of the distal radius or palmar displacement of bone fragments can cause compression of the MN. They are best evaluated by standard radiographs or CT. Nevertheless, they can also be assessed by US (Fig. 10). In chondrocalcinosis, calcified deposits in the volar capsule of the wrist joint can also result in a mass effect with secondary displacement of the MN (Fig. 10). A volar subluxed or dislocated semilunar is rapidly detected by US inside the CT by its characteristic outline. Neurogenic tumors located inside the CT are a rare cause of CTS. They appear as hypoechoic masses with well-defined borders located close to the MN. A definite differential diagnosis between Schwannomas and neurofibromas can be difficult, if not impossible, at US. Schwannomas are usually eccentric to the nerve and can show high internal vascular signals at color Doppler, while in neurofibromas nerve fascicle enter the relatively avascular tumor. Lipofibromatous is a fibrofatty mass that densely infiltrates and encases most commonly the MN. The enlarged nerve can be easily detected by either US or MRI (Toms et al. 2006).

US is useful in the assessment of post-operative PN lesions (Peer et al. 2001) and also has a role in recurrent symptoms or complications (Tagliafico et al. 2008) after CTS release and in the post-surgical follow-up (Smith et al. 2008). In well-performed surgical release of the TCL, the MN can be seen displaced anteriorly. Transverse images are best suited to assess the absence of persistent compression (Fig. 11). Recurrences are mainly related to thickening of the TCL due to local fibrosis (Fig. 12) or incomplete surgical section of the TCL. Incomplete sections of the proximal portion of the TCL are mostly seen in patients operated by an endoscopic approach. In these patients, US usually detects the swollen, interrupted distal TCL; while in a more proximal location, the ligament appear continuous (Fig. 13). The most common complications of endoscopic release are

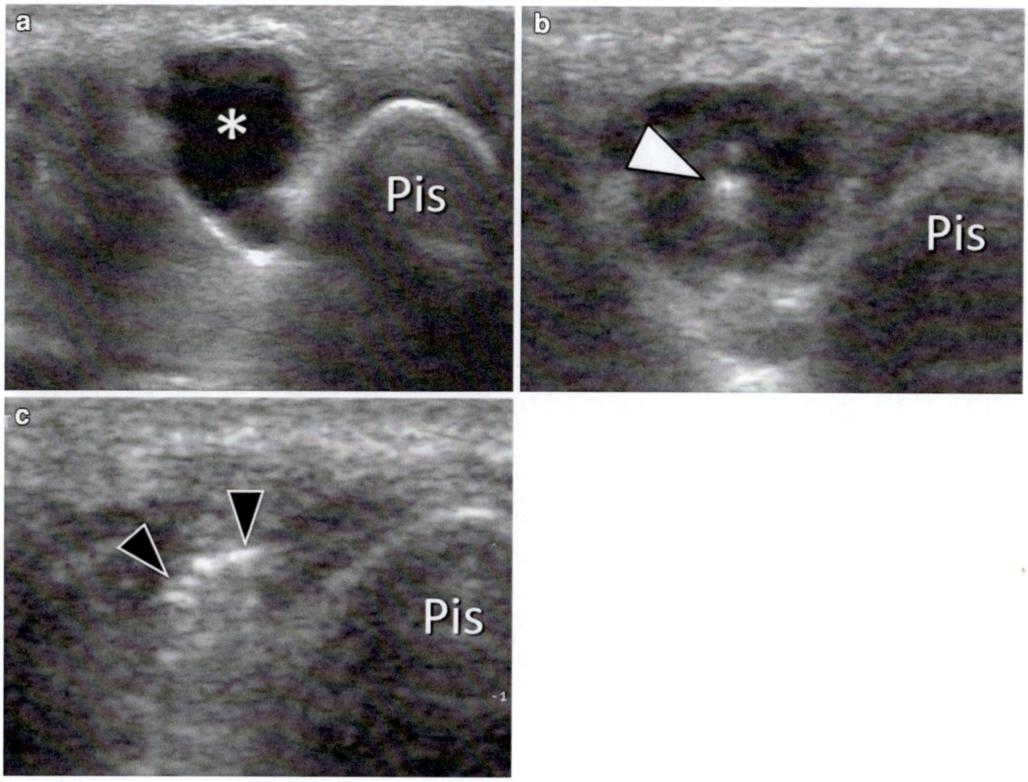

Fig. 19 Guyon's tunnel. Intracanalar ganglion cyst. Transverse sonograms obtained at the level of the Guyon's tunnel. **a** note the ganglion (*asterisk*) appearing as an anechoic cystic lesion located inside the tunnel. **b** US-guided needle puncture. Note the needle (*white arrowhead*) located in the center of the ganglion. **c** After aspiration of the mucoid content, the injected steroid presents as hyperechoic foci (*black arrowhead*). *Pis* pisiform

section of the MN. They are more commonly encountered in patients with bifid MN (Fig. 14). They appear as partial or complete interruption of the nerve that can show focal swelling due to amputation neuromas. Inadvertent section of distal branches of the MN at the palm of the hand can be also detected (Fig. 15). Cut of the palmar sensitive branch of the MN during sectioning of the TCL can be seen in open release of CTS (Tagliafico et al. 2008). In addition, the small branch can be injured in the post-operative course due to the development of local fibrosis of the perineural tissues (Fig. 16).

7 Guyon's Tunnel Syndrome

Compared to the common CTS, ulnar neuropathies at the Guyon's canal are rare. Depending on the site of compression (cranial or distal to nerve bifurcation), various syndromes due to the involvement of either the main nerve trunk or its motor and sensitive branches have been described.

Chronic external pressure caused by repetitive utilization of tools during manual work or sport activities (such as biking), in which chronic stress is applied on the ulnar aspect of the volar wrist, can cause a nerve entrapment. Focal masses are easily detected on transverse US scans. As mentioned before, anomalous muscles inside the GT are well depicted by US (Fig. 17). Since there are no muscles inside the tunnel in normal conditions, the diagnosis is straightforward in case of a mass located inside the tunnel, which presents the typical internal muscle architecture. Color Doppler does not show any internal flow signals. Contrasted abduction of the small finger during dynamic US examination reveals shortening and increase in the axial diameters of the muscle due to its contraction (Fig. 18). These muscles

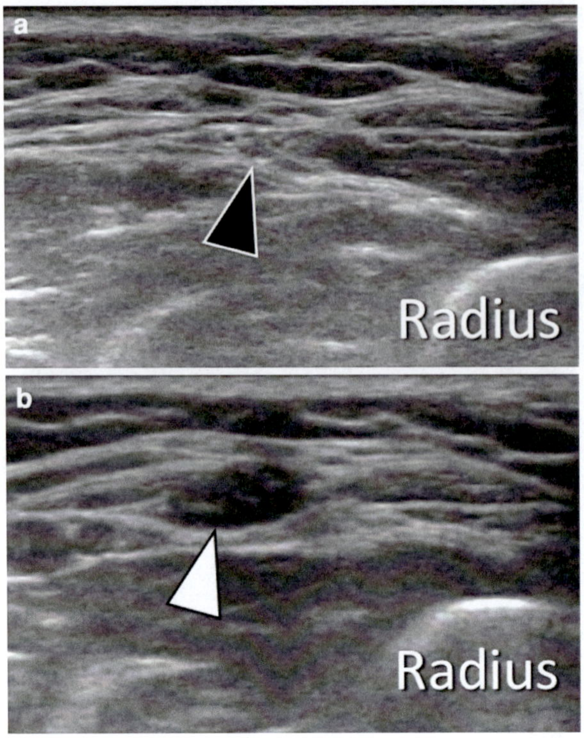

Fig. 20 Post-traumatic neuroma of the superficial branch of the radial nerve. Transverse images (**a**) A proximal image shows a normal branch (*white arrowhead*). More distally (**b**), the nerve is swollen and hypoechoic (*black arrowhead*) because of a post-traumatic neuroma

are however normally well tolerated. When hypertrophied, they can compress the UN (Patel et al.). Ganglion cysts usually related to the pisotriquetrum joint space can develop inside the GT. They present at US as anechoic cystic lesion with sharp borders (Fig. 19). US can effectively guide a real-time cystic puncture, thus avoiding inadvertent injury to the UA and UN. Steroid injection can also be guided by US (Fig. 19).

8 Disorders of the Superficial Branch of the RN

The superficial branch of the RN is rarely affected by CN at the wrist or hand. This small sensitive nerve can be compressed by local fibrosis of the tissues surrounding the retinaculum of the first extensor compartment in patients affected by De Quervain's tenosynovitis (Lanzetta and Foucher 1993). US shows aspecific thickening of the nerve associated with the typical findings of De Quervain's stenosing tenosynovitis. In rare cases, the superficial branch can be unintentionally injured during surgery (Fig. 20).

9 Key Points

US bone landmarks of the carpal tunnel
- Radial side proximal: tubercle of the scaphoid (rounded)
- Ulnar side proximal: pisiform (rounded)
- Radial side distal: trapezium (flat)
- Ulnar side distal: hook of the hamate (pointed)

US appearance in peripheral nerves entrapment
- Nerve swollen and hypoechoic proximal to the entrapment site
- Nerve thinned at the level of the entrapment
- Nerve swollen and hypoechoic distal to the entrapment site (less common)
- Internal vascular signals proximal to the entrapment site (less common)

Clinical utility of US in CTS
- Confirm the clinical diagnosis by showing changes in the MN
- Assess the cause of nerve compression
- Illustrate normal anatomic variants that can modify the surgical approach

Most common complication after CT release
- Incomplete resection of the transverse carpal ligament (endoscopic approach)
- Local fibrosis with thickening of the transverse carpal ligament
- Nerve injuries (bifid median nerve) (endoscopic approach)

References

Aagaard BD, Maravilla KR, Kliot M (1998) MR neurography. MR imaging of peripheral nerves. Magn Reson Imaging Clin North Am 6:179–194

Aleman L, Berna JD, Reus M et al (2008) Reproducibility of sonographic measurements of the median nerve. J Ultrasound Med 27:193–197

Ashraf AR, Jali R, Moghtaderi AR, Yazdani AH (2009) The diagnostic value of ultrasonography in patients with electrophysiologicaly confirmed carpal tunnel syndrome. Electromyogr Clin Neurophysiol 49:3–8

Bard H, Lioté F (2007) Les syndromes canalaires vus en rhumatologie. Rev Rhum Fr Ed 74:315–433
Bayrak IK, Bayrak AO, Kale M et al (2008) Bifid median nerve in patients with carpal tunnel syndrome. J Ultrasound Med 27:1129–1136
Beekman R, Visser LH (2002) Sonographic detection of diffuse peripheral nerve enlargement in hereditary neuropathy with liability to pressure palsies. J Clin Ultrasound 30:433–436
Beekman R, Visser LH (2004) High-resolution sonography of the peripheral nervous system—a review of the literature. Eur J Neurol 11:305–314
Bianchi S, Martinoli C (eds) (2007) Ultrasound of the musculoskeletal system. Springer, Berlin
Bianchi S, Martinoli C, Abdelwahab IF (1999) High-frequency ultrasound examination of the wrist and hand. Skeletal Radiol 28:121–129
Bianchi S, Martinoli C, Sureda D et al (2001) Ultrasound of the hand. Eur J Ultrasound 14:29–34
Bianchi S, Montet X, Martinoli C et al (2004) High-resolution sonography of compressive neuropathies of the wrist. J Clin Ultrasound 32:451–461
Bianchi S, Demondion X, Bard H et al (2007) Ultrasound of the median nerve (Echographie du nerf médian). Rev Rhum Ed Fr 74:376–383
Blancher A, Kubis N (2007) Physiopathogenie des syndromes canalaires. In: Les syndromes canalaires vus en rhumatologie. Revue du Rhumatisme 74:319–326
Boutte C, Gaudin P, Grange L et al (2009) [Sonography versus electrodiagnosis for the diagnosis of carpal tunnel syndrome in routine practice]. Rev Neurol 165:460–465
Buchberger W, Schon G, Strasser K et al (1991) High-resolution ultrasonography of the carpal tunnel. J Ultrasound Med 10:531–537
Buchberger W, Judmaier W, Birbamer G et al (1992) Carpal tunnel syndrome: diagnosis with high-resolution sonography. AJR Am J Roentgenol 159:793–798
Chen P, Maklad N, Redwine M et al (1997) Dynamic high-resolution sonography of the carpal tunnel. AJR Am J Roentgenol 168:533–537
Duncan I, Sullivan P, Lomas F (1999) Sonography in the diagnosis of carpal tunnel syndrome. AJR Am J Roentgenol 173:681–684
El Miedany Y, Ashour S, Youssef S et al (2008) Clinical diagnosis of carpal tunnel syndrome: old tests-new concepts. Joint Bone Spine 75:451–457
Fornage BD (1988) Peripheral nerves of the extremities: imaging with US. Radiology 167:179–182
Gassner EM, Schocke M, Peer S et al (2002) Persistent median artery in the carpal tunnel: color Doppler ultrasonographic findings. J Ultrasound Med 21:455–461
Graif M, Seton A, Nerubali J et al (1991) Sciatic nerve: sonographic evaluation and anatomic-pathologic considerations. Radiology 181:405–408
Hobson-Webb LD, Massey JM, Juel VC et al (2008) The ultrasonographic wrist-to-forearm median nerve area ratio in carpal tunnel syndrome. Clin Neurophysiol 119:1353–1357
Iannicelli A, Chianta GA, Salvini V et al (2000) Evaluation of bifid median nerve with sonography and MR imaging. J Ultrasound Med 19:481–485
Iannicelli E, Almberger M, Chianta GA et al (2001) Bifid median nerve in the carpal tunnel: integrated imaging. Radiol Med 101:456–458
Jamadar DA, Jacobson JA, Hayes CW (2001) Sonographic evaluation of the median nerve at the wrist. J Ultrasound Med 20:1011–1014
Kaymak B, Ozcakar L, Cetin A et al (2008) A comparison of the benefits of sonography and electrophysiologic measurements as predictors of symptom severity and functional status in patients with carpal tunnel syndrome. Arch Phys Med Rehabil 89:743–748
Kele H, Verheggen R, Reimers CD (2002) Carpal tunnel syndrome caused by thrombosis of the median artery: the importance of high-resolution ultrasonography for diagnosis. Case report. J Neurosurg 97:471–473
Klauser AS, Halpern EJ, De Zordo T et al (2009) Carpal tunnel syndrome assessment with US: value of additional cross-sectional area measurements of the median nerve in patients versus healthy volunteers. Radiology 250:171–177
Kwon BC, Jung KI, Baek GH (2008) Comparison of sonography and electrodiagnostic testing in the diagnosis of carpal tunnel syndrome. J Hand Surg Am 33:65–71
Lanzetta M, Foucher G (1993) Entrapment of the superficial branch of the radial nerve (Wartenberg's syndrome). A report of 52 cases. Int Orthop 17:342–345
Martinoli C, Serafini G, Bianchi S et al (1996) Ultrasonography of peripheral nerves. J Peripher Nerv Syst 1:169–178
Martinoli C, Bianchi S, Derchi LE (2000a) Ultrasonography of peripheral nerves. Semin US CT MR 21:205–213
Martinoli C, Bianchi S, Gandolfo N et al (2000b) US of nerve entrapments in osteofibrous tunnels of the upper and lower limbs. Radiographics 20(Spec No):S199–S213 Discussion S213-197
Martinoli C, Bianchi S, Cohen M et al (2005) Ultrasound of peripheral nerves. J Radiol 86:1869–1878
Mondelli M, Filippou G, Gallo A (2008) Diagnostic utility of ultrasonography versus nerve conduction studies in mild carpal tunnel syndrome. Arthritis Rheum 59:357–366
Padua L, Pazzaglia C, Caliandro P et al (2008) Carpal tunnel syndrome: ultrasound, neurophysiology, clinical and patient-oriented assessment. Clin Neurophysiol 119:2064–2069
Patel N, Harvie P, Ostlere SJ Ultrasound of accessory muscles at the Guyon canal. Session 6 European Society of musculoskeletal radiology, IX Annual Meeting. Abstract book, p 156
Peer S, Bodner G (eds) (2008) High-resolution sonography of the peripheral nervous system, 2nd edn. Berlin, Springer
Peer S, Bodner G, Meirer R et al (2001) Examination of postoperative peripheral nerve lesions with high-resolution sonography. AJR 177:415–419
Pinilla I, Martin-Hervas C, Sordo G et al (2008) The usefulness of ultrasonography in the diagnosis of carpal tunnel syndrome. J Hand Surg Eur Vol 33:435–439
Propeck T, Quinn TJ, Jacobson JA et al (2000) Sonography and MR imaging of bifid median nerve with anatomic and histologic correlation. AJR Am J Roentgenol 175:1721–1725
Sernik RA, Abicalaf CA, Pimentel BF et al (2008) Ultrasound features of carpal tunnel syndrome: a prospective case-control study. Skeletal Radiol 37:49–53

Silvestri E, Martinoli C, Derchi LE et al (1995) Echotexture of peripheral nerves: correlation between US and histologic findings and criteria to differentiate tendons. Radiology 197:291–296
Smith J, Wisniewski SJ, Finnoff JT et al (2008) Sonographically guided carpal tunnel injections: the ulnar approach. J Ultrasound Med 27:1485–1490
Spratt JD, Stanley AJ, Grainger AJ et al (2002) The role of diagnostic radiology in compressive and entrapment neuropathies. Eur Radiol 12:2352–2364
Stewart JD (1993) Compression and entrapment neuropathies. In: Dyck PJ, Thomas PK (eds) Peripheral neuropathy, 3rd edn. WB Saunders, Philadelphia, pp 1354–1379
Tagliafico A, Pugliese F, Bianchi S et al (2008) High-resolution sonography of the palmar cutaneous branch of the median nerve. AJR Am J Roentgenol 191:107–114
Taleisnik J (1973) The palmar cutaneous branch of the median nerve and the approach to the carpal tunnel. An anatomical study. J Bone Joint Surg Am 55:1212–1217
Toms AP, Anastakis D, Bleakney RR et al (2006) Lipofibromatous hamartoma of the upper extremity: a review of the radiologic findings for 15 patients. AJR Am J Roentgenol 186:805–811
Touborg-Jensen A (1970) Carpal-tunnel syndrome caused by an abnormal distribution of the lumbrical muscles. Case report. Scand J Plast Reconstr Surg 4:72–74
Valle M, Zamorani MP (2007) Nerve and vessels. In: Bianchi S, Martinoli C (eds) Ultrasound of the musculoskeletal system. Springer, Berlin, Heidelberg, pp 97–136
van Holsbeeck M, Introcaso JH (eds) (2001) Musculoskeletal ultrasound. Chicago, Mosby

Osteonecrosis and Osteochondrosis

Waqar A. Bhatti and Andrew J. Grainger

Contents

W. A. Bhatti (✉)
Consultant in Musculoskeletal and Sports Radiology,
University Hospital South Manchester,
South Manchester, UK
e-mail: Waqar.bhatti@uhsm.nhs.uk

A. J. Grainger
Department of Musculoskeletal Radiology,
Chapel Allerton Orthopaedic Centre,
Leeds, LS7 4SA, UK
e-mail: andrew.grainger@leedsth.nhs.uk

Abstract

This succinct chapter on osteonecrosis and osteochondrosis in the wrist and hand describes the aetiology and typical bones involved in these conditions. A description of the available of imaging modalities including plain radiographs, computed tomography, scintigraphy and Magnetic resonance imaging are described with their strengths and weaknesses. Detailed individual description and classification of carpal bone osteonecrois and osteochondrosis including Kienbock's disease of the lunate and the rarer Preiser's disease of the scaphoid are included.

1 Introduction

Osteonecrosis or avascular necrosis of the carpal bones is a common cause for chronic wrist pain, limiting movement and weakening grip strength. In the wrist osteonecrosis most frequently occurs as a result of disruption to the osseous blood supply as a result of trauma. While the scaphoid is the most frequently affected bone in the wrist, osteonecrosis of any of the carpal bones can occur and multiple carpal bone involvement is described (De Smet et al. 1993; Humphrey et al. 2006; Telfer et al. 1994; Zafra et al. 2004; Garcia and Vaca 2006).

The osteochondroses refer to a heterogenous group of conditions with a tendency to affect the immature skeleton. A variety of possible mechanisms have been proposed for these conditions, but those affecting the wrist and hand are characterized by features of osteonecrosis thought to occur through a process of microtrauma.

A. M. Davis et al. (eds.), *Imaging of the Hand and Wrist*, Medical Radiology. Diagnostic Imaging,
DOI: 10.1007/174_2011_392,

The most well recognized of these conditions in the hand and wrist is Kienböch's disease affecting the lunate.

Osteonecrosis from any cause can result in late complications, most commonly osteoarthritis and although surgical options meet with varied success, early diagnosis may limit these complications. Conventional radiographs are often the first line imaging investigation but it should be appreciated that the changes seen are relatively late in the disease process. MR imaging is extremely well suited to the detection of the early phases of avascular necrosis, permitting diagnosis before collapse of the carpal bones has occurred (Golimbu et al. 1995).

2 Aetiology

The term osteonecrosis by definition implies bone necrosis or bone death. Originally infection was thought to be the underlying cause but histopathological studies showed that the bone is aseptic and also avascular, implicating vascular insufficiency as the underlying aetiology. A variety of insults may lead to osseous vascular impairment and carpal bones are particularly vulnerable to such insults as they have a poor collateral circulation. Notably osteonecrosis occurs most often in the scaphoid, lunate and capitate bones which have particularly tenuous vascularity (Botte et al. 2004; Gelberman and Gross 1986).

Vascular impairment and therefore osteonecrosis may result from a variety of underlying causes including radiation, vascular, metabolic and systemic conditions. In the wrist the most common cause is trauma, with the scaphoid and capitate most frequently affected. A clear cause for osteonecrosis is not always established. This situation most commonly arises in the lunate where it is termed Kienböch's disease. Despite the absence of a history of trauma it is generally believed that the aetiology of these conditions is traumatic in nature, rather than relating to a primary vascular event (Resnick 2002). Other osteochondroses described in the hand and wrist are Preiser's disease (scaphoid), Thiemann's disease (phalanges) and Dieterich's disease (metacarpal head) (Botte et al. 2004; de Smet 2000; Ferlic and Morin 1989; Herbert and Lanzetta 1994; Tashjian et al. 2004).

The different cellular elements within bone (including osteocytes, osteoblasts and osteoclasts) differ in their susceptibilities to anoxia. After physical disruption of blood flow, the haemopoietic elements are generally acknowledged to be the first to undergo anoxic death followed by bone cells and subsequently bone marrow fat cells (Cruess 1986; Glimcher and Kenzora 1979a, b, c). This means that temporary anoxia can result in varying degrees of cell death potentially affecting the haemopoeitic elements without necessarily involving the other bone cells. It is generally recognised that once marrow fat cell death occurs the involved segment of bone can be labelled as infarcted. Marrow involvement is critical to the detection of bone infarction on MRI examination.

3 Imaging Techniques

3.1 Radiography

In most cases the X-ray findings lag behind the clinical manifestations, hence the initial radiographs may appear normal. The onset of fat necrosis brings with it vasodilation in the still vascularised surrounding bone resulting in an influx of inflammatory cells. Dead bone starts to undergo removal by osteoclasts and this means that potentially viable bone will become relatively osteopaenic. This comparatively radiolucent bone will be adjacent to non-viable necrotic bone which becomes relatively sclerotic (Fig. 1). As the process progresses increasing sclerosis followed by collapse and fragmentation of the avascular bone occurs.

3.2 Computed Tomography

Computerised tomography is rarely used in the primary assessment of carpal bone osteonecrosis. However the complex 3-D anatomy of the carpal bones means it can be useful for providing information relating to the extent of volume reduction of the affected bone and the detection of early subchondral collapse, along with the detection of secondary changes such as osteoarthritis. It can also prove more sensitive to the detection of an associated un-united fracture and sclerosis in the avascular bone.

The base of the hook of hamate is at a relatively high risk for avascular necrosis following fracture (Telfer et al. 1994). The complex anatomy of this bone means avascular necrosis is often best detected at CT.

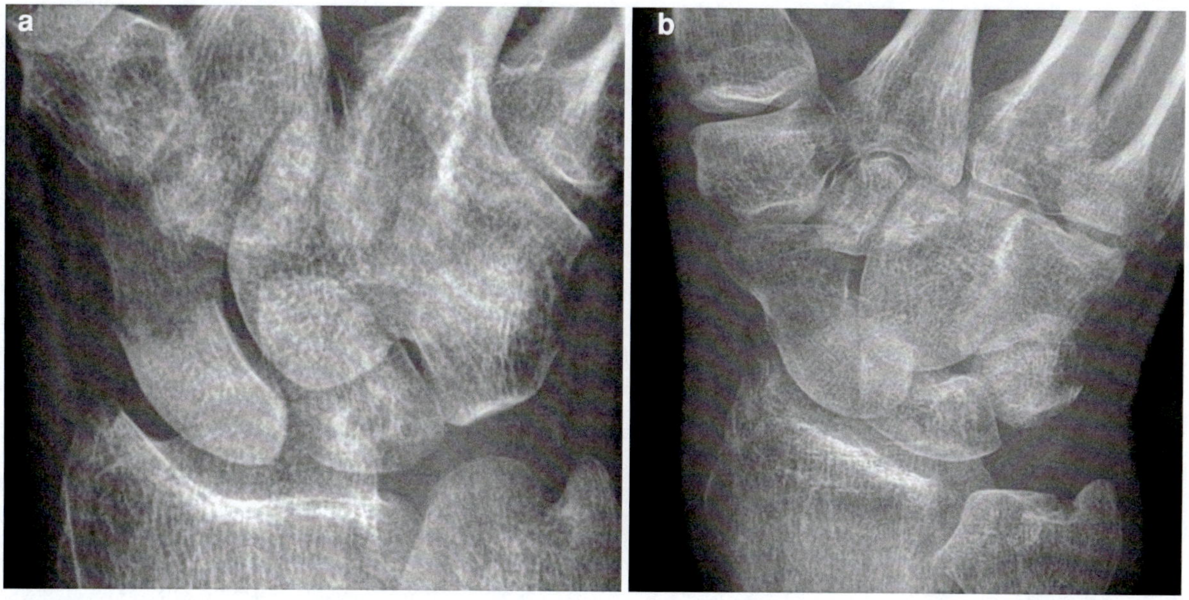

Fig. 1 Early avascular necrosis 8 weeks following a scaphoid fracture. **a** Ulnar deviated PA film with tube angulation and **b** Anterior Oblique shows a fracture line. The difference in density can be appreciated between the increased density of the proximal pole, accentuated by the relative osteopaenia of the distal pole

CT changes seen in osteonecrotic bone reflect the plain film findings of sclerosis, appreciated as increased attenuation and subsequent collapse and fragmentation (Fig. 2). Cystic change may be seen along the margins of an un-united fracture (Bush et al. 1987).

3.3 Magnetic Resonance Imaging

Magnetic resonance is the imaging modality of choice for the early detection of osteonecrosis, depicting marrow signal changes before changes are apparent using plain films and CT (Imhof et al. 1997). Although scintigraphy may offer similar sensitivity it shows less specificity when compared with MRI. The signal abnormality on MRI depends on alteration of the fat cells in the bone marrow, initially seen as oedema-like change within the marrow, appreciated as a reduction in the normal fat signal on T1 weighted imaging and increased signal on water sensitive sequences (Imhof et al. 1997; Mitchell et al. 1989) (Fig. 3). As the process progresses areas of reduced signal intensity on T2 weighted imaging emerge, surrounded by areas of increased signal intensity representing the interface between non-viable bone and reparative granulation tissue. At this stage MRI may show a characteristic serpiginous double line at the interface between the necrotic area and the fibrovascular granulation tissue. The double line represents the granulation tissue adjacent to reactive

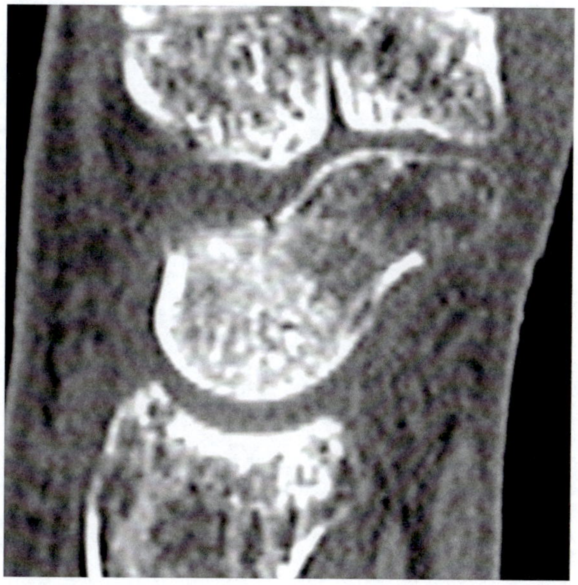

Fig. 2 Scaphoid fracture with early avascular necrosis. The sagittal CT reformat shows increased attenuation to the proximal pole of the scaphoid reflecting osteonecrotic bone with relative osteopaenia in the distal pole

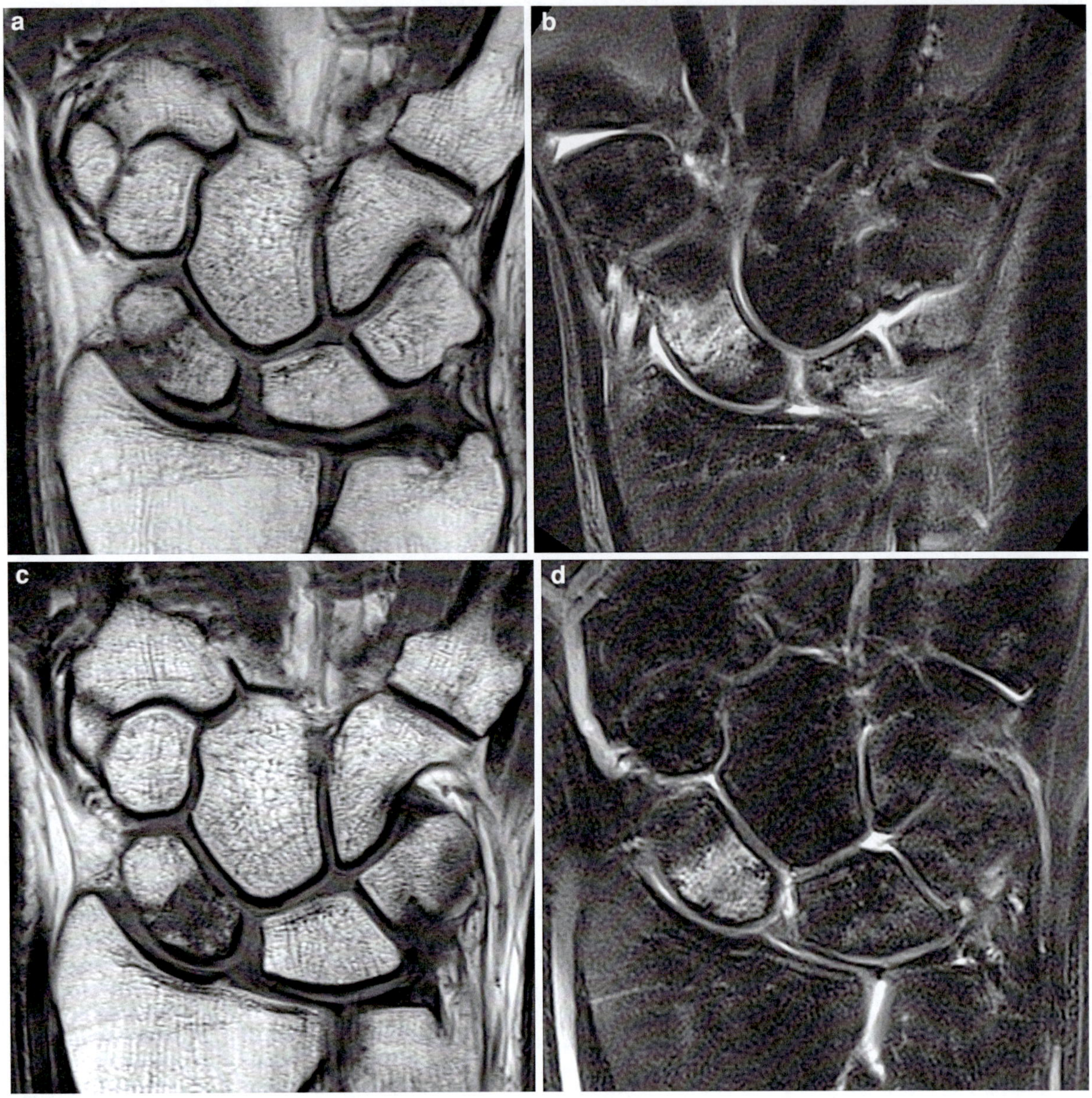

Fig. 3 **a** Coronal T1 and **b** Coronal Oblique T2 (fat sat) MR images obtained 18 days following scaphoid fracture. On the T1 the fracture line interrupts the marrow signal with patchy signal reduction around the fracture line seen as increased T2 signal (oedema) on the T2 image. Note the normal marrow signal at the proximal pole. Five weeks later (**c**) Coronal T1 MR image shows diffuse low signal and (**d**) Coronal T2 (fat sat) image shows diffuse increased signal in the proximal pole with normal signal in the distal pole. The appearances represent early AVN

bone formation (Imhof et al. 1997; Mitchell et al.1989). While the two lines may not always be distinguished a sharp line of demarcation is still a typical and helpful feature (Fig. 4). Contrast-enhanced imaging can be performed and may help distinguish viable from non-viable bone but should be interpreted with caution. See Sect. 4.1.

3.4 Bone Scintigraphy

The relative insensitivity of radiographs for detecting the early stages of avascular necrosis has led to the increased use of MRI for this role. Bone scintigraphy is also very sensitive to the early detection of osteonecrosis although it is relatively non-specific and

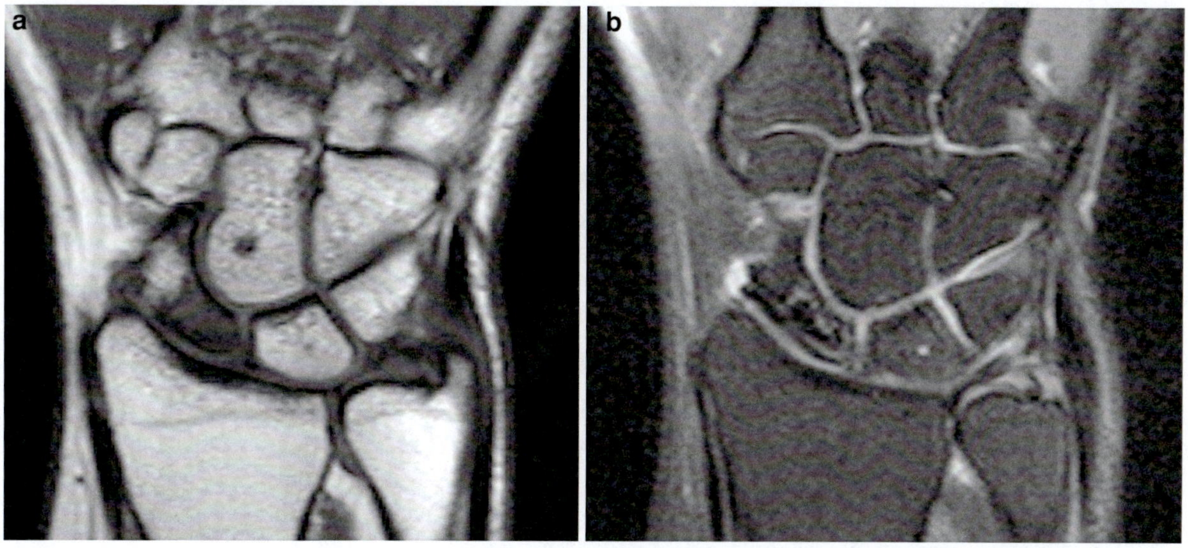

Fig. 4 **a** Coronal T1 W shows abnormal low signal within the proximal scaphoid bone **b** PD (fat sat) image also shows abnormal low signal delineated by a high signal serpiginous line. There is surrounding abnormal low signal within the proximal scaphoid bone demarcating the dead bone within the proximal pole and representing granulation tissue. There was no history of trauma in this case, which represents the partial form of Preiser's disease

should always be interpreted alongside conventional radiographic findings. In the early stages of avascular necrosis increased metabolic activity in the bone is seen as higher uptake in bone scintigraphy on early and late phase scanning. Later bone scintigraphy typically indicates an area of decreased radio-tracer uptake; a cold spot or photopenic region. This in isolation is not diagnostic of osteonecrosis as other conditions including myeloma, some skeletal metastases, irradiation, haemangiomas and infection can also result in reduced or impaired tracer uptake.

4 Scaphoid

The scaphoid is the most common site for osteonecrosis to occur in the wrist. This is because of its high susceptibility to trauma and precarious blood supply. The proximal pole of the scaphoid receives its blood supply in a retrograde fashion from small dorsal ridge vessels entering the waist of the scaphoid from the radial artery. These vessels provide around 70–80% of the internal vascularity of the bone, in particular to the proximal pole. A separate vascular supply from the palmar aspect supplies the remaining internal vascularity, all to the region of the distal pole (Botte et al. 2004). The consequent tenuous blood supply to the proximal pole makes it vulnerable to osteonecrosis following fracture. There is a reported frequency of proximal pole osteonecrosis of between 11 and 65% following scaphoid fracture (Mazet and Hohl 1963). However this varies according to the site of the fracture, with fractures of the proximal third having the highest incidence of osteonecrosis and a reducing incidence with more distally located fractures. Osteonecrosis has been reported as occurring in the distal pole of the scaphoid following fracture, but this is extremely rare (Sherman et al. 1983).

Plain radiographs of established cases show an increased bone density in the affected scaphoid seen at between 4 and 8 weeks and associated with non-union (Fig. 1). Later reduction in size, fragmentation and secondary degenerative changes can be seen (Fig. 5).

MR imaging is now the modality of choice for the detection of early avascular necrosis. Typically, MR will show low signal intensity within the bone marrow of the proximal pole on both the T1 and T2 weighted images. It has been suggested that high signal on T2 implies viability of bone but this is not the case (Cerezal et al. 2000) (Fig. 6a). Contrast enhancement significantly increases the detection of non-viable bone but the use of dynamic enhancement studies does not appear to improve sensitivity (Cerezal et al. 2000; Megerle et al. 2011; Donati et al.

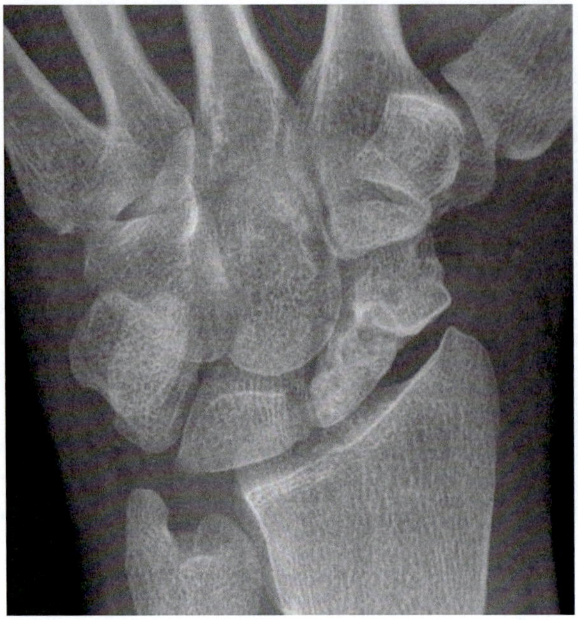

Fig. 5 Established proximal pole scaphoid osteonecrosis 6 months following fracture. There is fracture non-union with dense sclerosis and volume loss in the proximal pole. Cystic change is also seen about the fracture line

2011) (Fig. 6b). While studies do indicate that MRI provides a good assessment of the vascularity of the bone as assessed with punctate bleeding at the time of surgery; the general picture that is emerging suggests that MRI, even with gadolinium enhancement, is less good at predicting outcome of surgery in terms of union and revascularization (Cerezal et al. 2000; Megerle et al. 2011; Schmitt et al. 2011; Singh et al. 2004; Dawson et al. 2001).

4.1 Preiser's Disease

Preiser's disease is a rare condition which results in ischaemia of the scaphoid bone without a history of trauma. Rarely it can occur bilaterally and has also been described with Kienböch's disease (de Smet 2000; Ferlic and Morin 1989; Herbert and Lanzetta 1994) (Fig. 7). Risk factors may include excessive alcohol intake, corticosteroid administration, chemotherapy and other disease processes.

Histologically, there are empty bony lacunae, necrotic marrow and partly degenerated articular cartilage. Clinically, pain along the dorsal and radial aspects of the wrist is typical.

Conventional radiographic images and CT show the expected sclerosis, volume loss and cystic change which, with time progresses to collapse and fragmentation (Fig. 7 and 8). Using MRI two patterns can be identified, a partial or focal form with ischaemia of the proximal half of the scaphoid (Fig. 4) and a diffuse form with complete ischaemia and necrosis (Fig. 7) (Kalainov et al. 2003). The former, partial type has a better prognosis. Isolated non-traumatic osteonecrosis of the distal pole of the scaphoid has also been described (Garg et al. 2011).

Treatment protocols for Preiser's disease include wrist immobilization and cortisone injections. Surgical options include partial excision with replacement by non-vascularised or vascularised bone graft, proximal row carpectomy, scaphoid excision with midcarpal fusion and total wrist fusion.

5 Lunate

5.1 Kienböch's Disease

Kienböch's disease is most commonly observed in patients between the ages of 20 and 40 years, with a predilection for the right hand in persons engaged in manual labour. Some patients have an antecedent history of trauma but the majority of cases are idiopathic. There is a strong association between ulna minus variance and Kienböch's disease, which has led to the suggestion that abnormality in loading is an important aspect in the aetiology, although 40% of cases are seen in neutral ulna variance. Additionally, negative ulnar variance is usually bilateral and Kienböch's disease is rarely bilateral. Other theories that have been postulated include medialisation of the lunate, horizontalisation of the radial epiphysis or abnormal morphology of the lunate. In some individuals there is a variation in the blood supply of the lunate; a single dominant branch (8%) rather than a dual supply from volar and dorsal branches with an anastomosis potentially increasing the risk of osteonecrosis (Gelberman and Gross 1986).

5.1.1 Imaging

The appearances of established lunate osteonecrosis on conventional radiographs is initially sclerosis followed by progressive collapse of the lunate and fragmentation (Figs. 9 and 10). Associated findings such as ulnar negative variance may also be seen and in the later stages degenerative change may occur.

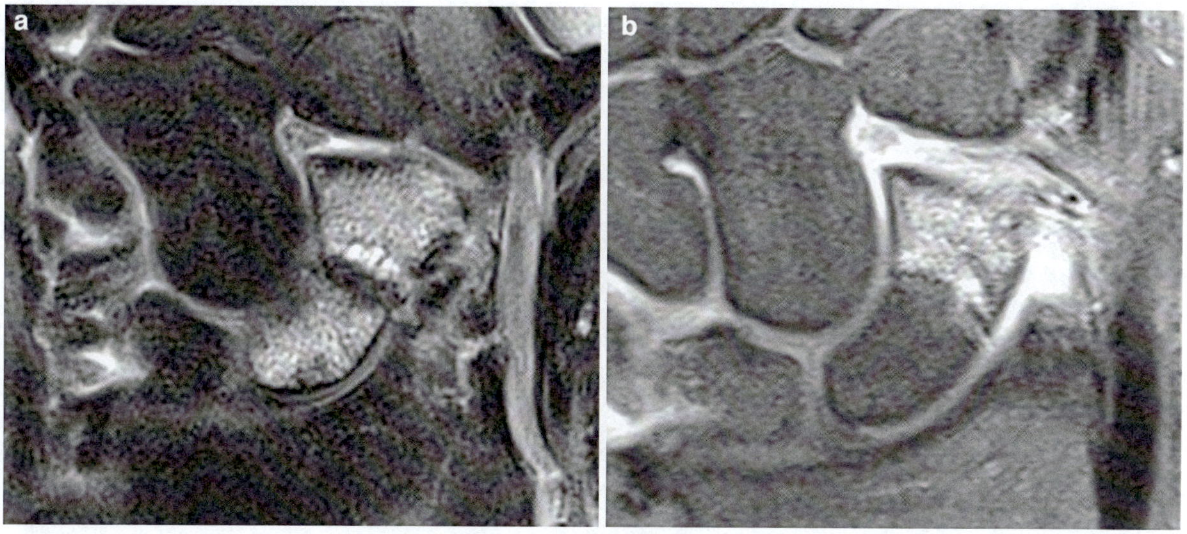

Fig. 6 **a** Coronal T2 W (fat sat) shows scaphoid fracture non-union. High signal oedema is seen in the marrow in both the proximal and distal fracture fragments. **b** Coronal T1 W (fat sat) post intravenous gadolinium shows oedema-induced enhancement in the distal pole with absent enhancement of the oedematous but avascular proximal pole despite the presence of oedematous change on T2 W imaging

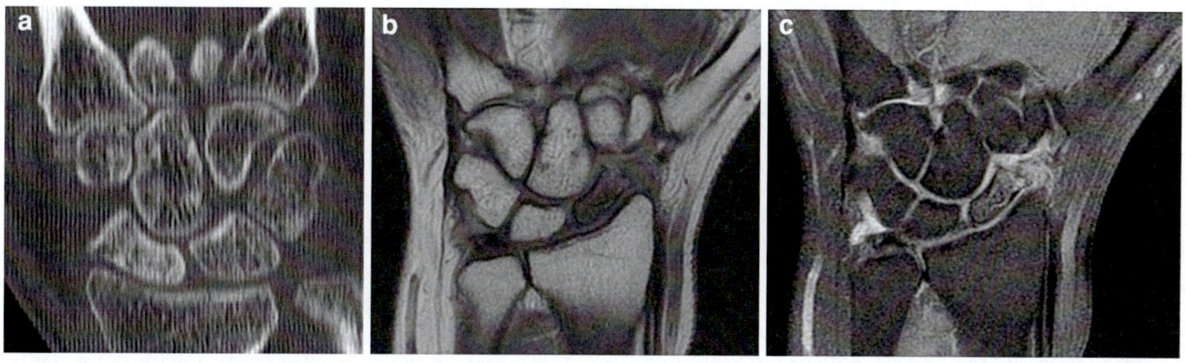

Fig. 7 Bilateral Preiser's disease. **a** Reformatted CT. There is sclerosis, fracturing and fragmentation with volume loss in the scaphoid of this patient without trauma. **b** T1 weighted and **c** T2 weighted (fat sat) MR images from the contralateral wrist show the condition is bilateral, with diffuse signal abnormality throughout the scaphoid with a serpiginous boundary between representing the interface between necrotic bone and granulation tissue Courtesy of Dr Phillip Tirman

Radiographs are important in differentiating osteonecrosis from other causes of wrist pain such as ulna-lunate abutment, fractures, carpal malalignment, instability and arthritis.

CT of the wrist is more sensitive than plain films for demonstrating structural change including sclerosis, compression and fractures of the lunate. Fractures are more common in Kienböch's disease than previously reported (Fig. 11). Earlier detection of fractures by CT, before collapse of the lunate occurs, may allow treatment to prevent the collapse (Friedman et al. 1991).

As with osteonecrosis at other sites, MRI and scintigraphy provide earlier evidence of Kienböch's disease and can help establish the diagnosis in the presence of normal conventional radiographs. Two patterns of abnormality have been defined on MRI, one involving only focal involvement of the radial half of the lunate, the second being a diffused reduction in T1 signal throughout the bone marrow (Sowa et al. 1989 Nov) (Fig. 12). In common with osteonecrosis elsewhere, marrow signal appears low on T2 imaging in the later stages of the disease, but initially high signal may

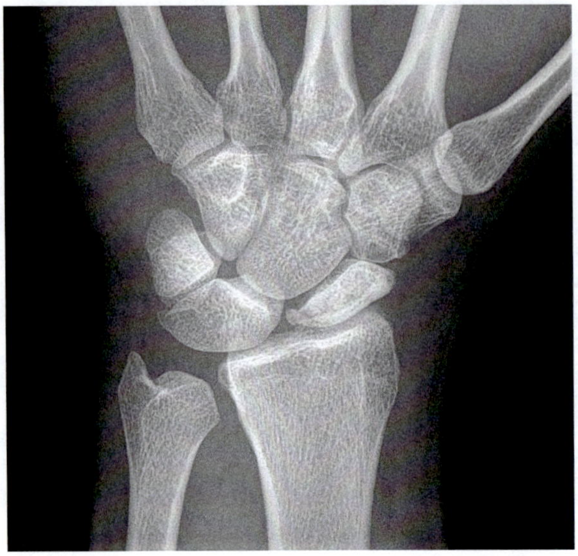

Fig. 8 Preiser's disease. The scaphoid shows sclerosis and volume loss due to osteonecrosis. There was no history of trauma in this 25-year-old male presenting with wrist pain and successfully treated with a vascularised graft Courtesy of Kimberly K. Amrami MD. Mayo Clinic, Rochester Minnesota, USA

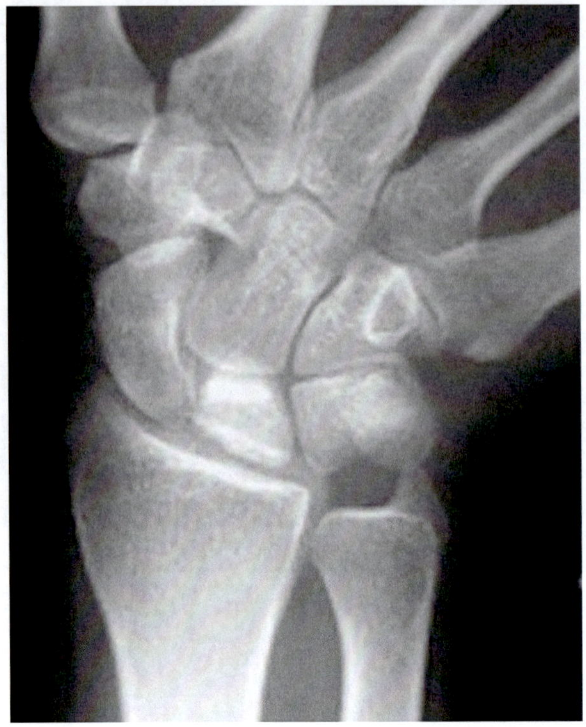

Fig. 9 Plain radiograph showing sclerosis of the lunate typical features of Kienböch's disease. Note the presence of ulnar negative variance, a typical but not exclusive association with Kienböch's disease

be seen, which may be focal or patchy in distribution. Cystic change and collapse/fragmentation may be seen in the later stages of the disease (Fig. 13).

5.1.2 Staging of Kienböch's Disease

Although many classifications have been proposed they are quite similar, four stages are recognised in the commonly used Lichtman classification (Lichtman et al. 1977).

Stage 1: Pre-radiological disease.

The plain radiograph is normal except for possible predisposing factors such as negative ulnar variance. Detection of stage 1 disease is by MRI where there is typically internal bone marrow signal change with low signal on T1 W and low or patchy high signal on T2 W imaging. Stage 1 disease can also be detected by bone scintigraphy.

Stage II: Sclerosis of the lunate bone without collapse (Fig. 9).

Stage III: Lunate fragmentation and collapse.

As a consequence of collapse there may be associated scapholunate dissociation and rotatory subluxation of the scaphoid. This has led to subdivision of stage III into stage IIIA: no rotatory subluxation and IIIB: associated scapholunate dissociation and rotatory subluxation.

Stage IV: Arthritis of the radiocarpal and mid carpal joints.

Although there is no difficulty in establishing the diagnosis of Kienböch's disease with MRI, many therapeutic options exist. Along with conservative management there are surgical options, including revascularisation of the lunate and lunate unloading by ulnar lengthening or radial shortening. However there is no strong consensus on the indications and results are variable (Kristensen et al. 1986; Weiss et al. 1991).

6 Capitate

Osteonecrosis of the capitate is recognised following fracture or more commonly following midcarpal fracture dislocations (scaphocapitate syndrome) (Tashjian et al. 2004). Although idiopathic osteonecrosis without a history of antecedent trauma is described it is rare (Kutty and Curtin 1995; Lapinsky and Mack 1992). The vascular anatomy of the capitate shares similar features

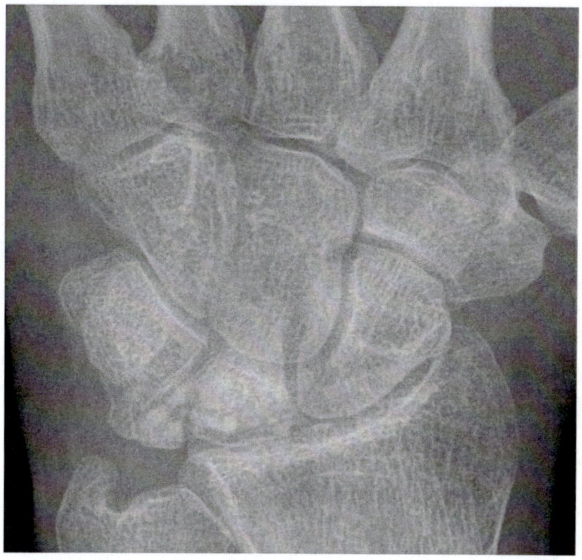

Fig. 10 Kienböch's disease at a more advanced stage than shown in Fig. 8, with subchondral fracturing and collapse at the proximal pole, again with ulnar minus variance

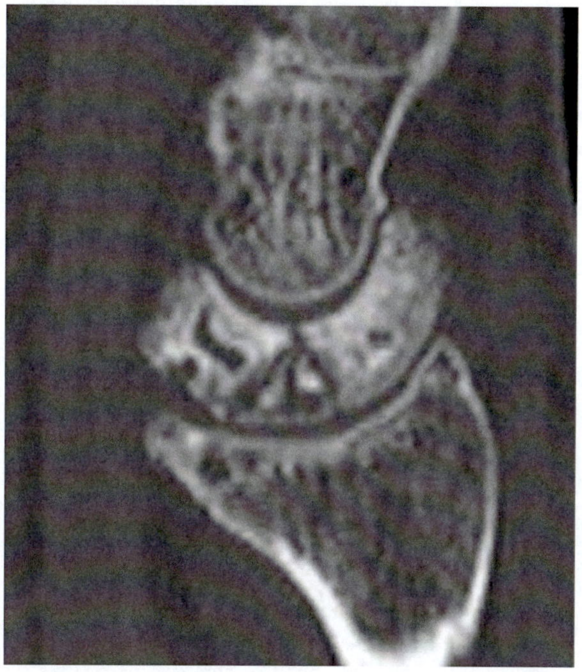

Fig. 11 Sagittal CT reformat shows advanced Kienböch's disease with sclerosis, fracture and fragmentation. Early secondary degenerative change at the radioulnar joint can be appreciated as irregular joint space loss and cystic change in the subchondral bone of the radius

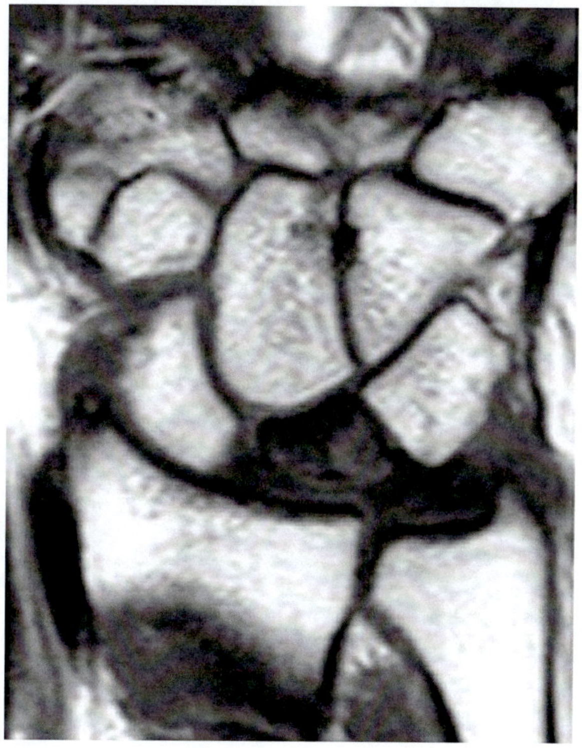

Fig. 12 Kienböch's Disease. Coronal T1 W image shows diffuse low signal change in the lunate, but there are focal regions of increased and intermediate signal intensity which are often observed in bone necrosis. Courtesy of Dr Muhammed Mubashar, University Hospital South Manchester, UK

to those of the scaphoid with a retrograde internal flow pattern which explains the predominant proximal pole pattern of necrosis.

The changes described on X-ray are of initial proximal pole osteopaenia followed by sclerosis. This may progress to complete fragmentation and collapse. MRI will show typical features of osteonecrosis as previously described.

Treatment often involves excision of the capitate bone with carpal fusion, revascularisation has also been successfully achieved (Murakami et al. 2002).

7 Hamate

Avascular necrosis of the hamate is relatively uncommon and in the cases reported follows trauma. Post-traumatic osteonecrosis of both the hook of hamate and body have been described (Telfer et al.

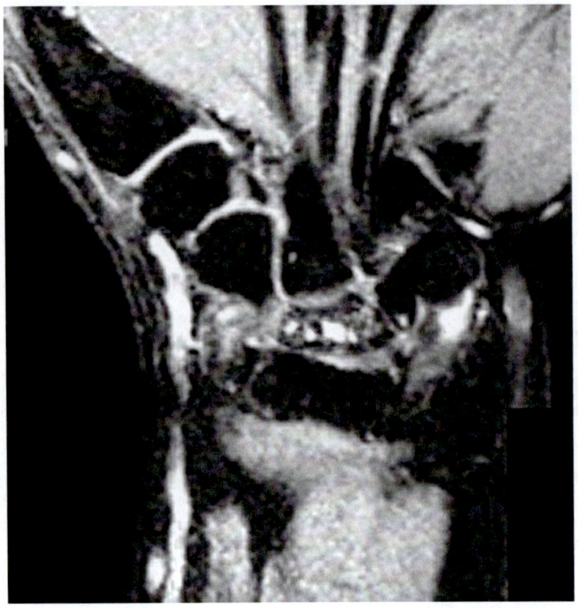

Fig. 13 Coronal T2 W image showing advanced Kienböch's disease. High signal change is seen associated with cystic change and volume loss

1994; Failla 1993). It has been noted that like the scaphoid and capitate the proximal pole is vascularised via a retrograde circulation and, as would be expected, the proximal pole seems to be more vulnerable (Botte et al. 2004; Tashjian et al. 2004).

8 The Hand

Osteonecrosis has been reported in a variety of bones in the hand, most commonly in the metacarpal heads and about the proximal interphalangeal (PIP) joints of the phalanges. Thiemann's disease is reported as a rare autosomal-dominant form of avascular necrosis affecting the PIP joint (Tashjian et al. 2004). The condition has also been termed juvenile osteochondropathy of the fingers and multiple phalangeal epiphysitis. It usually presents as progressive enlargement of the PIP joints, frequently starting with the middle finger before involving the index and ring fingers. There is often sparing of the little PIP and thumb IP joints. The condition is usually painless, but contractures, finger shortening and deformity are said to be features (Rubinstein 1975). As expected, radiographic features include flattening, sclerosis and fragmentation of the epiphyses.

Osteonecrosis of the metacarpal heads (Dieterich's disease) has been described in association with trauma, systemic lupus erthematosus and steroid use. Radiographs show sclerosis and fragmentation of the metacarpal head which may show features resembling periarticular erosion (Tashjian et al. 2004).

References

Botte MJ, Pacelli LL, Gelberman RH (2004) Vascularity and osteonecrosis of the wrist. Orthop Clin North Am 35(3): 405–421 xi

Bush C, Gillespy T, III, Dell P (1987) High-resolution CT of the wrist: initial experience with scaphoid disorders and surgical fusions. Am J Roentgenol 149(4):757–60

Cerezal L, Abascal F, Canga A, Garcia-Valtuille R, Bustamante M, Pinal Fd (2000) Usefulness of gadolinium-enhanced MR imaging in the evaluation of the vascularity of scaphoid nonunions. Am J Roentgenol 174(1):14–19

Cruess RL (1986) Osteonecrosis of bone. Current concepts as to etiology and pathogenesis. Clin Orthop Relat Res 208:30–9

Dawson JS, Martel AL, Davis TRC (2001) Scaphoid blood flow and acute fracture healing: a dynamic MRI study with enhancement with gadolinium. J Bone Joint Surg Br 83-B(6): 809–814

de Smet L (2000) Avascular nontraumatic necrosis of the scaphoid. Preiser's disease? Chir Main 19(2):82–5

De Smet L, Willemen D, Kimpe E, Fabry G (1993) Nontraumatic osteonecrosis of the capitate bone associated with gout. Ann Chir Main Memb Super 12(3):210–212

Donati OF, Zanetti M, Nagy L, Bode B, Schweizer A, Pfirrmann CWA (2011) Is dynamic gadolinium enhancement needed in MR imaging for the preoperative assessment of scaphoidal viability in patients with scaphoid nonunion? Radiology 28:808–816

Failla JM (1993) Hook of hamate vascularity: vulnerability to osteonecrosis and nonunion. J Hand Surg 18(6):1075–1079

Ferlic DC, Morin P (1989) Idiopathic avascular necrosis of the scaphoid: Preiser's disease? J Hand Surg Am 14(1):13–16

Friedman L, Yong-Hing K, Johnston GH (1991) The use of coronal computed tomography in the evaluation of Kienbock's disease. Clin Radiol 44(1):56–59

Garcia LA, Vaca JB (2006) Avascular necrosis of the pisiform. J Hand Surg Br 31(4):453–454

Garg B, Giupta H, Kotwal PP (2011) Nontraumatic osteonecrosis of the dista pole of the scaphoid. Indian Journal Orthop 45(2):185–187

Gelberman RH, Gross MS (1986) The vascularity of the wrist. Identification of arterial patterns at risk. Clin Orthop Relat Res 202:40–9

Glimcher MJ, Kenzora JE (1979a) The biology of osteonecrosis of the human femoral head and its clinical implications: I. Tissue biology. Clin Orthop Relat Res 138:284–309

Glimcher MJ, Kenzora JE (1979b) The biology of osteonecrosis of the human femoral head and its clinical implications: II. The pathological changes in the femoral head as an organ and in the hip joint. Clin Orthop Relat Res 139:283–312

Glimcher MJ, Kenzora JE (1979c) The biology of osteonecrosis of the human femoral head and its clinical implications. III. Discussion of the etiology and genesis of the pathological sequelae; commments on treatment. Clin Orthop Relat Res 140:273–312

Golimbu CN, Firooznia H, Rafii M (1995) Avascular necrosis of carpal bones. Magn Reson Imaging Clin N Am 3(2): 281–303

Herbert TJ, Lanzetta M (1994) Idiopathic avascular necrosis of the scaphoid. J Hand Surg Br 19(2):174–182

Humphrey CS, Izadi KD, Esposito PW (2006) Case reports: osteonecrosis of the capitate: a pediatric case report. Clin Orthop Relat Res 447:256–259

Imhof H, Breitenseher M, Trattnig S, Kramer J, Hofmann S, Plenk H et al (1997) Imaging of avascular necrosis of bone. Eur Radiol 7(2):180–186

Kalainov DM, Cohen MS, Hendrix RW, Sweet S, Culp RW, Osterman AL (2003) Preiser's disease: identification of two patterns. J Hand Surg Am 28(5):767–778

Kristensen SS, Thomassen E, Christensen F (1986) Kienbock's disease–late results by non-surgical treatment. A follow-up study. J Hand Surg Br 11(3):422–425

Kutty S, Curtin J (1995) Idiopathic avascular necrosis of the capitate. J Hand Surg Br 20(3):402–404

Lapinsky AS, Mack GR (1992) Avascular necrosis of the capitate: a case report. J Hand Surg (Case Reports Review). 17(6):1090–2

Lichtman DM, Mack GR, MacDonald RI, Gunther SF, Wilson JN (1977) Kienbock's disease: the role of silicone replacement arthroplasty. J Bone Joint Surg Am 59(7): 899–908

Mazet R Jr, Hohl M (1963) Fractures of the carpal navicular: analysis of ninety-one cases and review of the literature. J Bone Joint Surg Am 45-A:82–112

Megerle K, Worg H, Christopoulos G, Schmitt R, Krimmer H (2011) Gadolinium-enhanced preoperative MRI scans as a prognostic parameter in scaphoid nonunion. J Hand Surg (European Volume) 36(1):23–28

Mitchell DG, Steinberg ME, Dalinka MK, Rao VM, Fallon M, Kressel HY (1989) Magnetic resonance imaging of the ischemic hip. Alterations within the osteonecrotic, viable, and reactive zones. Clin Orthop Relat Res 244:60–77

Murakami H, Nishida J, Ehara S, Furumachi K, Shimamura T (2002) Revascularization of avascular necrosis of the capitate bone. Am J Roentgenol 179(3):664–666

Resnick D (2002) Osteochondroses. In: Resnick D (ed) Diagnosis of Bone and Joint Disorders, 4th edn. Saunders, Philadelphia, pp 3686–3741

Rubinstein HM (1975) Thiemann's disease. A brief reminder. Arthritis Rheum 18(4):357–360

Schmitt R, Christopoulos G, Wagner M, Krimmer H, Fodor S, van Schoonhoven J et al (2011) Avascular necrosis (AVN) of the proximal fragment in scaphoid nonunion: is intravenous contrast agent necessary in MRI? Eur J Radiol 77(2):222–227

Sherman SB, Greenspan A, Norman A (1983) Osteonecrosis of the distal pole of the carpal scaphoid following fracture–a rare complication. Skeletal Radiol 9(3):189–191

Singh AK, Davis TR, Dawson JS, Oni JA, Downing ND (2004) Gadolinium enhanced MR assessment of proximal fragment vascularity in nonunions after scaphoid fracture: does it predict the outcome of reconstructive surgery? J Hand Surg Br 29(5):444–448

Sowa DT, Holder LE, Patt PG, Weiland AJ (1989) Application of magnetic resonance imaging to ischemic necrosis of the lunate. J Hand Surg 14(6):1008–1016

Tashjian RZ, Patel A, Akelman E, Weiss A-pC (2004) Avascular necrosis of the wrist and hand excluding the scaphoid and lunate. J Am Soc Surg Hand 4(2):109–116

Telfer JR, Evans DM, Bingham JB (1994) Avascular necrosis of the hamate. J Hand Surg Br 19(3):389–392

Weiss AP, Weiland AJ, Moore JR, Wilgis EF (1991) Radial shortening for Kienbock disease. J Bone Joint Surg Am 73(3):384–391

Zafra M, Carpintero P, Cansino D (2004) Osteonecrosis of the trapezium treated with a vascularized distal radius bone graft. J Hand Surg Am 29(6):1098–1101

Metabolic and Endocrine Disorders

Giuseppe Guglielmi and Silvana Muscarella

Contents

G. Guglielmi (✉) · S. Muscarella
Department of Radiology, University of Foggia,
Viale L. Pinto 1, 71100 Foggia, Italy
e-mail: g.guglielmi@unifg.it

G. Guglielmi · S. Muscarella
Department of Radiology, Hospital "Casa Sollievo della Sofferenza", Viale Cappuccini 1, 71013 San Giovanni Rotondo, Italy

Abstract

Hand and wrist are well recognized as a mirror of disease for various metabolic and endocrine pathologic conditions. Among them, osteoporosis is the most common metabolic bone disorder. It is defined as "a skeletal disease, characterized by decreased bone mineral density (BMD) and micro-architectural deterioration of bone tissue, with a consequent increase in bone fragility and susceptibility to fracture" . As a disease of the elderly, its prevalence will increase as the population ages leading to a need to intensify and optimize the diagnostic techniques for its assessment. BMD is a measurement of bone mass and a reflection of the amount of calcium in bone. Currently, the *gold standard* for measuring BMD is Dual-energy X-ray Absorptiometry (DXA).

1 Introduction

Hand and wrist are well recognized as a mirror of disease for various metabolic and endocrine pathologic conditions (Theodorou et al. 2001). Among them, osteoporosis is the most common metabolic bone disorder. It is defined as "a skeletal disease, characterized by decreased bone mineral density (BMD) and micro-architectural deterioration of bone tissue, with a consequent increase in bone fragility and susceptibility to fracture" (Anonymous 2003). As a disease of the elderly, its prevalence will increase as the population ages leading to a need to intensify and optimize the diagnostic techniques for its assessment. BMD is a measurement of bone mass

A. M. Davis et al. (eds.), *Imaging of the Hand and Wrist*, Medical Radiology. Diagnostic Imaging,
DOI: 10.1007/174_2010_127,

and a reflection of the amount of calcium in bone. Currently, the *gold standard* for measuring BMD is Dual-energy X-ray Absorptiometry (DXA). On the basis of the T-score (the difference between the BMD of the patient under examination and the BMD of a standard young adult population) The World Health Organization (WHO) has defined as:

- *normal* T-score values of −1.0 or higher;
- *osteopenia* T-score values of less than −1.0 but higher than −2.5;
- *osteoporosis* T-score values of −2.5 or less;
- *severe osteoporosis* T-score values of −2.5 or less with a fragility fracture (Kanis JA, on behalf of the World Health Organization Scientific Group 2007).

Osteoporotic fractures may affect any part of the skeleton except the skull. Most commonly, fractures occur in the distal forearm (Colles' fracture), thoracic and lumbar vertebrae, and proximal femur (hip fracture). Fractures usually have substantial clinical and social impact. Following a fragility fracture, significant pain, disability, and deformity can ensue, compromising life quality and shorten life expectancy (Cockerill et al. 2004; Center et al. 1999). Moreover, if fracture union is not achieved, the patient may suffer long-term disability due also to degenerative joint disease distal to the fracture and to reflex sympathetic dystrophy (Cosman 2005). A prior fracture increases the risk of future fractures (Cummings et al. 1995). Moreover, fractures are often under-recognized and patients who sustain a fragility fracture often do not receive adequate or appropriate medical treatment for the underlying osteoporosis. Given the substantial impact of osteoporosis on both patients and the medical community, it is imperative that physicians improve awareness and knowledge of osteoporosis in the setting of low-energy fractures.

2 Classification of Osteoporosis

Osteoporosis is generally characterized into primary and secondary causes. Primary osteoporosis is divided into type I, postmenopausal osteoporosis, and type II, senile or age-related osteoporosis. Type I represents a high turnover state that occurs after menopause. Type II is largely a failure of osteoblastic bone to form (Lane et al. 2006). In "postmenopausal" osteoporosis there is an apparent excess loss of cancellous bone with relative sparing of cortical bone, and the clinical syndrome involves Colle's fracture and vertebral fracture. In "senile" osteoporosis there is a more simultaneous loss of both cortical and cancellous bone. The pathogenesis of senile osteoporosis is uncertain, but it is postulated to result from an age-related decline in renal production of 1,25-dihydroxyvitamin D and calcium malabsorption, with subsequent secondary hyperparathyroidism. Fracture syndrome often seen in the patient with senile osteoporosis characteristically involves the hip and pelvis (Ross 1998). Besides the above mentioned, other risk factors like presence of dementia, susceptibility to falling, history of fractures in adulthood, history of fractures in a first-degree relative, frailty, impaired eyesight, insufficient physical activity and low body weight can partly contribute to the development of osteoporosis and its complications (Guglielmi et al. 2008).

Secondary osteoporosis is caused by a multitude of factors, including endocrine disorders, hematopoietic diseases, immobilization, gastric disorders, medications (long-term oral glucocorticoid therapy), increased alcohol intake and smoking (Seeman et al. 1983).

3 Diagnosis of Osteoporosis

3.1 Conventional Radiography

Indications of bone loss on radiographs are generally a reduction in density and changes in morphology. It has been estimated that in most cases osteopenia becomes detectable on conventional radiographs only after a loss of at least 20–40% of the skeletal bone mass (Virtama 1960; Grampp et al. 1993). Nevertheless, conventional radiography is widely available, and it remains useful for the detection of specific alterations in certain instances (e.g., subperiosteal resorption in hyperparathyroidism). Alone and in conjunction with modern, computed-aided, imaging techniques, conventional radiography is widely used for the detection of fractures, for the differential diagnosis of osteopenia, or for follow-up examinations in specific clinical settings (Genant et al. 1996; Guglielmi et al. 1994). Moreover, conventional radiographies are predominantly performed at sites of the peripheral skeleton (calcaneus and distal radius) as surrounding soft tissue does not compromise image quality and standardization (Caligiuri et al. 1994; Vokes et al. 2006).

In osteoporosis a decrease in the mineralized bone volume results in a decrease of the total bone calcium and a decreased absorption of the X-ray beam. This phenomenon is then referred to as *increased radiolucency*. As bone mass is lost, changes in the bone structure occur. Bone is composed of two compartments: cortical bone and trabecular bone. The structural canes seen in the cortical bone represent bone resorption at different sites (e.g., the inner and outer surfaces of the cortex, or within the cortex in the Haversian and Volkmann channels). These three sites (endosteal, intracortical, and periosteal) may react differently to distinct metabolic stimuli. Cortical bone remodeling typically occurs in the endosteal "envelop", and the interpretation of subtle changes in this layer may be difficult. With increasing age there is a widening of the marrow canal due to an imbalance of endosteal bone formation and resorption that leads to a "trabeculization" of the inner surface of the cortex. Endosteal scalloping due to resorption of the inner bone surface can be seen in high-bone turnover states like reflex sympathetic dystrophy. Intracortical bone resorption may cause longitudinal striation or tunneling. These changes are seen in various high-turnover metabolic diseases affecting the bone like hyperparathyroidism, osteomalacia, renal osteodystrophy, and acute osteoporoses from disuse or reflex sympathetic dystrophy syndrome, but also rapidly evolving postmenopausal osteoporosis. It is usually not apparent in disease states with relatively low turnover like senile osteoporosis.

Accelerated endosteal and intracortical resorption, with intracortical tunneling and indistinct border of the inner cortical surface, is best depicted with high-resolution radiographic techniques with optical magnification.

Subperiosteal bone resorption is associated with an irregular definition of the outer bone surface. This finding is pronounced in diseases with high bone turn-over, principally primary and secondary hyperparathyroidism (Guglielmi et al. 2001, 2003).

In the appendicular skeleton, changes in the trabecular and cortical bone are first apparent at the ends of long and tubular bones due to the predominance of cancellous bone in these regions.

Radiologic imaging of the hand is a fundamental step in evaluating grade and type of osteoporosis, thanks to anatomic peculiarities of this anatomic region that allow a best detailed evaluation through high-resolution systems (e.g., industrial films).

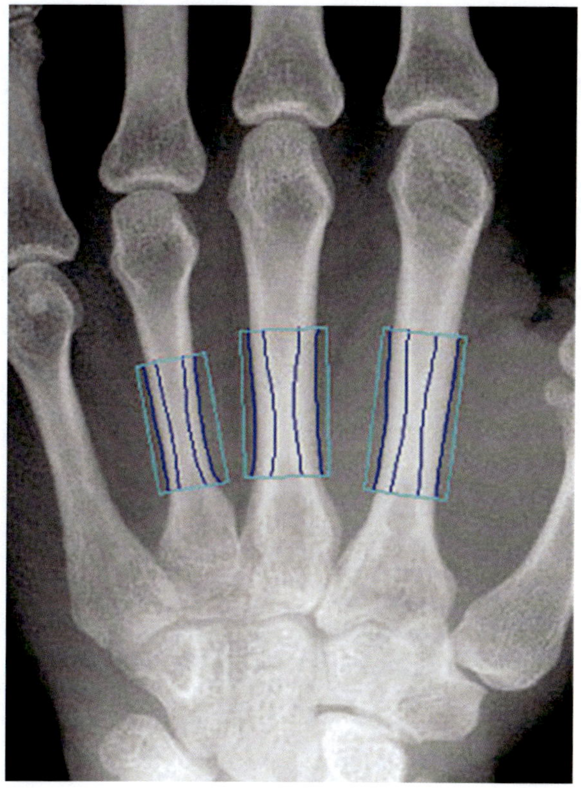

Fig. 1 Radiographs of the hand showing a detailed evaluation of II, III, and IV metacarpal bones. Spongious and cortical compartments are separately evaluated

Metacarpal bones (usually II, III, and IV) are investigated. Spongious and cortical compartments are separately evaluated (Fig. 1). The cortico-medullar index, based on the evaluation of the cortical thickness at II metacarpal bone, represented in the past a good semi-quantitative measure for grading osteoporosis at this site (Link et al. 1994).

3.2 Peripheral Dual-Energy X-Ray Absorptiometry

Bone mineral density is an important factor influencing bone strength and a key predictor of fracture risk in patients with osteoporosis and other metabolic bone diseases (Cummings et al. 2002; Grampp et al. 1997). DXA is the most widely used technique for diagnosis of osteoporosis (Cauley et al. 2005;

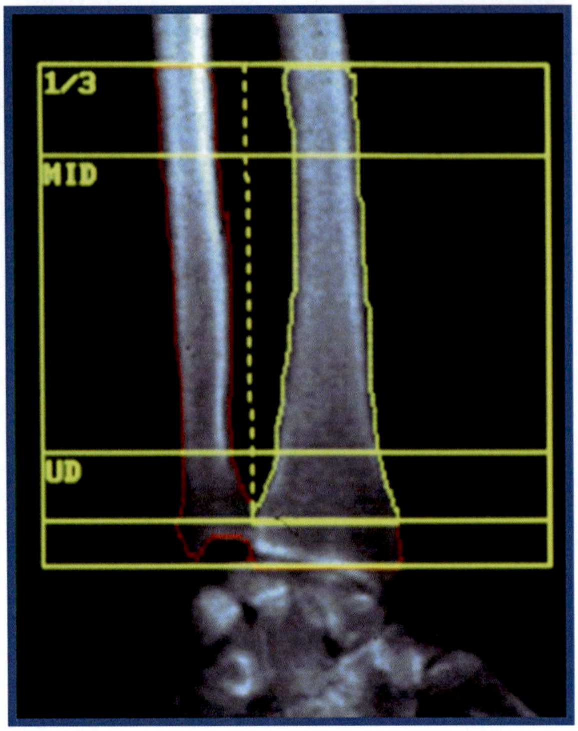

Fig. 2 DXA of the distal (87% cortical bone) and ultradistal (65% trabecular bone) forearm

Damilakis et al. 2006; Guglielmi et al. 2003). This technique determines an aerial density and BMD is therefore given as g/cm^2. It has a limited ability to evaluate bone geometry and cannot provide separate cortical and trabecular bone evaluations (Seeman and Delmas 2006).

An increasing number of small, portable DXA scanners are becoming available for application to peripheral sites (distal radius and calcaneus). Scanning of the forearm takes about 5 min to perform. The position of the forearm is standardized by the patient gripping a vertical rod. DXA allows an evaluation of weight-bearing and not weight-bearing bones. The scan is performed in a rectilinear fashion at a distal (87% cortical bone) and ultradistal (predominantly 65% trabecular bone) site (Fig. 2). Accuracy is 3%, precision is better than 1% and radiation dose is 0.1 μSv. Due to its composition, the forearm site is not a sensitive site for monitoring changes in BMD with respect to the calcaneus that is 95% trabecular bone and offers more potential for this purpose. The WHO criterion for the diagnosis of osteoporosis (T-score of −2.5 or less) is applicable to the forearm but the definitive threshold for diagnosis has still to be determined (Pacheco et al. 2002). By consequence, BMD changes in peripheral bones such as phalanx and forearm must be very carefully interpreted. In fact, screening individuals using peripheral sites and technologies is not completely supported by current evidences. Picard and collaborators (Picard et al. 2004) compared results of BMD obtained at the forearm and phalanges with those obtained at lumbar spine and femoral neck evaluated by DXA: even though the negative predictive value reached more than 95% of the true negatives, the positive predictive value was only ranged from 40 to 43% what is, again, distant from the ideal situation. In general, it is recognized that the elder the subject is, the more likely to have agreement between a peripheral and a central measurement (Deng et al. 1998).

Monitoring treatment could be a very specific applicability but, even in this case, distal sites are not completely accepted due, mainly, to the fact that the changes expected with the available therapies are also smaller than at central sites. As reviewed by the ORAG group (Guyatt et al. 2002), if the forearm was used for monitoring treatment, only the treatment with Hormonal Therapy and Alendronate for 2–4 years could be adequately monitored.

3.3 Peripheral Quantitative Computed Tomography

Bone strength and fracture risk are also influenced by parameters of bone quality such as micro-architecture and tissue properties, evaluable by developing techniques other than DXA. Peripheral Quantitative Computed Tomography (pQCT) has been proposed as a relatively inexpensive method to assess trabecular BMD in single-slice mode (Rüegsegger et al. 1976; Schneider and Börner 1991; Guglielmi and Lang 2002; Guglielmi et al. 1997). Dedicated peripheral CT scanners are available for assessing BMD in the radius and tibia. They are smaller, more mobile and less expensive that whole body CT scanners. pQCT measures the apparent volumetric BMD (mg/cm^3), in contrast to projection techniques such as DXA of the radius, and allows separate assessments of trabecular and cortical bone (Ito et al. 1997; Schneider and Reiners 1998) (Fig. 3). Peripheral QCT is most commonly applied to the non-dominant forearm.

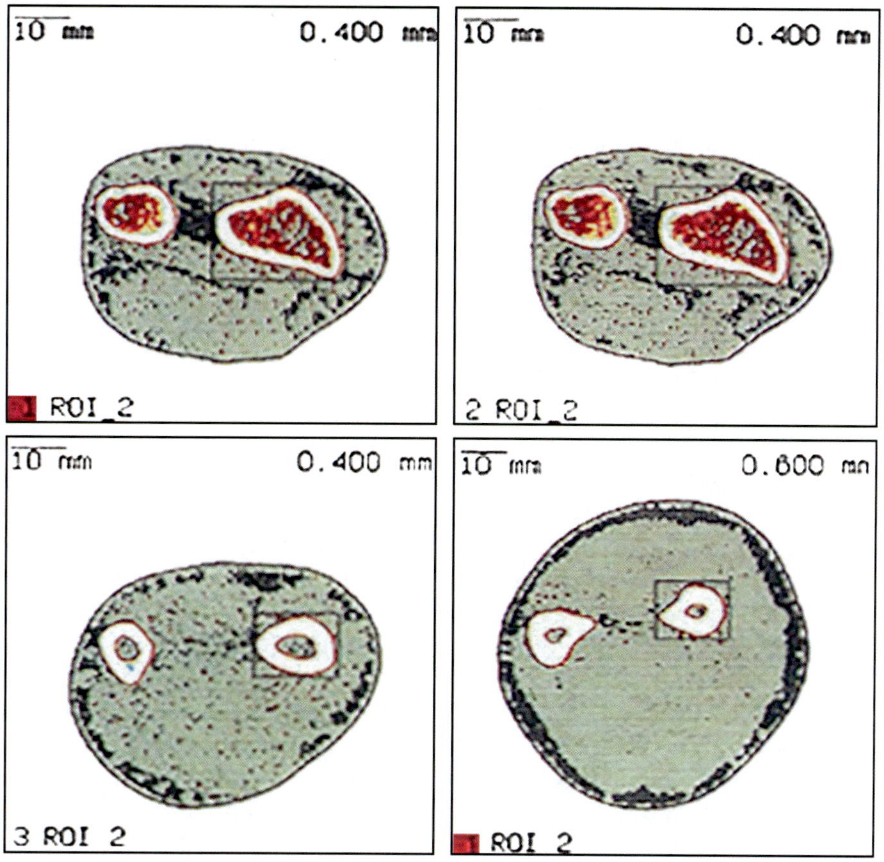

Fig. 3 Peripheral QCT of the distal radius allows separate measurement of trabecular bone, cortical bone, total and cortical area and marrow cross-sectional area

Initially the forearm length is measured as the distance between the tip of the ulnar styloid and the olecranon. The patient's forearm is placed pronated in the pQCT gantry with the elbow resting on a block and the hand gripping the hand fixture. The arm is secured with Velcro straps to prevent movement. A coronal scout scan is performed and a reference line is placed to bisect the medial border of the end of the distal radius. Accurate and consistent positioning of this reference line is essential in any longitudinal or multi-center studies for comparable results. The sites generally scanned in the radius are the 4% (distal), 50% (mid) and between 60 and 66% (proximal) shaft, but other sites (e.g., 38% distal) are also used. The parameters measured at the 4% site include total and trabecular bone mineral content (BMC), BMD and cross-sectional area (CSA); in the shaft cortical BMC and BMD are measured with many geometric parameters including total and cortical area (mm^2), cortical thickness (mm), marrow cross-sectional area (mm^2), periosteal and endosteal circumference (mm), (Adams 2009). The definition of osteoporosis given by the WHO (T-score of −2.5 or less), is applicable only to DXA of the lumbar spine, femoral neck, total hip and distal 33% radius. The definition does not apply to other anatomical sites (e.g., calcaneus) or to other densitometric techniques, such as Quantitative Ultrasound (QUS) or QCT, in either a central or peripheral QCT in the spine, and in distal radius and tibial sites.

Measurements of either total or trabecular BMD of the ultra-distal radius, by pQCT, predict fractures of the hip in post-menopausal women (Engelke et al. 2008). pQCT performs as well as, if not better than, DXA spine or QCT spine for prediction of wrist and hip fractures (Engelke et al. 2008).

Advantages of pQCT over axial QCT are that pQCT generates a lower radiation dose (1–2 μSv in pQCT compared with 50 μSv in spinal QCT), and that it provides substantially higher reproducibility (Guglielmi et al. 1997). Advantages of pQCT over DXA are high accuracy, separate measurement of cortical and trabecular bone, and cross-sectional bone imaging to offer additional information.

Recent advancements in another novel technology, volumetric QCT (vQCT), offers three-dimensional (3D) information, and cortical and trabecular bone can be separately analyzed. A particular challenge of volumetric BMD (vBMD) is the reproducible location of a given analysis volume of interest (VOI) in longitudinal scans. Most analysis software is experimental and only a few commercial programs are available. The overall advantages of this vQCT technique include high precision, on the order of 1–2% for BMD of the spine, hip and radius; nearly instant availability of data, in a matter of seconds to minutes; widespread access, with many thousands of systems available worldwide; and minimal user interaction. The major disadvantage for vBMD is the use of modest radiation exposure, which for the radius requires an effective dose <10 μSv (Genant et al. 2008). Guglielmi et al. found that pQCT of the ultradistal radius is a precise method for measuring the true volumetric BMD and for detecting age-related bone loss in the trabecular and total bone of female subjects encompassing the adult age range and menopausal status (Guglielmi et al. 2000).

Another area of active research is high-resolution peripheral QCT (HR-pQCT), that allows accurate and precise 3D evaluation of vBMD, quantitative trabecular structure analysis of the distal radius and also a separate assessment of cortical and trabecular BMD, although with longer scan times and increased likelihood of motion artifacts (Boutroy et al. 2008; Sornay-Rendu et al. 2009). The advancement of techniques allowing assessments of cortical bone is important. Indeed, non-vertebral fractures are a significant cause of morbidity and mortality in osteoporosis, and cortical bone can account for a significant amount of the likelihood for fracture in the peripheral skeleton. On the other hand, occurrence of a forearm fracture increases the risk of future hip, spine, and forearm fractures (Cuddihy et al. 1999). This is of particular importance if one thinks that although they are accepted as a major fracture type, forearm fractures remain under-recognized and under-treated as osteoporosis-related fractures (Endres et al. 2007). Spadaro et al. (1994) evaluated the contributions of the cortical and trabecular compartments to bone strength at the radius and found that the cortical shell contributes substantially to bone strength.

The structure or spatial arrangement of bone at the macroscopic and microscopic levels is thought to provide additional, independent information on mechanical properties and may help to better predict fracture risk and assess response to drug intervention. Boutroy and colleagues (Boutroy et al. 2005) gave the first indication that peripheral trabecular structure assessment is indeed useful to differentiate women with an osteoporotic fracture history from controls better than DXA at hip or spine. Khosla and colleagues (Khosla et al. 2006a; Khosla et al. 2006b) examined age- and sex-related bone loss cross-sectionally and speculated as to the different patterns of bone loss in men and women.

3.4 Quantitative Ultrasound

Quantitative sonography methods have been introduced in recent years for the assessment of skeletal status in osteoporosis (Guglielmi et al. 2009). QUS involves generating ultrasound impulses that are transmitted (transversally or longitudinally) through the bone under study. The frequency range employed in QUS of bone lies between 200 kHz and 1.5 MHz. The ultrasound wave is produced in the form of a sinusoid impulse by special piezoelectric probes, and is detected once it has passed through the medium; there are two distinct probes, emitting and receiving, and the skeletal segment for evaluation is placed between them (Guglielmi and de Terlizzi 2009).

The first ultrasound parameters employed for characterizing bone tissue were: Speed of Sound (SoS) and Broadband Ultrasound Attenuation (BUA). More complex parameters have been developed from combination of SoS and BUA: Amplitude Dependent Speed of Sound (AD-SoS), stiffness, Quantitative Ultrasound Index (QUI) (Gluer and the International Quantitative Ultrasound Consensus Group 1997; Guglielmi et al. 2003). The technique is usually applied at the calcaneus, tibia, and phalanges, but has also been used at the patella and distal radius (Gnudi et al. 2000). The phalanx is a long bone consisting of a trabecular component and a cortical component, the principal determinant of the mechanical resistance of the bone. The phalanx is measured by QUS at the metaphyseal site,

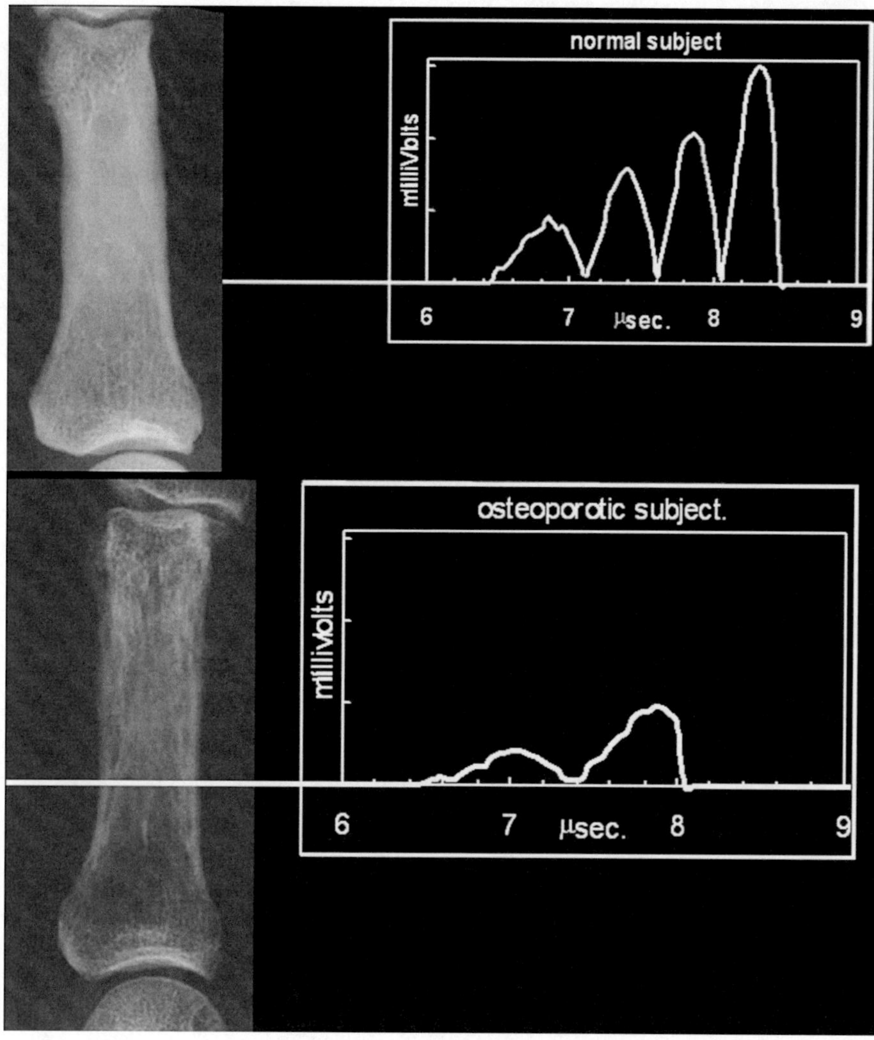

Fig. 4 Quantitative ultrasound at hand phalanges showing the different graphic traces in a normal subject and osteoporotic patient

where both trabecular (at about 40%) and cortical, bones are present. The metaphysis of the phalanx is, moreover, characterized by a high bone turnover and, therefore, extremely sensitive to changes in skeletal status due to natural causes (growth and aging), metabolic diseases (e.g., hyperparathyroidism), or drug-induced effects (treatment with glucocorticoids). When measurements are performed at the radius site, propagation occurs mainly along the external surface of the bone, and thus provides information mostly of cortical bone.

The European multi-center study (PhOS) (Wüster et al. 2000), performed on over 10.000 women, provided clinical validation of QUS at the phalanx. In this study the method could identify osteoporotic subjects with vertebral or hip fractures. Guglielmi et al. (1999) found no significant differences between phalangeal QUS and X-ray densitometric BMD methods (DXA and central QCT) in separating normal from osteoporotic subjects when using ROC analysis (Fig. 4). Hartl et al. (Hartl et al. 2002) showed that the diagnostic performance of QUS at the calcaneus and the phalanx were comparable with central DXA in assessing subjects with osteoporotic vertebral fractures. Krieg et al. (2003) studied an elderly (70–80 years) Swiss population, to assess the ability of QUS at the calcaneus and phalanx in discriminating subjects with, and without, hip fracture. An interesting Italian study demonstrated that QUS at the phalanx is more sensitive in discriminating subjects with, and without, vertebral fractures immediately post-menopause, prior to the age of

70 years, whereas QUS at the calcaneus is more sensitive in the subsequent period, at the age of 70 years and older (Camozzi et al. 2007).

Even if clinical studies demonstrated positive and statistically significant correlations between results from QUS and photon bone densitometric method, this is not sufficient to predict central BMD from QUS (Wüster et al. 2000; Guglielmi et al. 1999; Schott et al. 1995). These observations demonstrate that QUS cannot replace photon absorptiometric bone densitometry, but the two techniques can provide complementary information to improve estimates of vertebral fracture risk: low QUS values must be considered as a factor in fracture risk assessment which is independent of BMD and, therefore, emphasizes the clinical importance of QUS in appropriate clinical situations. Anyway, it is important to note that the WHO definition of osteoporosis based on densitometry terms (T-score of −2.5 or less) is not applicable to QUS. On the other hand, QUS for the study of post-menopausal osteoporosis is now completely validated: scientific societies of several European countries have included bone QUS in their national guidelines for the diagnosis and management of osteoporosis, particularly for the evaluation of fracture risk in post-menopausal women (National Osteoporosis Society 2002; Schattauer GmbH 2006). Ultrasound velocity has also been applied to monitor changes and response to treatment in women with osteoporosis. In particular, some studies show that treatment with alendronate (Ingle et al. 2005), raloxifene (Agostinelli and de Terlizzi 2007), and teriparatide (Gonnelli et al. 2006) can be monitored using phalanx QUS.

3.5 Magnetic Resonance

Magnetic resonance (MR) offers alternative ways of assessing skeletal properties. Trabecular bone is not visualized at MR imaging so that a trabecula appears as a signal void, surrounded by high-intensity fatty bone marrow. This signal void is due to the very short T2 relaxation time of bone and to the bone marrow interface (Link et al. 1999; Guglielmi et al. 2003). Due to technical advances, like optimized coil design, fast gradients and high field strength, clinical MR scanners provide an in vivo spatial resolution close to the diameter of a single trabecula (Sell et al. 2005; Wehrli 2007). Moreover, with the advent of parallel imaging, motion correction techniques and new sequences, the limits of spatial resolution and scan time can be further overcome (Banerjee et al. 2006; Techawiboonwong et al. 2005). Most in vivo studies focused on peripheral skeleton because the distal radius, distal tibia and the calcaneus are easily accessible with small coils, contain a high number of trabeculae and the bone marrow consists of fat, resulting in high bone–bone marrow contrast. Each stage needs to be standardized to ensure a high degree of reproducibility (Newitt et al. 2002). On the other hand, the processing of high-resolution MR (HR–MR) images generally consists of several stages (registration, segmentation, resolution enhancement and normalization or binarization), before measures of the trabecular architecture can be evaluated (Wehrli 2007; Newitt et al. 2002) (Fig. 5). The efficiency of these techniques was evaluated in terms of reproducibility (2–4%), (Gomberg et al. 2004) and different approaches have been applied successfully in several cross-sectional, and recently in longitudinal, studies (Wehrli et al. 2001; Majumdar et al. 1999; Cortet et al. 2000). MR imaging aims to quantification of the trabecular bone architecture trough five types of measures (describing scale; shape and orientation of the trabeculae; connectivity or complexity of the trabecular network and finite element models—FEM) directly characterizing mechanical properties.

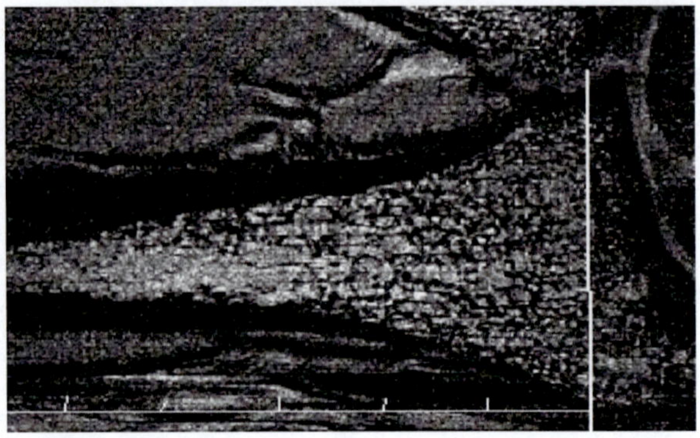

Fig. 5 High-resolution MR of the radius allows quantification of the trabecular bone architecture (scale, shape, orientation, connectivity and finite element models of the trabeculae)

Many Authors studied performances of MR in studying trabecular structure at distal radius and phalanges. Stampa et al. (2002) used phalanges, a convenient anatomic site particularly suitable for obtaining high signal-to-noise and high-spatial resolution images, to derive quantitative three-dimensional parameters based on an algorithm and model for defining trabecular rods and plates. To date the quantification of trabecular bone architecture by HR–MR imaging at distal radius aimed to assess the prevalence and incidence of osteoporotic fractures (Majumdar et al. 1999; Cortet et al. 2000; Majumdar et al. 1997). Early studies suggested that MR-based parameters of the trabecular architecture better separate patients with, and without, osteoporotic fractures compared to BMD (Cortet et al. 2000; Majumdar et al. 1997). Link et al. (1998), Majumdar et al. (Majumdar et al. 1997), and Wehrli et al. (Wehrli et al. 1998; Wehrli et al. 2001; Wehrli et al. 2002) have shown the ability to discriminate spine and/or hip fractures using trabecular structure or textural parameters from in vivo MR images of the radius. In measuring the effect of pharmacological therapies for osteoporosis, some studies shows that parameters of trabecular micro-architecture derived by MR could better monitor changes due to anti-resorptive treatment than BMD (Chesnut et al. 2005). One of the early longitudinal studies showed that salmon calcitonin had therapeutic benefit compared with placebo in maintaining trabecular micro-architecture at multiple skeletal sites (Chesnut et al. 2005).

4 Other Metabolic and Endocrine Disorders

4.1 Acromegaly and Gigantism

These conditions are characterized by excess production of growth hormone (GH) due to acidophilic adenomas of the anterior lobe of the pituitary gland or from diffuse hyperplasia of the acidofilic cells. GH excess, which can arise in children (gigantism) or in adult (acromegaly), leads to an overgrowth of bone in the skeleton. In the immature skeleton the disease is associated with extreme height and a large skeleton with normal bone age. In the mature skeleton, after physeal closure, excessive GH production causes an increase in width of bone and soft tissue enlargement manifested particularly in the acral parts of the skeleton.

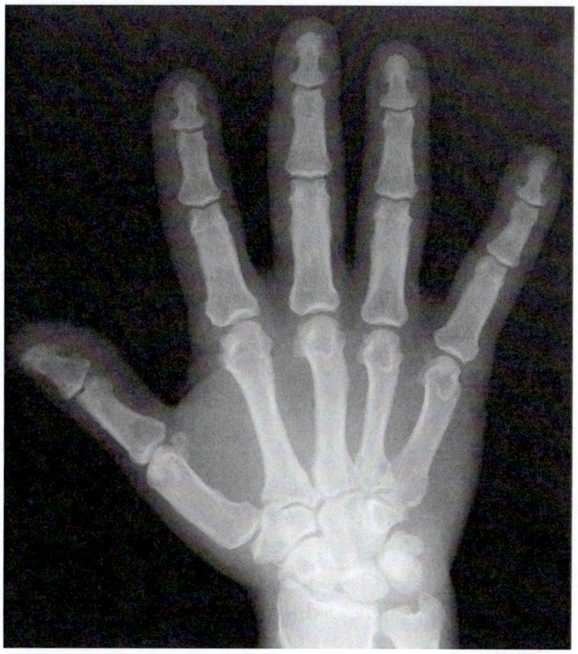

Fig. 6 Acromegaly showing bony overgrowth, joint widening, metacarpal hooking, and arrow-head terminal tufts

Radiographic manifestations of the hand in patients with acromegaly include soft tissue thickening of the digits, osseous enlargement and increased width by means of thickening and squaring of the phalanges and metacarpal bones, overconstrictions or overtubulation of the shafts of the phalanges with normal or increased cortical thickness, widening of the articular spaces due to thickening of the articular cartilage, bone proliferation at tendon and ligament attachment site (enthesopathy) (Fig. 6).

In diagnosing early acromegalic changes some indexes have been proposed. Among them the sesamoid index, proposed by Kleinberg et al. (1966). According to this method, the size of the medial sesamoid at the first metacarpophalangeal joint is measured. This index has, however, a limited reliability because of the significant overlap in measurements in acromegalic patients and controls. Besides bone proliferation, bone resorption can associate (Resnick 1995), leading to a decreased bone density, particularly in the late stages of disease (Sartoris 1971). In addition, osteoarthritis usually complicates the disease (Resnick 1995).

4.2 Hypopituitarism

Hypopituitarism can arise from many causative factors (neoplasms, surgery, irradiation, injury, vascular insult, infection, and granulomas of the pituitary gland or the hypothalamus). Familial pituitary deficiency is reported in 10% cases. Isolated GH deficiency during the period of skeletal growth leads to abnormality of osseous development as a delay in appearance and growth of ossification centers and a similar delay in their fusion and disappearance (Resnick 1995). Radiographic manifestations in the hand include shortening and broadening of the metacarpal bones and distal phalanges or, less commonly, a hypoplastic appearance of the distal phalanges, metaphyseal irregularity, flattening and absence of closure of the physes, and severe osteoporosis. Open epiphyses may be observed in the distal portions of the radius and ulna (Resnick 1995).

4.3 Thyroid Disorders

Thyroid hormone increases bone remodeling (Mosekilde et al. 1990). In cases of excessive thyroid hormone, osteoclastic activity predominates on osteoblastic one, with resultant bone resorption. In the hand, hyperthyroid osteopathy leads to bone loss that is manifested as a lattice-like appearance in the phalanges, and "flaky" cortices due to radiolucent intracortical striations (Resnick 1995). In hypothyroidism, bone abnormalities are more evident in neonates, children, and young adults, and result in retardation of skeletal maturation with subsequent retardation in growth. Delayed appearance and growth of epiphyseal ossification centers, and abnormality of physeal development accompanied by delayed physeal closure are observed. In the hand, arrest in growth is manifested as shortening and widening of the metacarpal bones, which present endosteal cortical thickening (Fig. 7) (Steinbach et al. 1975). Hypoplastic phalanges of fifth finger may be seen (Sartoris 1996). In affected epiphyses, ossification proceeds from multiple centers rather than from a single site (pseudoepiphyses). Abnormal epiphiseal ossification results in a characteristic irregular ad fragmented epiphyseal appearance recognized as epiphyseal dysgenesis (Borg et al. 1975; Parker 1981).

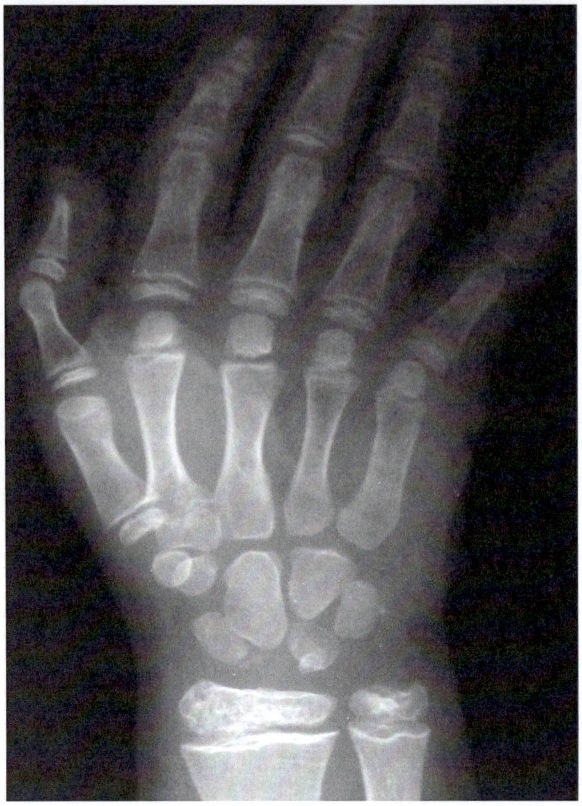

Fig. 7 Hypothyroidism (cretinism) in a child. There is retarded skeletal maturation with shortening of the metacarpals and squaring of the epiphyses

4.4 Hyperparathyroidism

Hyperparathyroidism, a clinical condition characterized by an elevation of serum parathyroid hormone concentration, may be primary, secondary, or tertiary. In primary hyperparathyroidism, hypersecretion of parathyroid hormone is due to abnormality in the parathyroid glands (single or multiple adenomas, diffuse hyperplasia, and carcinoma). Secondary hyperparathyroidism usually is secondary to chronic renal disease, or occasionally, malabsorption states. Tertiary hyperparathyroidism occurs in patients with chronic renal disease and secondary hyperparathyroidism who develop autonomous parathyroid function.

The hand is almost always involved in hyperparathyroidism. Subperiosteal bone resorption is most frequently observed along the radial aspect of the phalanges, particularly in the middle phalanges of the index and middle fingers (Fig. 8) (Resnick 1995).

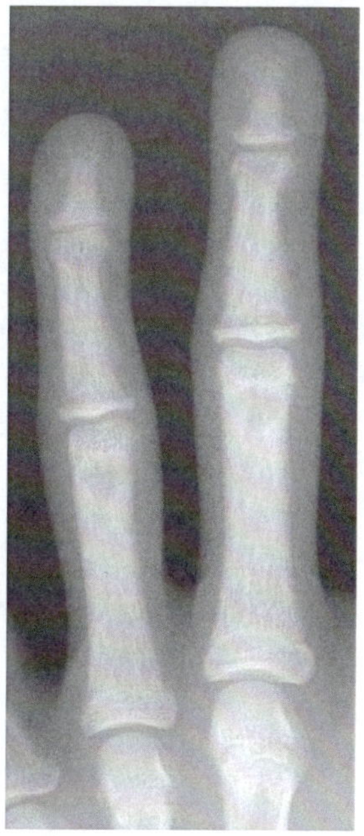

Fig. 8 Hyperparathyroidism. There is subperiosteal resorption along the middle phalanges with terminal phalangeal resorption (acro-osteolysis)

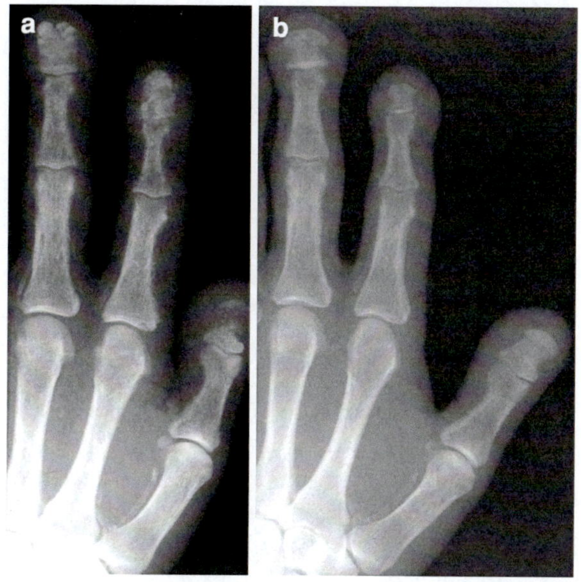

Fig. 9 Secondary hyperparathyroidism in an adult with chronic renal disease. **a** There is subperiosteal resorption along the phalanges, terminal phalangeal resorption with soft tissue and vascular calcification. **b** After successful renal transplantation the resorption has resolved as has the soft tissue but not the vascular calcification. The terminal phalanges remain stunted

Subperioteal bone resorption involves the phalangeal tufts as well, where loss of the cortical "white line" represents the earliest sign of the disease progressing to acro-osteolysis (Sundaram et al. 1979). Intracortical resorption always associates (Meema and Meema 1972) leading to development of pseudoperiostitis (Resnick 1995). Owing to rapid or severe bone loss multiple intracortical, radiolucent areas, in the form of linear striations or tunneling, may be observed in the metacarpal bone and appear more evident in the cortex of the second metacarpal bone (Meema and Meema 1972). In the hand, osteoclastic resorption occurs along the endosteal surface of bone causing localized scalloped or pocket-like defects along the endosteal margin of the cortex. In children with primary or secondary hyperparathyroidism, irregular radiolucent areas may be apparent in the metaphysis adjacent to the growth plate of tubular bones of the hand (Resnick 1995). In the hyperparathyroid state, osseous resorption may occur at sites of tendon and ligament attachment to bone also at the hand and the wrist (Resnick 1995). Trabecular resorption within medullary bone, particularly in the advanced stages of the disease, may involve the tubular bones of the hand that assume a characteristic granular appearance, with loss of distinct trabecular detail, and subsequent osseous deformities that may simulate the changes of osteomalacia (Resnick 1995). Brown tumors are also included among the radiographic manifestations of hyperparathyroidism and represent localized accumulations of osteoclasts, fibrous tissue, and giant cells, which can replace bone and occasionally produce osseous expansion. They appear as single or multiple well or poorly demarcated osteolytic lesions with an eccentric or cortical location (Resnick 1995). A prominent radiographic feature of hyperparathyroidism is generalized osteopenia. Nevertheless, as hyperparathyroidism may induce either bone resorption or formation, increased radiodensity of bones may become a prominent radiographic feature. There is a meaningful association between primary hyperparathyroidism and CPPD crystal deposition that may lead to the pseudogout syndrome. Renal osteodystrophy is the clinical term indicating bone disease in patients with chronic renal failure. The radiographic manifestations of renal osteodystrophy reflect hyperparathyroidism and deficiency of 1,25-dihydroxyvitamin D, rickets and osteomalacia, osteoporosis, soft tissue and vascular calcifications, and miscellaneous changes (Fig. 9) (gout arthritis due to hyperuricemia). Lytic, expansile lesions, the so-called brown tumor may occur in the long bones of the hand and will mimic a giant cell tumor both radiographically and histologically (Fig. 10). They are commoner in patients with chronic renal disease because of the larger numbers of patients surviving on dialysis and that most cases of primary hyperparathyroidism are now detected on serum biochemistry.

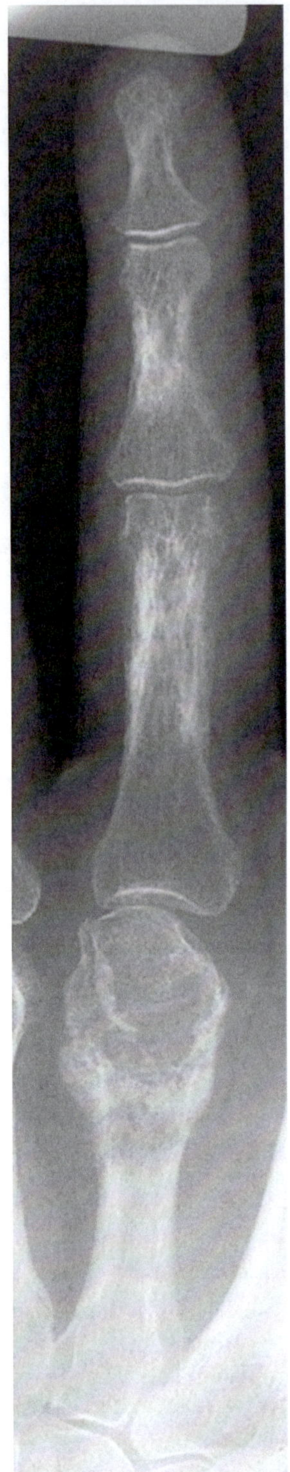

Fig. 10 Brown tumor in a patient with chronic renal disease. There is a pathological fracture developing through a lytic expansile lesion in the distal end of the metacarpal. There are features of hyperparathyroidism affecting the phalanges

4.5 Rickets and Osteomalacia

The terms rickets and osteomalacia refer to the same condition manifesting in the child and adult, respectively. The commonest cause worldwide is inadequate dietary intake of vitamin D. Other causes include inadequate sunshine, malabsorption states, anti-epileptic drug therapy, renal disease and rarely tumur related. This results in inadequate or delayed mineralization of osteoid in mature cortical and spongy bone (osteomalacia) and from an interruption in orderly development and mineralization of the growth plate (rickets) (Resnick 1995). As rachitic changes are more evident in regions of the most active bone growth, target sites of rickets include the distal ends of ulna and radius (Park 1932). General radiographic features of rickets include retardation in bone growth and osteopenia. Slight axial widening of the physis represents the earliest specific radiographic finding (Steinbach and Noetzli 1964). Disorganization and "fraying" of the spongy bone occur in the metaphyseal region, which eventually demonstrates widening and cupping (Fig. 11) (Resnick 1995). In the hand of the rachitic children, irregularities and widening of the physes seen in the metacarpals and phalanges also may be associated with bone resorption. In osteomalacia medullary bone shows a decrease in the total number of trabeculae, owing to a loss of secondary trabeculae. The remaining bone trabeculae are prominent and present a "coarsened" pattern with unsharp margins reflecting deposition of inadequately mineralized osteoid. Looser's zones, typical of osteomalacia elsewhere in the skeleton, are uncommon in the hands.

4.6 Hypoparathyroidism

Hypoparathyroidism is a general term describing a clinical state of parathyroid hormone deficiency, which results in hypocalcemia and neuromuscular

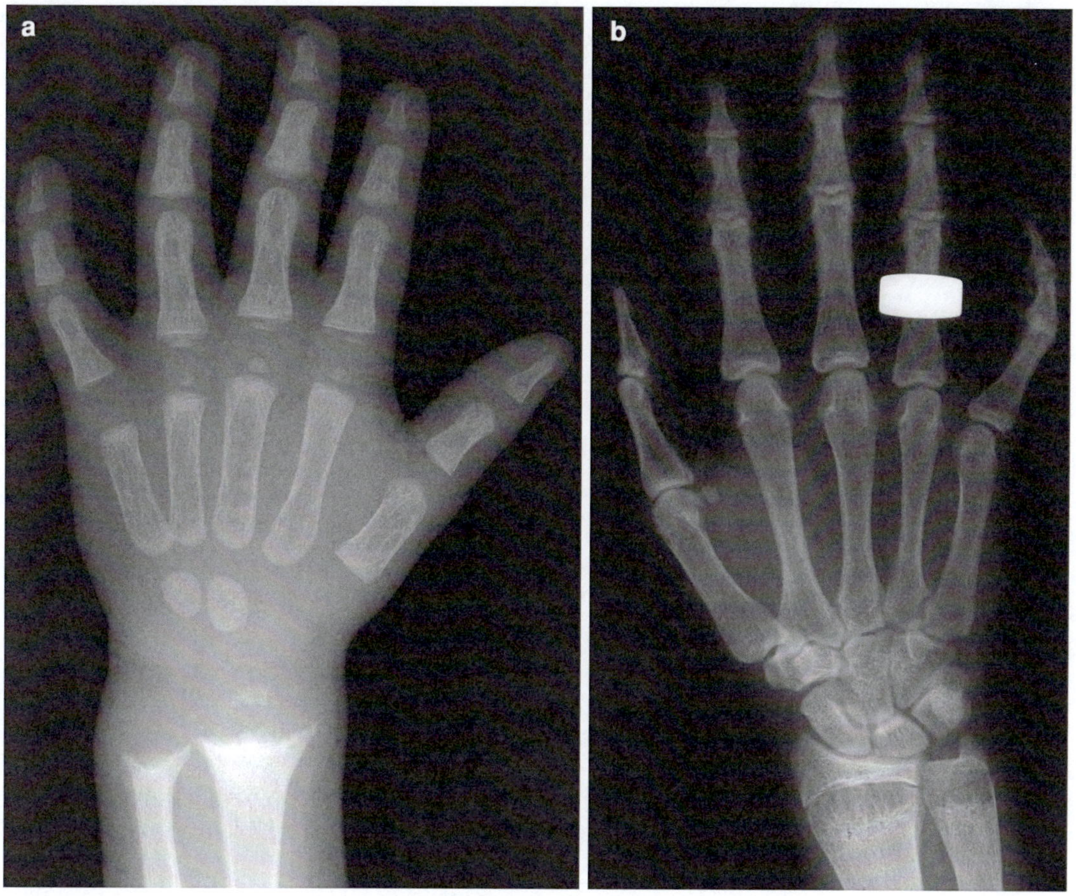

Fig. 11 Rickets. **a** In a young child there is generalized osteopenia with cupping, splaying, and fraying of the distal radial and ulnar metaphyses. **b** In an adolescent the only abnormalities are generalized osteopenia and relative demineralization of the distal radial and ulnar metaphyses

dysfunction. It can have many causes like surgery, congenital absence or atrophy of the parathyroid glands, and parathyroid gland destruction after radiation. The major radiographic manifestations of hypoparathyroidism are osteosclerosis, which may be generalized or localized, and soft tissue calcification. In the hand, radiographic findings of hypoparathyroidism are usually subtle and represented by subcutaneous, ligamentous and tendinous calcifications, premature fusion of the physes, entsopathy, and osteoporosis (Resnick 1995).

Pseudohypoparathyroidism (PHP) or Albright's hereditary osteodystrophy, is a congenital disorder characterized by hypocalcemia and hyperphosphatemia. Pseudopseudohypoparathyroidism (PPHP) is the normocalcemic form of PHP and is also caused by failure and end-organ response to parathyroid hormone. In the hand, radiographic findings of PHP and PPHT include shortening of the metacarpal bone and phalanges secondary to premature physeal closure, widening and shortening of the phalanges with presence of cone-shaped and pseudo-epiphyses, soft tissue calcification, and small diaphyseal exostoses that extend perpendicularly from the surface of the bone (Fig. 12). In most cases of PHP and PPHP, metacarpal shortening shows predilection for the first, fourth, and fifth rays and may lead to a positive metacarpal sign (the line drawn tangential to the heads of the fourth and fifth metacarpal bones intersects the end of the third metacarpal bone, indicating disproportionate shortening of the fourth and fifth metacarpal bones).

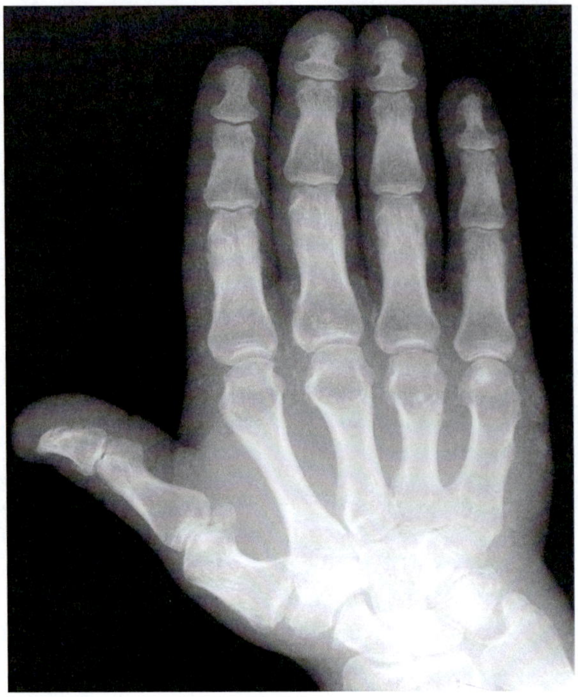

Fig. 12 Pseudohypoparathyroidism. There is shortening of the metacarpals with soft tissue calcifications

4.7 Scurvy

Scurvy is due to a deficiency, typically dietary, of vitamin C (ascorbic acid) which leads do a reduction in collagen formation in bone. The radiographic features include generalized osteopenia, thinned cortices with sparse trabeculae, dense metaphyseal line with an adjacent lucent line, metaphyseal spurs (Pelkan spurs) and finely pencilled dense epiphyseal margins (Wimburger's sign). Capillary fragility may lead to subperiosteal hemorrhage that in time may heal with exuberant periosteal ossification. All these features are more commonly seen in the lower limbs than the hand or wrist.

5 Conclusions

Several metabolic and endocrine disorders cause skeletal involving of hand and wrist. Among them osteoporosis is the most common metabolic bone disease. Besides traditional methods (conventional radiographs), new interesting techniques are developing and appear promising in the evaluation of peripheral osteoporosis. Many studies evaluate DXA application at distal radius; pQCT demonstrates promising results in studying bone microarchitecture thanks to new technologies like vQCT and HR-QCT; QUS are proving to be very useful in the evaluation of bone properties and showed good performances with respect to DXA; finally, HR-MR, on the basis of sophisticated software, is becoming a new challenging technique in the assessment of trabecular structure. Other metabolic and endocrine conditions may manifest with radiographic abnormalities in the hands including rickets and hyperparathyroidism.

6 Key Points

- Osteoporosis and other several metabolic and endocrine disorders cause skeletal involving of hand and wrist.
- DXA is the *gold standard* for measuring BMD in the axial skeleton, as defined by WHO.
- pDXA as well as pQCT are the methods of choice in the evaluation of peripheral osteoporosis.
- QUS is a useful tool in the evaluation of bone properties.
- vQCT, HR-QCT, and HR-MR, on the basis of sophisticated software, are challenging techniques in the assessment of trabecular structure.

References

Adams JE (2009) Quantitative computed tomography. Eur J Radiol 71:415–424

Agostinelli D, de Terlizzi F (2007) QUS in monitoring raloxifene and estrogen-progestogens: a 4-year longitudinal study. Ultrasound Med Biol 33:1184–1190

Anonymous (2003) Prevention and management of osteoporosis. World Health Organ Tech Rep Ser 921:1–164

Banerjee S, Choudhury S, Han ET, Brau AC, Morze CV, Vigneron DB, Majumdar S (2006) Autocalibrating parallel imaging of in vivo trabecular bone microarchitecture at 3 Tesla. Magn Reson Med 56:1075–1084

Borg SA, Fitzer PM, Young LW (1975) Roentgenologic aspects of adult cretinism. Two case reports and review of the literature. Am J Roentgenol Radium Ther Nucl Med 123:820–828

Boutroy S, Bouxsein ML, Munoz F, Delmas PD (2005) In vivo assessment of trabecular bone microarchitecture by high-resolution peripheral quantitative computed tomography. J Clin Endocrinol Metab 90:6508–6515

Boutroy S, Van Rietbergen B, Sornay-Rendu E, Munoz F, Bouxsein ML, Delmas PD (2008) Finite element analysis based on in vivo HR-pQCT images of the distal radius is associated with wrist fracture in postmenopausal women. J Bone Miner Res 23:392–399

Caligiuri P, Giger ML, Favus M (1994) Multifractal radiographic analysis of osteoporosis. Med Phys 21:503–508

Camozzi V, De Terlizzi F, Zangari M, Luisetto G (2007) Quantitative bone ultrasound at phalanges and calcaneus in osteoporotic postmenopausal women: influence of age and measurement site. Ultrasound Med Biol 33:1039–1045

Cauley JA, Lui LY, Ensrud KE, Zmuda JM, Stone KL, Hochberg MC, Cummings SR (2005) Bone mineral density and the risk of incident nonspinal fractures in black and white women. JAMA 293:2102–2108

Center JR, Nguyen TV, Schneider D, Sambrook PN, Eisman JA (1999) Mortality after all major types of osteoporotic fracture in men and women: an observational study. Lancet 353:878–882

Chesnut CH 3rd, Majumdar S, Newitt DC, Shields A, Van Pelt J, Laschansky E, Azria M, Kriegman A, Olson M, Eriksen EF, Mindeholm L (2005) Effects of salmon calcitonin on trabecular microarchitecture as determined by magnetic resonance imaging: results from the QUEST study. J Bone Miner Res 20:1548–1561

Cockerill W, Lunt M, Silman AJ, Cooper C, Lips P, Bhalla AK, Cannata JB, Eastell R, Felsenberg D, Gennari C, Johnell O, Kanis JA, Kiss C, Masaryk P, Naves M, Poor G, Raspe H, Reid DM, Reeve J, Stepan J, Todd C, Woolf AD, O'Neill TW (2004) Health-related quality of life and radiographic vertebral fracture. Osteoporos Int 15:113–119

Cortet B, Boutry N, Dubois P, Bourel P, Cotten A, Marchandise X (2000) In vivo comparison between computed tomography and magnetic resonance image analysis of the distal radius in the assessment of osteoporosis. J Clin Densitom 3:15–26

Cosman F (2005) The prevention and treatment of osteoporosis: a review. MedGenMed 7:73

Cuddihy MT, Gabriel SE, Crowson CS, O'Fallon WM, Melton LJ 3rd (1999) Forearm fractures as predictors of subsequent osteoporotic fractures. Osteoporos Int 9:469–475

Cummings SR, Nevitt MC, Browner WS, Stone K, Fox KM, Ensrud KE, Cauley J, Black D, Vogt TM (1995) Risk factors for hip fracture in white women. Study of Osteoporotic Fractures Research Group. N Engl J Med 332:767–773

Cummings SR, Bates D, Black DM (2002) Clinical use of bone densitometry: scientific review. JAMA 288:1889–1897

Damilakis J, Maris TG, Karantanas AH (2006) An update on the assessment of osteoporosis using radiologic techniques. Eur Radiol 17:1591–1602

Deng HW, Li JL, Li J, Davies KM, Recker RR (1998) Heterogeneity of bone mineral density across skeletal sites and its clinical implications. J Clin Densitom 1:339–353

Endres HG, Dasch B, Maier C, Lungenhausen M, Smektala R, Trampisch HJ, Pientka L (2007) Diagnosis and treatment of osteoporosis in postmenopausal women with distal radius fracture in Germany. Curr Med Res Opin 23:2171–2181

Engelke K, Adams JE, Armbrecht G, Augat P, Bogado CE, Bouxsein ML, Felsenberg D, Ito M, Prevrhal S, Hans DB, Lewiecki EM (2008) Clinical use of quantitative computed tomography and peripheral quantitative computed tomography in the management of osteoporosis in adults: the 2007 ISCD Official Positions. J Clin Densitom 11:123–162

Genant HK, Engelke K, Fuerst T, Glüer CC, Grampp S, Harris ST, Jergas M, Lang T, Lu Y, Majumdar S, Mathur A, Takada M (1996) Noninvasive assessment of bone mineral and structure: state of the art. J Bone Miner Res 11:707–730

Genant HK, Engelke K, Prevrhal S (2008) Advanced CT bone imaging in osteoporosis. Rheumatology 47:iv9–iv16

Gluer CC, The International Quantitative Ultrasound Consensus Group (1997) Quantitative ultrasound techniques for the assessment of osteoporosis: expert agreement on current status. J Bone Miner Res 12:1280–1288

Gnudi S, Ripamonti C, Malavolta N (2000) Quantitative ultrasound and bone densitometry to evaluate the risk of nonspine fractures: a prospective study. Osteoporos Int 11:518–523

Gomberg BR, Wehrli FW, Vasilić B, Weening RH, Saha PK, Song HK, Wright AC (2004) Reproducibility and error sources of micro-MRI-based trabecular bone structural parameters of the distal radius and tibia. Bone 35:266–276

Gonnelli S, Martini G, Caffarelli C, Salvadori S, Cadirni A, Montagnani A, Nuti R (2006) Teriparatide's effects on quantitative ultrasound parameters and bone density in women with established osteoporosis. Osteoporos Int 17:1524–1531

Grampp S, Jergas M, Glüer CC, Lang P, Brastow P, Genant HK (1993) Radiologic diagnosis of osteoporosis. Current methods and perspectives. Radiol Clin North Am 31:1133–1145

Grampp S, Genant HK, Mathur A, Lang P, Jergas M, Takada M, Glüer CC, Lu Y, Chavez M (1997) Comparisons of noninvasive bone mineral measurements in assessing age-related loss, fracture discrimination, and diagnostic classification. J Bone Miner Res 12:697–711

Guglielmi G, de Terlizzi F (2009) Quantitative ultrasound in the assessment of osteoporosis. Eur J Radiol 71:425–431

Guglielmi G, Lang TF (2002) Quantitative computed tomography. Semin Musculoskelet Radiol 6:219–227

Guglielmi G, Genant HK, Pacifici R, Giannatempo GM, Cammisa M (1994) The imaging diagnosis of osteoporosis. The state of the art and outlook. Radiol Med 88:535–546

Guglielmi G, Schneider P, Lang TF, Giannatempo GM, Cammisa M, Genant HK (1997a) Quantitative computed tomography at the axial and peripheral skeleton. Eur Radiol 7:32–42

Guglielmi G, Cammisa M, De Serio A, Giannatempo GM, Bagni B, Orlandi G, Russo CR (1997b) Long-term in vitro precision of single slice peripheral Quantitative Computed Tomography (pQCT): multicenter comparison. Technol Health Care 5:375–381

Guglielmi G, Cammisa M, De Serio A, Scillitani A, Chiodini I, Carnevale V, Fusilli S (1999) Phalangeal US velocity discriminates between normal and vertebrally fractured subjects. Eur Radiol 9:1632–1637

Guglielmi G, De Serio A, Fusilli S, Scillitani A, Chiodini I, Torlontano M, Cammisa M (2000) Age-related changes assessed by peripheral QCT in healthy Italian women. Eur Radiol 10:609–614

Guglielmi G, Cammisa M, De Serio A (2001) Bone densitometry and osteoporosis at the hand and wrist. In: Gulglielmi G, Van Kuijk C, Genant HK (eds) Fundamentals of hand and wrist imaging. Springer-Verlag, Heidelberg, pp 233–235

Guglielmi G, Perta A, Cammisa M (2003a) Plain radiographs in the study of osteoporotic syndrome. Radiol Med 105:1–5
Guglielmi G, Perta A, Palladino D, Crisetti N, Mischitelli F, Cammisa M (2003b) Bone densitometry in the diagnosis and follow-up of osteoporosis. Radiol Med 106:29–35
Guglielmi G, Crisetti N, Mischitelli F, Cammisa M (2003c) Quantitative ultrasound. Radiol Med 105:27–33
Guglielmi G, Toffanin R, Cova M, Cammisa M (2003d) Quantitative magnetic resonance of trabecular bone. Radiol Med 105:34–40
Guglielmi G, Muscarella S, Leone A, Peh WC (2008) Imaging of metabolic bone diseases. Radiol Clin North Am 46: 735–754
Guglielmi G, Adams J, Link TM (2009) Quantitative ultrasound in the assessment of skeletal status. Eur Radiol 19:1837–1848
Guyatt GH, Cranney A, Griffith L, Walter S, Krolicki N, Favus M, Rosen C (2002) Summary of meta-analyses of therapies for postmenopausal osteoporosis and the relationship between bone density and fractures. Endocrinol Metab Clin North Am 31:659–679
Hartl F, Tyndall A, Kraenzlin M, Bachmeier C, Gückel C, Senn U, Hans D, Theiler R (2002) Discriminatory ability of quantitative ultrasound parameters and bone mineral density in a population-based sample of postmenopausal women with vertebral fractures: results of the Basel Osteoporosis Study. J Bone Miner Res 17:321–330
Ingle BM, Machado AB, Pereda CA, Eastell R (2005) Monitoring alendronate and estradiol therapy with quantitative ultrasound and bone mineral density. J Clin Densitom 8:278–286
Ito M, Tsurusaki K, Hayashi K (1997) Peripheral QCT for the diagnosis of osteoporosis. Osteoporos Int 7:S120–S127
Kanis JA, on behalf of the World Health Organization Scientific Group (2007) Assessment of osteoporosis at the primary health-care level. Technical Report. World Health Organization Collaborating Centre for Metabolic Bone Diseases, University of Sheffield, UK, 2008
Khosla S, Riggs BL, Atkinson EJ, Oberg AL, McDaniel LJ, Holets M, Peterson JM, Melton LJ 3rd (2006a) Effects of sex and age on bone microstructure at the ultradistal radius: a population-based noninvasive in vivo assessment. J Bone Miner Res 21:124–131
Khosla S, Melton LJ 3rd, Achenbach SJ, Oberg AL, Riggs BL (2006b) Hormonal and biochemical determinants of trabecular microstructure at the ultradistal radius in women and men. J Clin Endocrinol Metab 91:885–891
Kleinberg DL, Young IS, Kupperman HS (1966) The sesamoid index. An aid in the diagnosis of acromegaly. Ann Intern Med 64:1075–1078
Krieg MA, Cornuz J, Ruffieux C, Sandini L, Büche D, Dambacher MA, Hartl F, Häuselmann HJ, Kraenzlin M, Lippuner K, Neff M, Pancaldi P, Rizzoli R, Tanzi F, Theiler R, Tyndall A, Wimpfheimer K, Burckhardt P (2003) Comparison of three bone ultrasounds for the discrimination of subjects with and without osteoporotic fractures among 7562 elderly women. J Bone Miner Res 18:1261–1266
Lane JM, Serota AC, Raphael B (2006) Osteoporosis: differences and similarities in male and female patients. Orthop Clin North Am 37:601–609
Link TM, Rummeny EJ, Lenzen H, Reuter I, Roos N, Peters PE (1994) Artificial bone erosions: detection with magnification radiography versus conventional high resolution radiography. Radiology 192:861–864
Link TM, Majumdar S, Augat P, Lin JC, Newitt D, Lu Y, Lane NE, Genant HK (1998) In vivo high resolution MRI of the calcaneus: differences in trabecular structure in osteoporosis patients. J Bone Miner Res 13:1175–1182
Link TM, Majumdar S, Grampp S, Guglielmi G, van Kuijk C, Imhof H, Glueer C, Adams JE (1999) Imaging of trabecular bone structure in osteoporosis. Eur Radiol 9: 1781–1788
Majumdar S, Genant HK, Grampp S, Newitt DC, Truong VH, Lin JC, Mathur A (1997) Correlation of trabecular bone structure with age, bone mineral density, and osteoporotic status: in vivo studies in the distal radius using high resolution magnetic resonance imaging. J Bone Miner Res 12:111–118
Majumdar S, Link TM, Augat P, Lin JC, Newitt D, Lane NE, Genant HK (1999) Trabecular bone architecture in the distal radius using magnetic resonance imaging in subjects with fractures of the proximal femur. Magnetic Resonance Science Center and Osteoporosis and Arthritis Research Group. Osteoporos Int 10:231–239
Meema HE, Meema S (1972) Comparison of microradioscopic and morphometric findings in the hand bones with densitometric findings in the proximal radius in thyrotoxicosis and in renal osteodystrophy. Invest Radiol 7:88–96
Mosekilde L, Eriksen EF, Charles P (1990) Effects of thyroid hormones on bone and mineral metabolism. Endocrinol Metab Clin North Am 19:35–63
National Osteoporosis Society (2002) The use of quantitative ultrasound in the management of osteoporosis. Position statement of 31 January 2002
Newitt DC, van Rietbergen B, Majumdar S (2002) Processing and analysis of in vivo high-resolution MR images of trabecular bone for longitudinal studies: reproducibility of structural measures and micro-finite element analysis derived mechanical properties. Osteoporos Int 13:278–287
Pacheco EM, Harrison EJ, Ward KA, Lunt M, Adams JE (2002) Detection of osteoporosis by dual X-ray absorptiometry (DXA) of the calcaneus: is the WHO criterion applicable? Calcif Tissue Int 70:475–482
Park EA (1932) The Blackader Lecture on some aspects of rickets. Can Med Assoc J 26:3–15
Parker BR (1981) Hypothyroidism with epiphysial dysgenesis. AJR Am J Roentgenol 136:1030
Picard D, Brown JP, Rosenthall L, Couturier M, Lévesque J, Dumont M, Ste-Marie LG, Tenenhouse A, Dodin S (2004) Ability of peripheral DXA measurement to diagnose osteoporosis as assessed by central DXA measurement. J Clin Densitom 7:111–118
Resnick D (1995a) Acromegaly and gigantism. In: Resnick D (ed) Diagnosis of bone and joint disorders. Saunders, Philadelphia, pp 1971–1992
Resnick D (1995b) Hypopituitarism. In: Resnick D (ed) Diagnosis of bone and joint disorders. Saunders, Philadelphia, pp 1992–1993
Resnick D (1995c) Hyperthyroidism. In: Resnick D (ed) Diagnosis of bone and joint disorders. Saunders, Philadelphia, pp 1995–1999

Resnick D (1995d) Hyperparathyroidism. In: Resnick D (ed) Diagnosis of bone and joint disorder. Saunders, Philadelphia, pp 2012–2036

Resnick D (1995e) Rickets and osteomalacia. In: Resnick D (ed) Diagnosis of bone and joint disorder. Saunders, Philadelphia, pp 1885–1922

Resnick D (1995f) Hypoparathyroidism. In: Resnick D (ed) Diagnosis of bone and joint disorder. Saunders, Philadelphia, pp 2061–2064

Ross PD (1998) Epidemiology of osteoporosis. In: Genant HK G, Jergas M (eds) Bone densitometry and osteoporosis. Springer, Heidelberg, pp 21–42

Rüegsegger P, Elsasser U, Anliker M, Gnehm H, Kind H, Prader A (1976) Quantification of bone mineralization using computed tomography. Radiology 121:93–97

Sartoris D (1971) Acromegaly. In: Sartoris D (ed) Musculoskeletal imaging. Mosby-Year Book, St. Louis, pp 302–303

Sartoris D (1996) Hypothyroidism. In: Sartoris D (ed) Muskuloskeletal imaging. Mosby-Year Book, St. Louis, pp 301–302

Schattauer GmbH (2006) Evidence-Based DVO Guidelines Osteoporosis in Germany; prophylaxis, diagnosis and therapy in postmenopausal women and men over 60 years. Verlag fur medizin und naturwissenschaften, 70174 Stuttgart

Schneider P, Börner W (1991) Peripheral quantitative computed tomography for bone mineral measurement using a new special QCT-scanner. Methodology, normal values, comparison with manifest osteoporosis. Rofo 154:292–299

Schneider P, Reiners C (1998) Peripheral quantitative computed tomography. In: Genant HK, Guglielmi G, Jergas M (eds) Bone densitometry and osteoporosis. Springer, Heidelberg, pp 349–363

Schott AM, Weill-Engerer S, Hans D, Duboeuf F, Delmas PD, Meunier PJ (1995) Ultrasound discriminates patients with hip fracture equally well as dual energy X-ray absorptiometry and independently of bone mineral density. J Bone Miner Res 10:243–249

Seeman E, Delmas PD (2006) Bone quality–the material and structural basis of bone strength and fragility. N Engl J Med 354:2250–2261

Seeman E, Melton LJ 3rd, O'Fallon WM, Riggs BL (1983) Risk factors for spinal osteoporosis in men. Am J Med 75:977–983

Sell CA, Masi JN, Burghardt A, Newitt D, Link TM, Majumdar S (2005) Quantification of trabecular bone structure using magnetic resonance imaging at 3 Tesla–calibration studies using microcomputed tomography as a standard of reference. Calcif Tissue Int 76:355–364

Sornay-Rendu E, Boutry S, Munoz F, Bouxsein ML (2009) Cortical and trabecular architecture are altered in postmenopausal women with fracture. Osteoporos Int 20:1291–1297

Spadaro JA, Werner FW, Brenner RA, Fortino MD, Fay LA, Edwards WT (1994) Cortical and trabecular bone contribute strength to the osteopenic distal radius. J Orthop Res 12:211–218

Stampa B, Kühn B, Liess C, Heller M, Glüer CC (2002) Characterization of the integrity of three-dimensional trabecular bone microstructure by connectivity and shape analysis using high-resolution magnetic resonance imaging in vivo. Top Magn Reson Imaging 13:357–363

Steinbach Hl, Noetzli M (1964) Roentgen appearance of the skeleton in osteomalacia and rickets. Am J Roentgenol Radium Ther Nucl Med 91:955–972

Steinbach H, Gold R, Preger L (1975) Congenital hypothyroidism (cretinoid epiphyseal dysplasia). In: Steinbach H, Gold R, Preger L (eds) Roentgen appearance of the hand in diffuse disease. Year Book Medical Publishers, Chicago, pp 239–241

Sundaram M, Joyce PF, Shields JB, Riaz MA, Sagar S (1979) Terminal phalangeal tufts: earliest site of renal osteodystrophy findings in hemodialysis patients. Am J Roentgenol 133:25–29

Techawiboonwong A, Song HK, Magland JF, Saha PK, Wehrli FW (2005) Implications of pulse sequence in structural imaging of trabecular bone. J Magn Reson Imaging 22:647–655

Theodorou DJ, Theodorou SJ, Resnick D (2001) The hand in endocrine disorders. In: Guglielmi G, Van Kuijk C, Genant HK (eds) Fundamentals of hand and wrist imaging. Springer-Verlag, Heidelberg, p 203

Virtama P (1960) Uneven distribution of bone minerals and covering effect of non-mineralized tissue as reasons for impaired detectability of bone density from roentgenograms. Ann Med Intern Fenn 49:57–65

Vokes TJ, Giger ML, Chinander MR, Karrison TG, Favus MJ, Dixon LB (2006) Radiographic texture analysis of densitometer-generated calcaneus images differentiates postmenopausal women with and without fractures. Osteoporos Int 17:1472–1482

Wehrli FW (2007) Structural and functional assessment of trabecular and cortical bone by micro magnetic resonance imaging. J Magn Reson Imaging 25:390–409

Wehrli FW, Hwang SN, Ma J, Song HK, Ford JC, Haddad JG (1998) Cancellous bone volume and structure in the forearm: noninvasive assessment with MR microimaging and image processing. Radiology 206:347–357

Wehrli F, Gomberg B, Saha P, Song H, Hwang S, Snyder P (2001) Digital topological analysis of in vivo magnetic resonance microimages of trabecular bone reveals structural implications of osteoporosis. J Bone Miner Res 16:1520–1531

Wehrli FW, Saha PK, Gomberg BR, Song HK, Snyder PJ, Benito M, Wright A, Weening R (2002) Role of magnetic resonance for assessing structure and function of trabecular bone. Top Magn Reson Imaging 13:335–355

Wüster C, Albanese C, De Aloysio D, Duboeuf F, Gambacciani M, Gonnelli S, Glüer CC, Hans D, Joly J, Reginster JY, De Terlizzi F, Cadossi R (2000) Phalangeal osteosonogrammetry study: age-related changes, diagnostic sensitivity, and discrimination power. The Phalangeal Osteosonogrammetry Study Group. J Bone Miner Res 15: 1603–1614

Arthritis

Andrew J. Grainger

Contents

A. J. Grainger (✉)
Department of Musculoskeletal Radiology,
Chapel Allerton Orthopaedic Centre,
Leeds, LS7 4SA, UK
e-mail: andrew.grainger@leedsth.nhs.uk

Abstract

Joint involvement in the hand and wrist is a feature of many forms of arthritis and because multiple joints are included, a view of both hands and wrists can provide important diagnostic information based on the pattern of disease involvement, even before the actual appearances of the changes are considered. Although for the most part this chapter focuses on plain film appearances, advanced imaging modalities, particularly ultrasound (US) and MRI, are increasingly finding applications in the mainstream clinical imaging of hand arthritis and are discussed in the appropriate sections.

1 Introduction

Joint involvement in the hand and wrist is a feature of many forms of arthritis and because multiple joints are included, a view of both hands and wrists can provide important diagnostic information based on the pattern of disease involvement, even before the actual appearances of the changes are considered. Although for the most part this chapter focuses on plain film appearances, advanced imaging modalities, particularly ultrasound (US) and MRI, are increasingly finding applications in the mainstream clinical imaging of hand arthritis and are discussed in the appropriate sections.

2 The Inflammatory Arthritides

The inflammatory arthritides include rheumatoid arthritis (RA), the seronegative arthritides and juvenile inflammatory arthritis (JIA). While it is recognised that

A. M. Davis et al. (eds.), *Imaging of the Hand and Wrist*, Medical Radiology. Diagnostic Imaging,
DOI: 10.1007/174_2010_65,

osteoarthritis (OA) has an inflammatory variant, the features of this condition will be discussed separately.

The management of inflammatory arthritis has changed dramatically in recent years with the advent of powerful biological therapies which, if instigated early, can prevent the severe joint destruction that used to be commonly seen. The use of such drugs means that imaging plays an increasingly important role in the management of these diseases. While CR shows characteristic features of inflammatory arthritis, these represent late findings in the disease process and the use of advanced imaging techniques is becoming more common as they allow early diagnosis before irreversible joint damage has occurred. Nevertheless CR continues to play an important role in the diagnosis and characterisation of hand and wrist arthritis and usually forms the initial imaging study.

2.1 Plain Film General Principles

The subtle changes seen in early inflammatory arthritis require high quality radiographs reviewed in optimal lighting conditions. The use of digital radiographic techniques is now prevalent and has been shown to provide similar accuracy to film-screen techniques in the diagnosis of arthritis (van der Jagt et al. 2000; Jonsson et al. 1994). Additional advantages over conventional films exist for the reader such as on-screen magnification and windowing (Paskins and Rai 2006).

A systematic approach to the review of the hand and wrist radiograph for arthritis is required. Important features to identify are:

- soft tissue swelling
- joint space loss
- bone changes
  - erosion
  - osteopaenia
  - enthesitis
- bone alignment.

Finally the distribution of joint disease provides important information when forming a differential diagnosis.

2.1.1 Soft Tissue Swelling

Soft tissue swelling is usually the earliest sign on CR of an inflammatory arthritis. It represents synovial hypertrophy, oedema in the adjacent soft tissues and joint effusion. When seen at the interphalangeal joints the swelling has a symmetrical spindle shape about the joint. This pattern of soft tissue swelling contrasts with that seen in gout which tends to show a more irregular asymmetrical 'lumpy' appearance. At the metacarpophalangeal (MCP) and wrist joints the soft tissue contour may not be significantly displaced and it is often the appreciation of an increased density to the periarticular soft tissues and effacement of the fat planes that suggests the presence of joint disease. At the MCP joints soft tissue swelling can be extremely subtle and it is useful to look for loss of the fat planes normally seen between the joints (Fig. 1). In the wrist the normal fat planes adjacent to the scaphoid and ulnar styloid are sensitive sites for the detection of soft tissue swelling.

2.1.2 Alteration in Joint Space

Loss of joint space as a result of cartilage destruction is a characteristic feature of many joint diseases. In inflammatory arthritis joint space loss is typically uniform, across the joint. In many joints this is helpful in distinguishing inflammatory from OA, which typically shows non-uniform joint space loss. However, it is less useful in the hands where the interphalangeal and MCP joints in both forms of arthritis can show uniform joint space loss.

As with soft tissue swelling joint space loss is an early plain film feature of inflammatory arthritis, but while soft tissue swelling can be subtle, the recognition of joint space loss is generally more straightforward (Fig. 1). It is important to recognise that once joint space loss is identified irreversible damage has occurred to the joint. So while it is an early plain film feature, it still represents a relatively late stage in the whole disease process.

Detection of joint space loss in the hands and wrists is usually straightforward because joint space can be easily compared to other similar joints on the radiograph. It is important to recognise that the joints between the carpal bones normally all show similar spaces. The observation of preserved joint space, in a joint which otherwise shows evidence of significant arthropathic change, is an important one and may help with the differential diagnosis. In particular gout characteristically preserves joint space until late in the disease.

In severe arthritic change bony ankylosis may occur. This is most commonly seen in the seronegative arthritides and in juvenile arthritis and represents end stage disease. Ankylosis may be bony or fibrous.

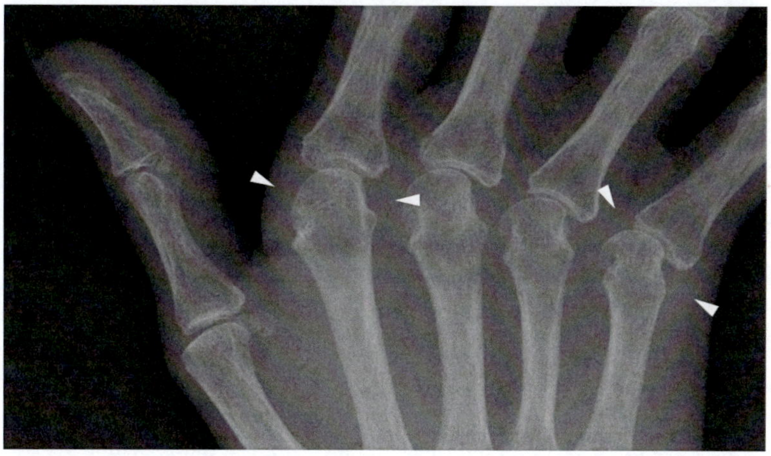

Fig. 1 Rheumatoid arthritis: there is joint space loss demonstrated at the middle, ring and little MCP joints. This is made more apparent by the relative preservation of joint space at the thumb and index MCP joints. There is also soft tissue swelling which is best appreciated at the index and little MCP joints (*arrowheads*). The joint space swelling at the MCP joints can also be appreciated by the loss of the normal fat plane between the joints. There is also malalignment of the MCP joints with ulnar deviation

Occasionally widening of the joint space may be seen in arthritis. This is rare and is usually the result of a tense effusion distending the joint and separating the bones.

2.1.3 Bone Changes

Osteopaenia

Periarticular osteopaenia is a well-recognised feature of some inflammatory arthritides but is perhaps the most difficult to reliably identify. It may be more obvious in cases of mono or pauciarticular joint involvement, where other joints are clearly normal for comparison, but can be more difficult to appreciate when there is polyarticular disease as is often the case in the inflammatory arthritides. Appearances can also be difficult to interpret if there is an element of generalised disuse osteoporosis. Often it is easier to identify that there is no evidence of osteopaenia, and this in itself is a useful observation when forming a differential diagnosis.

Erosion

Bone erosion is a hallmark of inflammatory arthritis and a sign of significant joint damage. Erosions can be subdivided into proliferative and non-proliferative erosions. Proliferative erosions are associated with new bone formation and are classically a feature of entheseal disease as discussed below. Non-proliferative erosions are a feature of seropositive (rheumatoid) arthritis. The distinction between these two types of erosion is an important one in the differentiation of seropositive and seronegative arthritis.

Erosions can be described by their relationship to the joint and can be categorised as central, marginal or juxta-articular. Marginal erosions occur at the edge of the joint line and involve the exposed bone between the edge of the articular cartilage and the joint capsule. They are a classical feature of RA. Central erosions occur, as their name suggests, into bone normally covered by the articular cartilage. They are less common and are classically seen in inflammatory (erosive) OA. Juxta-articular erosions occur further away from the joint and are typically seen in gout. They have characteristic features that are discussed later (see Sect. 3.1.1).

Erosions are seen as a discontinuity in the cortex of a bone. However, this is only the case when the eroded cortex is seen in profile on the radiograph. While this is frequently the case in the finger joints, wrist erosions are often seen en-face if they lie on the palmar or dorsal aspect of the carpal bones. En-face erosions are seen as focal lucencies within the bone without associated cortical breach and may be indistinguishable from cysts. The improved detection of these erosions, particularly when small, is one of the reasons cross-sectional imaging techniques such as US and MRI have a much greater sensitivity to erosive change than CR.

Entheseal Disease

Enthesitis is a characteristic feature of the seronegative arthritides. Entheses represent the bony attachment sites of ligaments, tendons and capsule. On plain film imaging the important bone changes that can be visualised in enthesitis are enthesophyte formation and erosion. Enthesophytes, which develop at, or immediately adjacent to the site of an enthesis are seen as bone proliferation. They may have a coarse appearance, with both cortical and medullary bone being apparent, or may have a finer 'whisker' like appearance.

MRI demonstrates intra-osseous bone changes, in enthesitis in the form of high T2 (oedema like) signal in the bone adjacent to the enthesis. MRI and US also show changes in the soft tissues about the enthesis including bursitis and alteration in the appearance of the ligament or tendon inserting at the affected enthesis. These will only be detected on plain films if there are adjacent fat planes that become effaced by a thickened tendon, or enlarged bursa.

2.1.4 Bone Alignment

Joint malalignment is a feature of many arthropathic processes and results from a variety of causes (Fig. 1). These include ligament degeneration or disruption, tendon rupture or subluxation, cartilage loss and bone attrition or erosion. In most cases the malalignment will be apparent clinically and may even be less apparent on the radiograph in the case of reversible subluxations, such as are seen with SLE, as the act of positioning the patient for the radiograph reduces the subluxation.

2.2 Rheumatoid Arthritis

The aetiology of RA remains unknown, but it is recognised that it is a chronic autoimmune disorder with the potential to affect multiple systems and has an incidence of approximately 1%. Women are more frequently affected than men and the joint disease is characterised by a polyarticular synovitis. The synovitis is initiated by cytokines including interleukin-1 and tumour necrosis factor (TNF) and occurs early in the disease process (Arend 2001). The later stages of the disease involve joint destruction as a result of bone erosion and cartilage loss. Synovitis is considered to be a strong predictor of bone erosion (McGonagle et al. 1999; McQueen et al. 1999). The majority of patients have polyarticular involvement at presentation although occasionally patients may present with single joint involvement. The hands and wrists are commonly affected and radiographs of the hand and wrist provide a valuable tool in being able to assess multiple joints in a single examination. In addition to joint involvement, synovitis may involve the tendon sheaths and rheumatoid nodules may occasionally be seen in the hands.

The clinical, and consequently radiological, picture of RA has changed over recent years due to dramatic advances in the way RA is treated clinically. Management now involves the use of powerful biologic agents, which can arrest joint damage early in the disease process preventing the development of the severely mutilated joints that were seen previously on CR (Villeneuve and Emery 2009). However, the effective use of these new treatments requires the early diagnosis of the disease, before plain film changes are evident. Increasingly US and MRI are finding roles in routine clinical practice for this purpose. Despite this plain films of the hands and wrists remain widely used in the diagnosis and management of the disease; and the need to detect early and subtle changes of RA is greater than ever. The hallmarks of RA on plain film imaging are soft tissue swelling, periarticular osteopaenia, joint space loss, erosion and malalignment. The classical plain film appearance of RA in the hands and wrists is of a symmetrical polyarthritis with a proximal distribution typically involving the wrists, MCP and proximal interphalangeal (PIP) joints. Characteristically the distal interphalangeal (DIP) joints are spared providing an important distinguishing feature from OA and psoriatic arthritis.

2.2.1 Soft Tissue Changes and Bone Density

The earliest plain film changes are soft tissue swelling and periarticular osteopaenia. At the MCP and PIP joints the soft tissue swelling is appreciated as spindle shaped thickening of the soft tissues developing symmetrically about the joint (Fig. 1). In the wrists, early changes of soft tissue swelling are best appreciated along the ulnar border of the joint and medial to the ulnar styloid and can be detected early by the loss of the normal fat planes (Fig. 2). As discussed above periarticular osteopaenia can be a difficult sign to evaluate, particularly with the polyarticular involvement seen in RA.

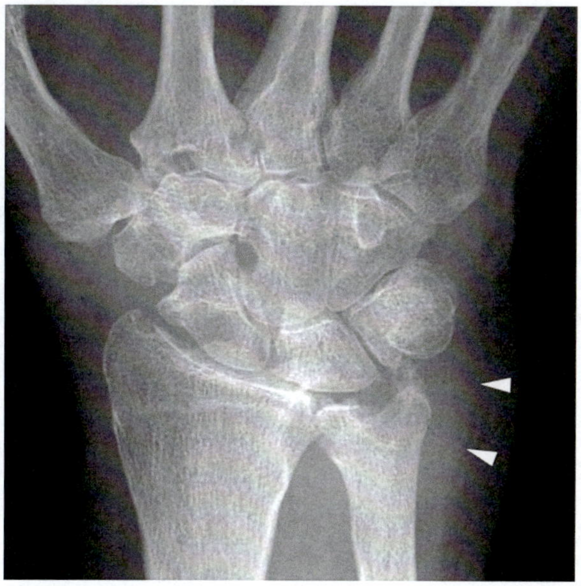

Fig. 2 Rheumatoid arthritis: there is soft tissue swelling about the distal ulnar seen as deviation of the fat planes (*arrowheads*). Note also the erosive change seen for example in the ulnar styloid, radial styloid and 2nd metacarpal base

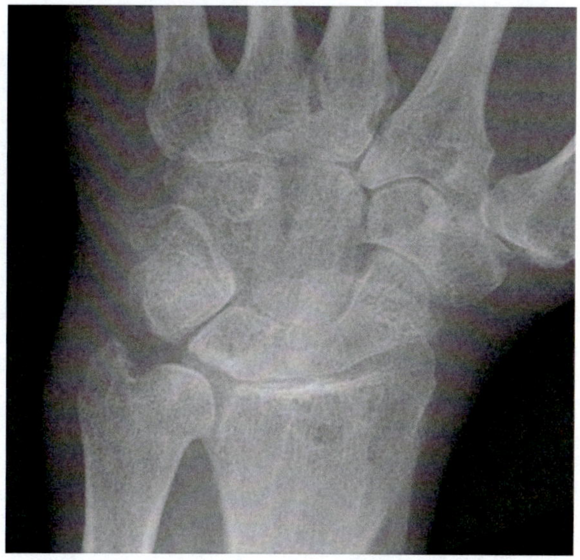

Fig. 3 Rheumatoid arthritis: there is joint space narrowing between the carpal bones and at the radiocarpal joint. The lucency in the distal radius represents an erosion seen en-face despite cystic appearance. There is also erosion of the ulnar styloid with soft tissue swelling. Note the radial deviation of the wrist typical of the malalignment pattern seen with rheumatoid arthritis

2.2.2 Joint Space Loss

As the disease progresses symmetrical joint space loss at involved joints becomes apparent (Fig. 1). In the wrist, the radiocarpal joint is usually the site where this is appreciated first, but with time the whole wrist becomes involved (Fig. 3). This is in contrast to OA with its classical isolated involvement of the thumb base in a trapeziocentric distribution.

2.2.3 Erosion

The earliest 'pre-erosive' changes of RA are typically seen on the radial aspect of the index and middle metacarpal heads (Fig. 4). Initially, cortical thinning develops, which then progresses to a 'skip' pattern or a 'dot-dash' type of deossification associated with localised osteopaenia. Subsequently, frank bone erosion is seen. Erosions in the finger joints are usually marginal in location, being seen in the first instance at sites within the joint that are unprotected by overlying articular cartilage (Fig. 5). In the wrist the earliest sites for erosion are typically along the ulnar aspect of the joint, on the ulnar styloid, trapezium and hamate (Figs. 3, 6). While erosion occurs at this site as a result of synovial proliferation on the ulnar aspect of the wrist joint, an important factor is also tenosynovitis of the extensor carpi ulnaris, an early site of soft tissue disease.

Cystic forms of RA have been described where cystic change develops, generally in the carpal bones, without radiographic or MRI evidence of erosion (Gubler et al. 1990). A form of the disease featuring large cystic areas, typically occurring in active men has been termed 'rheumatoid arthritis of the robust reaction type' (Fig. 7) (De Haas et al. 1974). Using CR it is not possible to reliably distinguish between cysts and en-face erosions, which also commonly occur in the carpal bones.

It is important to appreciate that erosive change is a dynamic process and involves healing as well as bone destruction. This can be appreciated on serial films where healing of erosions may be seen (Fig. 8). It also means that the morphology of erosions changes with the disease progress. In the later chronic stages of the disease, erosions become more clearly delineated with the development of sclerotic borders at the interface between the sites of bone destruction and healing (Fig. 9).

2.2.4 Malalignment and Ankylosis

Tendon and ligamentous dysfunction along with bone erosion results in deformity and malalignment in the later stages of the disease. 'Boutonniere' deformity describes a

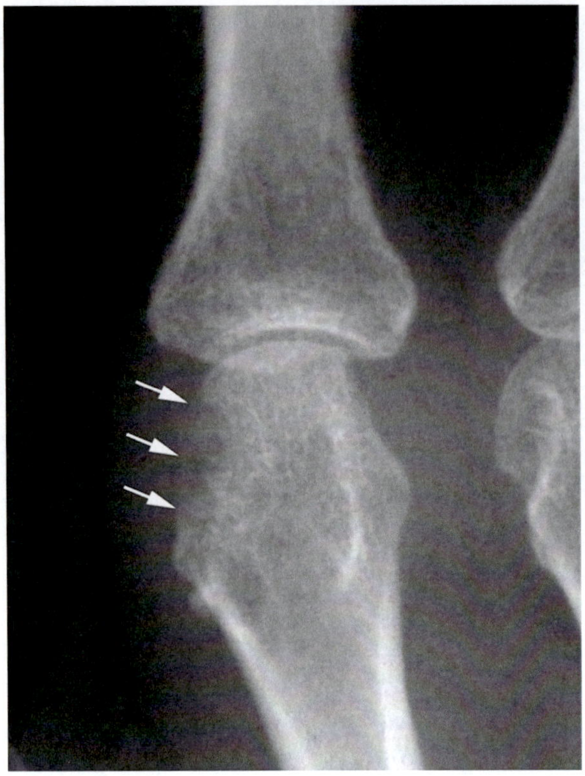

Fig. 4 Rheumatoid arthritis: early erosive change is seen along the radial border of this index metacarpal head. There is localised osteopaenia with a 'dot-dash' pattern of deossification (*arrows*). Note also the soft tissue swelling

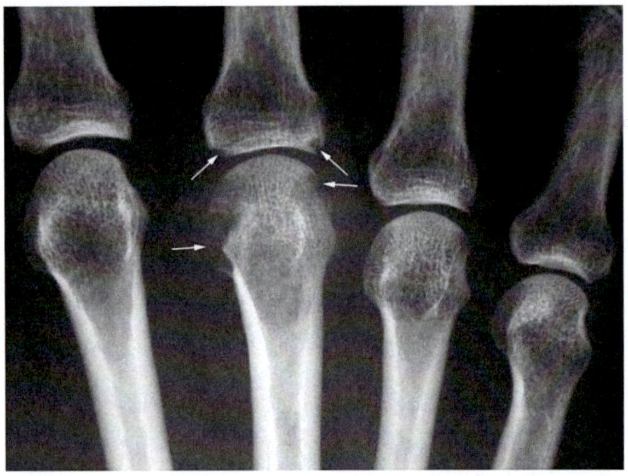

Fig. 5 Rheumatoid arthritis: marginal erosions are seen at the middle MCP joint (*arrows*). Note also the joint space loss compared with the adjacent MCP joints

pattern of malalignment produced by flexion of the PIP joint and extension of the DIP joint. This results from detachment of the extensor tendon from the middle phalanx, volar displacement and its subsequent action as a flexor. An opposite deformity referred to as the 'swan neck' deformity is seen as hyperextension of the PIP joint and flexion of the DIP joint. The cause is thought to be flexor tenosynovitis and/or synovitis in the PIP joint with resultant dysfunction of the stabilising effect of the volar plate. Mallet finger is a less common deformity resulting from disruption or dysfunction of the extensor tendon's action on the terminal phalanx. Ulnar deviation of the fingers and the radial deviation of the wrist giving a 'zigzag' deformity to the hand is typical for RA (Resnick 1976) (Figs. 1, 3, 10). This subluxation of the MCP and carpometacarpal joints seen in RA is irreversible.

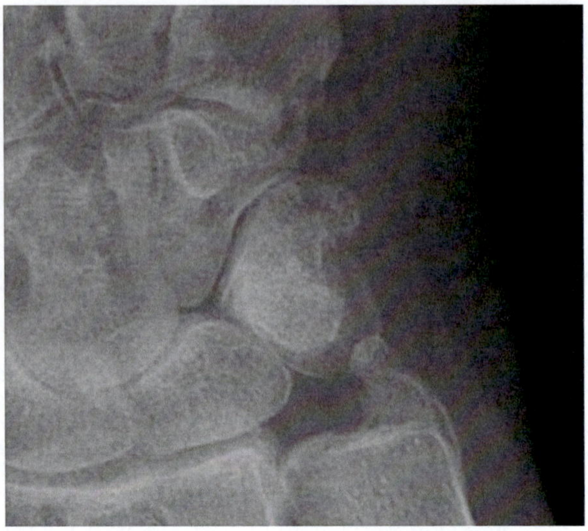

Fig. 6 Rheumatoid arthritis: erosive change is shown in the bones along the ulnar aspect of the wrist. In addition to erosions seen in the ulnar styloid, erosion is also seen in the triquetrum, hamate and base of 5th metacarpal. These represent early sites for the detection of erosions

In advanced disease, arthritis mutilans may develop where bony destruction leads to severe displacement with 'telescoping' of the phalanges. Ankylosis may also occur in the later stages of the disease. Typically this involves the wrist with intercarpal and carpometacarpal fusions but less commonly fusion may be seen at MCP and PIP joints, between the bases of the metacarpals or between the radius and ulna.

2.2.5 Secondary OA

As a result of the dysfunction of the joints, it is not uncommon for mechanical OA to develop in the later stages of the disease. Consequently a combination of

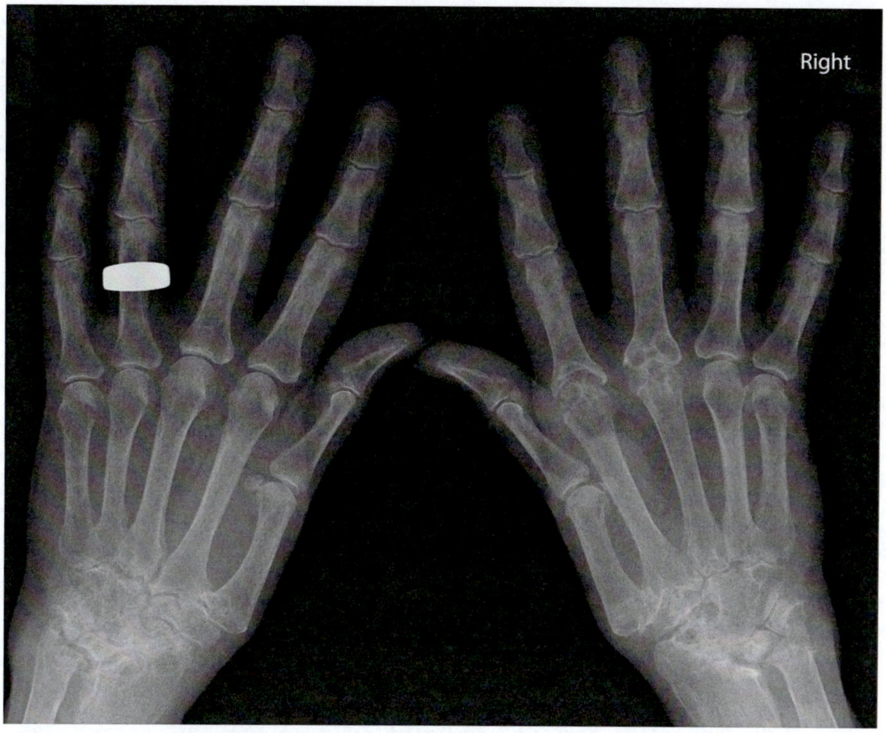

Fig. 7 'Robust' pattern of rheumatoid arthritis: this male patient shows severe bilateral wrist arthropathy with involvement also seen at the index and middle MCP joints on the right. Note the cystic changes seen in the wrist and MCP joints typical of the pattern of disease, which has been termed rheumatoid arthritis of robust reaction type

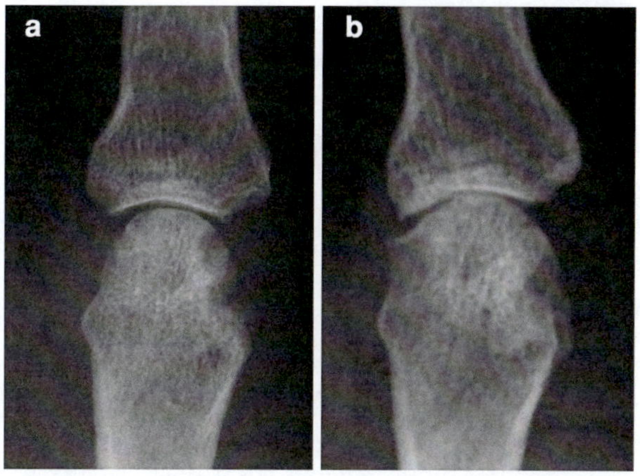

Fig. 8 Rheumatoid arthritis: **a** there are erosions seen at the MCP joint in both the metacarpal head and proximal phalangeal base. Two years later **b** there is evidence of healing of the erosions on both proximal and distal side of the joint. Despite this there is progressive joint space loss

both rheumatoid and OA may be seen in the hands and wrists, with typical subchondral sclerosis and marginal osteophyte formation being present alongside the RA changes described. However, the OA change does not usually overshadow the features of RA.

2.2.6 Other Soft Tissue Changes

The changes of RA are not confined to the joints and other synovial tissues may be affected. In the hand and wrist this is usually the flexor and extensor tendon sheaths, and the changes here contribute to the disability and deformities seen with the condition. Subcutaneous nodules are another common feature of the disease, seen in around 20% of patients. Nodules may also be seen within tendons and along with the tenosynovitis may be a cause of triggering. While soft tissue findings may be manifest as thickening or swelling on CR, they are better evaluated using US or MRI and will be discussed in Sect. 2.5 (el-Noueam et al. 1997; Fornage 1989; Gibbon and Wakefield 1999).

2.3 Seronegative Arthritis

The seronegative arthropathies comprise a group of multisystem inflammatory arthritides sharing common features. Chief among these is the characteristic involvement of the entheses with inflammation classically seen at the bony insertions of tendons and ligaments. Other important features are:

(a) an absence of rheumatoid factors,

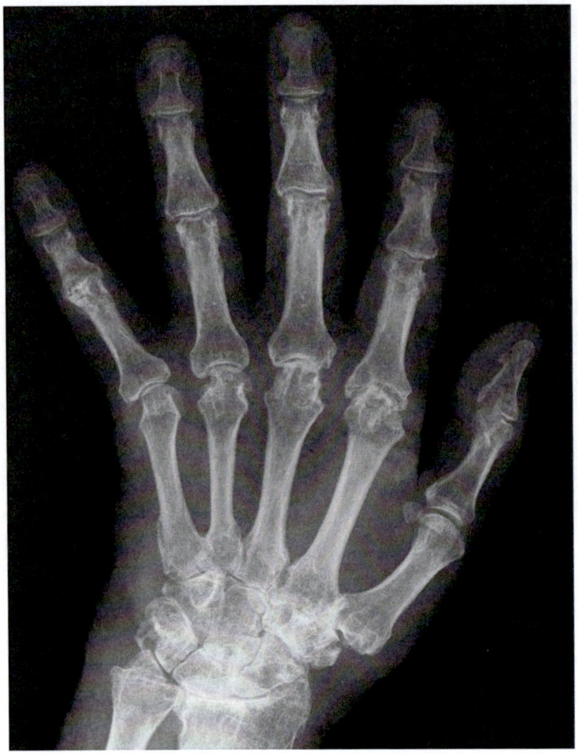

Fig. 9 Rheumatoid arthritis: this patient has long-standing RA with erosive involvement of multiple joints. Note the sclerotic margins of many of the erosions which is typical in the chronic stages of the disease

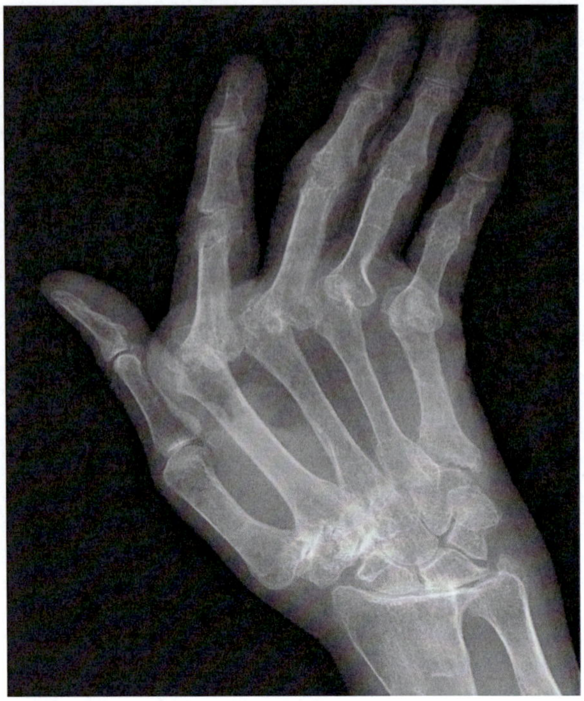

Fig. 10 Rheumatoid arthritis: the patient has severe polyarthritis and shows typical malalignment with radial deviation at the wrist and ulnar deviation at the MCP joints

(b) a strong association with the HLA-B27 histocompatibility antigen (although it is important to realise this is not necessary for the development of these diseases, or required for the diagnosis),
(c) a tendency for axial skeletal involvement.

The CR hallmark of these conditions as they affect the hand and wrist is the presence of proliferative erosive change representing erosive entheseal disease.

2.3.1 Psoriatic Arthritis

Hand involvement in the seronegative arthritides occurs most frequently and characteristically in psoriatic arthritis. The condition occurs in association with cutaneous psoriasis and there has often been a long history of skin psoriasis prior to development of the arthritis. However, in some cases (reports suggest up to 20%) the arthropathic changes may occur prior to the onset of the cutaneous disease (Scarpa et al. 1984). There is considerable variation in the reported incidence of psoriatic arthritis in patients with cutaneous psoriasis. One study has suggested psoriatic arthritis is seen in around 7% of patients with cutaneous psoriasis (Leczinsky 1948), while a more recent British study has suggested the figure may be as high as 40% (Green et al. 1981). Sacroiliac involvement is seen in 20–40% of patients and peripheral joint involvement is reported in around 15% of patients with psoriasis (Green et al. 1981; El-Khoury et al. 1996).

Five clinical subgroups of psoriatic arthritis are recognised:

1. Involvement of the DIP joints, usually asymmetrically often associated with dactylitis.
2. Arthritis mutilans.
3. A pattern of arthritis indistinguishable from RA but usually with a more benign course.
4. Oligo- (or mono-) arthritis distributed asymmetrically and involving any synovial joint.
5. A pattern of disease the same as ankylosing spondylitis (which may be associated with any of the above groups).

It is important to realise that patients with cutaneous psoriasis are susceptible to other arthropathies including RA and OA.

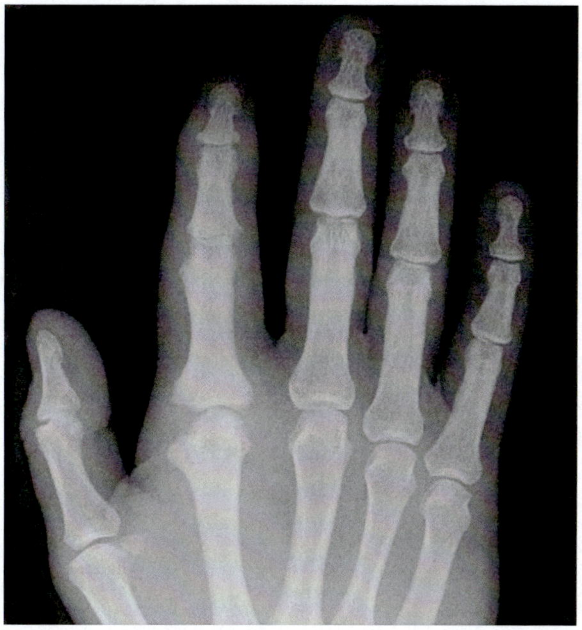

Fig. 11 Dactylitis in psoriatic arthritis: there is diffuse soft tissue swelling of the index finger with associated arthropathic change

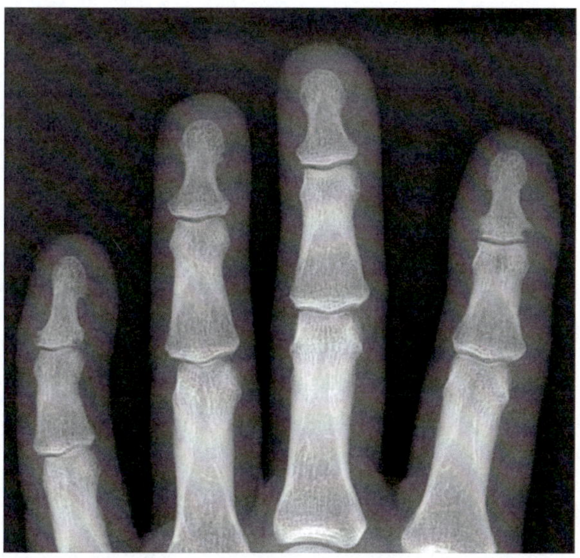

Fig. 12 Early psoriatic arthritis: marginal erosive changes are seen at the bases of the index and little distal phalanges, but note also the early enthesophyte formation adjacent to the erosions

In common with the other seronegative arthropathies the disease classically involves enthesis sites. It is suggested that inflammation in the multiple closely related entheseal sites in a digit is the cause of dactylitis seen in psoriatic arthritis (Benjamin and McGonagle 2001). The presence of nail dystrophy among psoriasis sufferers is a significant risk factor for the development of psoriatic arthritis and evidence suggests this may be because of the intimate relationship between the nail bed and the enthesis sites of the DIP joint (Wilson et al. 2009; McGonagle et al. 2009).

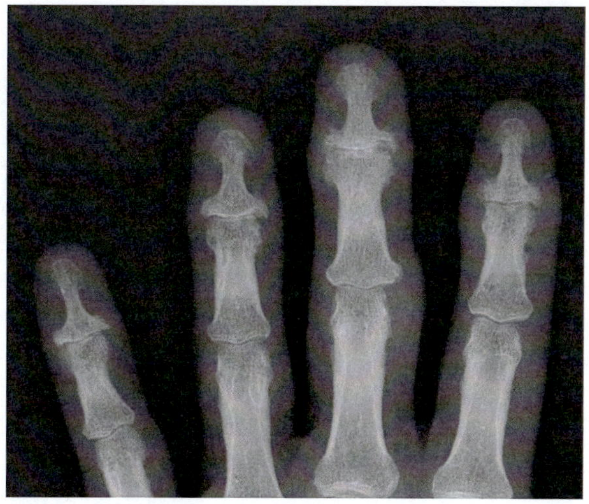

Fig. 13 Psoriatic arthritis: there is prominent fluffy enthesophyte formation seen both proximal and distal to the distal interphalangeal joints

The most significant pattern of joint disease seen in the hands is an erosive arthritis, which has a predominantly distal distribution with predilection for the DIP joints. The distal distribution helps distinguish it from RA, with its typically more proximal joint involvement. Joint involvement in RA tends to be symmetrical (similar joints involved in the two hands) while psoriatic arthritis tends to show a more asymmetrical distribution.

Soft Tissue Changes and Bone Density

Soft tissue joint swelling is seen as an early but non-specific radiographic feature of psoriatic arthritis. When seen global swelling of the digit in the form of dactylitis 'sausage digit', is virtually pathognomonic of the disease (Fig. 11). Periarticular osteopaenia is not a feature of psoriatic arthritis and can be useful in distinguishing it from RA.

Erosion, Bone Proliferation and Resorption

Bone erosion is seen most commonly at the joint margin and shows an entheseal pattern as discussed in "Entheseal Disease", with fluffy new bone formation at and adjacent to the erosion site (Figs. 12, 13). As the erosions develop they lose their initial marginal location and tend to coalesce. Classically, erosions on

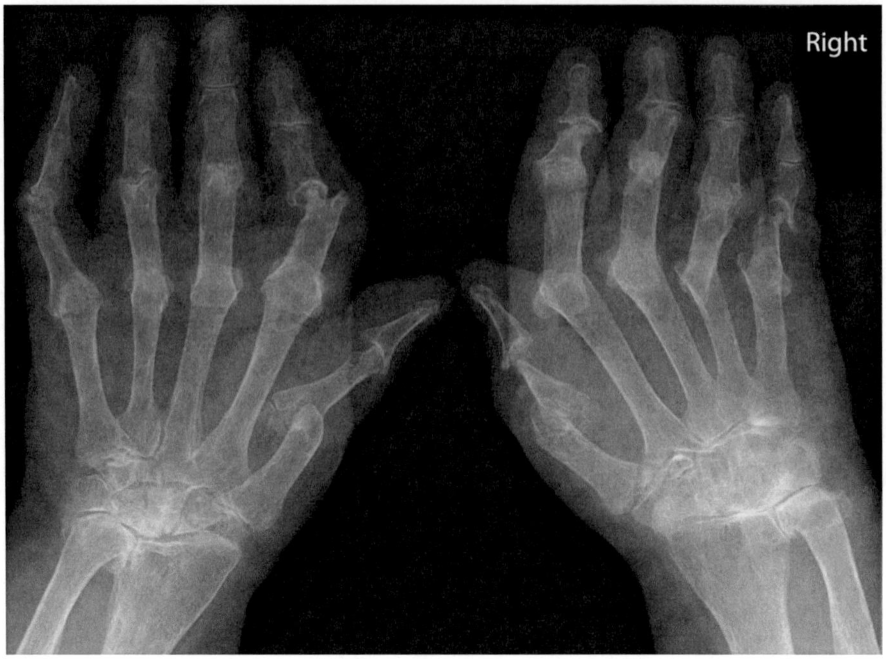

Fig. 14 Psoriatic arthritis: there is a severe mutilating polyarthritis with multiple subluxations and extensive erosive change. Note the 'pencil-in-cup' pattern of erosive change seen at the thumb interphalangeal joints. There has been extensive bone resorption, e.g. the right, little proximal and intermediate phalanges and there is bony ankylosis at the left little distal interphalangeal joint

the distal side of the joint merge together centrally to produce a concavity, which extends laterally as a result of enthesophyte formation, while the proximal erosions lead to a tapering of the bone. The effect is to produce the characteristic 'pencil in cup' appearance considered by some to be pathognomonic of the disease (Arnett 1987) (Fig. 14).

New bone formation is not confined to the enthesis sites and periosteal new bone may be seen relatively early in the disease occurring along the shaft of the phalanges (Fig. 15). This is frequently associated with a soft tissue swelling, and is probably related to tenosynovitis (El-Khoury et al. 1996; Olivieri et al. 1996).

A further feature of the entheseal disease seen on hand/wrist imaging can be noted at the sesamoid bones. Sesamoid bones lie within tendons and so a considerable portion of their surface area represents enthesis site. It has been noted that the sesamoid bone of the thumb may enlarge in patients with psoriatic arthritis giving an increased sesamoid index (length × width of the sesamoid) (Whitehouse et al. 2005).

Bone loss is not limited to periarticular erosion in psoriatic arthritis and acro-osteolysis (distal tuft resorption) is a well-recognised feature (Martel et al. 1980; Miller et al. 1971). It can help distinguish psoriatic arthritis from erosive OA, which may also cause erosive change at the DIP joints. Progressive osteolysis of the terminal phalanges may give them a 'peg like' appearance, although osteolysis may progress to involve the majority of the phalanx (Figs. 14, 16). When osteolysis is seen there is usually associated nail involvement. Acro-osteolysis may be seen in cases of psoriasis without arthritis (Miller et al. 1971).

Ankylosis

Bony ankylosis is a feature of psoriatic arthritis occurring later in the disease process (Fig. 14). The process commences as a result of fibrous tissue forming within the joint and this can give the impression of a widened joint space.

2.3.2 Other Seronegative Arthritides

Although hand and wrist involvement is seen in the other seronegative arthritides it is not as common or typical as the involvement of the hands in psoriatic arthritis.

Ankylosing Spondylitis

Ankylosing spondylitis primarily affects the axial skeleton but peripheral joint involvement is seen and this may involve hands and wrists (Resnick 1974; Vinje et al. 1985). Around 30% of patients with severe disease are reported to show hand and wrist

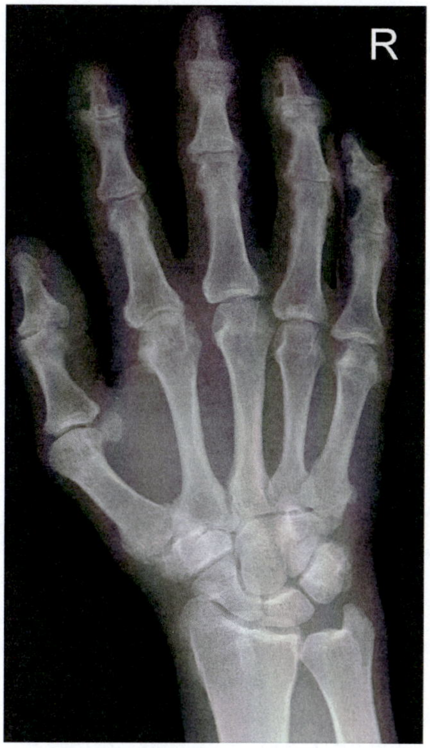

Fig. 15 Psoriatic arthritis: there is fluffy periostitis seen along the shafts of the proximal phalanges typical of psoriatic arthritis

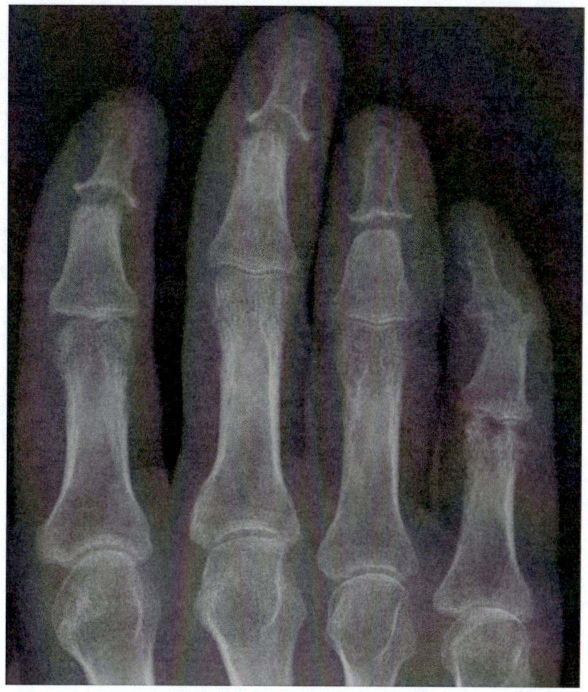

Fig. 16 Psoriatic arthritis: note the extensive bone destruction that has occurred about the distal interphalangeal joints. The cupped appearance to the bases of the distal phalanges is typical

involvement (Resnick 1974). An asymmetrical distribution is usually seen and features include periarticular osteoporosis, along with joint space narrowing, proliferative erosions and soft tissue swelling. Enthesophyte formation may be seen as part of the enthesitis (Fig. 17). Involvement may be seen in all compartments of the wrist and any of the small joints of the hands. Bony ankylosis may be seen and may have a relatively rapid onset.

Reactive Arthritis (previously Reiter's Syndrome)

Classically reactive arthritis involves the small and large joints of the lower limb, upper limb involvement is unusual. However, clinical and radiographic changes do occur in the hands and wrists with radiographic changes in the wrists being more common than changes in the hands (Lin et al. 1995; Mason et al. 1959). As with psoriatic arthritis, joint involvement tends to the asymmetrical. The changes seen in the hands are similar to those seen in psoriatic arthritis, with soft tissue swelling, joint space narrowing and proliferative marginal erosions. There may also be sesamoid enlargement as a result of the periostitis (Stadalnik and Dublin 1975). In contrast to psoriatic arthritis, where DIP joint involvement is most common, the PIP joints are more frequently involved in reactive arthritis than the DIP or MCP joints (Lin et al. 1995). While periarticular osteopaenia is not a typical feature of psoriatic arthritis, it is more widely recognised as occurring in the acute phases of reactive arthritis.

Wrist involvement may occasionally be severe in reactive arthritis. It can involve any of the wrist compartments and is typically asymmetrically distributed (Mason et al. 1959). Periosteal new bone formation is seen with erosions, osteopaenia and soft tissue swelling. Although the new bone formation has a fluffy configuration, more linear new bone may be seen, particularly alongside the radius and ulnar (Mason et al. 1959).

Arthritis Associated with Enteropathic Disease

Arthritis associated with inflammatory bowel disease is generally classified with the seronegative arthritides because the pattern of arthritis is very similar to that seen in ankylosing spondylitis. While axial involvement

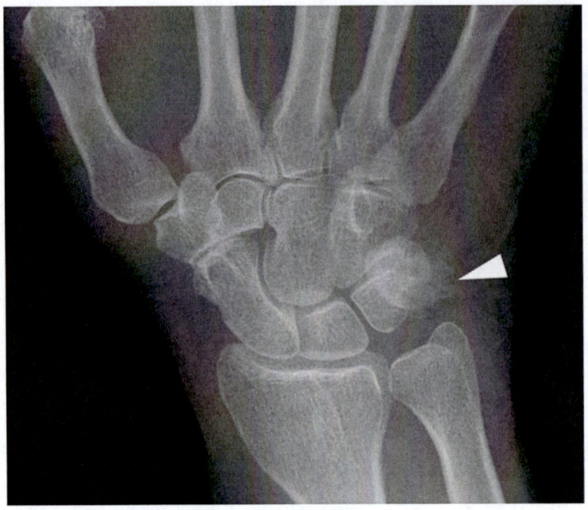

Fig. 17 Ankylosing spondylitis: there is exuberant enthesophyte formation at the insertion of the flexor carpi ulnaris tendon onto the pisiform (*arrowhead*). This represents an enthesitis, a typical feature of ankylosing spondylitis

predominates, 15–20% of patients with inflammatory bowel disease exhibit a peripheral arthritis, more frequently seen with Crohn's disease than ulcerative colitis (Gravallese and Kantrowitz 1988). Commonly this involves the wrists (along with the knees, ankles and elbows) and the condition occurs as transient arthritis. This is frequently asymmetric and occurrences tend to parallel flares of the inflammatory bowel disease. The arthritis is characteristically non-destructive and while CR may show soft tissue swelling and periarticular osteopaenia, erosions and joint space loss are not usually seen.

Destructive changes have been reported at peripheral joints in association with inflammatory bowel disease, but in this situation the findings are very similar to RA and distinction may not possible. Indeed the two conditions may coexist.

Hypertrophic osteoarthropathy has a well-recognised association with pulmonary disease, but there is also a rare association with inflammatory bowel disease. HPOA is typically seen as linear periosteal new bone formation at the wrist, involving the radius and ulna, but may also involve the metacarpals. There is some evidence that the periosteal new bone may fluctuate with the disease activity (Arlart et al. 1982).

Although not generally considered alongside the other spondyloarthropathies, an asymmetric erosive arthritis of the hands and wrists with predominantly distal distribution is recognised as occurring in association with primary biliary cirrhosis (Mills et al. 1981). Hypertrophic osteoarthropathy is also described with this condition.

2.4 Juvenile Idiopathic Arthritis

Juvenile idiopathic arthritis (JIA) is the term given to a heterogeneous group of conditions beginning in childhood and involving inflammation in one or more joints. By definition the term encompasses all forms of arthritis beginning before the age of 16 and persisting for more than 6 weeks when other known conditions have been excluded. The most recent classification has been determined by the International League of Associations for Rheumatology (ILAR) and unifies different classifications which previously existed in North America and Europe (Petty et al. 2004). Seven categories of JIA are recognised in the current classification (Table 1) (Petty et al. 2004; Ravelli and Martini 2007). The classification system is not without controversies and further developments may well occur (Ravelli and Martini 2007).

Early in the disease soft tissue swelling and osteopaenia may be seen in the hands and wrists of affected children. However, joint space loss is less frequently seen and often represents a later feature particularly in the oligoarthritis form of the disease. Erosion is also a relatively late radiographic finding in JIA. In patients with seropositive juvenile idiopathic polyarthritis more rapid joint space loss and erosion may be seen, a process similar to that seen in adult onset RA. Deformities may develop including boutonniere, flexion and swan neck deformities in the fingers. Radial deviation of the MCP joints in association with ulnar deviation of the wrist is recognised in JIA, and Resnick has noted the contrast between this pattern and the opposite finding of ulnar deviation of the MCP joints and radial deviation of the wrist commonly seen in adult onset RA (Granberry and Mangum 1980; Resnick 2002a).

Some radiographic findings are more specific to juvenile arthritis. In the late stages of the disease bony ankylosis is a common finding particularly at the wrist where radiographs may demonstrate union of the carpal bones to the metacarpals creating a solid ossific mass (Fig. 18). Periosteal new bone formation is also a common finding in the hands in JIA, typically

Table 1 Classification of Juvenile Idiopathic Arthritis (Petty et al. 2004; Ravelli and Martini 2007)

Category	Clinical features
Systemic arthritis	Arthritis in one or more joints associated with, or proceeded by fever and accompanied by one or more of the following: • rash • lymphadenopathy • hepatomegaly and/or splenomegaly • serositis
Oligoarthritis	Arthritis in 1–4 joints during the first 6 months of disease This typically occurs in early childhood and is more common in females. The oligoarthritis is usually asymmetric and predominantly affects the lower limbs
Rheumatoid-factor: positive polyarthritis	Arthritis affecting five or more joints during the first 6 months of disease with positive rheumatoid factor The disease typically affects the hands with a symmetric polyarthritis
Rheumatoid-factor: negative polyarthritis	Arthritis affecting five or more joints during the first 6 months of disease without rheumatoid factor
Enthesitis related arthritis	More common in male patients and characterised by the association of enthesitis and arthritis. The disease belongs to the group of spondyloarthropathies
Psoriatic arthritis	
Undifferentiated arthritis	

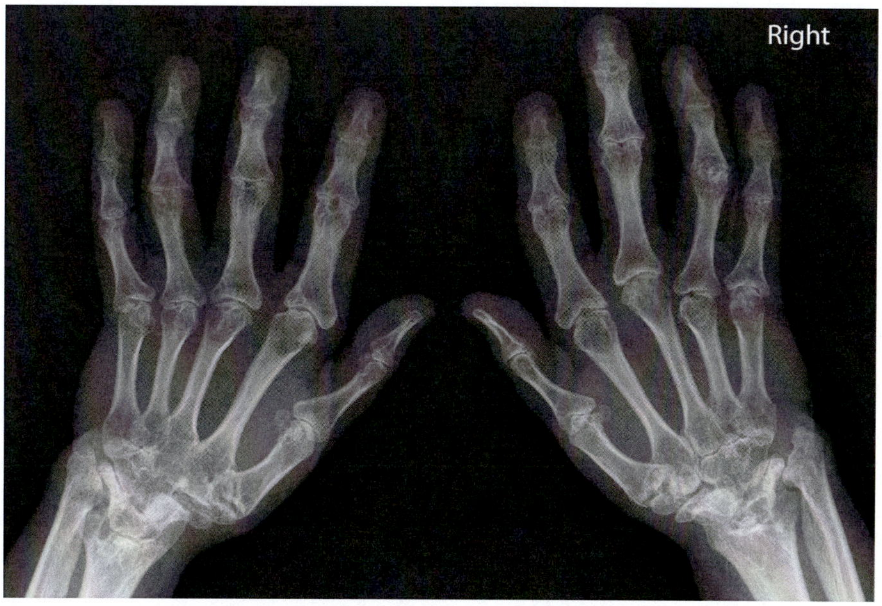

Fig. 18 JIA: this patient demonstrates many of the late features of JIA. Note the fusion of the carpal bones, cupping and deformity of the proximal phalangeal bases and epiphyseal deformities resulting from growth disturbance

occurring along the metacarpal and phalangeal shafts. Growth disturbances involving the epiphyses of long bones are a further feature of juvenile arthritis (Figs. 18, 19). In the wrists, abnormalities of bone growth are seen in the form of irregular or multiple ossification centres in the carpal bones. In the hands, short, widened phalanges and metacarpals may develop in the later stages of the disease as a result of growth disturbance and periosteal new bone formation (Fig. 19).

The osteoporotic bone seen in JIA may lead to epiphyseal collapse and deformity as a result of compression fractures due to abnormal stresses on the bone. Cupping of the proximal phalangeal bases as a result of compression by the metacarpals on the osteoporotic bone is described (Resnick 2002a) (Fig. 18).

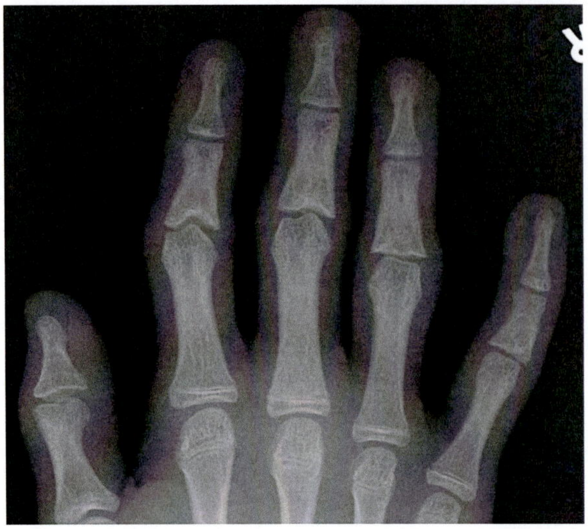

Fig. 19 JIA: there is epiphyseal deformity at the bases of the intermediate phalanges. There is corresponding deformity to the proximal phalangeal articular surface. Soft tissue swelling is also seen. Also note the widened intermediate phalanges typical of the disease

In common with adult onset RA, tenosynovitis is seen in JIA and may be observed as soft tissue swelling on plain radiographs. Rheumatoid nodules are also seen in JIA; these occur almost exclusively in the rheumatoid-factor-positive polyarthritis subcategory of the disease where they are seen in around one third of patients in the first year of disease (Ravelli and Martini 2007). Again on CR these may be seen as focal soft tissue lumps.

As with adult inflammatory arthritis, the majority of plain film findings represent late stages of the disease. While CR remains important in the assessment of the disease the role of more advanced imaging techniques, such as US and MRI, is increasing. In addition to allowing the visualisation of soft tissue changes such as synovitis, effusion and tenosynovitis; the cartilaginous bone ends of the immature skeleton, where early damage occurs are also demonstrated (Johnson and Gardner-Medwin 2002).

2.5 Advanced Imaging Techniques in Inflammatory Arthritis

Many of the features of inflammatory arthritis seen on CR represent late changes, which are often irreversible. Current guidelines in the management of these conditions emphasise the early and aggressive treatment of inflammatory arthritis to alter the long-term disease process, minimise joint damage and induce long-term remission.

2.5.1 Synovitis and Effusion

Synovitis is an early feature of many arthritic processes including the inflammatory arthritides and connective tissue disorders. Using plain films the earliest manifestation of synovitis is soft tissue swelling, which may be associated with periarticular osteopaenia. The soft tissue swelling is usually detectable clinically by the time it can be seen on CR. Both US and MRI are readily able to detect synovitis and effusion before changes are visible on CR or detectable at the clinical examination (Farrant et al. 2007a; Peterfy 2001).

Normally synovium is not visualised at US, but when it becomes thickened it is seen as abnormal intra articular soft tissue (Fig. 20a) (Wakefield et al. 2005). The echogenicity of synovitis varies depending on the extent of extracellular oedema, the more fluid present the darker the synovium appears. Generally it appears of low reflectivity when compared with adjacent subcutaneous fat, but it may appear anechoic or brightly hyperechoic. Vascularity will frequently be demonstrated in the synovium using colour or power Doppler (Fig. 20b). When anechoic or hypoechoic, synovitis may be difficult to distinguish from joint fluid, which may have similar echo characteristics. However, with probe pressure fluid will normally be displaced while synovium is non-displaceable and only poorly compressible. Effusion will also show no Doppler signal. The morphology of the inflamed synovium varies, but typically in the low capacity joints of the hand and wrist it appears as thickening of the joint lining or as a solid mass.

On MRI synovitis has been defined as an area in the synovial compartment that shows above normal, post gadolinium enhancement of a thickness greater than the width of normal synovium (Ostergaard et al. 2003). This definition emphasises the importance of post-gadolinium imaging in the detection of synovitis which readily enhances and is otherwise very difficult to distinguish from effusion using conventional T1, proton density and T2 weighted imaging (Fig. 21).

2.5.2 Bone Erosion and Marrow Oedema

US and MRI will demonstrate erosive change resulting from inflammatory arthritis. A defect in the cortical

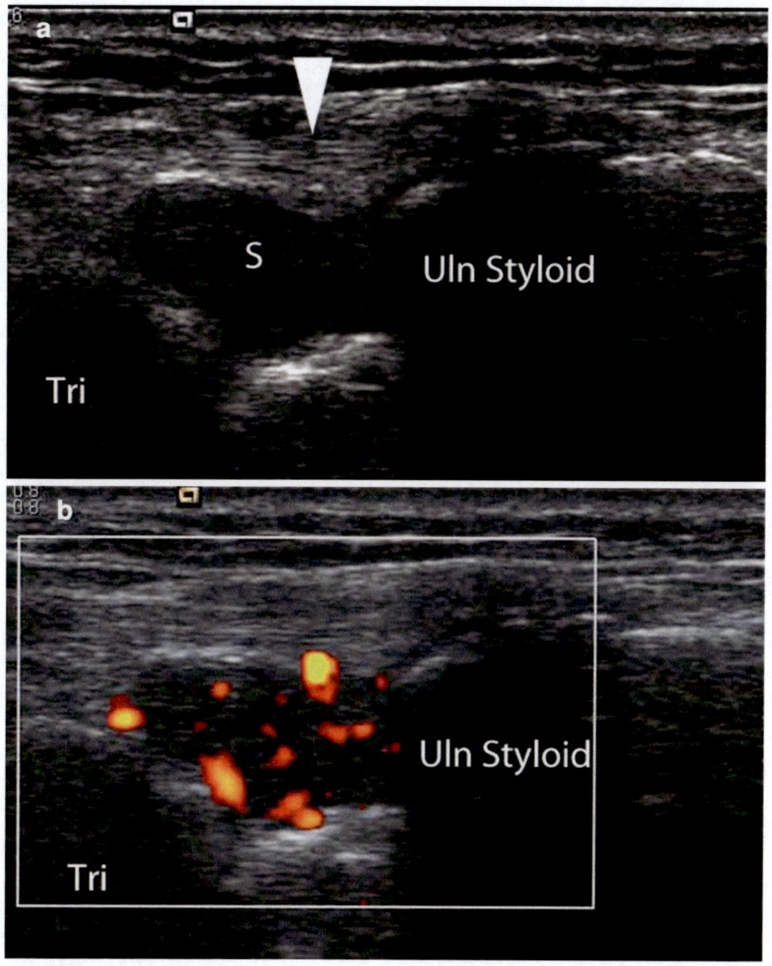

Fig. 20 Wrist synovitis shown on ultrasound in rheumatoid arthritis: **a** the synovitis is seen as a low reflective soft tissue mass lesion (*S*), in this case on the ulnar aspect of the wrist. Part of the extensor carpi ulnaris tendon can be appreciated just superficial to the synovitis (*arrowhead*). **b** Using power Doppler vascular flow can be demonstrated in the synovitis. *Uln Styloid* ulnar styloid process, *Tri* triquetrum

surface is identified which may contain synovium (Figs. 21, 22). With both techniques the erosion must be identified in two planes to avoid confusion with normal bone surface contours. It is also important to be aware of the normal shape of the bones and in particular the sites of ligament attachments and vascular channels both of which can be confused with erosions. US and MRI are both more sensitive than CR for erosion detection. While US will only show the surface defect of an erosion, MRI shows changes within the substance of the bone marrow at the erosion site in the form of high T2 signal consistent with increased water content and often described as bone marrow oedema (Fig. 21b, c) (Ostergaard et al. 2003). Bone marrow oedema is a common finding in RA reported in 39% of cases of less than 3 years duration and 68% of cases of longer established RA (Savnik et al. 2001). Marrow oedema may be seen in the absence of erosion and is potentially reversible; it is closely related to the extent of synovitis and may represent pre-erosive change, being strongly predictive of future erosion (McQueen et al. 2003; Haavardsholm et al. 2008; Hetland et al. 2009; Savnik et al. 2002).

2.5.3 Enthesitis

Enthesitis is a characteristic feature of the seronegative arthropathies and is seen in the hand and wrist as a common feature of psoriatic arthritis. MRI demonstrates changes within the bone, in the form of marrow oedema, erosion and enthesophyte, and within the inserting tendon or ligament and surrounding soft tissues in the form of high T2 signal change and thickening of the inserting structure. The changes seen in the inserting tendon or ligament are

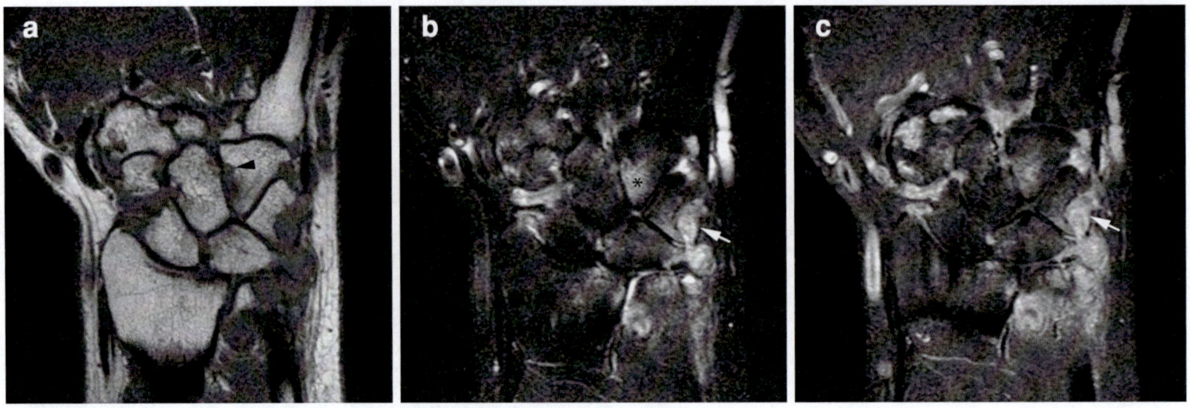

Fig. 21 Rheumatoid arthritis shown on coronal MRI: **a** T1 weighted, **b** T2 weighted with fat saturation. Extensive synovitis is seen at the wrist as intermediate signal soft tissue on T1 and high signal soft tissue on T2 weighted imaging. It is best appreciated on the ulnar aspects of the wrist (*arrow*) where it is seen eroding the triquetrum. **c** T1 fat saturated post i.v. gadolinium. Synovial enhancement is demonstrated. The T2 weighted and post gadolinium imaging demonstrates marrow oedema in the hamate (*asterisk*) and on T1 weighted imaging this is seen to be associated with bone erosion (*arrowhead*)

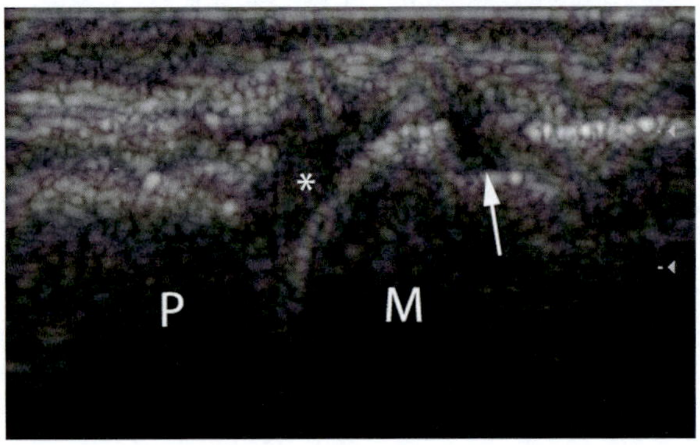

Fig. 22 Rheumatoid arthritis erosion on US: the index MCP joint is demonstrated in longitudinal section. There is synovitis within the joint (*asterisk*) and an erosion is seen in the metacarpal head (*arrow*). The erosion contains hypoechoic synovium. *M* metacarpal head, *P* proximal phalanx

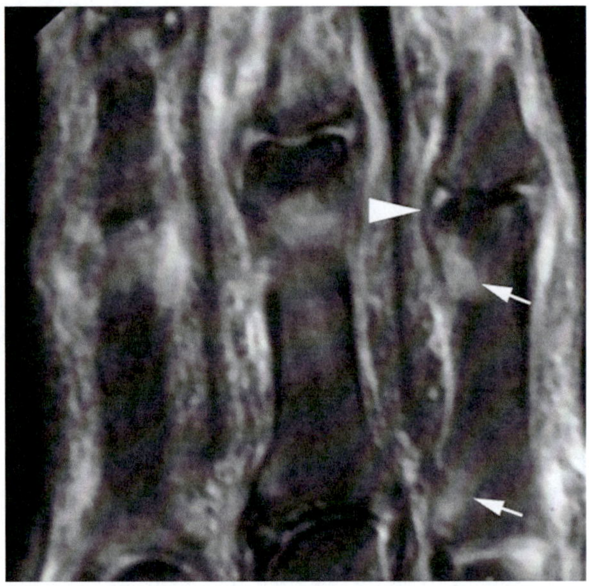

Fig. 23 Psoriatic arthritis: coronal T2 weighted fat saturated image showing dactylitis. Extensive soft tissue oedema is shown in the digits. Enthesitis is demonstrated as foci of marrow oedema associated with capsular and ligamentous insertion sites (*arrows*) such as the insertion of the collateral ligament of the proximal interphalangeal joint highlighted (*arrowhead*) (Image courtesy of Dr PJ O'Connor and Dr A Radjenovic)

similar to those seen in tendinopathic change. The fingers are sites of multiple entheses all in close proximity and a feature of psoriatic arthritis is dactylitis where widespread inflammatory changes seen throughout the digit which may reflect inflammation at the multiple enthesis sites (Fig. 23) (Benjamin and McGonagle 2001). The extensive high T2 signal soft tissue changes seen beyond the joints in psoriatic arthritis are an important distinguishing feature from RA (Jevtic et al. 1995). US will also detect changes at the enthesis sites in seronegative arthropathy, but will not show the associated marrow changes. Fine enthesophyte formation is particularly well shown at tendon and ligament insertions using US.

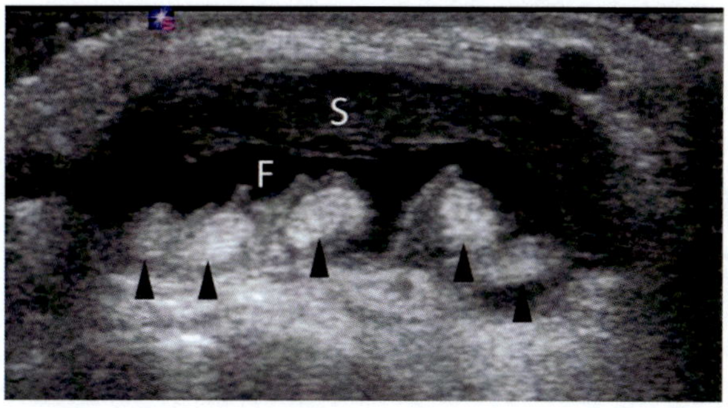

Fig. 24 Rheumatoid arthritis: a transverse ultrasound through the extensor digitorum compartment at the wrist shows tenosynovitis. The extensor tendons (*arrowheads*) are surrounded by fluid (*F*) and synovitis (*S*)

2.5.4 Tendon and Soft Tissue Disease

Tendon disease and tenosynovitis are both features of the inflammatory arthritides. Both US and MRI will demonstrate fluid in synovial sheaths and associated synovitis (Fig. 24). As in the case of joint disease gadolinium enhancement is helpful in distinguishing synovitis from fluid in tendon sheaths. Tendon rupture is a recognised complication of RA and may be due to tendon attrition resulting from adjacent osseous deformities or disease involvement of the tendon itself. Again US and MRI can demonstrate tendon rupture. The dynamic assessment of tendons that can be undertaken with US may help in identifying which tendons are torn and in establishing the location of the torn ends.

Rheumatoid nodules are a feature of RA. They most frequently occur in pressure bearing areas such as the elbow or heel, but are occasionally seen in the hand and wrist. They may occur in the subcutaneous soft tissues or adjacent or within tendons. Nodules typically appear on US as ovoid homogenous low reflective masses (Nalbant et al. 2003). On MRI nodules may have a solid appearance with a homogenous enhancement following gadolinium, but a cystic pattern may also be seen (el-Noueam et al. 1997). When nodules are seen adjacent to bone there may be associated cortical remodelling. The differential diagnosis for a rheumatoid nodule includes a gouty tophus. Bone remodelling is less frequently seen with rheumatoid nodules than with tophi, and tophi generally show increased density resulting in shadowing behind the lesion on US.

2.5.5 Application to Clinical Practice

Increasingly, US and MRI are being used in the early detection of inflammatory arthritis. US has clear advantages in being able to screen multiple joints in both hands and wrists rapidly and inexpensively while MRI is more time-consuming and requires intra-articular injection for the reliable assessment of synovitis. MRI has the advantage of being able to detect the early bone changes of bone marrow oedema along with synovitis and there is evidence to suggest that marrow oedema is the strongest predictor of future erosive damage (McQueen et al. 2003; Savnik et al. 2002). Most studies would suggest that US and MRI are of comparable sensitivity for the detection of synovitis and erosions, although US is limited around some joints, such as the MCP joints and in the wrist, by its inability to fully examine all bone surfaces (Farrant et al. 2007a, b).

2.5.6 Other Imaging Modalities

CT will demonstrate erosive change in bones, but at this time has not found routine clinical application in the investigation of the inflammatory arthritides. Scintigraphy will show increased uptake at inflamed joints using a variety of tracers including conventional 99mTc-MDP. Inflammatory arthritis will produce increased tracer activity on all three phases of the bone scan. The technique provides a means of observing disease distribution, which may help in indicating the type of arthropathy. It is also sensitive to early changes in the disease process and may give information about disease activity, but bone scintigraphy is not part of the routine investigation of inflammatory arthritis and generally MRI and US can provide similar information.

2.6 Monitoring Disease Progression

The monitoring of disease progression and response to treatment in inflammatory arthritis is currently a subject of intensive research. Plain film scoring methods exist such as those developed by Larsen and Sharp based on erosions, joint space loss and soft tissue changes (Larsen et al. 1977; Sharp 1996). However, in recent years attention has turned to the use of MRI and US for monitoring disease status.

The use of MRI and US to monitor disease progression has concentrated on the scoring of erosive change and synovitis and, on MRI, marrow oedema.

Techniques for monitoring synovitis fall into two broad groups, detection of change in synovial volume and detection of change in synovial vascularity. Both volume and vascularity are predictive of disease activity. Volume can be reliably assessed with MRI but there is considerable technical difficulty in producing reliable measurements of volume on US other than with the use of semiquantitative scores. Vascularity is assessed on MRI using dynamic scanning during gadolinium enhancement and evaluating the shape of the contrast uptake curve which is more rapid in more active disease. Doppler US imaging can be used to assess the vascularity of synovitis, which in RA is shown to increase with disease activity. At this time these techniques remain in the research environment and have not found their way into mainstream clinical practice.

3 The Crystal Arthritides

The crystal arthropathies all involve crystal deposition either in, or adjacent to an affected joint. This is a heterogeneous group of diseases resulting in a variety of radiographic findings. Common crystals implicated are monosodium urate (producing gout), calcium pyrophosphate dihydrate and hydroxyapatite (HA).

3.1 Gout

Although the radiological features of gout are well recognised, the pathophysiology of the disease is more complicated and remains the subject of research and controversy. Fundamental to the disease process is hyperuricaemia resulting either from decreased renal excretion or excess production of uric acid. The condition is frequently described as having four clinical phases (Monu and Pope 2004):

1. Asymptomatic hyperuricaemia: hyperuricaemia may exist in asymptomatic, but susceptible individuals, for years before the onset of clinical and radiographic findings.
2. Acute gouty arthritis: presentation with acute joint inflammation as a result of precipitation of urate crystals into the joint typifies this stage of the disease. While polyarticular disease is recognised, the acute inflammatory attacks are usually monoarticular and involve peripheral joints, usually in the lower limb and most commonly in the foot. Without treatment, progressive attacks result in more joints becoming involved and more chronic disease, which may affect any joint in the body.
3. Intercritical gout: this refers to the period without symptoms between acute attacks. It may last months or even years.
4. Chronic tophaceous gout: in this stage of the disease tophi develop in multiple tissues in the body as a result of urate crystal deposition with associated foreign body giant cell reaction. With the advent of effective antihyperuricaemic therapy this stage of the disease is becoming less common. Tophaceous deposits occur in a wide variety of tissues including tendons and ligaments, cartilage, bone and other soft tissues. Deposition in tendons and ligaments may lead to rupture (Moore and Weiland 1985) while mass effect may produce neural compression and gouty deposits are a recognised cause for carpal tunnel syndrome (Chen et al. 2000; Ogilvie and Kay 1988).

3.1.1 Imaging Findings

Gout arthritis may involve any of the joints in the hand and wrist, but the DIP and PIP joints are most frequently affected. In the acute stages of the disease the radiographic findings are often non-specific, soft tissue swelling may be evident. If US and MRI are undertaken an effusion may be evident. The bone and soft tissue changes become more characteristic and apparent in the chronic phase of the disease where soft tissue tophi develop. These are appreciated as asymmetrical soft tissue swellings and the hands are frequently involved. Although calcification of the soft tissue swellings may occur it is said to be an unusual finding, and is likely to reflect a disorder of calcium metabolism such as associated renal impairment (Fig. 25) (Watt and Middlemiss 1975).

Joint space usually remains well preserved until late in the disease despite extensive erosive change, and this is one of the key features of the disease helping to distinguish it from other arthritides (Fig. 26). Erosions

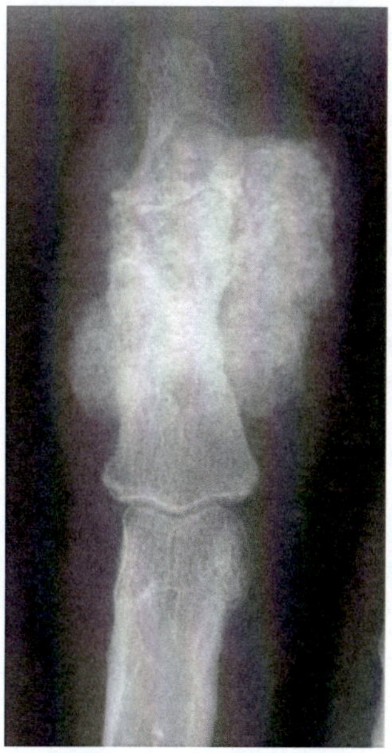

Fig. 25 Gout in patient with chronic renal failure: This patient has gout with large asymmetric soft tissue tophaceous masses about the distal interphalangeal joint which shows erosive change best appreciated in the terminal phalanx. The tophi are heavily calcified, a feature that is seen particularly in patients with renal impairment

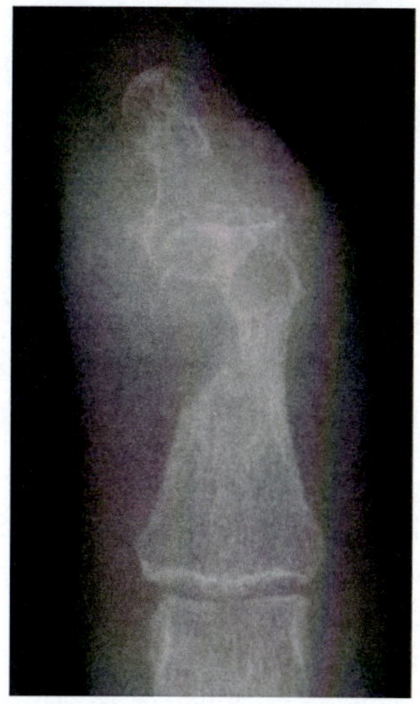

Fig. 26 Gout: this radiograph shows the typical 'punched-out' erosions with overhanging edges seen in gout. Note the marked soft tissue swelling and relative preservation of joint space, both features of this disease (Image courtesy of Dr PJ O'Connor)

result from tophi and may occur within joints, but are often seen some distance from the joint. The erosions have a characteristic circular or ovoid configuration and may have a sclerotic margin. Overhanging margins giving a 'punched out' appearance to the erosion are typical (Fig. 26) (Watt and Middlemiss 1975). Joint disease in the hand most commonly involves the interphalangeal joints in an asymmetrical distribution. All compartments in the wrist may be involved and extensive osseous erosion in the wrist is not uncommon.

US may detect crystal deposition on the articular cartilage and this has been reported in 92% of joints affected by gout (Thiele and Schlesinger 2007). The crystal deposition on the cartilage surface gives a double contour appearance to the joints. Both MRI and US will detect erosions due to gout and show tophaceous material associated with them. The tophi are seen as low reflective structures that are highly attenuating with shadowing behind the lesion. Crystal material within their substance varies from hypo- to hyperechoic. Lesions are clearly defined and may demonstrate marked hyperaemia. MRI shows tophi as structures of intermediate to low signal intensity on short TE imaging but with variable intensity on T2 weighted imaging, most frequently heterogenous intermediate to low signal. It has been postulated that the variation in T2 intensity may relate to differences in calcium concentration (Yu et al. 1997). Bone erosion by soft tissue tophi is more commonly seen in the feet than the hands. Tophaceous involvement of tendons in the hand may also be seen on US and MRI.

3.2 Calcium Pyrophosphate Crystal Deposition Disease (CPPD)

Calcium pyrophosphate dihydrate (CPPD) deposition disease may be a primary abnormality or may occur in association with other conditions. Given how common CPPD deposition disease is it has been pointed out that many of the suggested associations that have been described in the past may be simple chance occurrence of two disorders (Resnick 2002b).

The nomenclature of CPPD deposition disease is confusing and controversial. The following guidelines on terminology have been put forward and are helpful for the radiologist (Resnick 2002b; Steinbach 2004; Steinbach and Resnick 1996):

Chondrocalcinosis Refers to the presence of cartilage calcification identified radiologically or pathologically.

It can be due to a variety or combination of calcium crystals including calcium pyrophosphate dihydrate.

CPPD deposition disease A specific term indicating a disorder characterised by CPPD crystals in or around joints.

Pseudo-gout This is a clinical syndrome produced by CPPD crystals resulting in acute attacks of gout like symptoms. The diagnosis is clinical and cannot be made radiologically.

Pyrophosphate arthropathy This term describes a pattern of joint damage occurring in CPPD deposition disease. It resembles OA but has some distinct features. Chondrocalcinosis may or may not be present on radiographs demonstrating pyrophosphate arthropathy.

One of the reasons for the confusion is the highly variable presentation of the disease. Calcium pyrophosphate deposition may be completely asymptomatic or result in severe destructive arthropathy, its ability to mimic other arthritides has been emphasised (Steinbach 2004; Martel et al. 1970). Patients with symptomatic CPPD deposition disease generally present with an OA like arthropathy although an acute inflammatory component may be seen. Intermittent attacks of pseudogout are said to occur in 10–20% of symptomatic patients and result from the shedding of pyrophosphate crystals into the joint (Steinbach 2004). The wrist is a frequent site for attacks of pseudogout. Synovitis associated with CPPD crystal deposition disease is a recognised cause of carpal tunnel syndrome.

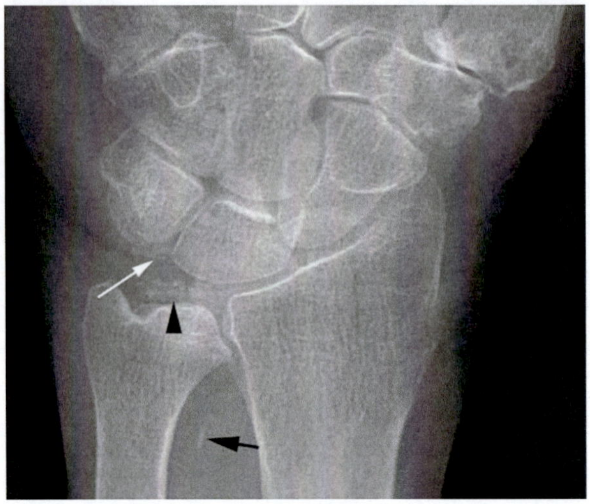

Fig. 27 Calcium pyrophosphate deposition: there is calcium crystal deposition in the triangular fibrocartilage (*arrowhead*). In addition crystal deposition is also seen in the lunotriquetral ligament (*white arrow*) and in the synovium of the distal radial the joint (*black arrow*)

3.2.1 Imaging Findings

The hallmark of CPPD deposition disease is the presence of CPPD crystals in or around a joint. This is most commonly seen in the form of chondrocalcinosis, but crystal deposition may also occur within synovium or capsular tissues. It is important to realise that the presence of these findings alone does not infer pyrophosphate arthropathy and pyrophosphate arthropathy does not require radiographic evidence of CPPD crystals. In the wrist chondrocalcinosis is frequently identified in the triangular fibrocartilage, although it has been shown that crystal deposition in the lunate-triquetral ligament is more common (Fig. 27) (Yang et al. 1995). Hyaline cartilage deposition may also be seen. Pyrophosphate arthropathy shows similar changes to OA with joint space narrowing along with subchondral sclerosis and cyst formation. However, the distribution of the changes in the wrist contrasts with the classic trapeziocentric distribution of OA with a strong predilection for the radiocarpal wrist compartment (Fig. 28a). Associated with crystal deposition there may be disruption of the triangular fibrocartilage and ligamentous dysfunction resulting in rotatory subluxation of the scaphoid and scapholunate disassociation; this gives rise to a pattern of dorsal intercalated segment instability (DISI) similar to that seen following trauma. This pattern of scapholunate advanced collapse of the wrist (SLAC wrist) was originally described as a feature of OA but studies indicate that CPPD deposition disease is also a major cause of SLAC wrist (Chen et al. 1990).

The pattern of joint disease in the hands is also different to that seen with generalised OA with relative sparing of the interphalangeal joints and involvement predominantly of the MCP joints, most frequently those of the index and middle fingers (Fig. 28b). Another typical feature of the disease is the presence of hook like osteophytes generally seen on the radial aspect of the metacarpal head; this pattern of osteophytosis is particularly seen in patients with haemochromatosis and pyrophosphate arthropathy, a recognised association. As with idiopathic pyrophosphate arthropathy, involvement of the index and middle MCPs is commonly seen with

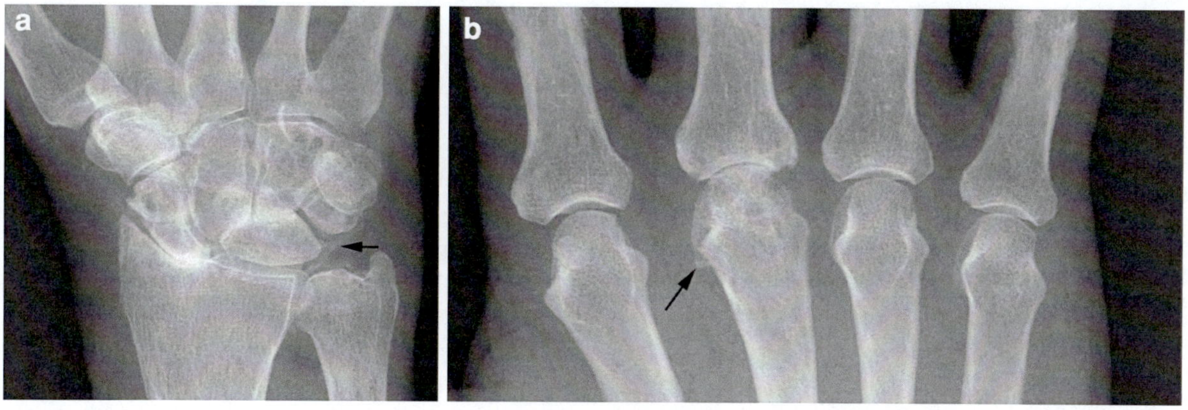

Fig. 28 Pyrophosphate arthropathy: **a** calcium pyrophosphate crystal deposition can be seen in the synovium about the triangular fibrocartilage and in the distal radial on the joint. There is also crystal deposition in the lunotriquetral ligament. This is associated with arthropathy. The distribution of arthritis in the wrist is not typical for osteoarthritis. There is involvement of the radioscaphoid and midcarpal joints, but note the preservation of the scaphotrapezial and thumb carpometacarpal joints. **b** In the same patient there is arthropathy involving the middle MCP joint with subchondral cyst formation, joint loss and early osteophyte formation (*arrow*)

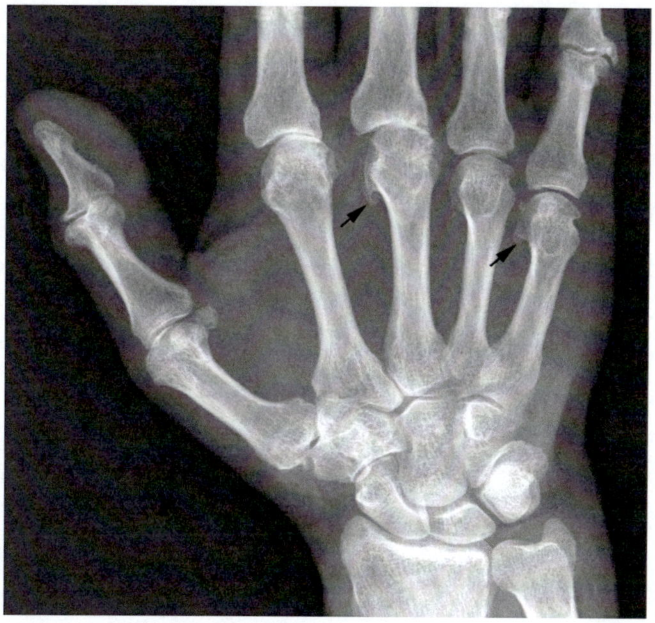

Fig. 29 Haemochromatosis arthropathy: there is joint space loss at the index and middle MCP joints with subchondral sclerosis. Involvement of the ring and little MCP joints and the little PIP joint can also be appreciated. Note the typical hook like osteophytes (*arrows*)

haemochromatosis; however, it has been observed that involvement of the ring and little finger MCP joints is also seen and is more common in patients with haemochromatosis than in those presenting with idiopathic pyrophosphate arthropathy (Fig. 29) (Steinbach 2004; Adamson et al. 1983).

Crystal deposition in cartilage and synovium and soft tissues including tendon is readily detected using US (Ciapetti et al. 2009). The position of crystals within the substance of cartilage is helpful in distinguishing pyrophosphate arthropathy from gout, where the crystals lie on the surface of the cartilage forming the double contour appearance.

3.3 Calcium Hydroxyapatite Crystal Deposition Disease

Hydroxyapatite (HA) deposition disease is the best characterised of a group of crystal deposition diseases

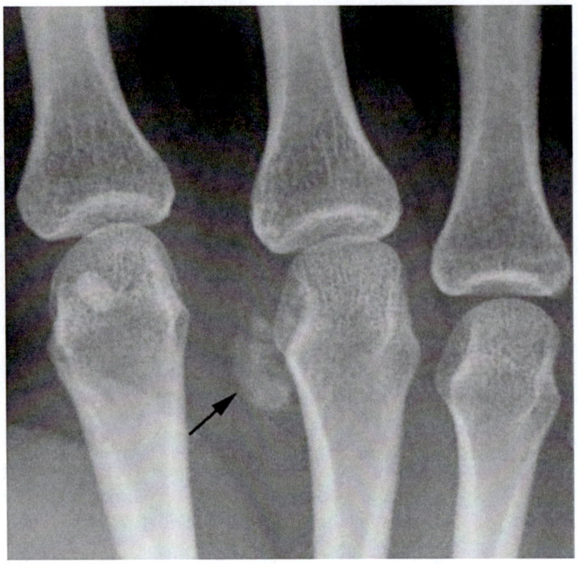

Fig. 30 Hydroxyapatite deposition: a large hydroxyapatite deposit is seen in the soft tissues adjacent to the middle MCP joint. Note the amorphous appearance. In this case the crystal deposition has a relatively well-defined margin

that may cause acute or chronic joint symptoms. The pathophysiology of the disease remains poorly understood. Crystal deposition may occur both in the periarticular tissues, most commonly tendons and ligaments, and within the joint itself and the disease can be usefully considered in two forms, periarticular disease and intra-articular disease (Uri and Dalinka 1996).

3.3.1 Periarticular HA Deposition Disease

The wrist and hand are common sites for HA crystal deposition and patients present with pain and swelling in the acute situation. When this occurs the pain may be particularly severe although in the more chronic situation the pain and tenderness is usually mild. Wrist involvement is more common than hand involvement, and crystal deposition usually occurs in tendons or ligaments, a particularly common site is in the flexor carpi ulnaris tendon on the ulnar aspect of the wrist (Gandee et al. 1979). In the hand the soft tissues around the MCP joints and the fingers are relatively common sites (Fig. 30). The calcification is seen on plain films and generally has an amorphous appearance without internal trabeculation. Deposits may have ill-defined borders or have a more well circumscribed appearance. While HA deposits may remain static on sequential radiographs, a notable feature is that the calcification may change in size becoming larger, smaller or even disappearing completely; and such changes may occur over a relatively short period of time. A definite history of trauma is rarely given, but there is some suggestion that HA deposition in soft tissues may be related to repetitive low grade trauma such as may occur with certain occupations and activities (Gandee et al. 1979).

3.3.2 Intra-Articular HA Deposition Disease

Intra-articular HA deposition can occur without visible changes on the radiograph. However, crystal deposition in the synovium or capsule may be seen and occasionally chondrocalcinosis is identified (Uri and Dalinka 1996). The hands and wrists are more frequently involved than the larger joints. A destructive arthropathy resembling OA may be seen with joint space loss and osteophyte formation.

4 Osteoarthritis (OA)

Despite its ubiquitous nature and increasing prevalence as a result of an ageing population, the pathophysiology of OA remains poorly understood and the subject of considerable research. The advent of advanced imaging modalities such as MRI and US has started to reveal that OA should be considered a disease of the whole joint and not just one of articular cartilage and bone, which is often the impression given by the plain film. Synovitis, effusion, marrow oedema and ligamentous and fibrocartilage abnormalities are now recognised imaging features of the disease and may play an important role in the pathogenesis of pain.

It is recognised that certain risk factors exist for the development of OA, including intrinsic problems with the joint such as previous trauma, laxity or bone deformity. However, other factors are also important, including gender and genetic susceptibility, along with extrinsic factors acting upon the joint such as obesity or joint overuse as a result of sporting or occupational activity (Felson 2004). OA may occur in one or more joints as a direct result of acute or chronic repetitive trauma; but the hand and wrist is an important site for the development of idiopathic OA. In this case, there is usually involvement of other larger joints such as the knees, hips and spine.

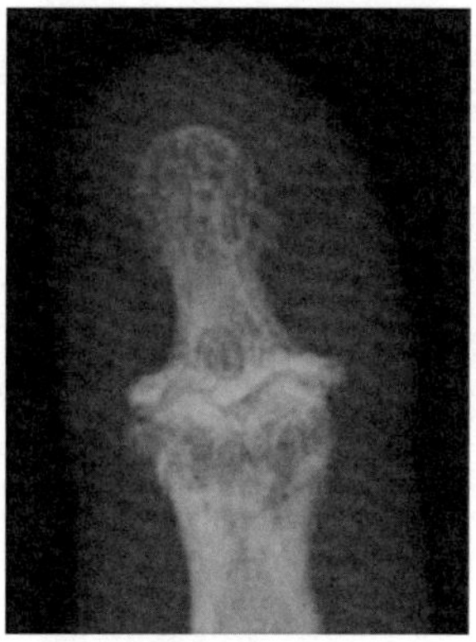

Fig. 31 Osteoarthritis: The typical 'saw-tooth' appearance of interphalangeal joint OA is seen. Note also the subchondral cyst formation and sclerosis

4.1 Plain Film Findings

The characteristic features of OA seen on CR are well recognised and reflect changes in the articular cartilage and subchondral bone along with osteophyte formation. Cartilage thinning and degradation is recognised as joint space narrowing. Subchondral bone change includes eburnation, sclerosis and cyst formation. Periarticular osteoporosis is not a feature of the disease.

In the hand the most commonly affected joints are the interphalangeal joints of the fingers and the thumb. Changes in both the PIP and DIP finger joints are frequently seen, but isolated involvement of the DIP joints may occur. Involvement of the PIP joints without DIP joint involvement is relatively unusual. Wrist involvement is almost always confined to the thumb base in a trapeziocentric distribution.

4.2 Findings at Specific Joints

4.2.1 Interphalangeal Joints

The classical features of OA described above are all seen at the interphalangeal joints. Subchondral cyst formation may be particularly prominent. In many joints cartilage loss in OA, seen as joint space narrowing, occurs asymmetrically within the joint favouring areas where the joint experiences particular pressure. In interphalangeal joints, joint space loss frequently occurs across the whole joint. Areas of eburnation and subchondral collapse may produce a characteristic 'saw-tooth' appearance to the articular surfaces (Fig. 31).

Osteophytes are often seen on the dorsal aspect of the interphalangeal joints where they may track proximally. The hands are usually evaluated radiographically with a dorsal-palmar view and on this single view the extent of such osteophytosis may not be appreciated. Osteophytes account in part for the palpable swellings appreciated at the DIP and PIP joints and termed Heberden's and Bouchard's nodes, respectively. However, it is also recognised that cystic distension of the joint capsule with gelatinous material and synovium is also seen, particularly at the DIP joints, and in some cases this may account for the nodes. Such cysts appear to extrude through points of weakness in the capsule, typically either side of the central extensor tendon (McGonagle et al. 2008; Tan et al. 2005).

4.2.2 Metacarpophalangeal Joints

Involvement of the MCP joints is not uncommon but usually only occurs in the presence of more distal disease involving the interphalangeal joints of the hand (Martel et al. 1973). In contrast, pyrophosphate arthropathy characteristically affects the MCP joints proving a useful distinguishing feature where otherwise, in the absence of any visible crystal deposition, it shows features similar to OA. In many cases joint space loss is the only finding and the presence of OA elsewhere and the absence of erosions and periarticular osteopaenia must be used to distinguish OA from inflammatory arthritis. Osteophytes when present are usually small, in comparison to the larger osteophytes seen in CPPD deposition disease.

4.2.3 The Wrist

Trapeziocentric Joints

The usual pattern of wrist OA involves the thumb base, occurring at the thumb carpometacarpal joint (trapeziometacarpal) and scaphotrapezotrapezoidal (STT) joint (between the scaphoid, trapezium and trapezoid). In the absence of trauma causing secondary OA, involvement of the other joint spaces in the wrist is uncommon and when seen, should suggest the possibility of an alternative diagnosis such as pyrophosphate arthropathy.

It is often helpful to think of the articulations between the scaphoid, trapezium, trapezoid and thumb metacarpal as a single unit and disease here can be summarised as trapeziocentric or pantrapezial. While either the STT joint or thumb carpometacarpal joint may show isolated OA changes, involvement in the two joints together is common (Fig. 32) (North and Eaton 1983). There is evidence that CR overestimates the

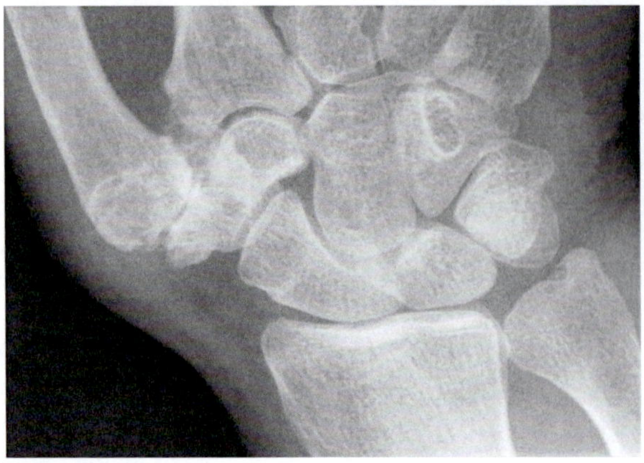

Fig. 32 Osteoarthritis: this example shows the typical appearances of thumb base OA involving the CMC joint. There is radial subluxation of the metacarpal base. In this case the STT joint is preserved. Also note the preservation of the remaining wrist joints typical of OA

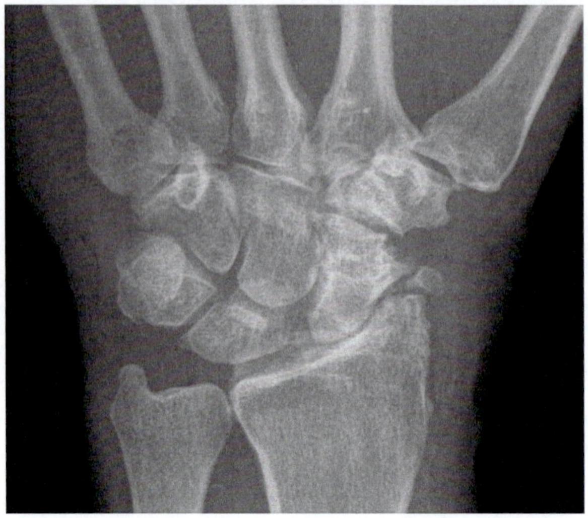

Fig. 33 SLAC wrist: osteoarthritis has developed following an injury with disruption of the scapholunate ligament (note widening of the scapholunate interval). Changes of OA are seen at the radioscaphoid joint, typical with this pattern of disease

extent of disease involving this unit. North and Eaten showed that while trapeziocentric OA was seen in 73% of cases radiographically it was found to be present in only 46% at anatomical dissection (North and Eaton 1983). Characteristic changes of sclerosis, osteophytosis, joint space loss and subchondral cyst formation are seen. Osteophytosis is particularly common at the thumb carpometacarpal joint where bony fragmentation may also be seen. It is thought that the pathogenesis of OA at the thumb carpometacarpal joint may result from abnormal joint laxity and radial subluxation of the metacarpal base at the carpometacarpal joint is a feature of advanced disease (Fig. 32) (Sicre et al. 1997). It has been noted that the saddle-shaped articulation between the trapezium and thumb metacarpal is generally flatter in women than men, and therefore inherently less stable (North and Rutledge 1983).

Other Wrist Joint Involvement

Injury to the wrist may result in secondary OA involving wrist joints other than those at the thumb base. Classically radiocarpal or midcarpal OA may be seen following scaphoid injury. If fracture occurs, secondary OA may develop, generally between the radial styloid and distal fragment of the scaphoid. This situation is known as scaphoid non-union advanced collapse (SNAC) and, in the later stages of the disease, involvement of the radio-scaphoid joint and subsequently the midcarpal joint is seen (Krimmer et al. 1997). Radioscaphoid disease progressing to midcarpal disease is also seen as a consequence of scapholunate disassociation and has been termed scapholunate advanced collapse (SLAC) (Fig. 33) (Watson and Ballet 1984). This pattern of joint disease is also seen as a consequence of pyrophosphate arthropathy and the distinction can only be reliably made if there is evidence of CPPD deposition disease (Chen et al. 1990).

A further pattern of wrist OA may be seen in association with positive ulnar variance leading to impingement across the ulna-lunate and ulna-triquetral joints. This has been termed the ulnocarpal impaction syndrome and results in findings typical of OA involving the ulna-lunate and ulna-triquetral joints. Dissociation of the lunate and triquetrum may be seen on CR as a consequence of lunate-triquetrum ligament disruption. MRI will also show this feature along with perforation of the triangular fibrocartilage, which is commonly associated.

4.3 Inflammatory OA

While OA is not generally viewed as an inflammatory arthritis, a subgroup of patients is recognised as having an inflammatory variant of the disease, which has been termed inflammatory OA (Ehrlich 1972a; Utsinger et al. 1978). Since these patients may show erosions the term erosive OA has also been used.

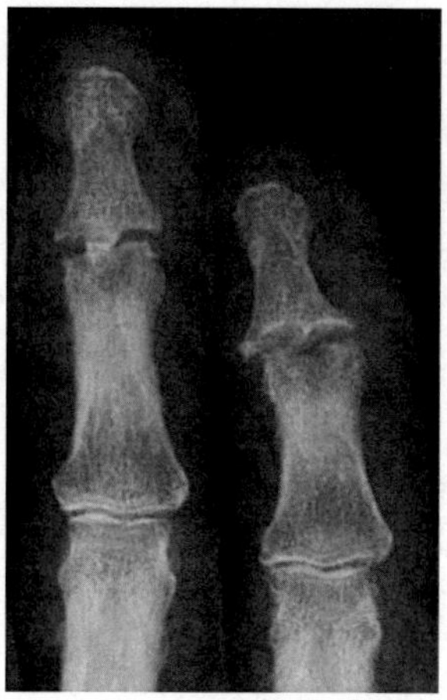

Fig. 34 Erosive OA: there is central (subchondral) erosion typical of erosive osteoarthritis

Although large joint involvement has been recognised, inflammatory OA characteristically affects the small joints of the hands. The relationship between conventional OA and erosive OA is unclear and authors have suggested on the one hand that the two arthropathies may constitute separate disease entities (Peter et al. 1966), while others suggest it may belong at one end of a disease spectrum (Grainger et al. 2007; Cobby et al. 1990). It has also been postulated that inflammatory OA represents a disease entity at an interface between OA and RA (Ehrlich 1972b). With the advent of more advanced imaging modalities it is apparent that cases not considered erosive using plain film criteria may show erosions with MRI (Tan et al. 2005; Grainger et al. 2007). These findings suggest that the division of OA into erosive and non-erosive forms on the basis of CR may be artificial.

4.3.1 Radiographic Features

The radiographic hallmark of erosive OA is the presence of erosive change alongside the expected findings in OA of joint space narrowing and proliferative change. Sites of involvement in the hand and wrist are the same as those seen in generalised primary OA although erosive change at the thumb base is rarely seen even in the presence of interphalangeal joint erosions. Erosions in inflammatory OA are typically central in location, which contrasts with the marginal erosions seen in rheumatoid and psoriatic arthropathy (Fig. 34). Nevertheless marginal erosions, indistinguishable from those seen in RA, may be demonstrated, particularly using MRI (Grainger et al. 2007; Kidd and Peter 1966). The central pattern of erosion may be due to synovial inflammation but it is also suggested it relates to collapse or pressure atrophy of the subchondral bone. Central erosions may lead to the characteristic 'seagull wing' appearance. Periosteal new bone formation may be seen although it is not usually as florid as that found in psoriatic arthritis. Bony ankylosis is a relatively frequent occurrence in inflammatory OA (Martel et al. 1980).

Distinguishing erosive OA from inflammatory arthropathy can be difficult. OA typically affects the PIP and DIP joints, which is useful in distinguishing it from RA with its generally more proximal distribution. The bone proliferation and sclerosis seen in OA also contrasts with the appearances of RA where osteopaenia is the typical finding. When seen in the wrist, erosive OA will usually show the characteristic thumb base distribution of OA while the inflammatory arthritides will show involvement in all wrist compartments. The distinction between erosive OA and psoriatic arthritis can be more difficult as the latter also shows bony proliferation in the form of enthesophyte formation and a distal distribution. The central pattern of erosion helps in distinguishing the two conditions, as does the more florid periosteal new bone seen in psoriatic arthritis. The presence of OA elsewhere such as the thumb base may also give clues, but it is important to remember that OA is a common condition and may coexist with seronegative arthritis or RA. This occurrence may account for some cases diagnosed as erosive OA.

4.4 Advanced Imaging Techniques

MRI has been used in a research capacity to look at OA in the hand and this has given valuable information on the potential aetiology of the disease (Tan et al. 2005, 2006a, b). However, as yet there are no mainstream applications for the routine use of MRI in hand and wrist OA. Similarly US is readily able to detect changes of OA, particularly synovitis, osteophyte and effusion (Keen et al. 2008a, b). While US appears to be more sensitive to the detection of osteophyte and joint space narrowing in hand and wrist OA than CR, its use as a diagnostic tool remains confined to the research environment (Keen et al. 2008b). US is useful as a technique for guiding therapeutic injection to the carpometacarpal joint in cases of trapeziocentric OA (Gregory et al. 2008).

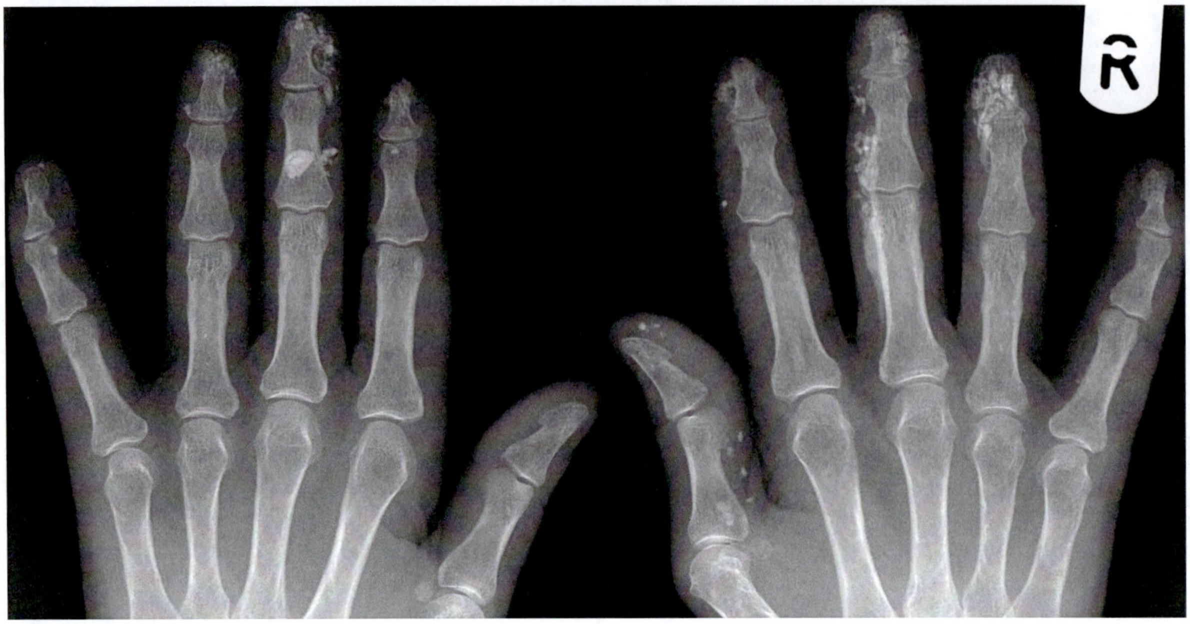

Fig. 35 Scleroderma: the study demonstrates extensive soft tissue calcification seen in subcutaneous tissues. Note also the soft tissue loss from the tips of the fingers

5 Connective Tissue Disease

5.1 Scleroderma

Scleroderma is a connective tissue disorder with characteristic radiographic abnormalities seen in the bones and soft tissues and frequently affecting the hands and wrists. Raynaud's syndrome (paroxysmal vasospasm of the digital arteries) is associated with the disease and may be the presenting feature. Joint involvement is an important component of the disease.

Radiographic features of scleroderma in the hands include:

- Soft tissue resorption at the fingertips: this is a common finding which may be visible on CR if the tissues overlying the distal tip of the terminal phalanx are examined (Fig. 35).
- Soft tissue calcification: The hand is the most common site for calcinosis seen in scleroderma and calcification may be seen in both of the subcutaneous tissues and periarticular capsular tissues. The calcification has an amorphous appearance (Fig. 35).
- Bone erosion and articular involvement: the most frequent pattern of bone loss in scleroderma involves resorption of the terminal tuft, which can result in complete destruction of the terminal phalanx. Patients may go on to develop an erosive arthropathy which generally favours the distal and PIP joints with sparing of the wrist; although it has been noted that involvement of the first carpometacarpal joint may be seen (Resnick et al. 1978). A pattern of erosive arthropathy has been reported in patients with scleroderma that much more closely resembles RA with a deforming arthropathy involving the hands and wrists (Armstrong and Gibson 1982; Baron et al. 1982). However, it has been emphasised that when these findings are seen they may represent part of an 'overlap syndrome' with features of both diseases, or indeed the coexistence of the two diseases (Armstrong and Gibson 1982).

5.2 Dermatomyositis and Polymyositis

Dermatomyositis and polymyositis are connective tissue disorders both characterised by muscle inflammation and weakness, and in the case of dermatomyositis, skin involvement. Both conditions may give rise to soft tissue calcification. Characteristically intramuscular calcification involves the proximal limb muscles, but subcutaneous calcification similar to that seen in scleroderma may be seen in the hands, as may distal phalangeal resorption. Joint involvement may also occur clinically although radiographs are normally unremarkable or show subtle changes such as periarticular osteopaenia and soft tissue swelling. Occasional reports of destructive joint changes exist (Bunch et al. 1976).

5.3 Systemic Lupus Erthematosus

Systemic lupus erthematosus (SLE) is a connective tissue disorder predominantly affecting women during childbearing years. Early clinical manifestations include systemic malaise and fever, skin rash and articular symptoms. In the later stages of the disease more severe multisystem involvement may be seen. Articular symptoms are common and have been reported in 76% of patients (Labowitz and Schumacher 1971), although the figure may be as high as 90% (Resnick 2002c). Symmetrical, bilateral involvement of the small joints of the hands is common. The most frequent finding is synovitis, and radiographs may show soft tissue swelling and osteopaenia (Weissman et al. 1978). At this stage MRI and US will demonstrate the effusion and synovial thickening. Erosive change is not typical of the disease and has only occasionally been reported (Weissman et al. 1978). This provides an important distinguishing feature from RA. It remains unclear whether those cases showing erosions in fact represent a group of patients with both SLE and RA.

A distinctive feature of SLE is a deforming nonerosive arthropathy, which may develop early in the disease course, but is more common later in the disease (Fig. 36) (Resnick 2002c; Weissman et al. 1978). Involvement is usually symmetrical involving multiple digits with a combination of deformities and subluxations that are commonly reducible. Swan-neck and Boutonniere deformities typical of those seen in RA are seen, but joint space loss and erosion are rarely seen even with severe deformities. Hyperextension at the thumb interphalangeal joint is said to be characteristic. It has been noted that the deformity may disappear when the hand is positioned for radiography (Resnick 2002c). These changes may also be seen in children where they may mimic JIA (Martini et al. 1987).

Some patients may demonstrate soft tissue calcification, and terminal phalangeal sclerosis has also been reported. The latter can occur in the absence of associated Raynaud's phenomenon (Weissman et al. 1978). Osteonecrosis is a well-recognised feature in SLE and may occur in the hands where its presence (typically in the MCP heads) should raise the question of possible SLE (Weissman et al. 1978; Fishel et al. 1987). Other features that have been reported include subchondral cyst formation, typically in the metacarpal heads and carpal bones, and occasionally 'hook erosions' seen as bony defects usually on the radial aspect of the metacarpal heads (Resnick 2002c).

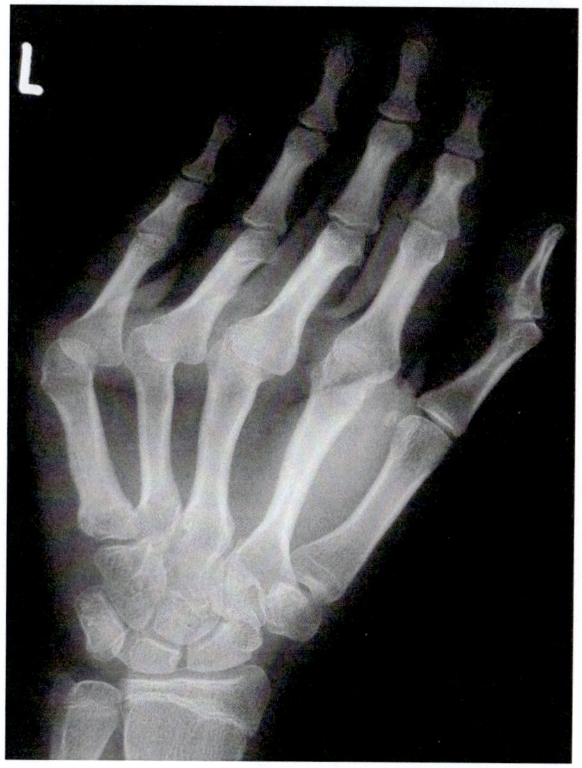

Fig. 36 SLE: subluxations, which were reversible, are seen at the MCP joints. However, note the absence of erosions and the preservation of joint spaces

5.4 Rheumatic Fever (Jaccoud's Arthropathy)

A deforming hand arthropathy associated with rheumatic fever is well recognised and is radiologically indistinguishable from the deforming non-erosive arthropathy of SLE. It has been termed Jaccoud's arthropathy. This usually occurs after repeated attacks of rheumatic arthritis.

Joint involvement is commonly seen in the course of an acute attack of rheumatic fever where multiple joints may be involved either simultaneously or successively. This joint inflammation may be seen as soft tissue swelling on CR. US and MRI may detect small joint effusions and occasionally tenosynovitis.

5.5 Mixed Connective Tissue Disease

Mixed connective tissue disease, as its name suggests, combines overlapping features of the connective tissue diseases and RA. A wide range of articular and soft tissue abnormalities may be seen on hand and wrist radiographs including osseous erosions, bone deformity, soft tissue calcification and atrophy and resorption of the terminal phalanges. Articular changes are most commonly seen in a proximal distribution similar to that seen in RA, involving PIP and MCP joints and the wrist.

References

Adamson TC 3rd, Resnik CS, Guerra J Jr, Vint VC, Weisman MH, Resnick D (1983) Hand and wrist arthropathies of hemochromatosis and calcium pyrophosphate deposition disease: distinct radiographic features. Radiology 147(2):377–381

Arend WP (2001) Physiology of cytokine pathways in rheumatoid arthritis. Arthritis Rheum 45(1):101–106

Arlart IP, Maier W, Leupold D, Wolf A (1982) Massive periosteal new bone formation in ulcerative colitis. Radiology 144(3):507–508

Armstrong RD, Gibson T (1982) Scleroderma and erosive polyarthritis: a disease entity? Ann Rheum Dis 41(2):141–146

Arnett FC (1987) Seronegative spondylarthropathies. Bull Rheum Dis 37(1):1–12

Baron M, Lee P, Keystone EC (1982) The articular manifestations of progressive systemic sclerosis (scleroderma). Ann Rheum Dis 41(2):147–152

Benjamin M, McGonagle D (2001) The anatomical basis for disease localisation in seronegative spondyloarthropathy at entheses and related sites. J Anat 199(Pt 5):503–526

Bunch TW, O'Duffy JD, McLeod RA (1976) Deforming arthritis of the hands in polymyositis. Arthritis Rheum 19(2):243–248

Chen C, Chandnani VP, Kang HS, Resnick D, Sartoris DJ, Haller J (1990) Scapholunate advanced collapse: a common wrist abnormality in calcium pyrophosphate dihydrate crystal deposition disease. Radiology 177(2):459–461

Chen CK, Chung CB, Yeh L, Pan HB, Yang CF, Lai PH et al (2000) Carpal tunnel syndrome caused by tophaceous gout: CT and MR imaging features in 20 patients. AJR Am J Roentgenol 175(3):655–659

Ciapetti A, Filippucci E, Gutierrez M, Grassi W (2009) Calcium pyrophosphate dihydrate crystal deposition disease: sonographic findings. Clin Rheumatol 28(3):271–276

Cobby M, Cushnaghan J, Creamer P, Dieppe P, Watt I (1990) Erosive osteoarthritis: is it a separate disease entity? Clin Radiol 42(4):258–263

De Haas WH, De Boer W, Griffioen F, Oosten-Elst P (1974) Rheumatoid arthritis of the robust reaction type. Ann Rheum Dis 33(1):81–85

Ehrlich GE (1972a) Inflammatory osteoarthritis. I. The clinical syndrome. J Chronic Dis 25(6):317–328

Ehrlich GE (1972b) Inflammatory osteoarthritis. II. The superimposition of rheumatoid arthritis. J Chronic Dis 25(10):635–643

El-Khoury GY, Kathol MH, Brandser EA (1996) Seronegative spondyloarthropathies. Radiol Clin N Am 34(2):343–357 xi

el-Noueam KI, Giuliano V, Schweitzer ME, O'Hara BJ (1997) Rheumatoid nodules: MR/pathological correlation. J Comput Assist Tomogr 21(5):796–799

Farrant JM, O'Connor PJ, Grainger AJ (2007a) Advanced imaging in rheumatoid arthritis. Part 1: synovitis. Skeletal Radiol 36(4):269–279

Farrant JM, Grainger AJ, O'Connor PJ (2007b) Advanced imaging in rheumatoid arthritis: part 2: erosions. Skeletal Radiol 36(5):381–389

Felson DT (2004) An update on the pathogenesis and epidemiology of osteoarthritis. Radiol Clin N Am 42(1):1–9

Fishel B, Caspi D, Eventov I, Avrahami E, Yaron M (1987) Multiple osteonecrotic lesions in systemic lupus erythematosus. J Rheumatol 14(3):601–604

Fornage BD (1989) Soft-tissue changes in the hand in rheumatoid arthritis: evaluation with US. Radiology 173(3):735–737

Gandee R, Harrison R, Dee P (1979) Peritendinitis calcaria of flexor carpi ulnaris. Am J Roentgenol 133(6):1139–1141

Gibbon WW, Wakefield RJ (1999) Ultrasound in inflammatory disease. Radiol Clin N Am 37(4):633–651

Grainger AJ, Farrant JM, O'Connor PJ, Tan AL, Tanner S, Emery P et al (2007) MR imaging of erosions in interphalangeal joint osteoarthritis: is all osteoarthritis erosive? Skeletal Radiol 36(8):737–745

Granberry WM, Mangum GL (1980) The hand in the child with juvenile rheumatoid arthritis. J Hand Surg Am 5(2):105–113

Gravallese EM, Kantrowitz FG (1988) Arthritic manifestations of inflammatory bowel disease. Am J Gastroenterol 83(7):703–709

Green L, Meyers OL, Gordon W, Briggs B (1981) Arthritis in psoriasis. Ann Rheum Dis 40(4):366–369

Gregory LU, Jeff SB, Mark-Friedrich BH, Jay S (2008) Ultrasound-guided intra-articular injection of the trapeziometacarpal joint: description of technique. Arch Phys Med Rehabil 89(1):153–156

Gubler FM, Maas M, Dijkstra PF, de Jongh HR (1990) Cystic rheumatoid arthritis: description of a nonerosive form. Radiology 177(3):829–834

Haavardsholm EA, Boyesen P, Ostergaard M, Schildvold A, Kvien TK (2008) Magnetic resonance imaging findings in 84 patients with early rheumatoid arthritis: bone marrow oedema predicts erosive progression. Ann Rheum Dis 67(6):794–800

Hetland ML, Ejbjerg B, Horslev-Petersen K, Jacobsen S, Vestergaard A, Jurik AG et al (2009) MRI bone oedema is the strongest predictor of subsequent radiographic progression in early rheumatoid arthritis. Results from a 2-year randomised controlled trial (CIMESTRA). Ann Rheum Dis 68(3):384–390

Jevtic V, Watt I, Rozman B, Kos-Golja M, Demsar F, Jarh O (1995) Distinctive radiological features of small hand joints in rheumatoid arthritis and seronegative spondyloarthritis demonstrated by contrast-enhanced (Gd-DTPA) magnetic resonance imaging. Skeletal Radiol 24(5):351–355

Johnson K, Gardner-Medwin J (2002) Childhood arthritis: classification and radiology. Clin Radiol 57(1):47–58

Jonsson A, Borg A, Hannesson P, Herrlin K, Jonsson K, Sloth M et al (1994) Film-screen vs. digital radiography in rheumatoid arthritis of the hand. An ROC analysis. Acta Radiol 35(4):311–318

Keen HI, Wakefield RJ, Grainger AJ, Hensor EM, Emery P, Conaghan PG (2008a) An ultrasonographic study of osteoarthritis of the hand: synovitis and its relationship to structural pathology and symptoms. Arthritis Rheum 59(12):1756–1763

Keen HI, Wakefield RJ, Grainger AJ, Hensor EM, Emery P, Conaghan PG (2008b) Can ultrasonography improve on radiographic assessment in osteoarthritis of the hands? A comparison between radiographic and ultrasonographic detected pathology. Ann Rheum Dis 67(8):1116–1120

Kidd KL, Peter JB (1966) Erosive osteoarthritis. Radiology 86(4):640–647

Krimmer H, Krapohl B, Sauerbier M, Hahn P (1997) Post-traumatic carpal collapse (SLAC- and SNAC-wrist)—stage classification and therapeutic possibilities. Handchir Mikrochir Plast Chir 29(5):228–233

Labowitz R, Schumacher HR Jr (1971) Articular manifestations of systemic lupus erythematosus. Ann Intern Med 74(6):911–921

Larsen A, Dale K, Eek M (1977) Radiographic evaluation of rheumatoid arthritis and related conditions by standard reference films. Acta Radiol Diagn (Stockh) 18(4):481–491

Leczinsky CG (1948) The incidence of arthropathy in a 10 year series of psoriasis cases. Acta Derm Venereol 28(5):483–487

Lin WY, Wang SJ, Lan JL (1995) Evaluation of arthritis in Reiter's disease by bone scintigraphy and radiography. Clin Rheumatol 14(4):441–444

Martel W, Champion CK, Thompson GR, Carter TL (1970) A roentgenologically distinctive arthropathy in some patients with the pseudogout syndrome. Am J Roentgenol Radium Ther Nucl Med 109(3):587–605

Martel W, Snarr JW, Horn JR (1973) The metacarpophalangeal joints in interphalangeal osteoarthritis. Radiology 108(1):1–7

Martel W, Stuck KJ, Dworin AM, Hylland RG (1980) Erosive osteoarthritis and psoriatic arthritis: a radiologic comparison in the hand, wrist, and foot. AJR Am J Roentgenol 134(1):125–135

Martini A, Ravelli A, Viola S, Burgio RG (1987) Systemic lupus erythematosus with Jaccoud's arthropathy mimicking juvenile rheumatoid arthritis. Arthritis Rheum 30(9):1062–1064

Mason RM, Murray RS, Oates JK, Young AC (1959) A comparative radiological study of Reiter's disease, rheumatoid arthritis and ankylosing spondylitis. J Bone Joint Surg Br 41-B(1):137–148

McGonagle D, Conaghan PG, O'Connor P, Gibbon W, Green M, Wakefield R et al (1999) The relationship between synovitis and bone changes in early untreated rheumatoid arthritis: a controlled magnetic resonance imaging study. Arthritis Rheum 42(8):1706–1711

McGonagle D, Tan AL, Grainger AJ, Benjamin M (2008) Heberden's nodes and what Heberden could not see: the pivotal role of ligaments in the pathogenesis of early nodal osteoarthritis and beyond. Rheumatology (Oxford) 47(9):1278–1285

McGonagle D, Benjamin M, Tan AL (2009) The pathogenesis of psoriatic arthritis and associated nail disease: not autoimmune after all? Curr Opin Rheumatol 21(4):340–347

McQueen FM, Stewart N, Crabbe J, Robinson E, Yeoman S, Tan PL et al (1999) Magnetic resonance imaging of the wrist in early rheumatoid arthritis reveals progression of erosions despite clinical improvement. Ann Rheum Dis 58(3):156–163

McQueen FM, Benton N, Perry D, Crabbe J, Robinson E, Yeoman S et al (2003) Bone edema scored on magnetic resonance imaging scans of the dominant carpus at presentation predicts radiographic joint damage of the hands and feet six years later in patients with rheumatoid arthritis. Arthritis Rheum 48(7):1814–1827

Miller JL, Soltani K, Tourtellotte CD (1971) Psoriatic acro-osteolysis without arthritis. A case study. J Bone Joint Surg Am 53(2):371–374

Mills PR, Vallance R, Birnie G, Quigley EM, Main AN, Morgan RJ et al (1981) A prospective survey of radiological bone and joint changes in primary biliary cirrhosis. Clin Radiol 32(3):297–302

Monu JU, Pope TL Jr (2004) Gout: a clinical and radiologic review. Radiol Clin N Am 42(1):169–184

Moore JR, Weiland AJ (1985) Gouty tenosynovitis in the hand. J Hand Surg Am 10(2):291–295

Nalbant S, Corominas H, Hsu B, Chen LX, Schumacher HR, Kitumnuaypong T (2003) Ultrasonography for assessment of subcutaneous nodules. J Rheumatol 30(6):1191–1195

North ER, Eaton RG (1983) Degenerative joint disease of the trapezium: a comparative radiographic and anatomic study. J Hand Surg Am 8(2):160–166

North ER, Rutledge WM (1983) The trapezium-thumb metacarpal joint: the relationship of joint shape and degenerative joint disease. Hand 15(2):201–206

Ogilvie C, Kay NR (1988) Fulminating carpal tunnel syndrome due to gout. J Hand Surg Br 13(1):42–43

Olivieri I, Barozzi L, Favaro L, Pierro A, de Matteis M, Borghi C et al (1996) Dactylitis in patients with seronegative spondylarthropathy. Assessment by ultrasonography and magnetic resonance imaging. Arthritis Rheum 39(9):1524–1528

Ostergaard M, Peterfy C, Conaghan P, McQueen F, Bird P, Ejbjerg B et al (2003) OMERACT rheumatoid arthritis magnetic resonance imaging studies. Core set of MRI acquisitions, joint pathology definitions, and the OMERACT RA-MRI scoring system. J Rheumatol 30(6):1385–1386

Paskins Z, Rai A (2006) The impact of picture archiving and communication systems (PACS) implementation in rheumatology. Rheumatology (Oxford) 45(3):354–355

Peter JB, Pearson CM, Marmor L (1966) Erosive osteoarthritis of the hands. Arthritis Rheum 9(3):365–388

Peterfy CG (2001) Magnetic resonance imaging in rheumatoid arthritis: current status and future directions. J Rheumatol 28(5):1134–1142

Petty RE, Southwood TR, Manners P, Baum J, Glass DN, Goldenberg J et al (2004) International League of Associations for Rheumatology classification of juvenile idiopathic arthritis: second revision, Edmonton, 2001. J Rheumatol 31(2):390–392

Ravelli A, Martini A (2007) Juvenile idiopathic arthritis. Lancet 369(9563):767–778

Resnick D (1974) Patterns of peripheral joint disease in ankylosing spondylitis. Radiology 110(3):523–532

Resnick D (1976) Inter-relationship between radiocarpal and metacarpophalangeal joint deformities in rheumatoid arthritis. J Can Assoc Radiol 27(1):29–36

Resnick D (2002a) Chapter 22: Juvenile chronic arthritis. In: Resnick D (ed) Diagnosis of bone and joint disorders. W.B. Saunders Co, Philadelphia, PA, pp 988–1022

Resnick D (2002b) Chapter 39: calcium pyrophosphate dihydrate crystal deposition disease. In: Resnick D (ed) Diagnosis of bone and joint disorders. W.B. Saunders Co, Philadelphia, PA, pp 1560–1618

Resnick D (2002c) Chapter 28: Systemic lupus erthematosus. In: Resnick D (ed) Diagnosis of bone and joint disorders. W.B. Saunders Co, Philadelphia, PA, pp 1171–1193

Resnick D, Greenway G, Vint VC, Robinson CA, Piper S (1978) Selective involvement of the first carpometacarpal joint in scleroderma. AJR Am J Roentgenol 131(2):283–286

Savnik A, Malmskov H, Thomsen HS, Graff LB, Nielsen H, Danneskiold-Samsoe B et al (2001) Magnetic resonance imaging of the wrist and finger joints in patients with inflammatory joint diseases. J Rheumatol 28(10):2193–2200

Savnik A, Malmskov H, Thomsen HS, Graff LB, Nielsen H, Danneskiold-Samsoe B et al (2002) MRI of the wrist and finger joints in inflammatory joint diseases at 1-year interval: MRI features to predict bone erosions. Eur Radiol 12(5):1203–1210

Scarpa R, Oriente P, Pucino A, Torella M, Vignone L, Riccio A et al (1984) Psoriatic arthritis in psoriatic patients. Br J Rheumatol 23(4):246–250

Sharp JT (1996) Scoring radiographic abnormalities in rheumatoid arthritis. Radiol Clin N Am 34(2):233–241, x

Sicre G, Laulan J, Rouleau B (1997) Scaphotrapeziotrapezoid osteoarthritis after scaphotrapezial ligament injury. J Hand Surg Br 22(2):189–190

Stadalnik RC, Dublin AB (1975) Sesamoid periostitis in the thumb in Reiter's syndrome. Case report. J Bone Joint Surg Am 57(2):279

Steinbach LS (2004) Calcium pyrophosphate dihydrate and calcium hydroxyapatite crystal deposition diseases: imaging perspectives. Radiol Clin N Am 42(1):185–205 vii

Steinbach LS, Resnick D (1996) Calcium pyrophosphate dihydrate crystal deposition disease revisited. Radiology 200(1):1–9

Tan AL, Grainger AJ, Tanner SF, Shelley DM, Pease C, Emery P et al (2005) High-resolution magnetic resonance imaging for the assessment of hand osteoarthritis. Arthritis Rheum 52(8):2355–2365

Tan AL, Grainger AJ, Tanner SF, Emery P, McGonagle D (2006a) A high-resolution magnetic resonance imaging study of distal interphalangeal joint arthropathy in psoriatic arthritis and osteoarthritis: are they the same? Arthritis Rheum 54(4):1328–1333

Tan AL, Toumi H, Benjamin M, Grainger AJ, Tanner SF, Emery P et al (2006b) Combined high-resolution magnetic resonance imaging and histological examination to explore the role of ligaments and tendons in the phenotypic expression of early hand osteoarthritis. Ann Rheum Dis 65(10):1267–1272

Thiele RG, Schlesinger N (2007) Diagnosis of gout by ultrasound. Rheumatology (Oxford) 46(7):1116–1121

Uri DS, Dalinka MK (1996) Imaging of arthropathies. Crystal disease. Radiol Clin N Am 34(2):359–374 xi

Utsinger PD, Resnick D, Shapiro RF, Wiesner KB (1978) Roentgenologic, immunologic, and therapeutic study of erosive (inflammatory) osteoarthritis. Arch Intern Med 138(5):693–697

van der Jagt EJ, Hofman S, Kraft BM, van Leeuwen MA (2000) Can we see enough? A comparative study of film-screen vs digital radiographs in small lesions in rheumatoid arthritis. Eur Radiol 10(2):304–307

Villeneuve E, Emery P (2009) Rheumatoid arthritis: what has changed? Skeletal Radiol 38(2):109–112

Vinje O, Dale K, Moller P (1985) Radiographic evaluation of patients with Bechterew's syndrome (ankylosing spondylitis). Findings in peripheral joints, tendon insertions and the pubic symphysis and relations to non-radiographic findings. Scand J Rheumatol 14(3):279–288

Wakefield RJ, Balint PV, Szkudlarek M, Filippucci E, Backhaus M, D'Agostino MA et al (2005) Musculoskeletal ultrasound including definitions for ultrasonographic pathology. J Rheumatol 32(12):2485–2487

Watson HK, Ballet FL (1984) The SLAC wrist: scapholunate advanced collapse pattern of degenerative arthritis. J Hand Surg Am 9(3):358–365

Watt I, Middlemiss H (1975) The radiology of gout. Review article. Clin Radiol 26(1):27–36

Weissman BN, Rappoport AS, Sosman JL, Schur PH (1978) Radiographic findings in the hands in patients with systemic lupus erythematosus. Radiology 126(2):313–317

Whitehouse RW, Aslam R, Bukhari M, Groves C, Cassar-Pullicino V (2005) The sesamoid index in psoriatic arthropathy. Skeletal Radiol 34(4):217–220

Wilson FC, Icen M, Crowson CS, McEvoy MT, Gabriel SE, Kremers HM (2009) Incidence and clinical predictors of psoriatic arthritis in patients with psoriasis: a population-based study. Arthritis Rheum 61(2):233–239

Yang BY, Sartoris DJ, Djukic S, Resnick D, Clopton P (1995) Distribution of calcification in the triangular fibrocartilage region in 181 patients with calcium pyrophosphate dihydrate crystal deposition disease. Radiology 196(2):547–550

Yu JS, Chung C, Recht M, Dailiana T, Jurdi R (1997) MR imaging of tophaceous gout. AJR Am J Roentgenol 168(2):523–527

Soft Tissue and Bone Infections

Rainer R. Schmitt and Georgios Christopoulos

Contents

R. R. Schmitt (✉) · G. Christopoulos
Institut für Diagnostische und Interventionelle Radiologie, Herz- und Gefäss-Klinik GmbH, Salzburger Leite 1, 97616 Bad Neustadt an der Saale, Germany
e-mail: schmitt.radiologie@herzchirurgie.de

Abstract

Penetrating injuries and staphylococceal pathogens are the most frequent causes of infections at the hand, with the soft tissues involved in about 95%, and the bones and joints in 5%, only. In soft tissue infections, MRI is mostly necessary for depicting infections of the deep palmar spaces, whereas finger infections are prome to clinical examination. Typically, bone and joint infections are first visible in radiograms two weeks after clinical onset. MRI is powerful in early detection and in the assessment of spreading of both osteomyelitis and infectious arthritis, the adjacent soft tissues included. CT imaging is the modality of choice in the search of sequestra and cloaca when the superficial soft tissues and the skin are involved in chronic osteomyelitis. At the hands, rare infections are of tuberculous, syphilitic, leprous, viral, fungal, and parasitic orgin.

1 General Aspects

1.1 Introduction

Infectious diseases of the hand affect the soft tissues, the bones, and the joints solely or in combination. In the past, the final diagnosis was made by clinical, laboratory findings, and radiographic survey views (Hausman and Lisser 1992). However, the approach toward dedicated diagnostic imaging has changed for several reasons in the last decade (Pineda et al. 2009; Santiago-Restrepo et al. 2003): First, imaging accuracy has significantly improved with the introduction of the high-resolution techniques of ultrasound, CT,

A. M. Davis et al. (eds.), *Imaging of the Hand and Wrist*, Medical Radiology. Diagnostic Imaging,
DOI: 10.1007/174_2010_112,

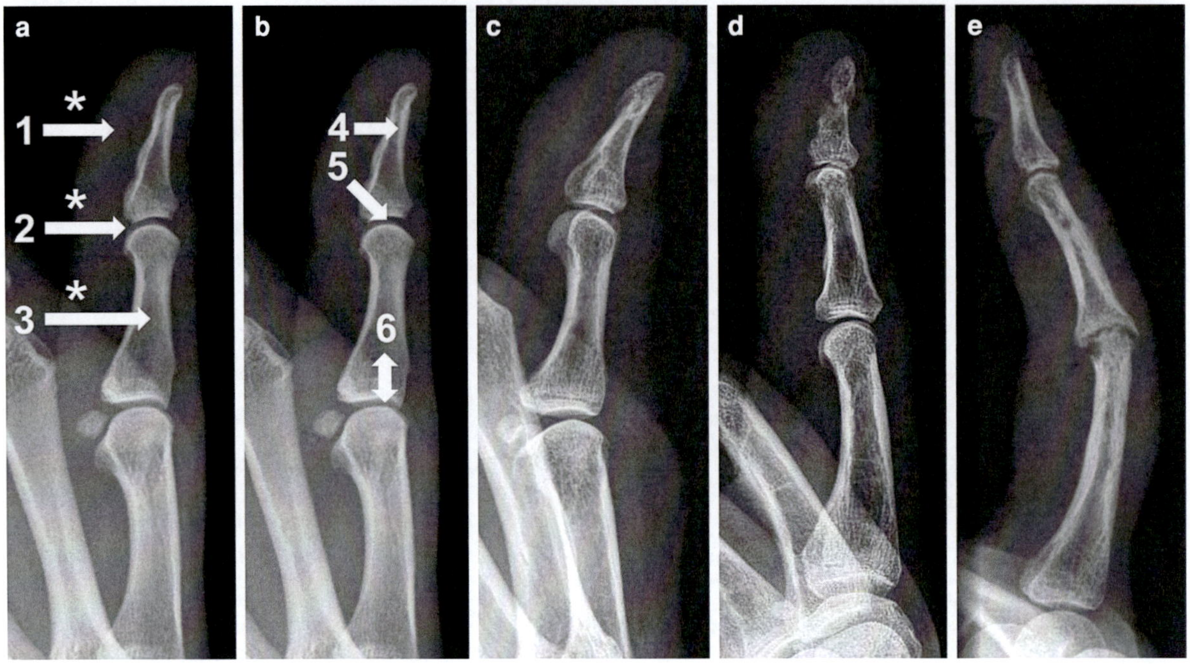

Fig. 1 Synopsis of the infectious pathways at the hand skeleton. **a** Direct pathways of infection with implantation or hematogenous spread of pathogens into the soft tissue (*1*), the joint (*2*), and the bone (*3*). *Stars* are used for symbolizing both the direct and hematogenous infection routes. **b** Indirect pathways comprising spreads of an infection from the soft tissues into the bone (*4*) or into the joint (*5*), and finally from the bone marrow into the adjacent joint and vice versa (*6*). **c** Marked thickening of the palmar digital bulb in the presence of a felon. The bony terminal phalanx is not involved. **d** In another case, infectious spread of a felon from the palmar soft tissues to the terminal phalanx is evident and has caused infectious bone destruction. **e** Subacute bacterial arthritis of the proximal interphalangeal joint immediately following a penetrating stab injury. There are deep erosions of the subchondral plates aside onset of sclerosing bone reaction

and MRI. Second, the advance of refined surgical and medical treatment options has increased the pretension according to detailed wrist and hand imaging. Third, the spectrum of hand infections has changed over the years with the expansion of the worldwide travel and the increasing number of surviving individuals suffering from immunodeficiency diseases.

Early diagnosis of hand infections is essential to prevent functional impairment or even destruction disease which usually remains secondary to delayed or insufficient treatment.

1.2 Routes of Infection

The soft tissues, bones, and joints of the hand can be contaminated by different routes (Fig. 1) (Tsai and Failla 1999; Resnick 1976):

- *Direct implantation of pathogens*: The infection arises directly after penetrating injuries with disruption of the overlying skin. This route is by far most frequent at the hands. In a similar pathway, pathogens can be incidentally inoculated during arthrography and arthroscopy, in open surgery as well as in transcutaneous insertion of pins.
- *Spread from a neighbored source of infection*: An infectious focus extends from one tissue layer to another, e.g. from the subcutis to the bones or joints, or from the bone marrow to an adjacent joint and the surrounding soft tissues, or from one to another communicating tendon sheath.
- *Hematogenous spread of infection*: Pathogens are inoculated via the blood circulation. Common sources of transient bacteremia are the respiratory, genitourinary, and gastrointestinal systems asides others and equivocal cases. This pathway is infrequent at the hands.

1.3 Imaging Techniques

Conventional radiograms (CR) complimented by fluoroscopic spot views in equivocal cases are exposed to exclude or confirm inflammatory involvement of the hand skeleton. Eight to ten days usually pass before signs of osteomyelitis are visible. Early signs of acute osteomyelitis include subtle periosteal reaction and focal subperiosteal osteopenia (Capitanio and Kirkpatrick 1970). Osteolyses follow within the next weeks, and osteosclerosis appears in the chronic stage. Obliteration and swelling of the periarticular soft-tissue planes ("soft-tissue sign of arthritis"), periarticular osteopenia ("collateral sign of arthritis") as well as articular destruction ("direct signs of arthritis") appear in acute pyogenic arthritis and will progress in days to weeks. Soft-tissue calcifications are sometimes seen in tuberculosis of the tendon sheath.

Nuclear scintigraphy (NUC) with ^{99m}Tc phosphonates provides information about local hyperemia when using the three-phase technique (angiographic, blood pool, and delayed phases). For early detection of an infectious source, this technique is useful days and weeks before abnormalities become visible in radiograms (Gold et al. 1991). If scintigraphic results are unremarkable, an acute infection of the hand skeleton can be excluded. Soft-tissue infections lead to regional hyperemia with a diffuse nuclide uptake in the area involved and the contiguous bone skeleton. If soft-tissue infection directly spreads to the adjacent bones and joints, a marked nuclide uptake indicating hyperemic bone metabolism is mostly evident in three-phase scintigrams. However, positive scintigraphy does not allow differentiation between posttraumatic bone remodeling and infection, because an increased formation of fibrous bone, and therefore, an increased binding of ^{99m}Tc phosphonates is seen in both disease entities (Schauwecker 1989). This is also the case in chronic osteomyelitis. Differentiation can be tried with gallium scintigraphy which is sensitive to active bone disease (Pineda et al. 2009; Gold et al. 1991).

Scintigraphy with ^{99m}Tc-HMPAO-labeled leukocytes and ^{99m}Tc-nanocolloids as well as immunoscintigraphy with ^{99m}Tc-labeled monoclonal granulocytes or human unspecific immunoglobulin selectively demonstrates acute granulocyte-induced inflammations (Schauwecker 1989). There are some limitations: First, in the early months after an injury, leukocytic scintigraphy cannot differentiate between reparative remodeling and inflammatory processes. Second, in aseptic arthritis such as rheumatoid arthritis and chronic infections such as tuberculous or leprous arthritis, uptake of labeled granulocytes can simulate findings of active osteomyelitis and pyogenic arthritis.

Ultrasonography (US) is the first-line imaging method when a fluid or abscess collection is assumed in the soft tissues and joint spaces (Kothari et al. 2001). For high-resolution US of the hands, probes of 10 MHz or more must be used. An important indication of US is the search for foreign bodies that are invisible in radiograms (Peterson et al. 2002). In the presence of osteomyelitis, involvement of the contiguous soft tissues can be screened with US.

Computed tomography (CT) is well suited to delineate the destructive bone processes in osteomyelitis, i.e. the sequestrum, the surrounding granulation tissue, and the involucrum. A sequestrum can be reliably detected in CT imaging by means of its dense eburnization and its location within the granulation tissue (Pineda et al. 2009; Santiago-Restrepo et al. 2003; Gold et al. 1991). Due to less sensitivity in comparison with MRI, CT is applied in the evaluation of soft-tissue inflammation in equivocal cases only for the search of foreign bodies and intraosseous or intraarticular air collections. Because osteomyelitis is often associated with soft-tissue infection, intravenous administration of a contrast agent is recommended for proper detection. The imaging features of an abscess are the peripheral enhancement and the semi-liquid abscess center (Kothari et al. 2001). Retrograde contrast-filling of a sinus tract (sinography) can be combined with CT scanning to depict the course of a sinus tract from the cutaneous orifice back to its medullary origin (Santiago-Restrepo et al. 2003). Finally, CT imaging—and also ultrasonography—is used for guiding percutaneous punctures of soft tissues, bones, and joints to obtain fluid for bacteriologic evaluation.

Magnetic resonance imaging (MRI) is very sensitive in detecting infections of the soft tissues, the bones, and joints and in depicting the extension of the inflammation (Pineda et al. 2009; Gold et al. 1991; Hopkins et al. 1995; Towers 1997; Morrison et al. 1993). The use of a dedicated surface coils or phased-array multi-channel coils is premise for MRI of the hand to obtain high-resolution images. In literature, the necessity of intravenous gadolinium is controversially discussed. According to the authors' experience, the administration of gadolinium is mandatory for further characterizing infectious bone, joint, and soft-tissue edema. Differentiation between vascularized inflammatory tissue and central abscess colliquation zone is facilitated with the use of gadolinium (Hopkins et al. 1995; Towers 1997; Morrison et al. 1993). However, it must be mentioned that MRI is inferior to CT imaging in detecting sequestra (Pineda et al. 2009; Gold et al. 1991). The T2-weighted fat-saturated FSE sequence (alternatively, the STIR-FSE sequence) and the T1-weighted fat-saturated SE sequence after gadolinium—both acquired in the transaxial plane—are most suitable to determine extra- and intraosseous inflammatory processes. The other imaging planes are crucial to determine the extent of the infection in the longitudinal direction.

2 Soft-Tissue Infections

In about 95% of all infections of the hand, exclusively the soft tissues are involved, namely the cutaneous, subcutaneous, fascial, tendinous, ligamentous, muscular, and synovial structures, whereas bones and/or joints are affected in only about 5% (Hausman and Lisser 1992; Tsai and Failla 1999). The heterogeneous spectrum comprises paronychia, felons, suppurative tenosynovitis, deep space infections, and gangrenous infections. The most common cause in etiology is a penetrating injury, while hematogenous spread is less frequent (Tsai and Failla 1999; Resnick 1976). Even the tiniest injury, such as a paronychial tear during nail care, is sufficient to inoculate pathogenic organisms. Individuals with a compromised immune system and/or sensory deficiency (e.g. patients suffering from diabetes mellitus or severe carpal tunnel syndrome) are predisposed to infections. In initial stages, infections mostly remain at the site of origin, since there are a number of anatomically defined compartments, like the subcutaneous space, the deep palmar spaces, the tendon sheaths, and the joint compartments. Clinical symptoms are local redness, hyperthermia, swelling, pain, and functional impairment.

Physical examination is usually sufficient for final diagnosis. However, when clinical uncertainty exists, diagnostic imaging can provide essential information for treatment decision, e.g. if an abscess in the deep spaces must be excluded or localized precisely (Beltran 1995). Furthermore, the pathogens can be identified with ultrasound-guided aspiration to specifically initiate antibiotic medication.

2.1 Soft-Tissue Infections at the Fingers and Midcarpus

The following types of soft-tissue infection can be differentiated by location:

A *paronychia* is an acute infection of the space surrounding the eponychial fold, mostly caused by *Staphylococcus aureus*, less frequently by anaerobic or fungal pathogens (Jebson 1998a). Paronychial infections often begin after nail care and immediately spread around the eponychium to develop a purulent drainage. Lymphadenitis can be present. Chronic courses of paronychia caused by *Candida albicans* are seen in diabetic individuals.

A *felon* is a closed space infection of the palmar digital bulb which can easily follow a skin lesion or a bagatelle injury (Jebson 1998a). The terminal phalanx is swollen, red, and painful.

A *collar button abscess* is a purulent infection of the interdigital subfascial web space (Jebson 1998b). Symptoms include painful swelling, redness, fluctuance, and tenderness of the web space with neighbored fingers being in an abducted posture.

A pyogenic *dumbbell infection* is located at the dorsoradial aspect and involves the thenar space, the first web and interosseous spaces, and the abductor pollicis muscle (Jebson 1998b). Mostly, the infection begins at the thenar space before extending into the peripheral and deep spaces.

Suppurative flexor tenosynovitis is a pyogenic infection of one or several flexor tendon sheaths which mostly is not only located at the digits but also in the midcarpal palm (Langer 2009).

In *radiograms*, swelling and obliteration of the tissue planes are characteristic. Bubbly gas inclusions are derived either from skin disruption or from gas-forming pathogens. Radiograms should always be ordered in the presence of phalangeal soft-tissue infection to confirm or exclude accompanying osteitis, osteomyelitis or even infective arthritis. Other than in paronychia, bone involvement is frequent in felons (Fig. 1c, d). When the infection has spread into the depth down to the osseous and/or articular surfaces, radiologic signs of osteitis include subtle periosteal thickening, indistinctly demarcated erosions,

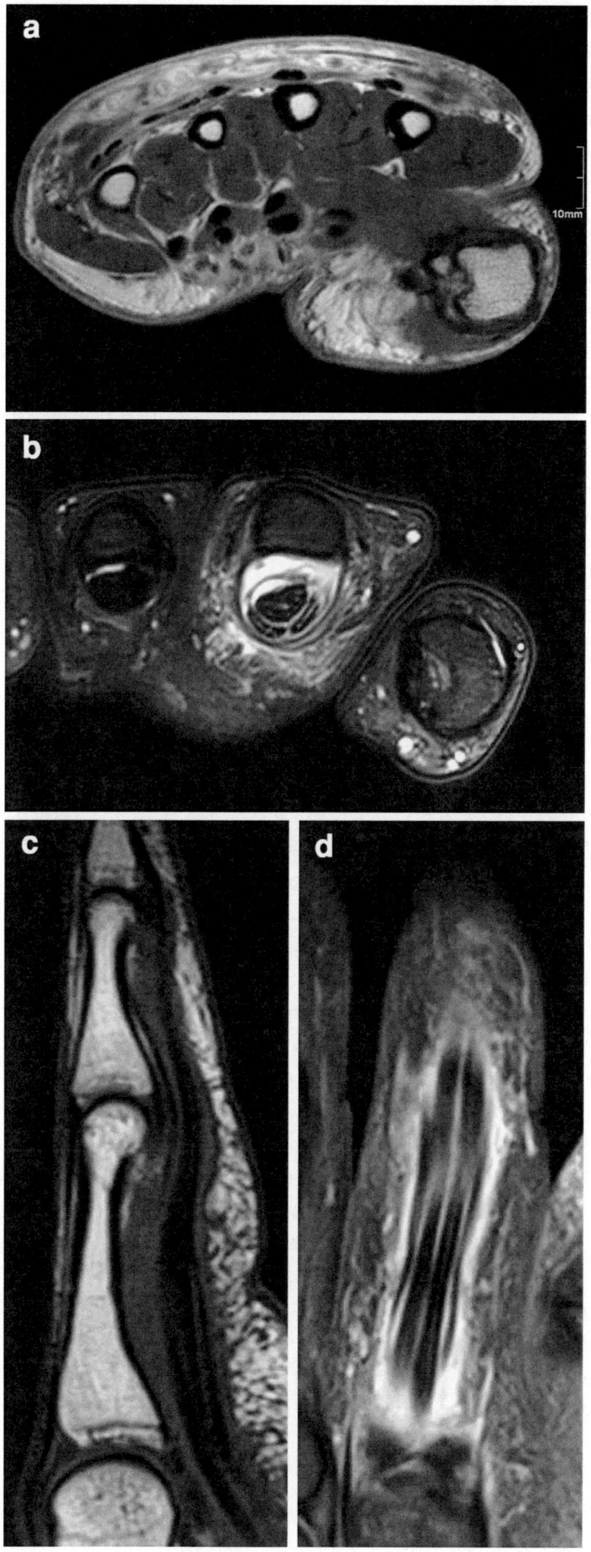

◄ **Fig. 2** Contrast-enhanced MRI of suppurative soft infections. **a** Massive phlegmon (cellulitis) at the dorsum of the metacarpus. In the T1-weighted SE image after gadolinium, the subcutaneous layer appears thickened and presents with increased contrast enhancement. Areas of low signal intensity are included and are suspicious of initial abscess. **b–d** Suppurative flexor tenosynovitis of the index finger following an open cut injury. The flexor tendon sheath is semi-circumferentially thickened. After application of gadolinium, marked contrast enhancement of the tendon sheath is evident on the T1-weighted SE images with fat-saturation (**b** and **d**) when compared with the non-enhanced image (**c**). Areas of low signal intensity are not included, and therefore, abscess formation must not be assumed. Inflammation of the adjacent soft tissues is accompanying

and focal subperiosteal osteopenia (Capitanio and Kirkpatrick 1970). After progressing to osteomyelitis, sharp osteolyses appear. When subtle osteopenia of the subchondral articular bone plate becomes visible, concomitant arthritis of the metacarpophalangeal and interphalangeal joints must be assumed. Radiograms are also needed for the search of radiodense foreign bodies. Both US and MRI are useful tools for differentiating cellulitis from abscess formation in the soft tissues (Fig. 2a).

2.2 Supporative Flexor Tenosynovitis

Supporative tenosynovitis is caused by spread from a subcutaneous abscess or by a penetrating injury with inoculation of pathogens from which most common are *Staphylococcus aureus* and Streptococci (Langer 2009). The proximal interphalangeal joint and the middle phalanx are preferred sites of puncture wounds. Symptoms are summarized by the Kanavel's signs: Flexed posture and swelling of the affected digit, tenderness over the flexor sheath, and pain on passive extension of the digit. Lymphadenitis is usually present. Rarely, a V-shaped phlegmon involving two or more fingers can develop due to communicating tendon sheaths. More frequent is a phlegmon that migrates from the thumb proximally into the carpal tunnel thereby causing a hyperacute carpal tunnel syndrome.

Radiograms serve to exclude concomitant osteomyelitis and/or arthritis and to detect foreign bodies (Resnick 1976; Capitanio and Kirkpatrick 1970; Kothari et al. 2001). Osteopenia and cortical erosions at the neighbored bone may be evident. Infectious tenosynovitis can nicely be demonstrated with US

(Jeffrey et al. 1997). There is a thickened, moderately hyperechoic tendon sheath directly aside the hypo- to anechoic synovial fluid. An enclosed foreign body is detectable by means of its hyperechoic pattern and its distal acoustic shadow. Foreign bodies are usually found in the center of infections. The same diagnostic criteria apply for tenosynovitis in MRI (Fig. 2). The inflamed tendon sheath is thickened, hyperintense in T2-weighted sequences, and presents an intense, peripheral contrast enhancement in T1-weighted, fat-saturated sequences after gadolinium (Towers 1997; Beltran 1995). Intravenous gadolinium is helpful in differentiating encapsulated synovial fluid in tendon overuse from suppurative tenosynovitis, both presenting with a thickened synovium. The transaxial imaging plane is most important for detection, whereas both the coronal and sagittal planes enable precise assessment of the longitudinal extension of tenosynovitis. Often, secondary edema in the adjacent soft tissues and in the tendon itself (tendinitis) is accompanying.

2.3 Tuberculosis of the Tendon Sheaths

Musculoskeletal tuberculosis is currently beginning to rise again. *Mycobacterium marinum*, avium or kansasii are the pathogens (Hausman and Lisser 1992; Hoffman et al. 1996). Clinical symptoms are mild and inconclusive. Only a doughy, painless swelling along the flexor tendons can be present at clinical examination. Thus, the "great masquerader" of tuberculosis should always be taken into consideration when a palmar, indolent soft-tissue swelling of unknown origin fails to medical and surgical treatment.

Radiograms are usually normal in soft-tissue tuberculosis. Infrequently, foggy and indistinct spots of calcification can be found, but can be hidden by bony structures in standard views. CT is usually not indicated to search for these calcifications, but when performed for other reasons, peritendinous location of foggy calcifications is highly suggestive of tuberculosis. In the differential diagnosis, an acute inflammatory onset is suspicious for hydroxyapatite deposition disease, whereas a chronic, insidious course is characteristic of soft-tissue tuberculosis or sarcoidosis. In US, tuberculous tenosynovitis can be assessed by means of a synovial fluid and the thickened tendon sheaths, which is hyperechoic in comparison with non-tuberculous tenosynovitis. In MRI, the tuberculous tendon sheaths appear distended and swollen and show a marked synovial contrast enhancement (Hoffman et al. 1996; Jaovisidha et al. 1996). These findings often contradict the minor patient's symptoms and are therefore guiding for the final diagnosis (Fig. 3a). The differential diagnosis includes chronic tenosynovitis of other origin, e.g. tenosynovial sarcoidosis.

Aside the tendon sheaths, other soft-tissue compartment of the hands can be infected by atypical mycobacterial bacilli in individuals with impaired resistance (Hoyen et al. 1998). *Mycobacterium marinum* is seen in soft-tissue infections of fishermen and aquarium workers and *Mycobacterium terrae* in infections of gardeners (Fig. 3b).

2.4 Infections of the Deep Palmar Spaces

Superficial infections can continuously spread into the deep compartments of the palm, often with the primary infection already healed when the deep abscess becomes symptomatic. Pain and function impairment are almost always present. However, redness and swelling can be missed because superficial tissue is covering the affected spaces. In the depth, there are anatomically defined compartments (Fig. 4a) (Jebson 1998b): (1) the thenar space (built by the short muscles of the thumb), (2) the hypothenar space (built by the short muscles of the little finger), (3) the carpal tunnel (bordered by the palmar flexor retinaculum), (4) the Guyon's canal (superficial and ulnar-sided to the carpal tunnel), (5) the Parona's space (deep to the flexor tendons at the distal forearm), and (6) the metacarpal space (deep to the flexor tendons at the metacarpus).

Radiograms are only performed to exclude concomitant osteomyelitis. This is also possible with the use of skeletal scintigraphy (*NUC*). An abscess is classically visualized in US by means of an anechoic or hypoechoic center associated with distal acoustic shadowing, and a hyperechoic wall of granulation tissue (Jeffrey et al. 1997). Membranous septa are often seen within the abscess. However, there are some diagnostic limitations: While huge and focal abscesses are reliably detectable with US, small abscesses deep in the carpal tunnel remain difficult to visualize due to acoustic absorption phenomena of the superficially traversing flexor tendons. Furthermore, it is difficult to depict the entire extent of a

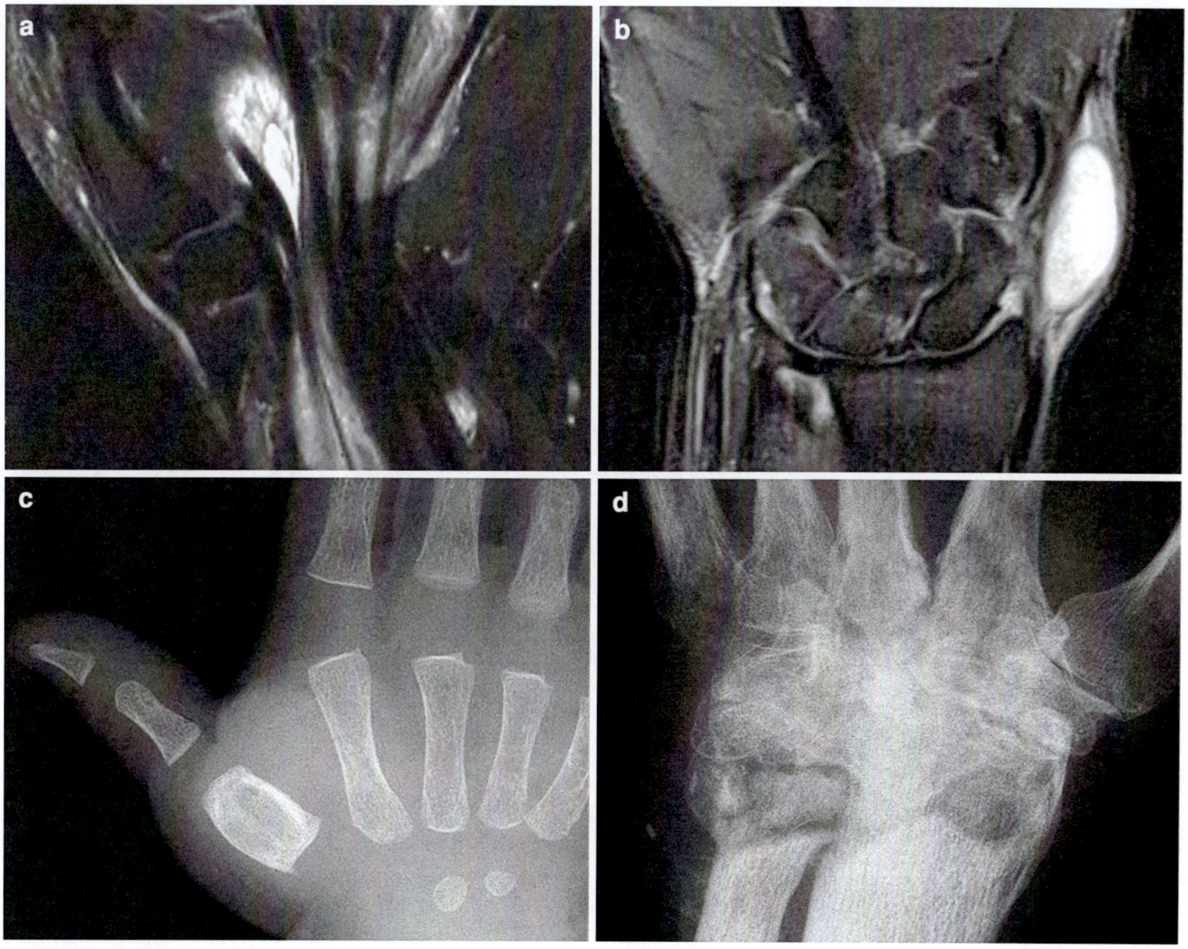

Fig. 3 Synopsis of the different sites of tuberculosis at the soft tissues and bones of the hand. **a** Tuberculous tenosynovitis in a female presenting with a doughty, painless swelling of her palm. In the contrast-enhanced T1-weighted SE scan with fat = saturation, there is a communicating tenosynovitis of the flexor pollicis longus and the flexor digitorum tendons at the levels of the Parona's space, the carpal tunnel, and the metacarpal space. **b** Tuberculous abscess in the subcutaneous layer of the thenar space (fat-saturated PD-weighted FSE image). Surprisingly, micro-bacterial evaluation revealed *Mycobacterium marinum* in this patient who was retrospectively identified as a hobby angler. **c** Tuberculous dactylitis of the thumb in a 1-year-old infant. There is the characteristic spina ventosa of the first metacarpal bone with increased volume, central osteolysis, and thickened compact bone. **d** Tuberculous arthritis of the wrist in an advanced stage with destruction, collapse, and ankylosis of the carpus. The ongoing inflammatory process is indicated by cystic radiolucencies, indistinct joint contours, and soft-tissue swelling. Calcifications in the soft tissues are also seen. Figures **a**, **c**, and **d** with permission from Schmitt R, Lanz U. Diagnostic imaging of the hand and wrist. Thieme International. Stuttgart, New York 2008

multi-compartmental abscess formation and to differentiate it from a sympathetic effusion. Abscesses can also be detected and determined in size by using CT imaging, although its capability is inferior to that of MRI. In CT, the signs of an abscess are the semi-liquid center of about 30–50 HU and the peripheral, contrast-enhancing wall (Jaovisidha et al. 1996). Preferentially, MRI should be applied if an abscess of the deep palmar spaces is suspected (Fig. 4b, c). MRI provides the most precise information for these purposes (Hopkins et al. 1995; Towers 1997; Beltran 1995). The semi-liquid center of an abscess is hyperintense in T2-weighted sequences and hypointense in T1-weighted sequences, in the latter with a strong peripheral enhancement seen after intravenous application of gadolinium. This pattern of contrast enhancement differentiates an abscess from a phlegmon as well as from a serous fluid collection.

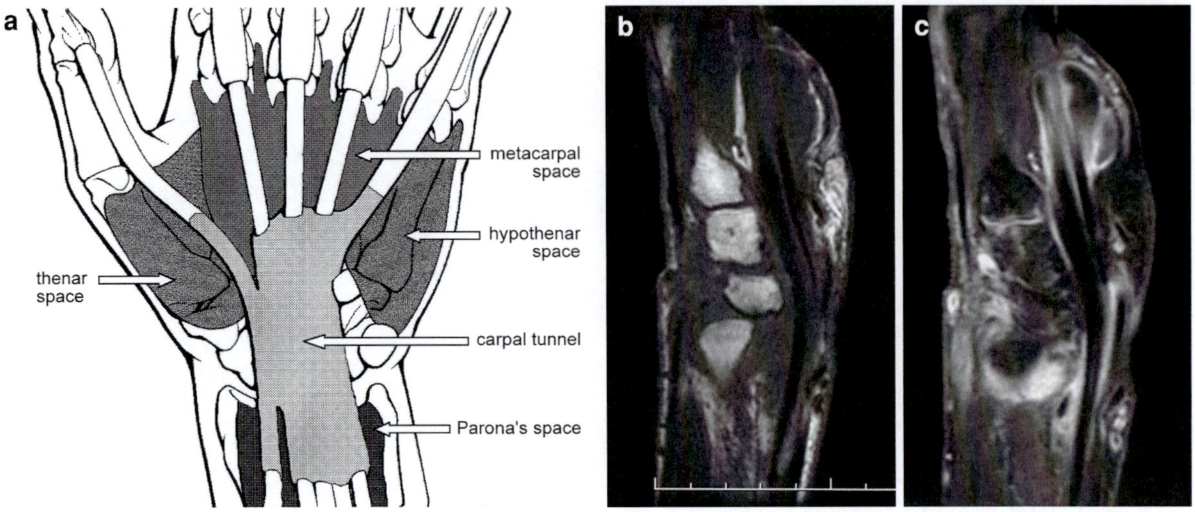

Fig. 4 Infections of the deep palmar spaces. **a** Schematic illustration of the deep palmar spaces (view into the palm). Indicated are the thenar and hypothenar spaces, the Parona's space (deep to the flexor tendons), the carpal tunnel, and the metacarpal space (deep to the flexor tendons). The Guyon's tunnel that is located ulnar-sided to the carpal tunnel is not depicted. **b–c** Deep palmar abscess extending over several deep spaces. Sagittal T1-weighted SE images before (**b**) and after (**c**) application of gadolinium. The contrast-enhanced images comprehensively depict suppurative tenosynovitis of the flexor tendons in the Parona's space, the carpal tunnel, and the metacarpal space. Central areas of low signal intensity in the Parona's and metacarpal spaces are typical of an abscess formation

2.5 Gangrenous Infection

Gangrene is a rare anaerobic infection of the soft tissues caused by gas- and toxin-producing anaerobic pathogens (Hausman and Lisser 1992; Hoyen et al. 1998). The most common pathogen is *Clostridium perfringens*. The infection spreads in the subcutaneous space and within the compartments along the fasciae. Muscle ischemia and devitalized tissues may proceed and are considered as predisposing factors. The initial symptom can solely be local tenderness, followed by rapidly spreading inflammation. Cutaneous crepitation can be present, but does not confirm gangrenous infection. Life-threatening impairment of the general condition soon develops.

Survey *radiograms* characteristically show patchy gas inclusions in the soft tissues, especially in the subcutaneous and subfascial layers. Low-kilovoltage radiograms and CT imaging can be advantageous in equivocal cases.

2.6 Pyomyositis and Necrotizing Fasciitis

These infection types are extremely rare at the distal forearm and hand and are mentioned here for completeness only.

Pyomyositis is a muscle infection mostly caused by *Staphylococcus aureus* in immunodeficient patients (Gonzales 1998). The intra-muscular mass is characterized by an abscess formation in contrast-enhanced MRI (or CT imaging).

Necrotizing fasciitis is a serious, life-threatening infection of the superficial and deep fasciae in the absence of muscular and cutaneous infections (Gonzales 1998). Pathogens are *Streptococcus pyogenes* alone or in combination with *Staphylococcus aureus*. In imaging, the fasciae appear thickened and inflamed. Gas bubbles and fluid collections can be included.

3 Osteomyelitis

Osteomyelitis of the hand is usually the result of a soft-tissue infection caused by penetrating injuries with implantation of pathogens into the soft tissues and contiguous spread to the bone via the tendon sheaths, fasciae, and lymphatic vessels (Hausman and Lisser 1992; Tsai and Failla 1999; Resnick 1976; Barbieri and Freeland 1998). In open fractures, pathogens can be directly inoculated into the bone. These "secondary" types of osteomyelitis are

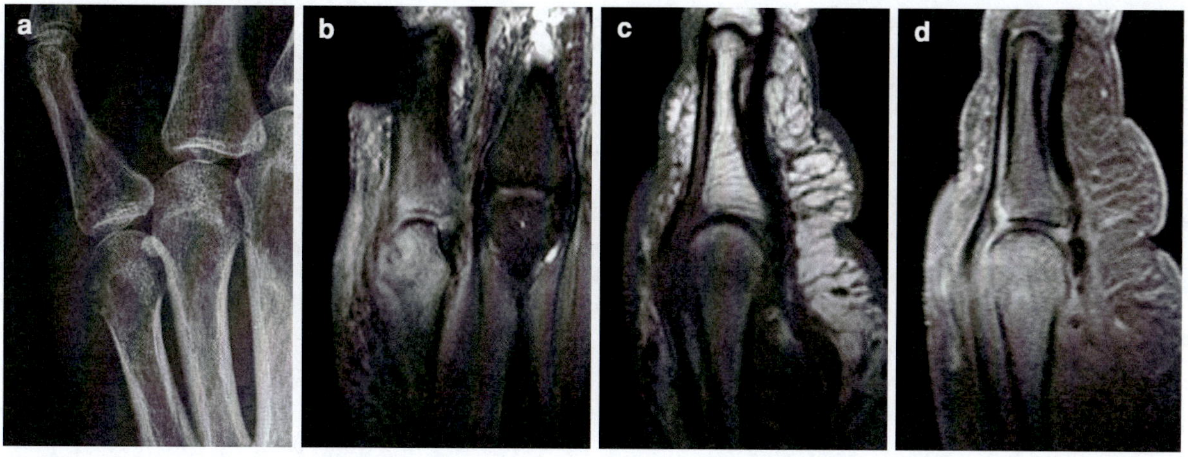

Fig. 5 Osteomyelitis and initial bacterial arthritis of the metacarpophalangeal joint of the little finger following a fist blow. **a** Obliteration of the soft-tissue planes and focal, subchondral demineralization at the dorso-ulnar segment of the fifth metacarpal head, depicted on a semi-pronated, oblique X-ray view. **b** Diffuse edema is present in the periarticular soft tissues as well as in the metacarpal head and the base of the proximal phalanx (coronal, fat-saturated PD-weighted image). **c** and **d** Sagittal T1-weighted SE images before and after application of gadolinium without and with fat saturation show hyperenhancement of the dorsal soft tissues with the joint capsule and synovia included and in the inflamed bone marrow of the metacarpal head

frequent because the hands are predisposed to injuries in workaday life. On the contrary, the hematogenous spread of ("primary") osteomyelitis is rare at the hand skeleton. The spectrum of pathogens includes *Staphylococcus aureus*, *Streptococcus pyogenes* and group B streptococci, and *Escherichia coli* (Tsai and Failla 1999; Barbieri and Freeland 1998; Reilly et al. 1997). Haemophilus influenza is a frequent pathogen in childhood, while fungal and tuberculous pathogens are more often seen in adulthood (Hoyen et al. 1998).

Osteomyelitis is defined as an infection of the bone marrow and the ossified bone substance itself (Pineda et al. 2009; Barbieri and Freeland 1998). Subcategories imply the osteitis (infection of the bone cortex) and the infectious periostitis (infection of the periosteal cloak). Further classification is based on the time course with differentiation of acute, subacute, and chronic osteomyelitis, all of them with fluent and non-definitive transitions (Pineda et al. 2009).

3.1 Time Course of Osteomyelitis

3.1.1 Acute Osteomyelitis

Acute osteomyelitis presents with acute redness, swelling, pain, and functional impairment of the hand area affected aside fever and general complaints (Tsai and Failla 1999; Barbieri and Freeland 1998). Acute osteomyelitis leads to progressive bone destruction.

Radiograms provide the imaging basis of acute osteomyelitis (Pineda et al. 2009; Resnick 1976; Gold et al. 1991; Schauwecker 1989). However, one should keep in mind that radiologic findings lag behind the onset of the infection by about 8–10 days. The earliest signs include obliteration of the parossal soft tissue fat planes and a focal area of decreased bone density (Capitanio and Kirkpatrick 1970). In the next days, aggressive bone destruction follows in a permeative pattern. Radiolucent, poorly defined osteolyses appear at the infectious focus (Fig. 5a). Finally, the infection leads to endosteal scalloping and cortical disintegration, and subtle or marked periosteal lesions at the metaphyseal level. In the acute phase of osteomyelitis, MRI is the imaging method of choice for two reasons (Pineda et al. 2009; Santiago-Restrepo et al. 2003; Gold et al. 1991; Hopkins et al. 1995; Towers 1997; Morrison et al. 1993): First, inflammatory bone marrow edema is the earliest finding which can be appreciated with MRI as early as 3 days after the onset of infection. The edema and exudates within the medullary space produce ill-defined high signals on fat-suppressed T2-weighted or STIR images and a low signal on T1-weighted images (Figs. 5b, 6a). Second, contrast-enhanced T1-weighted images

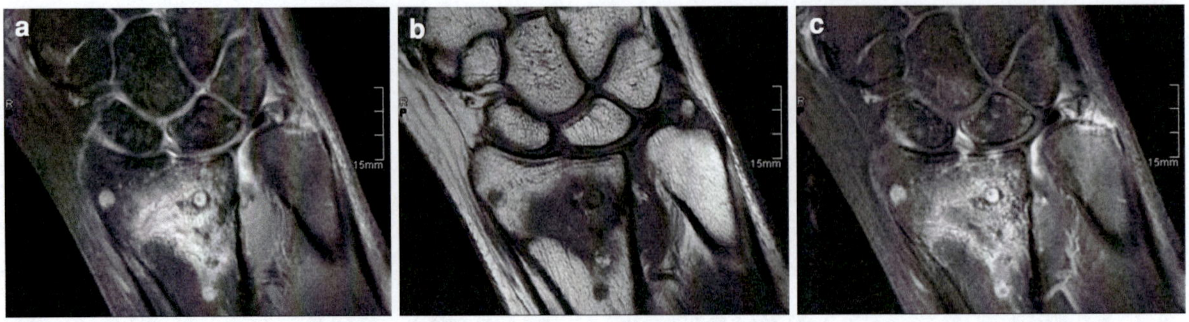

Fig. 6 Acute osteomyelitis of the distal end of the radius following 3 months after palmar plate osteosynthesis. After plate removal, X-ray views were completely unremarkable with regard to osteomyelitis. In MRI, a territorial zone of bone marrow edema (**a** and **b**) and peripheral contrast enhancement (**c**) is visible at the meta-epiphyseal section of the radius, and a parossal abscess located in the soft tissues between the radius and ulna is also recognizable. PD-weighted FSE sequence with fat-saturation (**a**), non-enhanced T1-weighted SE sequence (**b**), and contrast-enhanced T1-weighted SE sequence with fat-suppression (**c**), all acquired in the coronal plane

acquired in 3 planes allow a comprehensive assessment of the osteomyelitic extent by better differentiation of hypervascularized areas from non-viable and edematous areas in the affected bone and the soft tissues (Figs. 5d, 6c).

Complete clinical information is required for the differential diagnosis of permeative ("moth-eaten") bone lesions (Santiago-Restrepo et al. 2003; Resnick 1976; Capitanio and Kirkpatrick 1970). With this respect, healing of osteomyelitis can be correctly assessed only when judging both the clinical and imaging findings, because in the healing phase bone resorption is still continuing and simulating progressive osteomyelitis in radiograms, although the clinical symptoms are already improving (Erdman et al. 1991). The differential diagnosis includes malignant bone tumors, such as osteosarcoma, Ewing's sarcoma, and bone lymphoma. In most cases, bone destruction in acute osteomyelitis is more rapid and extensive in comparison with the malignant tumors mentioned.

3.1.2 Subacute Osteomyelitis

Brodie's Abscess

In staphylococcal osteomyelitis, an intra-osseous abscess can develop in individuals with immunologic deficiency, mainly in young boys. At the hand and forearm, there is a predilection for the distal ends of the radius and ulna. In *radiograms*, a round or elongated radiolucency with surrounding osteosclerosis, tortuous shape, and a connection to the growth plate is characteristic of a Brodie's abscess (Pineda et al. 2009; Miller et al. 1979). In MRI, the so-called "penumbra sign" is indicative. This sign describes a well-defined lesion which is composed of a central colliquation zone and a small peripheral zone of increased contrast enhancement surrounded by bone marrow edema in T1-weighted images (Grey et al. 1998). Mostly, Brodie's abscesses are located in the metaphysis, less frequently in the epiphysis (Fig. 6). However, locations in the diaphysis and cortex have been describted making differentiation to osteoid osteoma difficult even with the use of CT and MRI.

Plasma-Cell Osteomyelitis and Garré's Sclerosing Osteomyelitis

These special forms of osteomyelitis are infrequently found at the hands (Reilly et al. 1997). They are characterized by the appearance of osteosclerosis and the tendency of a chronic course. A pathogen usually cannot be isolated, both entities are non-purulent. A pathogenetic association to chronic recurrent multifocal osteomyelitis has been assumed. The diagnosis of Garré's osteomyelitis should be restricted to those cases of sclerosing osteomyelitis in which no sequestrum and granulation tissue can be found.

3.1.3 Chronic Osteomyelitis

The chronic stage is characterized by the development of sequestra, the formation of involucrum, and the deformation of the bone affected (Barbieri and Freeland 1998; Kaim et al. 2002). A *sequestrum* is a necrotic bone fragment which has developed from destruction of the cortical or cancellous bone (Pineda et al. 2009). Often, pathogens are harbored inside the sequestrum maintaining chronic osteomyelitis and flare-up acute episodes. Surrounding *granulation tissue* separates the sequestrum from the viable bone. New bone formation is induced by the periostitis and is therefore located peripherally around the altered cortex and the necrotic tissue, the so-called *involucrum*. In many cases, infection-induced channels (so-called *sinus tracts*) are connecting the area of dead bone with the cutaneous surface composed of an osseous break (so-called *cloaca*) (Pineda et al. 2009).

In *radiograms*, a sequestrum has an increased radiodensity, sharp margins, and is located within the medullary bone (Pineda et al. 2009; Santiago-Restrepo et al. 2003; Gold et al. 1991; Kaim et al. 2002). The size varies from sub-millimeter to several millimeters. New bone formation, the involucrum, leads to contour irregularities, bone deformation, and increased radiodensity (Fig. 8). Differential diagnosis includes the osteoid osteoma which is frequently found at the hand, and the rare fibrous dysplasia. MRI is helping to assess the devitalized tissue in chronic osteomyelitis. A sequestrum is of low signal intensity in all sequences, whereas the surrounding granulation tissue is of high signal intensity in STIR or T2-weighted sequences, and of intermediate to low signal intensity on T1-weighted images. After application of gadolinium, the granulation tissue is enhancing, whereas the sequestrum remains low signal (Hopkins et al. 1995; Towers 1997; Morrison et al. 1993). The involucrum has low signal intensity on all pulse sequences and is separated from the cortical bone by a periosteal reaction zone which is of intermediate signal intensity on T2-weighted or STIR images (Pineda et al. 2009; Gold et al. 1991). The periosteal reaction zone is highly suspicious of containing infectious material, when presenting as a mass of high signal intensity on T2-weighted images. In this area of infection, a break traversing both the cortical bone and the involucrum is characteristic of a cloaca. Often, a sinus tract extends from the cloaca and appears with a tram track-like enhancement in the adjacent soft tissues before reaching the cutaneous surface with an orifice (Santiago-Restrepo et al. 2003). In chronic osteomyelitis, CT is particularly useful to identify a sequestrum and to differentiate between granulation tissue and an involucrum (Fig. 8c, d). Therefore, CT is essential for planning surgical therapy, and—most importantly—for detecting sequestra which must be excised (Pineda et al. 2009; Santiago-Restrepo et al. 2003; Gold et al. 1991).

Differentiation of active from inactive osteomyelitis is of high clinical importance, but challenging in diagnostic imaging (Erdman et al. 1991). Ongoing activity of infection must be assumed when the radiologic appearance has changed in follow-up studies, and when a sequestrum or a subperiosteal cloaca is still provable. A disadvantage of MRI is the inability to distinguish infectious from reactive inflammation (Pineda et al. 2009).

3.2 Etiology of Osteomyelitis

3.2.1 "Primary" (Hematogenous) Osteomyelitis

In septicemia, the respiratory, genitourinary, gastrointestinal systems, and the skin serve as infectious sources which however remains unknown in up to 50% of the cases (Hausman and Lisser 1992; Pineda et al. 2009; Barbieri and Freeland 1998). Infrequently, hematogenous spread of pathogens leads either to acute osteomyelitis of the distal sections of the radius and ulna (Gold et al. 1991; Reilly et al. 1997) or to acute pyogenic arthritis of the wrist (Murray 1998). Hematogenous osteomyelitis usually originates in the metaphysis, where bacterial implantation is facilitated by the slow blood flow in the venous sinusoids. Both bone marrow edema and accumulation of pus increases the bone pressure and promote further osteomyelitic extension which follows an age-dependent pattern (Resnick 1976): (a) In infants up to 1 year, only a few metaphyseal vessels penetrate the bone plate to reach the epiphysis and therefore being responsible for simultane osteomyelitis and purulent arthritis in infancy. However, the combined infection is difficult to detect due to the unossified epiphyses at this age. (b) In children and adolescents, the metaphyseal vessels turn sharply at the open growth plate without penetrating them. This unique pattern of vascularity explains the predilection of juvenile osteomyelitis to affect the dia-metaphysis only. (c) In adulthood, many metaphyseal vessels are connected to the epiphyseal vessels via the closed bone plate. This free vascular communication allows metaphyseal osteomyelitis to migrate to the epiphysis.

Radiograms show "moth-eaten" osteolyses and less often sequestra (Resnick 1976; Capitanio and Kirkpatrick 1970). Later in the course, periostitis and periosteal bone formation is more extended when compared

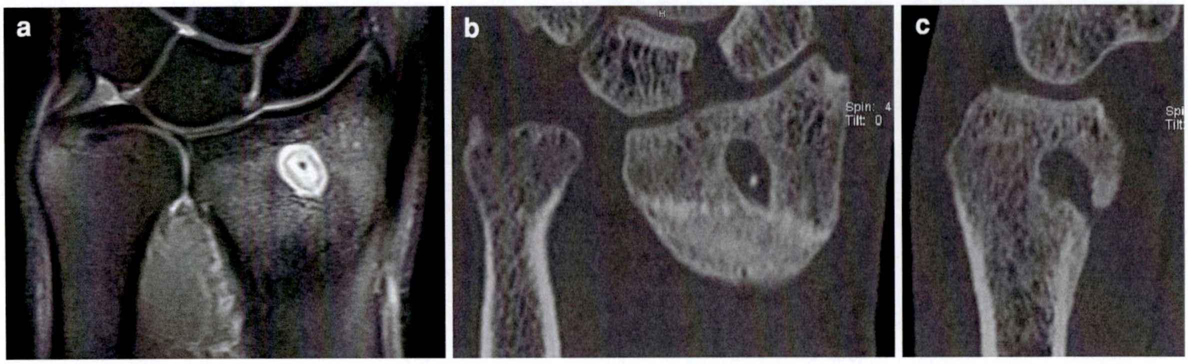

Fig. 7 Brodie's abscess in the distal end of the radius in a young man with no history of trauma or bone surgery. At the meta-epiphyseal junction, a sequestrum surrounded by an abscess and the so-called "double-line sign" are seen in a coronal PD-weighted sequence with fat-saturation (**a**). Reformatted CT images in the coronal (**b**) and sagittal (**c**) planes confirm the sequestrum and prove the presence of a cloaca on the palmar site of the radius

to secondary osteomyelitis spread from soft-tissue infection. Chronic osteomyelitis is characterized in radiograms by bone remodeling with more or less intense osteosclerotic areas. Even the primary development of chronic sclerosing osteomyelitis is possible. MRI is the modality of choice for early diagnosis, therapy planning, and the follow-up (Hopkins et al. 1995; Towers 1997; Morrison et al. 1993). It provides all the information about the extension of osteomyelitis, particularly about soft-tissue complications. Osteomyelitic abscesses and osteonecrosis can be detected with fat-saturated T1-weighted sequences after intravenous administration of gadolinium. *Skeletal scintigraphy* is suitable to exclude or confirm the presence of osteomyelitis before lesions can be detected in plain radiograms, especially if MRI is not available (Pineda et al. 2009; Schauwecker 1989).

3.2.2 "Secondary" (Spread From Soft Tissues) Osteomyelitis

Secondary forms of osteomyelitis develop from the adjacent soft tissues. At the hand, secondary osteomyelitis is much more frequent in comparison with primary osteomyelitis (Hausman and Lisser 1992; Tsai and Failla 1999; Resnick 1976).

Osteomyelitis of the Fingers

Phalangeal manifestation is by far the most common form of osteomyelitis at the hands with the distal phalanx being most often affected. The inoculation of pathogens is caused by two different ways: First, the organisms reach directly the periosteum or bone via the disrupted skin and the deep tissue layers. With this respect, even surgery can result in osteomyelitis, e.g. the pin tract infection (Tsai and Failla 1999). Second, there is initially a soft-tissue infection like a felon or suppurative flexor tenosynovitis after a puncture wound (Hausman and Lisser 1992; Beltran 1995; Jeffrey et al. 1997). These soft-tissue infections do not only extend longitudinally via the tendon sheaths and the fascial planes but also invade into the depth. The soft-tissue focus causes initial periostitis, then infectious invasion of the cortex, and finally osteomyelitis after invading the medullary bone via the cortical haversian and Volkmann's canals (Resnick 1976). Frequently, the formation of sequestra can result and maintain chronic fistulae.

In *radiograms*, positive findings cannot be expected in the first 10 days after an injury (Resnick 1976; Capitanio and Kirkpatrick 1970; Gold et al. 1991). As the result of the inward migrating infection from the soft tissues, discrete focal osteopenia and mild periostitis are the initial signs in osteomyelitis of the digits (Fig. 5a). Bone destruction with "moth-eaten" and permeative osteolyses subsequently follows. Finally, osteosclerotic transformation is typical of chronic osteomyelitis (Fig. 8). The radiologic examination should always include the search for foreign bodies which can cause and maintain infections of the fingers (Peterson et al. 2002). MRI is useful for depicting the infected soft tissues—particularly to prove or rule out an abscess (Fig. 6)—and for assessing the extension of osteomyelitis (Hopkins et al. 1995; Towers 1997; Morrison et al. 1993). However, the vast majority of paronychias and felons

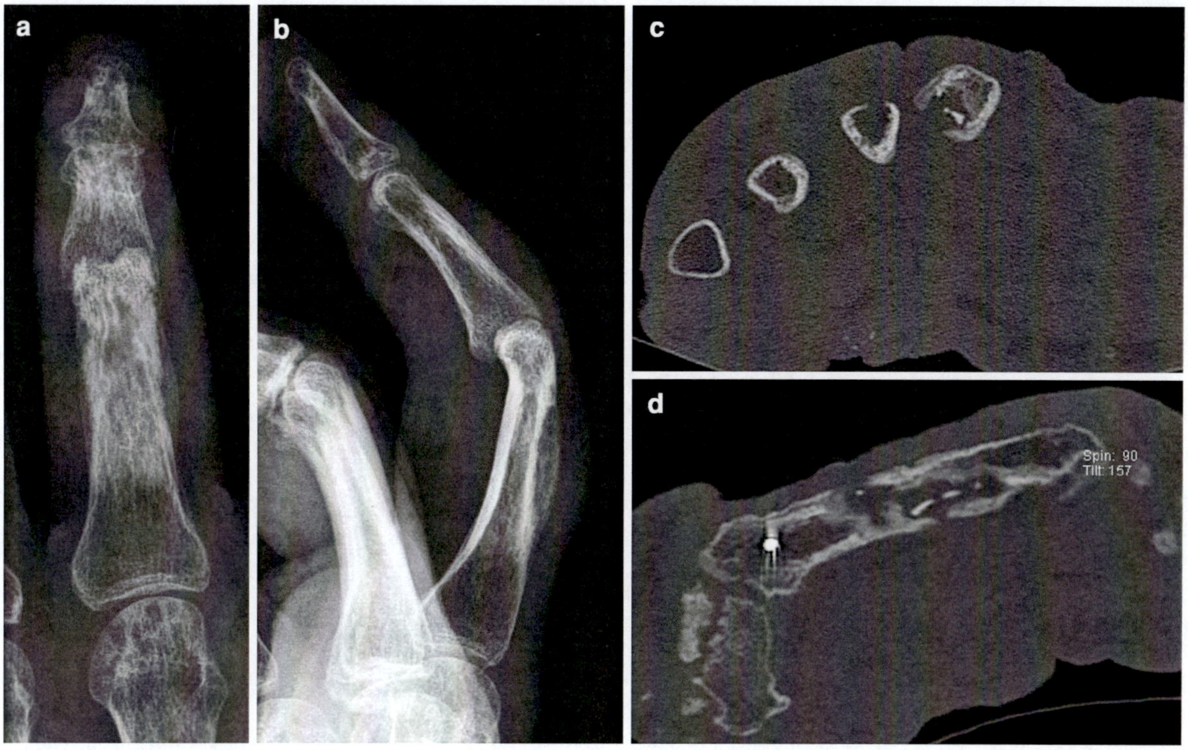

Fig. 8 Two patients suffering from chronic osteomyelitis of the finger skeleton. **a** and **b** In the first patient, X-rays show increased bone density of the proximal phalanx due to marked periosteal reaction with initial development of an involucrum and a cloaca. The periosteum is elevated at the dorsum. **c** and **d** In the second patient, all signs of chronic osteomyelitis are present in the index finger. In the metacarpal bone, several sequestra surrounded by granulation tissue, cloacae at the palmar and dorsal sites and an involucrum can be depicted in the transaxial (**c**) and sagittal (**d**) CT images. A *pin* has been introduced in the metacarpal base

do not involve the bone of the distal phalanx, and therefore, the role of MRI is mainly to exclude osteomyelitis. The use of CT is limited mainly for detecting sequestra (Figs. 7, 8) and intra-osseous abscesses (Kothari et al. 2001).

Bites

Bites at the hands are mostly caused by domestic animals, less frequent by humans, e.g. a fist blow to the mouth of the opponent (Gonzalez et al. 1993). Staphylococcal or streptococcal species are inoculated through the wound, particularly *Eikenella corrodens* in human bites, and *Pasteurella multocida* in cat bites (Resnick 1976). The rate of infectious complications such as soft-tissue infection, bacterial arthritis, and osteomyelitis is up to 50%. Symptoms are dominated by diffuse soft-tissue swelling, redness, impairment or loss of function and the local bite defect.

In *radiograms*, foreign bodies in the soft tissues must be excluded. In oblique views, subtle cortical lesions can sometimes be detected at the injury site after a deep bite down to the bone surface (Resnick 1976; Capitanio and Kirkpatrick 1970). Mostly, however, radiologic signs of osteomyelitis and/or bacterial arthritis appear first in about 8–10 days after the injury.

3.2.3 Special Forms of Osteomyelitis

Tuberculous Osteomyelitis

Skeletal tuberculosis that is a hematogenous infection caused by the Mycobacterium tuberculosis complex develops in the post-primary stage of tuberculosis. Pulmonary tuberculosis is evident in about half of the cases, but mostly inactive at the time of skeletal manifestation. Overall, the hands are involved only in about 5% of musculoskeletal tuberculosis with two age groups (Hoyen et al. 1998; Benkeddache and Gottesman 1982; Hsu et al. 2004): Tuberculous osteomyelitis is more common in children under 5 years, while tuberculous arthritis is mostly manifested in adults. However, transition of tuberculous osteomyelitis to tuberculous arthritis has been observed, and also the reversed infection route. Other than in pyogenic infections, meta-epiphyseal spread of tuberculous osteomyelitis is possible in childhood. Clinical presentation at the hand skeleton is characterized by a chronic course and by a wide range of symptoms (Benkeddache and Gottesman 1982). It is not unusual that painless swelling, focal tenderness, and a draining sinus are noticed over months to years before the final diagnosis is found. One should consider that incidence of tuberculosis is currently increasing.

Radiologic signs of tuberculous osteomyelitis are heterogeneous. They include soft-tissue swelling, diffuse osteopenia, "moth-eaten" osteolyses, and marked bone expansion when periosteal bone formation has been induced (Benkeddache and Gottesman 1982). One metacarpal or phalangeal bone is affected in about 70% of tuberculous infections, two or several bones in the remaining cases. The affected bones appear thickened and with increased radiodensity. Both tuberculous bone thickening and soft-tissue swelling leads to a sausage-like deformity of the ray affected. The clinical condition is termed "tuberculous dactylitis", and the radiographic appearance is the "spina ventosa" presenting with characteristic cyst-like bone expansion (Fig. 3c). Differential diagnosis of dactylitis also includes osteomyelitis of pyogenic, syphilitic, fungal, and leprous origin as well as fibrous dysplasia, sarcoidosis, hyperparathyreoidism, and sickle cell anemia. Sequestra are uncommon in skeletal tuberculosis. Osteosclerotic bone is seen at the thickened periosteum and at the borders of marginal erosions in case of concomitant tuberculous arthritis. In contrast-enhanced MRI, an intense, ring-shaped enhancement is observed at the small tubular bone(s) affected in tuberculous osteomyelitis (Hsu et al. 2004).

Chronic Recurrent Multifocal Osteomyelitis

Chronic recurrent multifocal osteomyelitis (CMRO) is a rare, aseptic condition of osteomyelitis seen in children and adolescents and is characterized by a prolonged or fluctuating course. Aside psoriatic skin lesions, osteomyelitic lesions of unknown origin appear synchronously (Kothari et al. 2001). Causative organisms are usually not identified, and therefore, both immunologic phenomena and a genetic predisposition have been discussed in the pathogenesis. Probably, there is an association to the entities of plasma-cell osteomyelitis and Garre's sclerosing osteomyelitis.

In *radiograms*, involved bones have findings typical of osteomyelitis and/or Brodie abscess with osteosclerotic lesions side by side with osteolytic destruction. The clavicles and the bones of the lower extremity are preferred locations. *Scintigraphy* is useful in identifying the multifocal involvement of CRMO (Kothari et al. 2001). Contrast-enhanced MRI is well suited for the follow-up.

3.3 Differential Diagnosis

Osteosarcoma and Ewing's sarcoma are very rare at the hand skeleton. These malignant bone tumors must be taken into differential diagnostic consideration, when moth-eaten or permeative lesions are found in the metaphysis or diaphysis of the short tubular bones of the hand and when typical inflammatory signs are initially absent in osteomyelitis. Furthermore, advanced soft-tissue sarcomas can also lead to bone destruction and can simulate the radiographic pattern of osteomyelitis. However, soft-tissue sarcomas as well as their osseous spread are rare at the hands.

4 Infectious Arthritis

Infectious arthritis is an acute joint disease which is either caused by the articular implantation of a pathogen ("primary infectious arthritis") or is triggered as an immunologic answer ("reactive post-infectious arthritis") following a nasopharyngeal, respiratory, urogenital or intestinal infection, e.g. acute rheumatic fever following streptococcal tonsillitis (Resnick 1976; Murray 1998). The discussion of whether infectious arthritis manifests in parallel with or complementary to an immunologically induced bacterial arthritis is ongoing.

Staphylococci are the most common pathogens in about 70% of all bacterial joint infections (Hausman and Lisser 1992; Murray 1998; Graif et al. 1999). Some group preferences are evident: Streptococci and *Haemophilus influenzae* are frequently seen in children, *Neisseria gonorrhoeae* in young women, and gram-negative rods in patients with immune deficiency. Tuberculous, viral or parasitic pathogens can be isolated less commonly (Hoyen et al. 1998). Chlamydia, *Borrelia burgdorferi* (Lyme disease), *Mycobacterium leprae*, *Schistosoma haematobium* as well as hepatitis B and rubella viruses have been identified aside others in the synovial fluid recently. Risk factors of acquiring septic arthritis include diabetes mellitus, liver cirrhosis, alcohol or drug abuse, malignancy, and the advanced age.

4.1 Bacterial Arthritis

Three different pathways (Tsai and Failla 1999; Resnick 1976) are possible in pyogenic joint inflammation (Figs. 1a, b): First, bacterial arthritis is caused by spread of soft-tissue infection or by osteomyelitic transmission from a neighbored bone. This pathway is mostly seen at the finger joints. Second, pathogens can be directly inoculated via a penetrating injury as occurring in cuts, stabs and bites, and artificially during a diagnostic or surgical procedure at the joint. All joints of the hand can be involved in this pathway, but the metacarpophalangeal and proximal interphalangeal regions are clearly preferred (Resnick 1976). Third, bacterial arthritis arises from hematogenous seeding of pathogens in patients suffering from severe sepsis or severe immunologic deficiency. The carpal joints are mostly affected by hematogenous arthritis (Murray 1998).

The distribution pattern of pyogenic arthritis is usually monoarticular (Resnick 1976). The symptoms comprise low-grade fever, chills, and the focal signs of infection (swelling, redness, heat, arthralgia, tenderness). The classical disease course begins at the synovial membrane which becomes thickened and edematous, thereby producing synovial fluid and pus. The inflamed, pannus-like synovium initially induces cartilage destruction, and then leads to deep erosions at the subchondral bone plate. Depending on the violence of the pathogen, the infected joint is progressively destroyed.

In *radiograms*, signs of pyogenic arthritis follow a time-dependent pattern (Resnick 1976; Murray 1998; Gonzalez et al. 1993). Initially, obliteration of the periarticular soft-tissue planes (so-called "soft-tissue sign") and a widened joint space caused by an infectious joint effusion are seen. Intra-articular gas formation is occasionally recognizable in gram-negative bacterial arthritis. Hyperemia-induced osteopenia is evident in about 8–10 days later (Fig. 9a), at first in the subchondral bone plate, then covering the entire epiphyseal area (so-called "collateral sign"). Synovial inflammation (Figs. 9b, e) leads subsequently to focal bone erosions at the bare areas and soon involves the entire articular space with poorly defined margins and progressive destruction of the joint (so-called "direct sign of arthritis"). The joint space narrows progressively with advanced destruction of the articular cartilage. Coarse erosions and destructive joint collapse are characteristic radiographic findings in bacterial arthritis (Fig. 9d–f). Finally, fibrous or bony ankylosis can develop at the end of the healing process. Another complication is the development of secondary osteoarthritis.

Most cases of infectious arthritis at the hand can be assessed clinically. At the wrist, the differential diagnosis includes rheumatoid arthritis, which however presents with a typical articular distribution pattern at the hands, and tuberculous arthritis, which progresses more slowly compared to bacterial arthritis (Graif et al. 1999). However, differential diagnosis can be challenging when other joint diseases like the calcium pyrophosphate dehydrate (CPPD) deposition disease, gout arthropathy or rheumatoid arthritis precede the joint infection (Murray 1998). In this situation, indium- or technetium-labeled leukocyte bone scans may be useful for differentiation (Pineda et al. 2009; Schauwecker 1989).

4.2 Tuberculous Arthritis

Tuberculosis osteomyelitis is commonly seen in children, while tuberculous arthritis is mostly affecting adults suffering from other underlying disorders (Hoyen et al. 1998; Benkeddache and Gottesman 1982; Hsu et al. 2004). The pathways of tuberculous arthritis comprise either primary joint infection or initial osteomyelitis followed by secondary spread to the joint(s). Typically, the latter is characterized by a

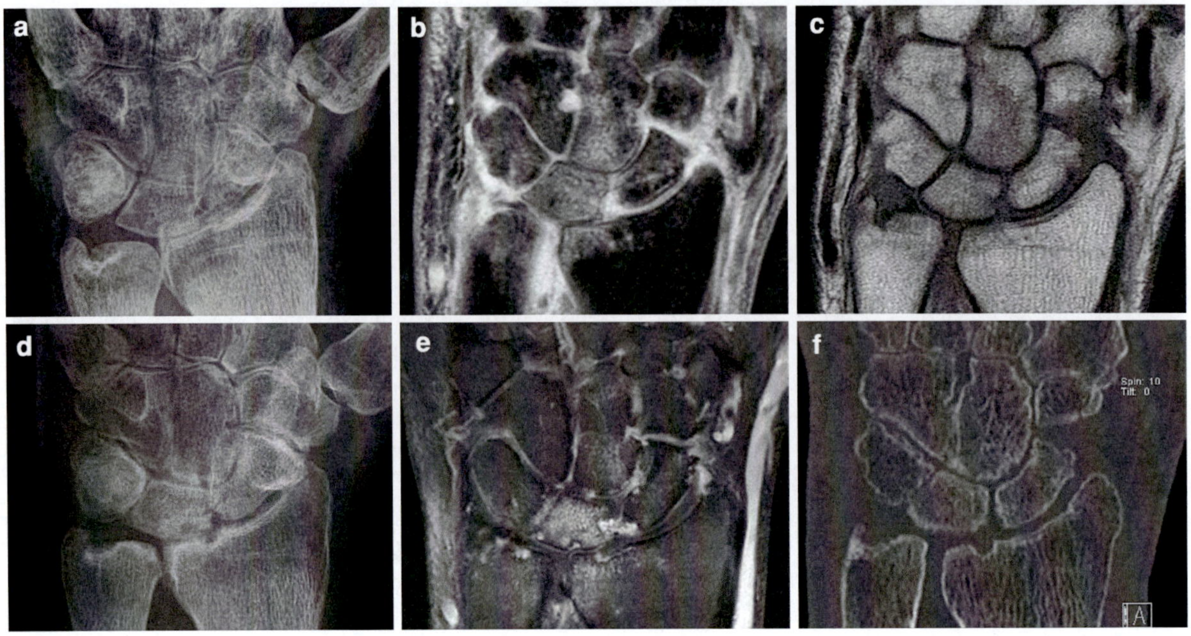

Fig. 9 Hematogenous arthritis of the wrist in a 52-year-old woman. Probably, the staphylococceal dissemination originated from an acute maxillary sinusitis. The image collection includes the initial imaging findings **a–c** 15 days after onset of the symptoms, and a follow-up examination **d–f** 4 weeks later for monitoring the antibiotic therapy response. **a–c** Initial imaging findings: diffuse osteopenia of the wrist, no erosions detectable (**a**). In the PD-weighted FSE sequence with fat-saturation (**b**) and in the non-enhanced T1-weighted SE image (**c**), diffuse bone marrow edema, carpal joint effusions, and synovitis are evident. **d–f** Follow-up imaging findings: multi-locular erosions have developed at the wrist bones and the distal forearm. While deep erosions can already be seen in the dorso-palmar X-ray view (**d**), the finest erosions are only detectable in the contrast-enhanced T1-weighted SE sequence with fat-saturation (**e**) and in high-resolution CT (**f**)

less destructive course. The stages from articular swelling to final joint destruction are passed through slowly over a period of months to years.

In *radiograms*, signs of tuberculous arthritis are first seen in about 2–4 months after the onset of symptoms (Hoyen et al. 1998; Benkeddache and Gottesman 1982). The radial side of the wrist and midcarpus are mainly affected. The radiographic features are best summarized by the Phemister's triad consisting of periarticular osteopenia, peripheral erosions, and mild joint space narrowing (Fig. 3d): The initial signs are soft-tissue swelling and periarticular osteopenia. The joint space is preserved over a long time, but is finally narrowing as the tuberculous synovitis progresses. Fine erosions at the subchondral bone plate lead to delineation of the articular contours. In contrast, marginal punched-out defects and central defects caused by granulomatous proliferation are characteristic of the cystic form of carpal tuberculosis which presents with a "nibbling of cheese" pattern. Extensive bone destruction and fibrous or bony ankylosis can develop if antituberculous medication is delayed or insufficient. Calcifications are observed in concomitant soft-tissue abscesses and during healing. In early stage of tuberculous arthritis, the differential diagnoses include non-infectious arthropathy such as rheumatoid arthritis, skeletal sarcoidosis in case of cystic tuberculosis, and more unlikely the pyogenic arthritis.

5 Rare Infections of the Hand Skeleton

5.1 Syphilis

The spirochete Treponema pallidum is the pathogen of congenital syphilis as well as in acquired syphilis (Hoyen et al. 1998; Sachdev and Bery 1982). Symptoms of the survived congenital infection include saber shins, a saddle nose, palate perforation, and the

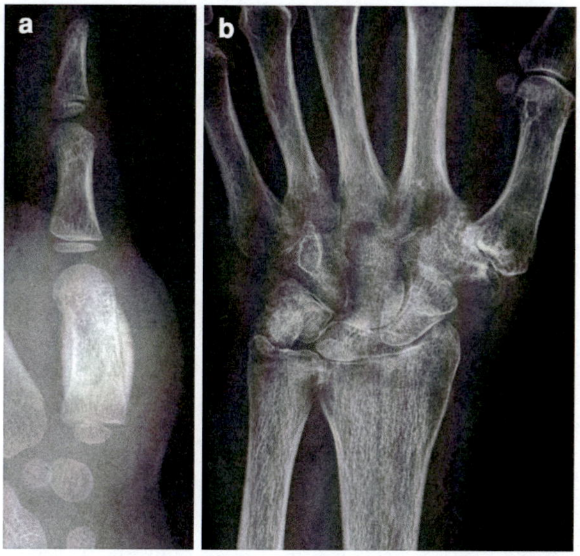

Fig. 10 Venereal infections of the hand. **a** Characteristic syphilitic dactylitis. In this child, dactylitis was limited to the metacarpal bone of the left thumb. The affected bone is increased in volume and radiodensity due to massive periosteal hyperostosis. Courtesy of Dr. A.M. Davies, Birmingham, UK. **b** Very rare case of an acquired gonococcal arthritis of the wrist in a 63-year-old woman. Marked osteopenia of the carpal, distal forearm, and the proximal metacarpal bones is evident. The heights of the radiocarpal and midcarpal cartilage are decreased, although there is a joint effusion with displaced soft-tissue planes. Pre-existing osteoarthritis of the trapezio-metacarpal joint

Hutchinson's triad (barrel-like teeth, keratitis, and nerve deafness). Three stages are discernable in the acquired disease: Focal skin ulceration develops at the site of infection (primary syphilis), followed by generalized skin eruption several weeks later (secondary syphilis). After healing, there is a prolonged syphilitic dissemination in almost all organ systems with the patients mostly being symptom-free. Many years later, about half of the patients develop cutaneous, cardiovascular, neurologic, and/or musculoskeletal symptoms due to granulomatous ("gummatous") lesions (tertiary syphilis). The hand skeleton is rarely involved.

Initially, the *radiographs* of newborns suffering from congenital syphilis reveal erosive irregularities at the epi-metaphyseal junctions induced by osteochondritis (Sachdev and Bery 1982). After these findings have disappeared, inflammatory enchondral and periosteal hyperostosis is causative of dense and thickened tubular bones. Bilateral and symmetric involvement of the metacarpals or phalanges is characteristic of syphilitic dactylitis in childhood. The radiographic appearance resembles that of osteoidosteoma and tuberculous dactylitis (Fig. 10a). In tertiary syphilis, both the pathogenesis (osteochondritis, periostitis, and osteomyelitis) as well as the radiologic appearance is similar to that of tuberculosis, however, with the joints being less severely involved. The main finding is periosteal proliferation leading to significant enlargement of the tubular bones.

5.2 Gonococcal Arthritis

Gonococcal arthritis develops about 2 weeks after the venereal infection with Neisseria gonorrhoeae. Polyarticular symptoms are observed in gonococcal sepsis only. Thus, gonococcal infection should be considered in sexually active patients presenting with migratory polyarthralgias. Mostly, however, there is a monoarticular infection with the carpal joints being predominantly affected among other joints (Hoyen et al. 1998) (Fig. 10b). If no gonococci can be proved in the joint fluid, differential diagnosis should include reactive arthritis and the postgonococcal Reiter's syndrome.

5.3 Leprosy (Hansen's Disease)

In Africa, South America and Asia, leprosy is a chronic infection caused by Mycobacterium leprae. The clinical presentation is determined by an incubation period over months and combinations of neural, osseous, and dermal leprosy (Hoyen et al. 1998). Lymphadenopathy is seen in most cases. Involvement of peripheral nerves is characteristic, particularly with implantation of pathogens in Schwann's cells of the ulnar and peroneal nerves. Subsequently, progressive denervation with sensory and motor impairment leads to repetitive traumatic lesions and extensive superinfections. Leprous arthritis is either of hematogenous origin or spread from the leprous bone marrow and the soft tissues. The joint infection is located at the carpal, metacarpophalangeal, and proximal interphalangeal joints. Finally, reactive arthritis can follow

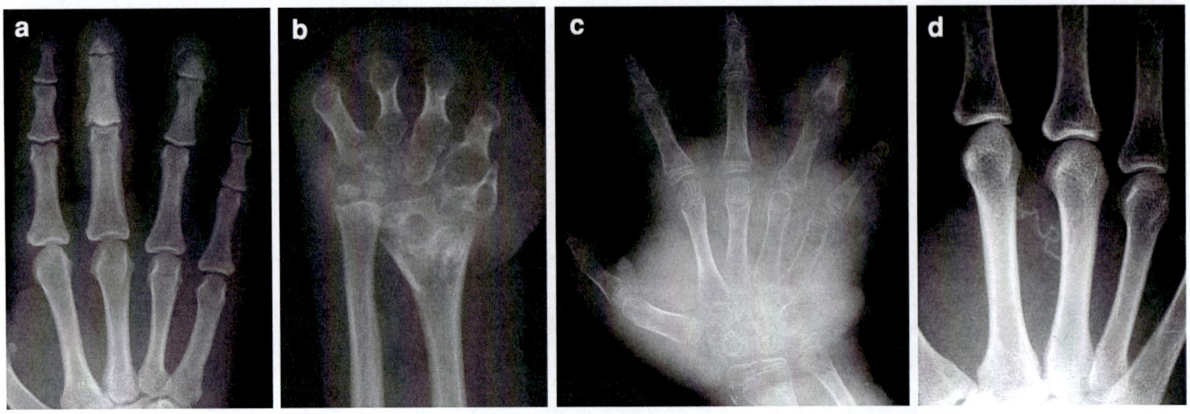

Fig. 11 Rare bacterial, fungal, and parasitic infections at the hand. **a** Leprosy. There are acro-osteolyses at the terminal phalanges leading to the "candystick" deformity of the middle and ring fingers. Additionally, sclerosing osteomyelitis of the middle phalanx of the middle finger is visible. Courtesy of Dr. A.M. Davies, Birmingham, UK. **b** Mutilation stage of meningococcal infection in an infant with osteomyelitic destruction of the distal radial section and of the entire wrist. All fingers have been amputated before because of severe septic embolism. Courtesy of Dr. A.M. Davies, Birmingham, UK. **c** Mycetoma of the hand in a child presenting with multi-locular soft-tissue masses and advanced osteopenia. Manifestation of mycetoma at the hand is very rare. Courtesy of Dr. A.M. Davies, Birmingham, UK. **d** Filariasis with detection of a calcified worm remnant in the soft tissue of metacarpus. This was an incidental finding in a woman suffering from known filariasis of her breasts. Courtesy of Dr. M. Langen, Würzburg/Germany

leprosy in a typically symmetric pattern and is associated with erythema nodosum.

Two different groups of leprous abnormalities are visible in *radiograms* (Enna et al. 1971): First, specific granulomatous lesions directly induced by the pathogens are found at the metacarpal and phalangeal bones in less than 10% of musculoskeletal leprosy (osteitis leprosa multiplex cystica). Initially, soft-tissue swelling is evident followed by periostitis as the infection extends to the bones. Signs of leprous osteomyelitis are focal osteopenia, enlarged nutrient channels, and finally advanced bone destruction. Second, unspecific neuropathic lesions account for the great majority of leprosy. Progressive bone destruction is the result of neuropathic articular malfunction, repetitive injuries, and additional superinfections. Neuropathic leprosy is associated with significant bone resorption and acro-osteolyses leading to the characteristic "candystick appearance" of the metacarpals and phalanges with the index finger predominantly affected (Fig. 11a). However, this radiographic appearance is also seen in Charcot's osteoarthropathy as found in syringomyelia, syphilis, and diabetes mellitus. Due to limited access to advanced imaging techniques in the non-developed countries, US and MRI are applied only in rare cases of neural leprosy for depicting the enlarged or compressed nerves (Martinoli et al. 2000). Finally, neural calcifications have been reported.

5.4 Rare and Atypical Infections of Bacterial Origin

These infections comprise a heterogeneous group with the hand skeleton being rarely involved (Hausman and Lisser 1992; Hoyen et al. 1998). The radiographic appearance is unspecific in most diseases. Occasionally, clinical or imaging findings can guide for final diagnosis, like the "doigt en lorgnette" aspect (shortened phalanges due to infectious bone resorption) in yaws (Jones 1972), or the late, but fulminant ball-and-socket destruction of the digits secondary to septic emboli in meningococcemia (Patriquin et al. 1981) (Fig. 11b). Some infections do not affect the hand skeleton although the site of inoculation has been there, as seen in rickettsial-induced cat-scratch disease which is characterized by chronic lymphadenopathy proximally to the elbows. Essential information is summarized in Table 1.

Table 1 Rare and atypical infections of bacterial origin at the musculoskeletal system

Type of infection	Pathogen	Occurrence	Imaging findings
Yaws	*Treponema pertenue*	Africa South America South Pacific Islands West Indies	Similar to those of syphilis in secondary and tertiary yaws Phalanges thickened ("dactylitis") or shortened ("doigt en lorgnette") Distal phalanges spared
Meningococcemia	*Neisseria meningitidis*	Ubiquitous	Fulminant in childhood late after meningococcal sepsis Ball-and-socket deformities of the fingers as the result of septic emboli
Lyme disease	*Borrelia burgdorferi* transmitted by the Ixodes ricinus tick	Ubiquitous Northeastern United States preferred	Joint effusions only No radiographic findings in the presence of intermittent and migrating arthralgia Chronic oligoarthritis very rarely
Brucellosis	*Brucella abortus*, melitensis or suis	Midwestern United States Saudi Arabia South America Southern Europe	Septic arthritis and osteomyelitis No specific manifestations on imaging Like "atypical" tuberculosis
Actinomycosis	*Actinomycis israelii*	Ubiquitous	Most frequent at mandible, spine and lung Hand very rarely affected Combination of osteolysis, sclerosis, and abscess

5.5 Viral Infections

Synovial infections have been observed in hepatitis B, rubella (measles), mumps, variola (smallpox), parvo-B19-infection, in vaccinia and others. The carpal, metacarpophalangeal, and proximal interphalangeal joints can be involved. Episodic, symmetric polyarthritis is observed which usually heals out. However, in adolescents growth disturbance can be associated. Carpal involvement can result in carpal tunnel syndrome.

Infections with *rubella* viruses can occur before birth (intrauterine rubella), or after birth (postnatal rubella), the latter induced either by contagious infection or by active immunization. The carpal and phalangeal joints are affected mostly by migratory symptoms, and only in rare cases erosive arthropathy resembling on juvenile chronic arthritis develops.

Variola (smallpox) is frequently manifested at the elbow joints, whereas the hands are typically spared. In the acute infection phase, radiographic signs are similar to those of purulent osteomyelitis or arthritis. The articular spread of variola tends to become chronic.

Patients suffering from the *human immunodeficiency virus (HIV)* infection do not provide a specific infection pattern at the hands (Eustace et al. 1996). However, these individuals are often affected by opportunistic bacterial infections (septic osteomyelitis and/or arthritis, and pyomyositis), by seronegative spondylarthropathic diseases, and by the development of Kaposi's sarcoma.

5.6 Fungal Infections

Fungal infections of the deep body layers and the musculoskeletal system are rare in comparison with their cutaneous manifestation (Amadio 1998). Almost always, individuals suffering from immunosuppression, malignant or chronic renal diseases are affected. Notably, candidiasis of the joints and bones is extremely rare, although Candida organisms reside on the human mucosal membranes. Fungal infections can be transmitted by traumatic inoculation of pathogens from the cutis into the depth or by hematogenous dissemination. Histoplasmosis, mycetoma (Fig. 11c), sporotrichosis, and coccidioidomycosis are tropical diseases which can induce polyostotic bone infections. None of the fungal diseases present with a

Table 2 Fungal infections at the musculoskeletal system

Type of infection	Pathogen	Occurrence	Imaging findings
Candidiasis (Moniliasis)	*Candida albicans*	Immunosuppression, antibiotic therapy, or diabetes mellitus common	Oral candidiasis, and disseminated abscesses In systemic candidiasis, osteomyelitis and arthritis extremely rare at the hand skeleton
Aspergillosis	*Aspergillus fumigatus*	Immunosuppression common	Mostly lung and chest wall affected Musculoskeletal system and hands rarely involved Localized bone destruction and soft-tissue mass
Coccidioidomycosis	*Coccidiodes immitis*	United States Mexico South America	Lung and visceral dissemination Protuberances preferred in skeletal manifestation Well-defined osteolyses
Sporotrichosis	*Sporothrix schenckii*	Ubiquitous Immunosuppressed individuals preferred	Primary infection of the skin and lymph nodes Carpal and phalangeal joints often involved Marginal erosions and osteomyelitis
Histoplasmosis	*Histoplasma capsulatum* *Histoplasma dubosii*	United States Africa	Visceral and bone involvement common Cystic bone lesions at the wrist and hand skeleton
Mycetoma (Maduromycosis)	Mixed infection with Actinomyces, Nocardia, and Streptomyces pathogens	India Tropical climates Africa	Madura foot most common Chronic granulomatous infection of the subcutis and underlying bones Hand very rarely affected
Blastomycosis	*Blastomyces dermatitidis*	North America Central America South America	Lung, lymph nodes, and skin affected Skeleton involved in 50% of cases, the carpus included Unspecific bone destruction (erosions, osteomyelitis, osteoclerotic margins)
Cryptococcosis (Torulosis)	*Cryptococcus neoformans*	Ubiquitous	Predilection for the CNS Osteolytic foci at the axial skeleton and long bones, hand very rarely affected

specific radiographic appearance at the hand skeleton. The various symptoms range from self-limiting arthralgia over acute polyarthritis to mutilating joint destruction (Amadio 1998). The radiologic appearance is cystic or honey-combed or even erosive (Comstock and Wolson 1975). As a rule, fungal arthritis has a slow course when compared to acute pyogenic arthritis. As in other bone and joint infections, MRI provides detailed information about the extent of bone and soft-tissue involvement. Table 2 summarizes possible fungal infectious disease of the musculoskeletal system.

5.7 Parasitic Infections

Parasitic infections are extremely rare at the hands. Late in the natural disease course, dead parasites can cause bizarre calcifications in the soft tissues (Samuel 1950) (Fig. 11d). The form of these calcified remnants is either cystic (echinococcosis), spotty (cysticercosis) or linear and curled (filariasis, *Loa loa*, Guinea worm disease). When such atypical calcifications are detected and equivocal in origin, one should consider the presence of one of these rare parasitic infections.

6 Key Points

- Approximately 95% of all hand infections are located within the soft tissues, with only 5% involving bone or joint.
- The majority of superficial soft-tissue infections can be managed clinically without the need of imaging. However, radiographs, CT or MRI is required in two clinical settings: First, if spread of infection from the soft tissues to the adjacent bones or joints is suspected. Second, if a deep palmar abscess is suspected.
- In acute osteomyelitis, radiographic signs typically lag behind the onset of the infection by 8–10 days. In the majority of cases, initial findings are very subtle, before marked and poorly defined bone destruction appears.
- MRI is the most powerful imaging tool in detecting and comprehensively staging soft tissue and bone infections. Intravenous gadolinium is recommended for better differentiating abscesses from diffuse infections and the surrounding edema.
- CT imaging is best suited in chronic osteomyelitis for depicting the osseous structures, particularly for detecting sequestra that should be surgically removed to reduce the risk of reactivation of the osteomyelitis.
- Tuberculosis of the flexor tendon sheaths, the bones or the joints of the hands should be considered with slowly progressive infections associated with painless swelling and/or a draining sinus.
- Full clinical information is required for correct interpretation of the destructive bone and joint changes. Identification of the causative pathogen is mandatory to indicate the appropriate antibiotic therapy. Imaging-guided aspiration can be useful for this purpose.

References

Amadio PC (1998) Fungal infections of the hand. Hand Clin 14:605–612

Barbieri RA, Freeland AE (1998) Osteomyelitis of the hand. Hand Clin 14:589–603

Beltran J (1995) MR imaging of soft tissue infection. MRI Clin North Am 3:743–751

Benkeddache Y, Gottesman H (1982) Skeletal tuberculosis of the wrist and hand: a study of 27 cases. J Hand Surg 7:593–600

Capitanio MA, Kirkpatrick JA (1970) Early roentgen observations in acute osteomyelitis. Am J Roentgenol 108:488–496

Comstock C, Wolson AM (1975) Roentgenology of sporotrichosis. Am J Roentgenol 125:651–655

Enna CD, Jacobson RB, Rausch RO (1971) Bone changes in leprosy: a correlation of clinical and radiologic features. Radiology 100:295–299

Erdman WA, Tamburro F, Jayson HT, Weatherall PT, Ferry KB, Peshock RM (1991) Osteomyelitis: characteristics and pitfalls of diagnosis with MR imaging. Radiology 180:533–539

Eustace SJ, Lan HH, Katz J et al (1996) HIV arthritis. Radiol Clin North Am 34:450–453

Gold RH, Hawkins RA, Katz RD (1991) Bacterial osteomyelitis: findings on plain radiographs, CT, MR, and scintigraphy. Am J Roentgenol 157:365–370

Gonzales MH (1998) Necrotizing fasciitis and gangreane of the upper extremity. Hand Clin 14:635–645

Gonzalez MH, Papierski P, Hall RF (1993) Osteomyelitis of the hand after a human bite. J Hand Surg 18A:520–522

Graif M, Schweitzer ME, Deely D et al (1999) The septic versus nonseptic inflamed joint. MR characteristics. Skeletal Radiol 28:616–620

Grey AC, Davies AM, Mangham DC et al (1998) The "penumbra sign" on T1-weighted MR imaging in subacute osteomyelitis: frequency, cause and significance. Clin Radiol 53:587–592

Hausman MR, Lisser SP (1992) Hand infections. Orthop Clin North Am 23:171–185

Hoffman KL, Bergman AG, Hoffman DK et al (1996) Tuberculous tenosynovitis of the flexor tendons of the wrist: MR imaging with pathologic correlation. Skeletal Radiol 25:186–188

Hopkins KL, Li KCP, Bergman G (1995) Gadolinium-DTPA-enhanced magnetic resonance imaging of musculoskeletal infectious processes. Skeletal Radiol 24:325–330

Hoyen HA, Lacey SH, Graham TJ (1998) Atypical hand infections. Hand Clin 14:613–634

Hsu CY, Lu HC, Shih TT (2004) Tuberculous infection of the wrist: MRI features. Am J Roentgenol 183:623–628

Jaovisidha S, Chen C, Ryu KN et al (1996) Tuberculous tenosynovitis and bursitis: imaging findings in 21 cases. Radiology 201:507–513

Jebson PJL (1998a) Infections of the fingertip. Hand Clin 14:547–555

Jebson PJL (1998b) Deep subfascial space infections. Hand Clin 14:557–566

Jeffrey RB Jr, Laing FC, Schechter WP et al (1997) Acute suppurative tendosynovitis of the hand: diagnosis with US. Radiology 162:471–472

Jones WP (1972) Doigt en lorgnette and concentric bone atrophy associated with healed yaws osteitis. J Bone Joint Surg Br 54:341–345

Kaim AH, Gross T, von Schulthess GK (2002) Imaging of chronic posttraumatic osteomyelitis. Eur Radiol 12:1193–1202

Kothari NA, Pelchovitz DJ, Meyer JS (2001) Imaging of musculoskeletal infections. Radiol Clin North Am 39:653–671

Langer MF (2009) Pyogenic flexor tendon sheath infection: a comprehensive review. Handchir Mikrocir Plast Chir 41:256–270

Martinoli C, Derchi LE, Bertolotto M et al (2000) US and MR imaging of peripheral nerves in leprosy. Skeletal Radiol 29:142–150

Miller WB, Murphy WA, Gilula LA (1979) Brodie abscess: reappraisal. Radiology 132:15–23

Morrison WB, Schweitzer ME, Bock GW et al (1993) Diagnosis of osteomyelitis. Utility of fat-suppressed contrast-enhanced MR imaging. Radiology 189:251–257

Murray PM (1998) Septic arthritis of the hand and wrist. Hand Clin 14:579–587

Patriquin HB, Trias A, Jecquier S et al (1981) Late sequelae of infantile meningococcemia in growing bones of children. Radiology 141:77–82

Peterson JJ, Bancroft LW, Kransdorf MJ (2002) Wooden foreign bodies: imaging appearance. Am J Roentgenol 178:557–562

Pineda C, Espinosa R, Pena A (2009) Radiographic imaging in osteomyelitis: the role of plain radiography, computed tomography, ultrasonography, magnetic resonance imaging, and scintigraphy. Semin Plast Surg 23:80–89

Reilly KE, Linz JC, Stern PJ, Giza E, Wyrick JD (1997) Osteomyelitis of the tubular bones of the hand. J Hand Surg Am 22:539–644

Resnick D (1976) Osteomyelitis and septic arthritis complicating hand injuries and infections: pathogenesis of roentgenographic abnormalities. J Can Assoc Radiol 27:21–28

Sachdev M, Bery K, Chawla S (1982) Osseous manifestations in congenital syphilis: a study of 55 cases. Clin Radiol 33:319–323

Samuel E (1950) Roentgenology of parasitic calcification. Am J Roentgenol 63:512–522

Santiago-Restrepo C, Giménez CR, McCarthy K (2003) Imaging of osteomyelitis and musculoskeletal soft tissue infections: current concepts. Rheum Dis Clin North Am 29:89–109

Schauwecker DS (1989) Osteomyelitis: diagnosis with In-111-labeled leukocytes. Radiology 171:141–146

Towers JD (1997) The use of intravenous contrast in MRI of extremity infection. Semin Ultrasound CT MR 18:269–275

Tsai E, Failla JM (1999) Hand infections in the trauma patient. Hand Clin 15:373–386

Tumours and Tumour-Like Lesions of Bone

Nikhil A. Kotnis, A. Mark Davies, and Steven L. J. James

Contents

N. A. Kotnis (✉) · A. M. Davies · S. L. J. James
Department of Radiology,
Royal Orthopaedic Hospital,
Birmingham, B31 2AP, UK
e-mail: nkotnis@hotmail.com

A. M. Davies
e-mail: wendy.turner1@nhs.net

Abstract

Bone tumours affecting the hand and wrist are rare. Only 2% of a series of 4,277 bone tumours were located in the hand or wrist. Furthermore, primary bone tumours are uncommon when compared with tumours arising in the soft tissues of the hand. Haber described 2,321 tumours of the hand with only 38 cases involving bone.

1 Introduction

Bone tumours affecting the hand and wrist are rare. Only 2% of a series of 4,277 bone tumours were located in the hand or wrist (Dahlin 1995). Furthermore, primary bone tumours are uncommon when compared with tumours arising in the soft tissues of the hand. Haber described 2,321 tumours of the hand with only 38 cases involving bone (cited by Garcia and Bianchi 2001).

The majority of bone tumours that affect the hand are benign. Of a series of 469 cases reported by Campanacci and Laus (cited by Garcia and Bianchi 2001), only ten were malignant tumours, six of which were metastases. The most frequent benign lesion is enchondroma and the most common malignant lesion is chondrosarcoma (Wilner 1982; Campbell et al. 1995). In Campbell et al. series of 80 bone tumours of the hand and wrist, gender distribution was equal and there was no left- or right-sided predominance (Campbell et al. 1995). The proximal phalanges and metacarpals are the most commonly affected locations (Wilner 1982; Campbell et al. 1995). Radiographs are sufficient to allow accurate diagnosis in the majority

A. M. Davis et al. (eds.), *Imaging of the Hand and Wrist*, Medical Radiology. Diagnostic Imaging,
DOI: 10.1007/174_2010_121, © Springer-Verlag Berlin Heidelberg 2013

of bone tumours of the hand and wrist. Computed tomography (CT) allows characterization of tumour matrix and presence of bone destruction. Magnetic resonance imaging (MRI) provides information regarding the extent of marrow involvement and soft tissue invasion.

This chapter reviews the most common benign and malignant bone neoplasms of the hand and wrist. The incidence, demographics, clinical presentation, distribution and imaging characteristics of these tumours specific to this location are discussed.

2 Benign Bone Tumours of the Hand and Wrist

2.1 Benign Cartilaginous Tumours

2.1.1 Enchondroma

Enchondromas are located more frequently in the hand and wrist than any other part of the body, accounting for up to 54% of all cases (Unni 1996). It is believed that the tumour develops from fragments of cartilage that originate from the central physis (O'Connor and Bancroft 2004). They most frequently occur in the proximal phalanx, followed by the metacarpal and middle phalanx (Takigawa 1971). Carpal enchondromas are rare and account for approximately 2% of hand enchondromas (Takigawa 1971).

Typically, patients present with a pathological fracture following minor trauma. Alternatively, the tumour presents as a slowly enlarging mass or is discovered incidentally on radiographs obtained for other reasons (Fig. 1). Multiple hand enchondromas may be encountered in association with either Ollier disease or Maffucci syndrome. Ollier disease is characterized by multiple enchondromas (Fig. 2), whereas the presence of multiple enchondromas in association with soft tissue haemangiomas is termed Maffucci syndrome (Fig. 3). The distribution of lesions tends to be in either a monomelic or hemimelic fashion. Both conditions are usually associated with bone deformity. Several authors have reported an association between enchondromatosis and chondrosarcoma of the hand (Fig. 4). Jaffe found malignant change in 50% of his cases of Ollier disease (cited by Liu et al. 1987). Liu et al. found the incidence of chondrosarcoma developing in Ollier disease to be 30% (Liu et al. 1987). Schwartz et al. estimated that development of chondrosarcoma in Mafucci syndrome was an 'almost certainty' (cited by O'Connor and Bancroft 2004). To the best of our knowledge, there are only 7 reports in the literature of chondrosarcoma of the hand arising from a pre-existent

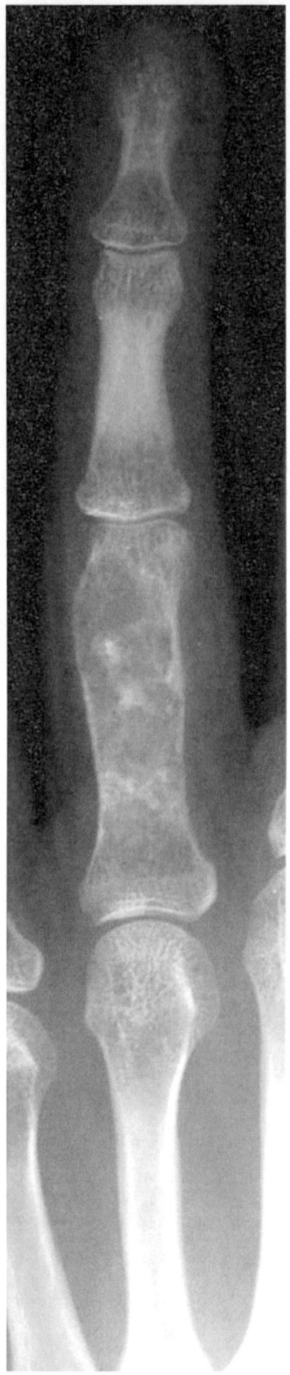

Fig. 1 Enchondroma. There is a lytic, mildly expansile tumour in the proximal phalanx containing punctate cartilage calcification

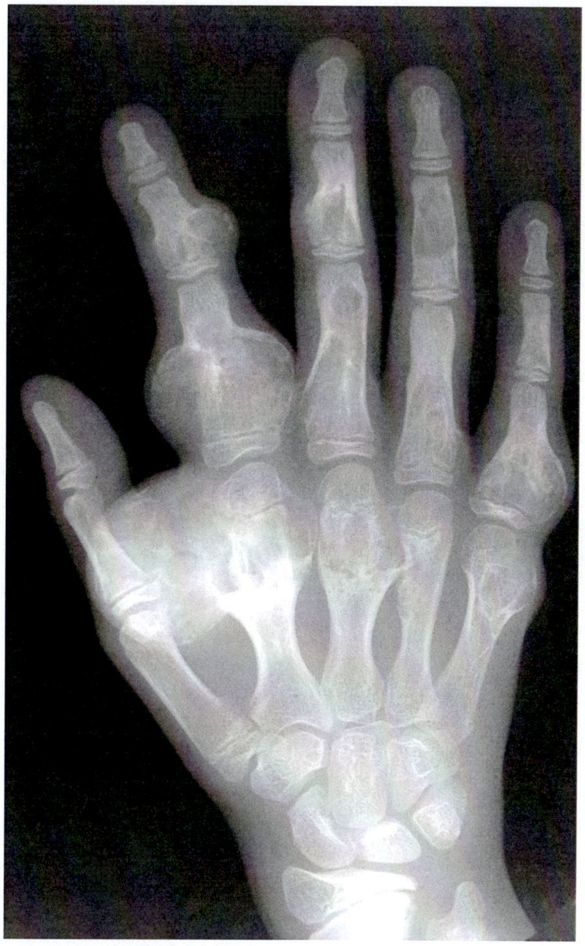

Fig. 2 Ollier disease. Multiple enchondromas arising in the metacarpals and phalanges

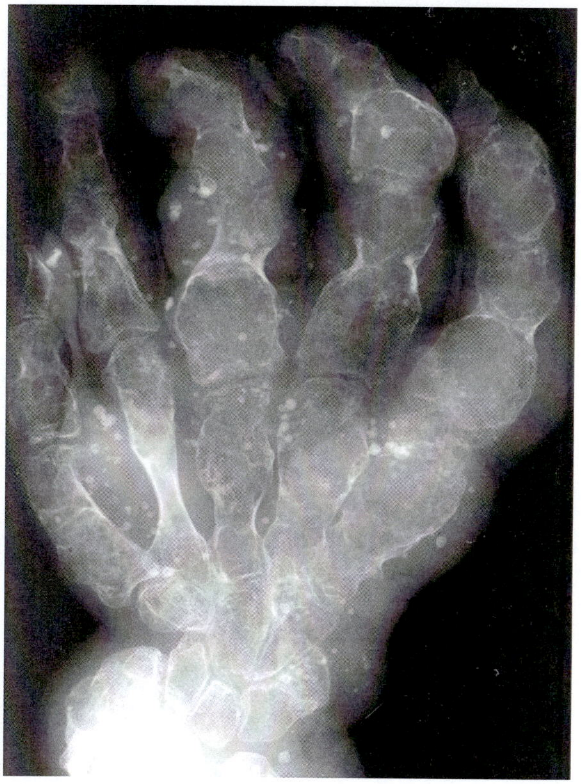

Fig. 3 Maffucci syndrome. Multiple enchondromas in association with soft tissue angiomas. Multiple calcified phleboliths are present

benign solitary enchondroma, confirmed on histology and radiology (Culver et al. 1975, Justis and Dart. 1983, Nelson et al. 1990, Sbarbaro and Straub. 1960, Trias et al. 1978, Wu et al. 1983). This may relate more to the difficulty of establishing the presence of a pre-existing unequivocally benign lesion when a relatively small calibre bone is involved.

Radiographs show the enchondroma to be typically located in the meta-diaphyseal region of the tubular bones of the hand. It is classically a well-defined radiolucent intramedullary lesion containing thin internal trabeculations (Fig. 1). Endosteal scalloping, cortical thinning and expansion of the bone are commonly identified (O'Connor and Bancroft 2004). Associated chondroid calcifications are noted less often in enchondromas of the hand than at other skeletal locations. Cross-sectional imaging is rarely required to make the diagnosis but CT helps clarify the presence of chondroid matrix and is superior to MRI at delineating endosteal scalloping. Enchondroma has a distinctive appearance on MR imaging, with multiple lobules of high signal intensity on T2W, fat suppressed and STIR sequences. The high signal characteristic is due to the hyaline cartilage content in these lesions. Low signal septae are often seen separating the lobules. Low signal foci corresponding to chondroid matrix may also be apparent. Radiographic features concerning for malignant transformation include cortical destruction and an associated soft tissue mass. A zone of lucency developing in a previously mineralized cartilage lesion is also suspicious for malignancy (Sun et al. 1985). MR imaging is useful in evaluating the extent of soft tissue extension in cases where malignant transformation is suspected.

2.1.2 Periosteal Chondroma

Periosteal chondroma (also termed juxtacortical chondroma) is a solitary, benign cartilaginous lesion

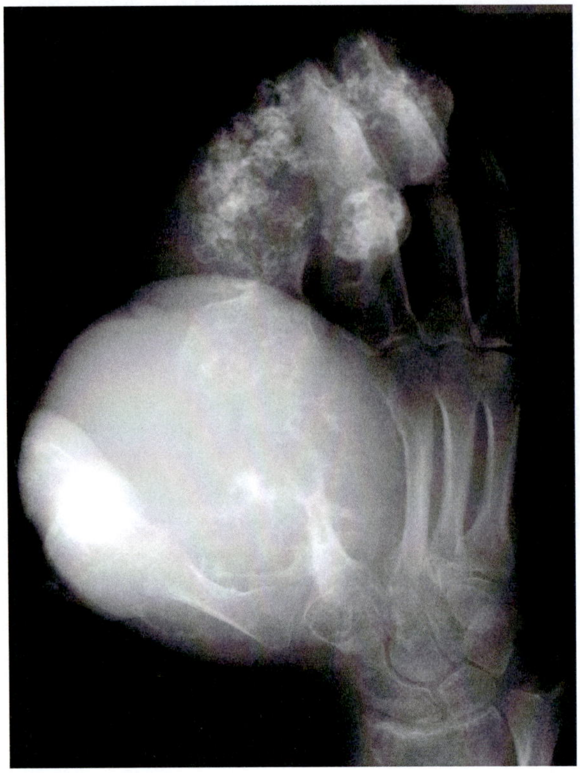

Fig. 4 Malignant transformation in Ollier disease. Multiple enchondromas with a large chondrosarcoma arising in the second metacarpal

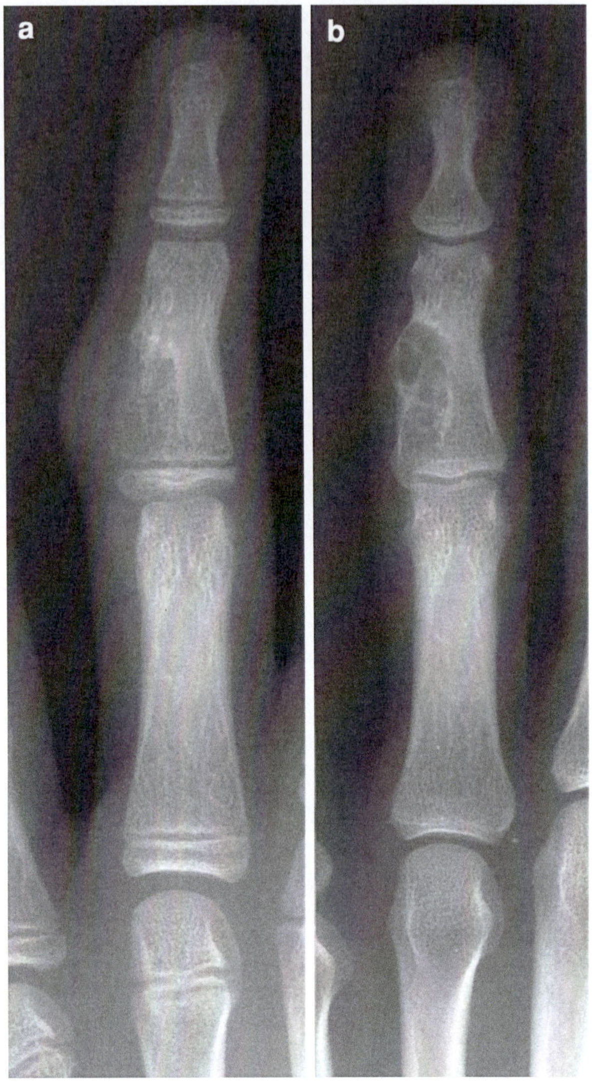

Fig. 5 Periosteal chondroma. **a** There is an eccentric lytic lesion arising in the base of the middle phalanx in a child. **b** 11 years later, the lesion extends down to the subarticular margin

that arises in the periosteum or adjacent soft tissues (O'Connor and Bancroft 2004). It is a rare tumour that was first described by Liechtenstein and Hall in (1952). It represents less than 2% of bone neoplasms (Robbin and Murphey 2000). The lesion is most common in males usually presenting in the second decade of life but the age range is broad (de Santos and Spjut 1981). While the lesion most commonly affects the metaphyses or metadiaphyses of the long bones, between 25 and 29% involve the hands and feet (deSantos and Spjut 1981; Boriani et al. 1983).

Scalloping of the cortex is a typical radiographic feature and can range from minimal change to displacement of cortex into the medullary cavity (Fig. 5). Sclerosis is typically present at the base of the lesion. Overhanging edges are seen at the margin which may completely or partially encircle the lesion. A visible soft tissue mass with associated chondroid matrix is seen in about 50% of cases and is more commonly associated with small lesions of the hands and feet (deSantos and Spjut 1981; Robbin and Murphey 2000). CT and MRI are useful in demonstrating the presence of an outer periosteal shell, soft tissue mass and calcified matrix. MRI demonstrates a juxtacortical mass of low to intermediate T1 and high T2 signal reflecting the hyaline cartilage content of the lesion. Robinson et al. found that size was the most reliable criteria for differentiating periosteal chondrosarcoma from periosteal chondroma (Robinson et al. 2001). In their series, periosteal chondrosarcomas were larger and never less than 3 cm in size. Other features such as intramedullary extension on radiographs and intramedullary oedema on MRI were less specific.

2.1.3 Osteochondroma

Osteochondromas are benign bony projections that are capped by cartilaginous tissue. They typically arise in long tubular bones that develop by enchondral ossification. The lesion is believed to originate from an aberrant focus of cartilage. Although osteochondromas are the most common benign bone tumour, occurrence in the bones of the hands and feet is uncommon. In Ostrowski and Spjut's series of 240 lesions of the hand and feet, only 3% were osteochondromas (Ostrowski and Spjut 1997). Only 4% of osteochondromas involve the hands (Unni 1996).

The proximal phalanx is the most common location of solitary hand osteochondroma (O'Connor and Bancroft 2004i, Kamath et al. 2007). The metacarpals are a less common location (Fig. 6). In Unni's series of 1,024 solitary osteochondromas, only 4 (0.39%) were present in the metacarpals (Unni 1996). Solitary osteochondroma of the carpus is even rarer. It most frequently affects the scaphoid but has been reported in the capitate, hamate, lunate and trapezium (Heiple 1961; Malhotra et al. 1992; Van Alphen et al. 1996; Takagi et al. 2005; Koti et al. 2009). Since solitary osteochondroma of the hand is rare, patients should be assessed for hereditary multiple exostoses (HME).

Osteochondromas are usually asymptomatic in the hand unless they lie in a position that interferes with function. Trigger finger due to impingement of the flexor tendons by an osteochondroma has been reported (Al-Harthy and Rayan 2003). Growth around a joint may lead to blocking of motion at the joint or a pseudomallet deformity (Karr et al. 1984; Murase et al. 2002). In children, osteochondroma may be extremely small and difficult to identify as a cause of finger deformity (Moore et al. 1983). Fracture at the base of the lesion may occur (O'Connor and Bancroft 2004).

HME is an autosomal dominant skeletal disorder affecting the enchondral skeleton during growth, characterized by thickening and deformity of the growing bone with formation of numerous cartilage-capped exostoses. The overall incidence of hand lesions in HME is 79% (Solomon 1967). In this condition, the ulnar metacarpals and proximal phalanges are most commonly affected, with the thumb,

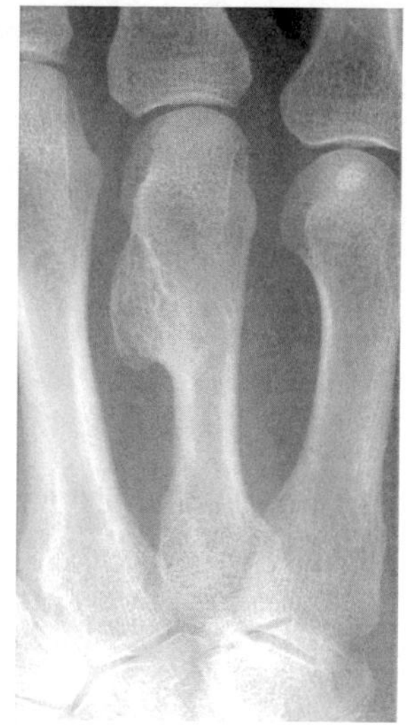

Fig. 6 Osteochondroma. It is arising from the surface of the distal 4th metacarpal. Note that there is continuity of trabeculae within the lesion and the underlying medullary bone

distal phalanges and carpal bones less commonly involved. Shortening of the 4th and 5th metacarpals is also a characteristic feature of the condition. Multiple lesions are typical in these patients with an average of 11.6 exostoses per hand (Fig. 7) (Cates and Burgess 1991). They affect the forearm (40–60%) more commonly than the upper arm. It has been concluded that an increasing distal radius involvement in HME is associated with a greater severity of the disease process overall (Taniguchi 1995). Disruption of the normal epiphyseal growth plate in HME leads to limb length discrepancies and angular deformity at the ends of long bones. This can present around the hip, knee, elbow and wrist. At the wrist, ulnar shortening leads to secondary bowing deformity of the distal radius giving rise to a pseudo-Madelung deformity (Fig. 7) (Vanhoenacker et al. 2001).

The risk of developing chondrosarcoma in a solitary osteochondroma is between 2 and 3% rising to 5–25% in patients with HME (Crandall et al. 1984, Garrison et al. 1982). However, these risks may be overstated as most series originate from tertiary orthopaedic oncology referral centres. The mean age of malignant transformation is 30 years and the most common site is the ilium (Garrison et al. 1982). To our knowledge, only one chondrosarcoma of the hand developing from a solitary osteochondroma has been reported in the literature (Cash and Habermann 1988). As with solitary osteochondromas, more peripherally located tumours are less likely to undergo malignant transformation in patients with HME. A chondrosarcoma of the hand arising in a

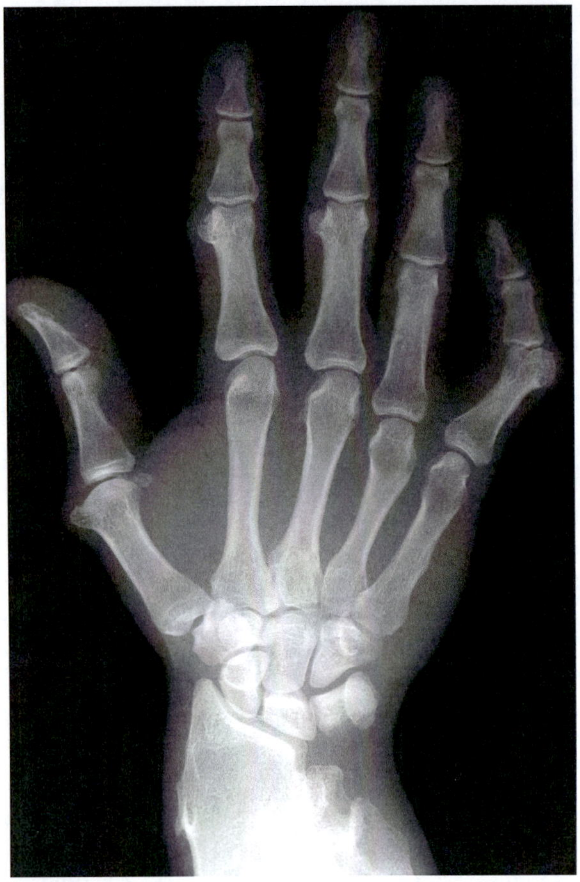

Fig. 7 Hereditary multiple exostoses (diaphyseal aclasis). Multiple small osteochondromas and a pseudo-Madelung deformity of the wrist

patient with HME has only twice been reported in the literature (Fig. 8) (Ostlere et al. 1991; Saunders et al. 1997).

Osteochondromas of the hand are typically sessile lesions which show continuity with the underlying medullary cavity of the bone of origin (Fig. 6). Most osteochondromas related to HME are juxta-epiphyseal in location (Fig. 7); the non-epiphyseal end of bone being the next most common and the diaphysis the least common location. Radiographs aid in demonstrating complications of osteochondromas such as fracture, growth disturbance, osseous deformity or malignant change. Any increase in size of a lesion after skeletal maturity is concerning for sarcomatous change and necessitates further evaluation. Loss of a previously well-defined margin, lucency within a previously mineralized area in the cartilage cap and a cap thickness of 2 cm or above are also concerning features (Fig. 8b) (Ostlere et al. 1991). MR imaging provides precise information about thickness of the cartilage cap that has high signal intensity on T2 spin echo sequences and is important when assessing potential malignant transformation. It also provides information regarding complications such as reactive bursa formation, neural impingement and vascular compromise.

Two cases of dysplasia epiphysealis hemimelica (Trevor's disease) have been reported in the hand both arising at a proximal interphalangeal joint (De Smet 2004). This condition is characterized by asymmetric overgrowth of epiphyseal cartilage or an accessory eiphyseal ossification centre. This leads to excessive growth of the epiphysis with resultant bony protrusion. Though a distinct condition from osteochondroma, radiographs demonstrate an osteochondroma-like protruberans arising from an epiphysis (Fig. 9).

2.2 Giant Cell Tumour of Bone and Giant Cell Reparative Granuloma

Giant cell tumour of bone (GCTOB) is a benign, locally aggressive primary tumour of bone. Histologically, the tumour is characterized by the diffuse presence of osteoclastic, multinucleated giant cells in a background of mononuclear cells (Murphey et al. 2001). It accounts for 4.5% of primary bone tumours (Murphey et al. 2001) and 21% of benign skeletal tumours (Moser et al. 1990). The tumour most commonly occurs in the distal femur, proximal tibia and distal radius of skeletally mature individuals (Fig. 10). Only 2–3% of tumours arise in the bones of the hand (Minguella 1982; Athanasian 2004). A review of 1,228 cases of GCTOB found almost 1% occurred in the metacarpals (Fig. 11) and 1% in the phalanges (Averill et al. 1980). In a series of 452 cases of GCTOB, 57 occurred in the hand and wrist (James and Davies 2005). In this series, 11 (2%) cases were located in a metacarpal and 3 (1%) in a phalanx, the rest comprising lesions of the distal radius and ulna. Involvement of the carpal bones is very rare. In a literature review of GCTOB published in 2006, Shigematsu et al. found only 29 of 193 (15%) reported cases of GCTOB of the hand occurred in the carpus (Shigematsu et al. 2006). With the exception of the pisiform, all the carpal bones were represented with the hamate being the most common location.

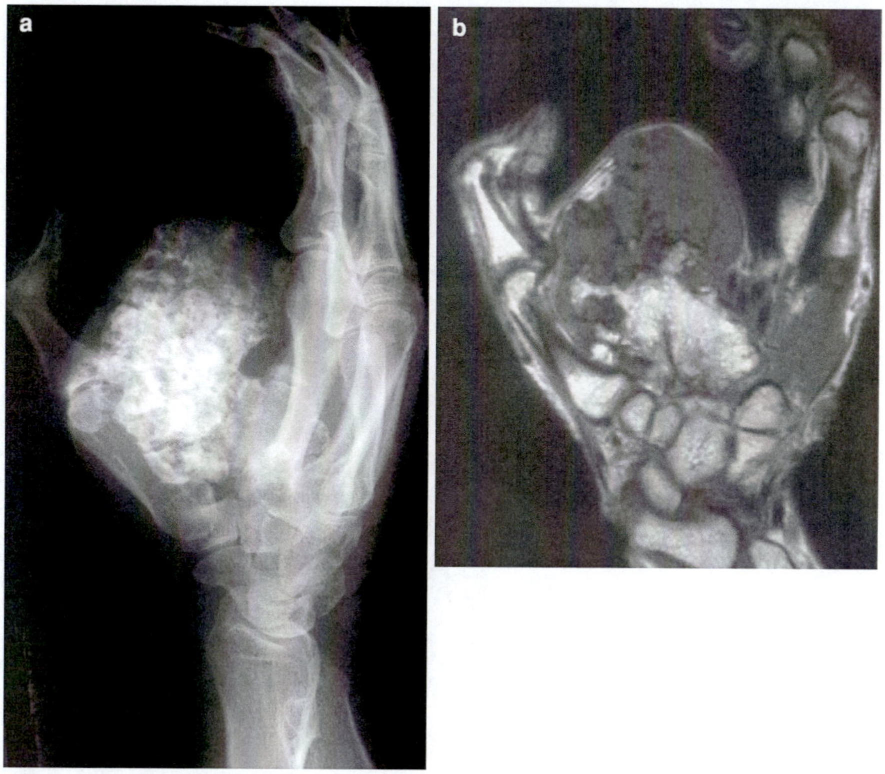

Fig. 8 Malignant transformation in hereditary multiple exostoses. **a** PA oblique radiograph and **b** coronal T1-weighted MR image showing a large peripheral low-grade chondrosarcoma arising from the second metacarpal. Note the thick cartilaginous cap in the MR image (>2 cm)

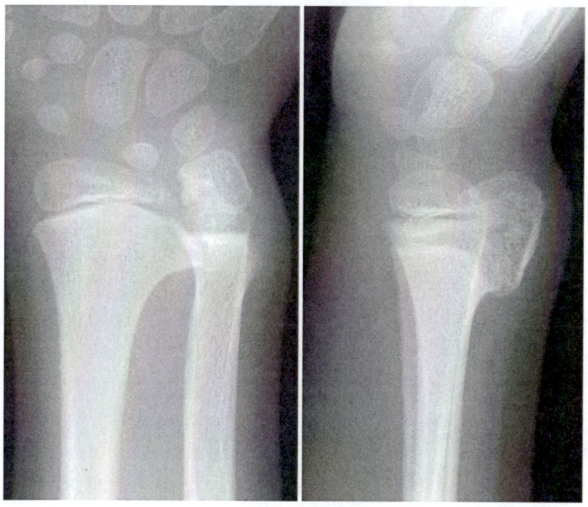

Fig. 9 Dysplasia epiphysealis hemimelica (Trevor disease). There is a modelling deformity with an osteochondroma-like mass arising from the distal ulnar epiphysis

There is a slight female preponderance in cases of GCTOB arising in the small bones of the hand (Athanasian et al. 1997; Biscaglia et al. 2000). The age range is similar to that of GCTOB at other locations, occurring most commonly in the third decade though the age range is wide (Athanasian et al. 1997; James and Davies 2005). Lesions in skeletally immature individuals account for between 2 and 6% of all GCTOB (Picci et al. 1983 Kransdorf et al. 1992). When arising in the small bones of the hand and wrist, patients usually present with pain and swelling but may also present with a pathological fracture (Biscaglia et al. 2000). The average duration of symptoms is between 6 and 8 months (Sanjay et al. 1996; Biscaglia et al. 2000).

GCTOB is usually monostotic, but multicentric cases have been described. The rate of multicentric GCTOB in the hand and wrist is between 7 and 18% (James and Davies 2005; Wold and Swee 1984; Sanjay et al. 1996) compared to less than 1% at other locations. GCTOB is generally considered a benign lesion but does have metastatic potential with risk of spread to the lungs. The overall risk of metastasis in GCTOB is between 1 and 9% (Harness and Mankin 2004; Jaffe 1935; Jaffe et al. 1940; Rock et al. 1984). Of a series of 21 cases occurring in the hand, 5% developed pulmonary metastases (Averill et al. 1980). Tumours of the distal radius have been implicated in the literature as the most common primary site in

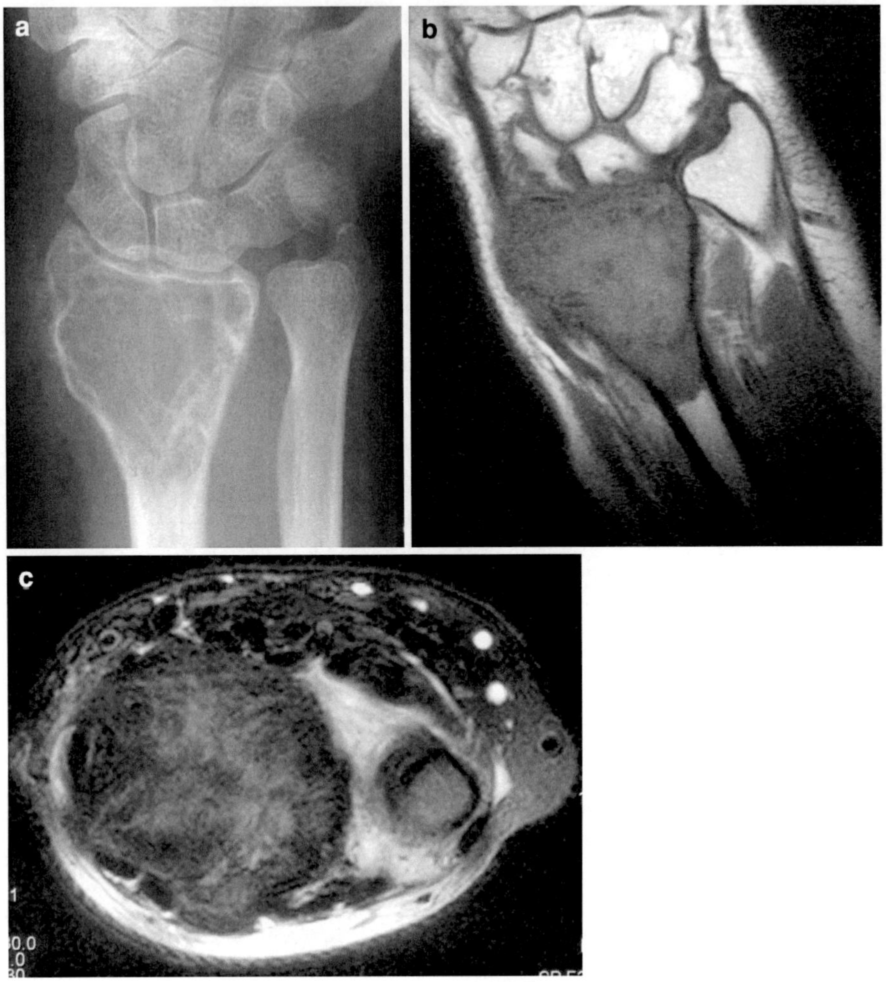

Fig. 10 Giant cell tumour. **a** PA radiograph showing a subarticular, expansile, lytic lesion in the distal radius with a trabeculated contour. **b** Coronal T1-weighted and **c** Axial T2-weighted MR images showing the extent of the lesion and low signal areas due to the presence of haemosiderin

patients with pulmonary metastases (Athanasian et al. 1997). Earlier and higher rates of recurrence in GCTOB of the hand, compared to the tumour at other sites, have been reported (Patel et al. 1987). The risk of recurrence in the hand is reported as 83% (Averill et al. 1980) compared to 25% at other locations (O'Donnell et al. 1994; McDonald et al. 1986). Malignant GCTOB is known to occur and may be primary but usually occurs as a secondary tumour, usually due to sarcomatous transformation following radiotherapy. Malignant GCTOB of the distal radius has been reported (Pho 1981), but to the best of our knowledge, it has not been reported in the small bones of the hand and wrist.

Lesions in the distal radius demonstrate an eccentric, expansile, lytic lesion located in a subarticular position involving the epiphysis and metaphysis as is typically seen elsewhere in the skeleton (Fig. 10a). In skeletally immature patients, the tumour is typically metaphyseal though extension across the growth plate into the epiphysis is rarely observed (Kransdorf et al. 1992; Picci et al. 1983). The metacarpals and phalanges effectively represent the equivalent of a long bone in the hand (Fig. 11). The tumour occurs in a more central location in the bones of the hand probably due to the limited volume of bone (James and Davies 2005). A narrow zone of transition is seen at the metaphyseal margin of the lesion, and there is typically no matrix mineralization. Internal trabeculation is common but the pattern may vary from fine striations to coarse trabeculation (Fig. 10a). Periosteal reaction is unusual unless there is a complicating fracture (James and Davies 2005). Thinning of the cortex and extension into the soft tissues is well recognized in GCTOB. Campanacci et al. described a grading system based on radiographic findings: Stage I

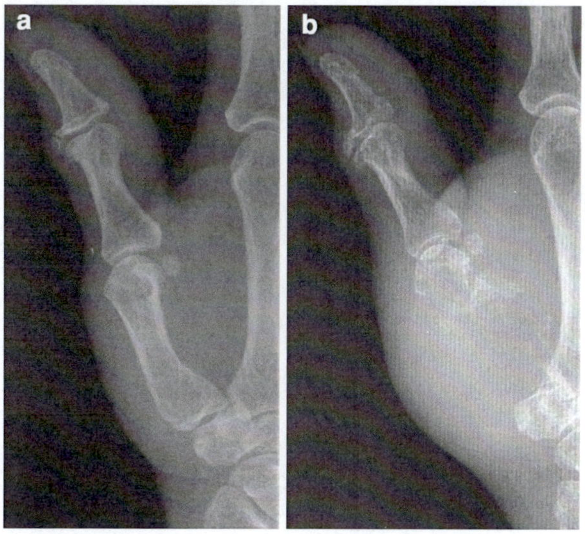

Fig. 11 Giant cell tumour. **a** PA radiograph at presentation showing a small area of permeative bone destruction in the proximal 1st metacarpal. **b** 4 months later without treatment the tumour has enlarged dramatically and is destroying much of the metacarpal

where lesions do not distort of perforate the cortex; Stage II where lesions expand or distort the cortex but do not extend into soft tissues; and Stage III where there is cortical destruction and soft tissue extension (Campanacci et al. 1979). Stage III tumours are associated with a higher rate of recurrence (O'Donnell et al. 1994). Technetium 99-m bone scintigraphy may demonstrate a classic "doughnut" configuration with avid uptake at the periphery of the tumour and a relatively photopenic centre. The routine use of bone scintigraphy has been advocated by some authors where hand lesions are identified given the higher frequency of multicentric lesions at this location (Averill et al. 1980; Wold and Swee 1984; Peimer et al. 1980).

Lesions in the hand and wrist show similar MR imaging characteristics to GCTOB elsewhere in the body (Fig. 10b). MRI defines the intra- and extra-osseous extent of the tumour. Low signal intensity on all sequences can be seen which is indicative of chronic haemosiderin deposition in GCTOB (Fig. 10c) (Aoki et al. 1996). Fluid–fluid levels may be demonstrated within the tumour mass, indicating the presence of secondary aneurysmal bone cyst (ABC) formation.

Giant-cell reparative granuloma (GCRG) is a reactive process that most commonly involves the mandible, maxilla and small bones of the hands and feet. It has been suggested that this lesion may be morphologically related or may constitute the same clinical entity as GCTOB (Gouin et al. 2003). Others have however expressed a differing opinion (Murphey et al. 2001). Histologically, GCRG is characterized by fibroblasts and clusters of multinucleated giant cells surrounded by foci of haemorrhage which may also contain areas of osteoid matrix and aneurysmal bone cyst formation (Yamaguchi and Dorfman 2001; Murphey et al. 2001; Macdonald et al. 2003). In general, GCRG affects a younger age group than GCTOB, with presentation often seen in skeletally immature patients. Sex distribution is equal in GCRG of the hands and feet (Ratner and Dorfman 1990). As with GCTOB, clinical presentation may be non-specific. GCRG most commonly affects the phalanges, followed by the metacarpals and carpal bones (Fig. 12) (Yamaguchi and Dorfman 2001). The tumours are metaphyseal in location, and unlike in GCTOB, involvement of the epiphysis is rare (Murphey et al. 2001). To our knowledge, extension of GCRG across an unfused physis has not been reported. The tumours may have an expansile, lytic radiographic appearance and may demonstrate cortical destruction (Fig. 11). Pathological fracture and periosteal reaction are rarely seen (Wold et al. 1986).

2.3 Bone Cysts

Aneurysmal bone cyst (ABC) is rare accounting for between 5 and 6% of benign bone tumours (Huvos 1991). ABCs are composed histologically of blood-filled cavities lined by giant cell osteoclasts, fibrous tissue and woven bone. The most common locations of ABC are the proximal tibia, humerus and pelvis. ABC of the hand is rare. In a series of 516 ABCs, only 17 lesions occurred in the hand (Fuhr and Hendron 1979). Of 95 cases reviewed by Tillman et al., only 3 were in the hand (Tillman et al. 1968).

ABC most commonly presents in the second decade of life and has an equal distribution among males and females. In a review of the literature, Platt and Klugman concluded that ABC of the hand most commonly involves the metacarpals (52%) followed by the phalanges (36%) and carpal bones 4% (Platt and Klugman 1995). An unusual case of ABC arising in a sesamoid bone of the hand has been reported

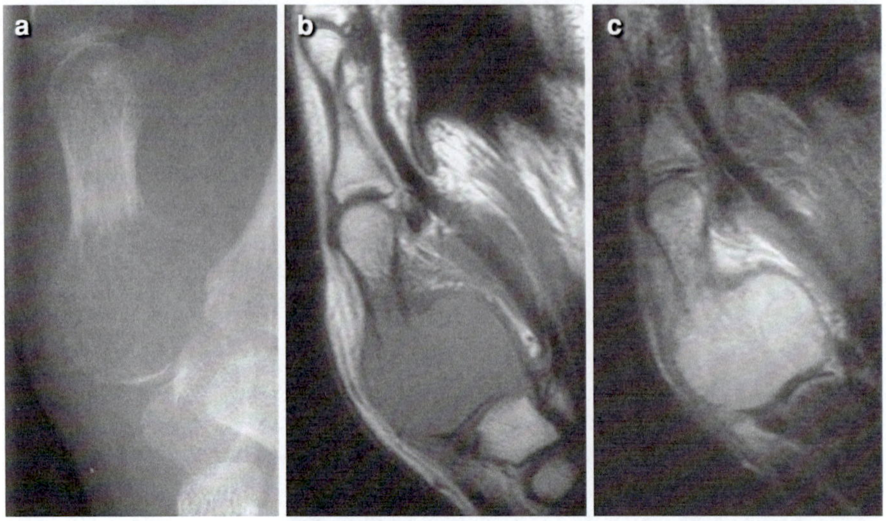

Fig. 12 Giant cell reparative granuloma. **a** PA radiograph **b** Coronal T1-weighted and **c** Coronal STIR MR images showing a lytic, expansile lesion destroying the proximal third of the first metacarpal

(Havulinna et al. 2005). Trauma is implicated in association with almost half of the published cases of hand ABC; however, many authors suggest this is coincidental and has simply drawn attention to a pre-existing lesion. Typically, the patient presents with a slowly enlarging mass that may or may not be painful (Athanasian 2004). On examination, there may be extensive swelling and warmth. Patients may present with a pathological fracture.

Radiographs of the hand demonstrate a central, expansile, lytic lesion that causes cortical thinning. ABCs are normally epiphyseal or metaphyseal in location (Fig. 13). Subperiosteal ABCs are eccentrically located and tend to involve the metaphysis or metadiaphysis. These lesions grow outside the confine of normal bone but are limited externally by periosteum and internally by endosteum (James and Davies 2006). Only two cases of subperiosteal ABC have been reported in the hand, one in a metacarpal and the other in a phalanx (Fig. 14a) (Alnot et al. 1983; Maiya et al. 2002). ABCs may be surrounded by a sclerotic margin. Matrix trabeculations are sometimes observed and may be mixed or lytic. Pathological cortical fractures are associated with a periosteal reaction. When the lesion presents in the distal phalanx, significant bone destruction may occur. The natural history of ABC is that of progressive enlargement and bone destruction though some authors have noted spontaneous healing or healing following minor disturbance such as fracture or biopsy (Chalmers 1981; Leeson et al. 1988). MR and CT imaging, as in other skeletal locations, may demonstrate fluid–fluid levels which are suggestive but not diagnostic of ABC (Fig. 14b, c). The possibility of secondary ABC formation in a pre-existing lesion should always be considered. Both radiologically and histologically the lesion may be confused with telangiectatic osteosarcoma; however, the latter entity is rarer than ABC in the hand. Although ABC can be locally aggressive, it is not known to have

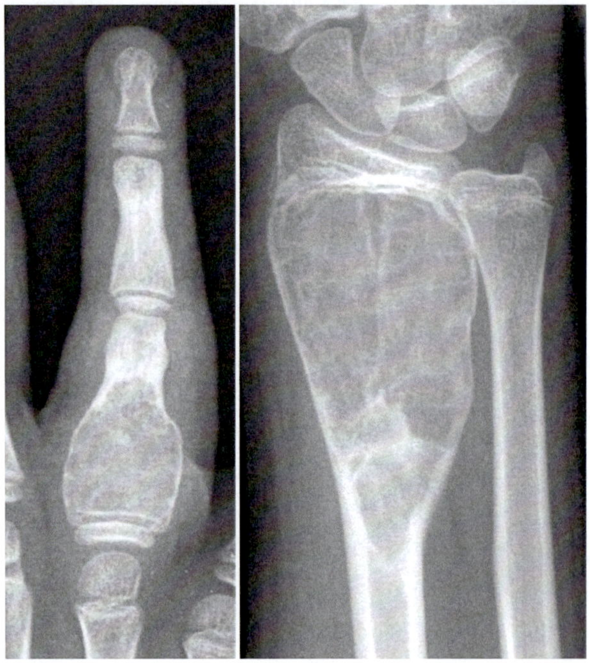

Fig. 13 Aneurysmal bone cyst. Two different cases both in children. There a lytic, expansile, juxta-epiphyseal lesions arising in the proximal phalanx and distal radius

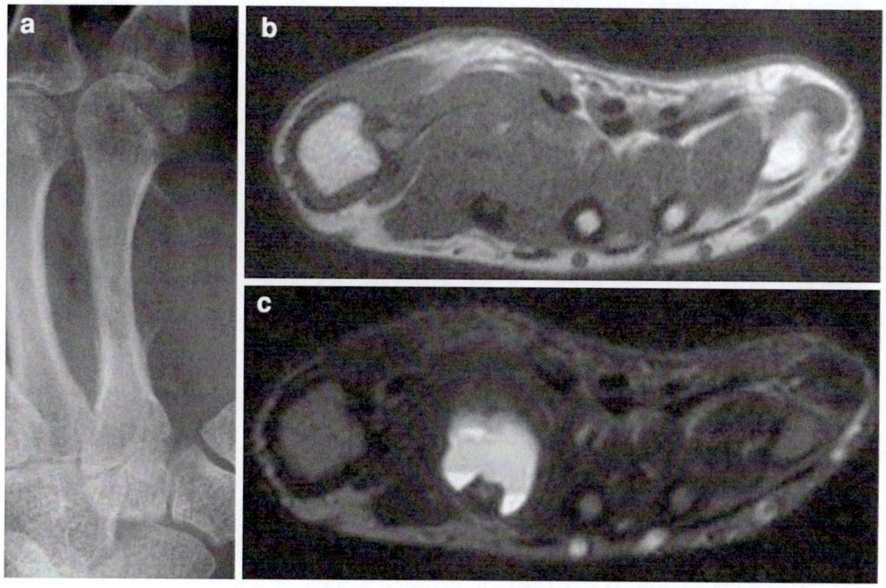

Fig. 14 Subperiosteal aneurysmal bone cyst. **a** Oblique radiograph showing a thin shell of periosteal new bone arising from the second metacarpal. **b** Axial T1- and **c** Axial T2-weighted fat suppressed MR images showing an eccentric lesion with fluid–fluid levels

metastatic potential. Local recurrence after curettage has been widely reported.

Simple bone cyst, also termed unicameral bone cyst, is a tumour-like lesion of unknown cause. It consists of a bony cavity, lined by a thin membrane and filled with fluid. It most commonly arises in the proximal humerus and proximal femur with 85% occurring pre-skeletal fusion. Involvement of the hand and wrist is rare. Radiographic features, irrespective of site, are those of a benign looking, lytic lesion arising in the metaphysis of a long bone. Frequently, cases present with a pathological fracture following only minor trauma (Fig. 15a). In time the cyst will grow away from physis with the laying down of normal intervening trabecular bone (Fig. 15b).

Intraosseous ganglia are benign non-neoplastic bone lesions that are histologically similar to their soft tissue counterpart. The terms intraosseous ganglion, subchondral cyst or geode are often applied interchangeably, although the latter are more frequently used to describe juxta-articular lesions associated with degenerative or inflammatory joint disease (Williams et al. 2004). They appear as well-defined subarticular lytic lesions. When not associated with degenerative joint disease, they can mimic other juxta-articular lesions such as giant cell tumour (Fig. 16). Cases arising in the carpal bones are not uncommon, can be multiple and bilateral (Logan et al. 1992; Lorente et al. 1992).

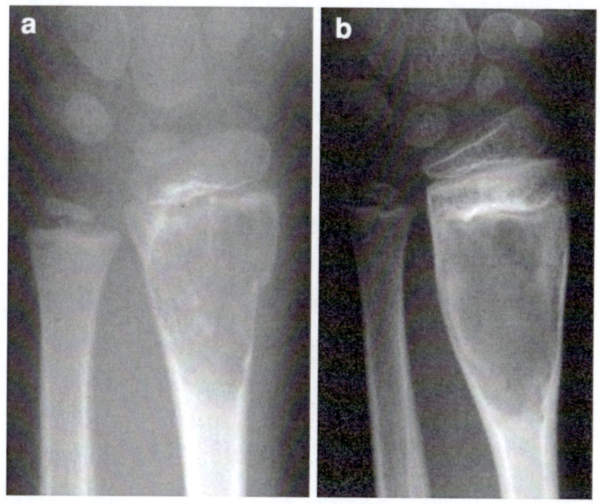

Fig. 15 Simple bone cyst. **a** PA radiograph showing a pathological fracture through a lytic lesion in the distal radial metaphysis. **b** 2 years later the fracture has healed. The lesion is mildly expansile and has started to grow away from the distal radial growth plate

2.4 Osteoid Osteoma

Osteoid osteoma is a benign osteoblastic tumour that was first described in 1935 (Jaffe 1935). The tumour consists of an area of variably calcified osteoid tissue within a stroma of relatively loose vascular connective tissue. A rim of sclerotic reactive bone, less than 2 cm in diameter, surrounds the lesion and there may be a

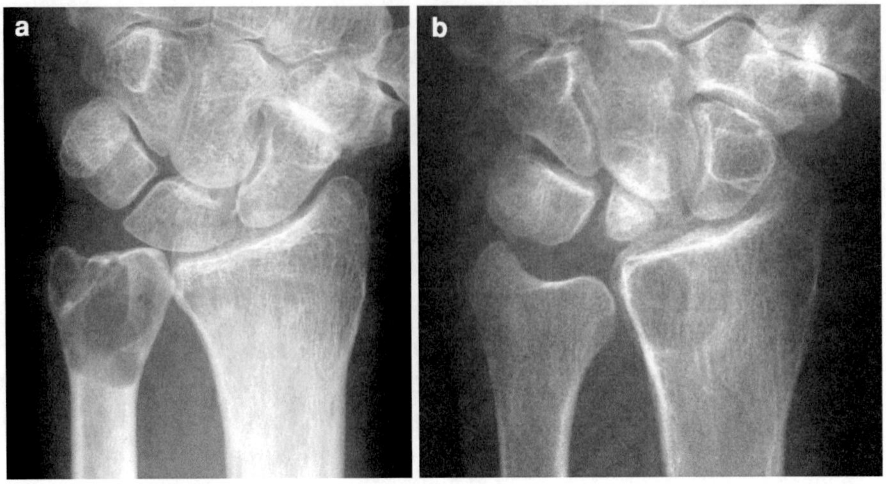

Fig. 16 Intraosseous ganglion. Two different cases showing subarticular lytic lesions involving **a** the distal ulna and **b** the distal radius. This second case also shows scapho-lunate disassociation

periosteal reaction. Approximately 10% of cases of osteoid osteoma involve the hand and wrist: 6% the phalanges, 2% the metacarpals and 2% the carpal bones (Jackson et al. 1977). The middle phalanges are the least commonly affected bones in the hand (Bednar et al. 1993; Ambrosia et al. 1987; Marcuzzi et al. 2002; Rex et al. 1997).

In general, osteoid osteoma most commonly presents in the second decade of life and has a 2:1 male to female ratio (Jackson et al. 1977). In Marcuzzi et al. series of 18 cases of osteoid osteomas of the hand and wrist, the male: female ratio was equal and the average age at presentation was 27 years (Marcuzzi et al. 2002). Typical clinical symptoms are of gradually increasing pain and swelling. Juxta-articular location can lead to restriction of movement. Physical signs often vary depending on the site of clinical symptoms. Proximal and middle phalanx involvement may be associated with a grossly enlarged phalanx with hypertrophy of the soft tissues, while distal phalanx involvement may lead to finger clubbing and hypertrophy of the nail (Marcuzzi et al. 2002; Rosborough 1966). The average duration of symptoms for osteoid osteoma of the hand and wrist before diagnosis is between 13 and 15 months (Bednar et al. 1993; Doyle et al. 1985; Marcuzzi et al. 2002). However based on reports in the literature, painless osteoid osteoma appears to occur in the digits more frequently than in any other skeletal location (Basu et al. 1999; Lawrie et al. 1970; Rex et al. 1997; Wiss and Reid 1983).

Osteoid osteomas may arise centrally in the medulla, in the cortex or in a subperiosteal location. As with other skeletal sites, the cortex is the most common location for osteoid osteomas of the hand and wrist.

Subperiosteal lesions are extremely rare in the hand, with only limited reported cases (Crosby and Murphy 1988; Kayser et al. 1998; Shankman et al. 1997). The typical radiographic appearance is that of a small, radiolucent lesion or nidus surrounded by an area of bone sclerosis (Fig. 17). Lesions noted in the subperiosteum have atypical radiographic findings (Fig. 18). Of 18 hand and wrist osteoid osteomas reported by Marcuzzi et al., only two had characteristic appearances on radiographs (Marcuzzi et al. 2002). Initially, these were normal in almost all patients, with bony abnormality becoming visible from 6 to up to 25 months. As with other skeletal locations, bone scintigraphy of osteoid osteoma of the hand and wrist shows a well-defined focal area of increased activity during all three phases of a technetium-99 MDP scan. Findings can be non-specific with diffuse uptake of radionuclide in the area of the lesion. CT is the most specific investigation (Fig. 18b) (Assoun et al. 1994). This characteristically shows a lytic lesion with a central granular opacity surrounded by a sclerotic margin. While MRI is the most sensitive imaging modality, it lacks specificity and can be misleading in the absence of radiographs and radionuclide scans (Assoun et al. 1994). The typical MRI pattern is that of a lesion composed of a hypointense, sclerotic centre with a high T2 signal rim surrounded by marrow oedema (Kreitner et al. 1999). Soft tissue oedema is also commonly present. MRI however is often non-specific particularly when there is diffuse oedema. It is also non-specific in differentiating osseous neoplasms

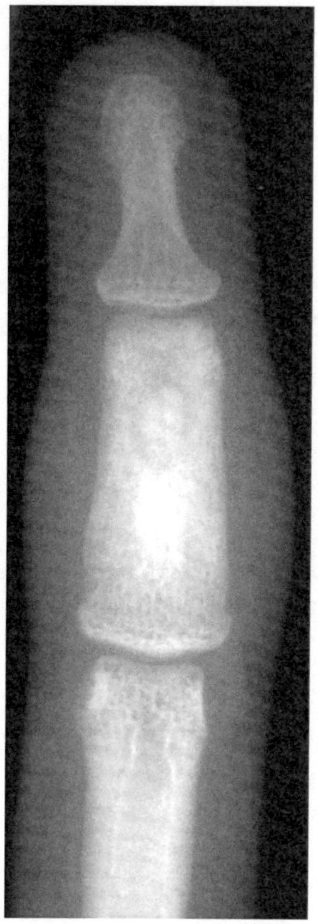

Fig. 17 Osteoid osteoma. There is sclerosis and thickening of the middle phalanx with a faint lucent cavity containing a focus of calcification representing the nidus of the lesion

like osteoid osteoma from low-grade infection and florid reactive periostitis (Ehara et al. 1994).

2.5 Focal Proliferative Periosteal Processes

Florid reactive periostitis (FRP) was first reported in 1933 by Mallory (cited by Jambhekar et al. 2004). Subsequently, bizarre parosteal osteochondromatous proliferation (BPOP) of the phalanges was described as a new radiopathological entity by Nora et al. (1983). Initially, these two conditions were considered to represent two distinct processes. Yuen et al. proposed a hypothesis that the two entities, along with turret exostosis, are part of a continuous spectrum of the same process (Yuen et al. 1992). They suggested that initial subperiosteal haemorrhage causes a localized fusiform periostitis consistent with FRP. Later the periostitis becomes incorporated into cortex and remodelling leads to a broad-based cancellous protruberance that is characteristic for BPOP. Sundaram et al. reported a series of three cases where a presumptive radiographic diagnosis of FRP was made, biopsy withheld and the patients closely followed-up with serial radiographs (Sundaram et al. 2001). They observed maturing of the periosteal reaction as expected in BPOP, leading them to also conclude that FRP can progress to BPOP.

2.5.1 Florid Reactive Periostitis

The term Florid reactive periostitis was first used by Spjut and Dorfman in their series of 12 cases (Spjut and Dorfman 1981). Because of its histological resemblance to nodular fasciitis, other names used to describe the entity have included Fasciitis ossificans and Parosteal fasciitis (Hutter et al. 1962; Kwittken and Branche 1969). Dupree and Enzinger, in a series of 21 cases, used the term Fibro-Osseous pseudotumour of the digits. They dispute its periosteal origin suggesting it arises from soft tissues and surrounding fibrous structures (Dupree and Enzinger 1986).

FRP is more frequent in the second and third decades of life (Callahan et al. 1985; Rogers et al. 1999). According to Flechner and Mills, there is a slight female preponderance (quoted by Solana et al. 2003). An antecedent history of trauma is present in between 10 and 50% of cases of FRP (Spjut and Dorfman 1981; Michelsen et al. 2004). The majority of cases involve the proximal phalanx, followed by the middle phalanx, metacarpal and distal phalanx in decreasing order of frequency (Rogers et al.1999). Radiographs typically demonstrate soft tissue swelling with intralesional calcification (Howard et al. 1996). Periosteal reaction is present in approximately 50% of cases and can either be lamellated or mature (Fig. 35.20a) (Howard et al. 1996; Spjut and Dorfman 1981). Cortical erosions associated with FRP have been described in several series (Spjut and Dorfman 1981; Dupree and Enzinger 1986; Landsman et al. 1990; Jongewood et al. 1985; Howard et al. 1996). All were successfully managed with marginal resection which led Howard et al. to conclude that lesions with cortical erosion should not be considered an aggressive form of the disease. The main radiological differential diagnoses include osteomyelitis and parosteal osteosarcoma. Concern regarding a delay in treatment for potential malignancy often leads to hastily performed surgical procedures (Jambhekar et al. 2004). Sundaram et al. advocate more prospective radiological diagnosis of FRP with close

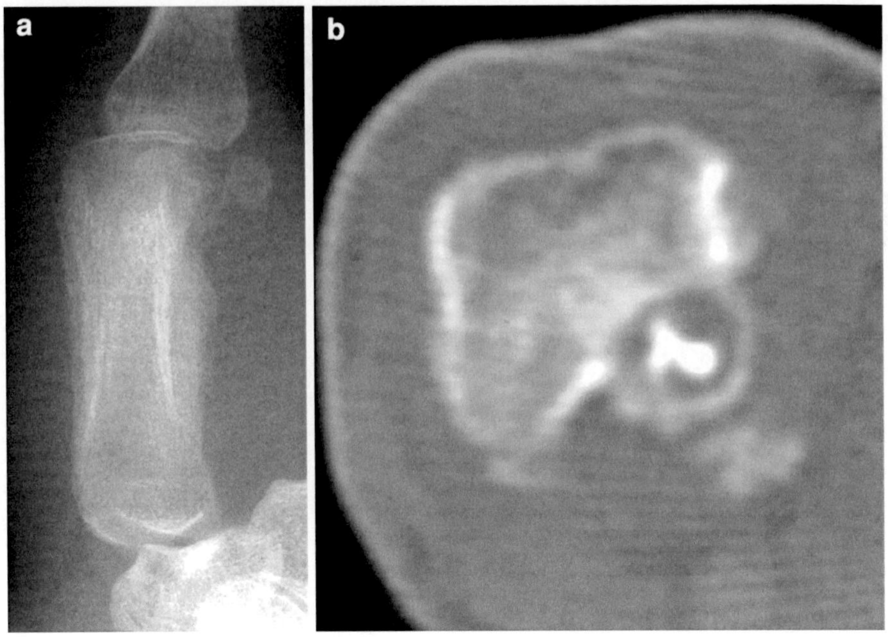

Fig. 18 Subperiosteal osteoid osteoma. **a** Radiograph showing periosteal new bone formation along the 1st metacarpal with a faint eccentric nidus located distally. **b** Axial CT reveals the nidus formed by the subperiosteal cavity and containing a small focus of calcification

clinical and radiographic follow-up to allow more appropriate and timely intervention (Sundaram et al. 2001).

2.5.2 Bizarre Parosteal Osteochondromatous Proliferation

Since its initial description by Nora, several case series and case reports of BPOP have been published. Of 65 cases in Meneses series, 36 (55%) were located in the hand (Meneses et al. 1993). Though the age at which presentation occurs is wide, peak incidence tends to be in the third and fourth decades (Meneses et al. 1993). There is no sex predilection. An antecedent history of trauma is uncommon but is reported by some authors (Meneses et al. 1993; Michelsen et al. 2004). Typically, presentation is insidious and characterized by a slow-growing, usually painless mass. Radiographs demonstrate a well-marginated mineralized mass arising from the cortical surface of the affected bone (Fig. 19b) (Nora et al. 1983). Though the cortex is classically unaffected, one case report describes cortical erosion in association with BPOP, but this was in the distal radius (Helliwell et al. 2001). The lesion can measure from 0.4 to 4 cm (Nora et al. 1983; Dhondt et al. 2006). Occurrence is 4 times more common in the hand than the foot. Fifty percent of cases affect the proximal phalanges with the remainder evenly distributed between the middle phalanges and metacarpals (Bednar et al. 1995 quoted by Torreggiani et al. 2001). The distal phalanx tends not to be involved. The characteristic radiological findings that differentiate BPOP from osteochondroma are the lack of cortical flaring at the margin of the protruberance and the absence of continuity of the lesion with medulla of underlying bone. Rybak et al. however have reported a series of histologically proven BPOP cases where medullary communication was demonstrated leading them to hypothesize that a continuum also exists between BPOP and osteochondroma (Rybak et al. 2007). None of the cases in this series were in the hand.

CT is of value in demonstrating the relationship between the lesion and underlying cortex and establishing that there is not continuity with the medullary cavity. There are a number of reports of the characteristic MRI appearances of BPOP (Tannenbaum and Biermann 1997; Torreggiani et al. 2001; Orui et al. 2001). The lesion is of low signal intensity on T1-weighted images and high signal intensity on T2 and STIR-weighted images (Torreggiani et al. 2001). The medulla and surrounding soft tissues are usually normal in appearance though Orui reported a case with oedema in both medulla and surrounding soft tissues (Orui et al. 2001).

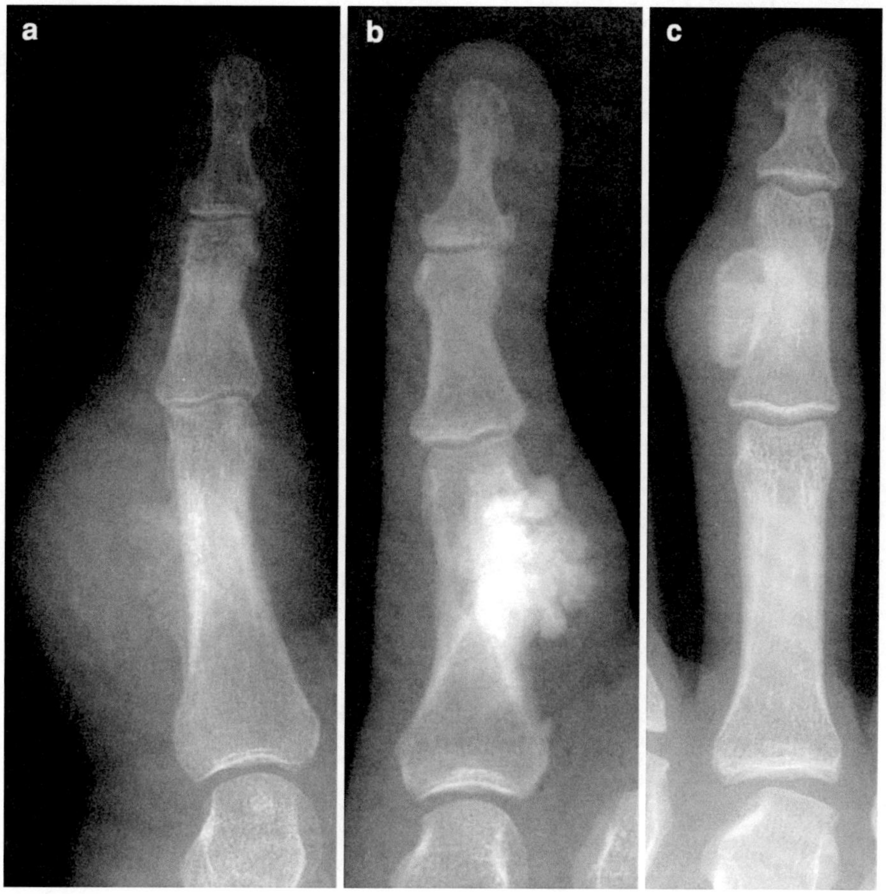

Fig. 19 Focal proliferative periosteal processes. **a** Florid reactive periostitis, **b** bizarre parosteal osteochondromatous proliferation and **c** turret exostosis

Definitive treatment is surgical excision. The recurrence rate is however high. There was recurrence in 18 of the 35 cases in Nora's series and 22 of 40 cases where follow-up was available in Meneses series. A case of fibrosarcoma in association with BPOP has been reported in the distal fibula (Choi et al. 2001) To the authors knowledge, this is the only reported case of malignancy associated with BPOP. There have been no reported cases of metastatic disease.

2.5.3 Turret Exotosis

Turret exostosis is a rare complication of trauma to the fingers. It is thought to result from breach of the periosteum with formation and subsequent ossification of subperiosteal haemorrhage. The index and little finger digits are most frequently involved (Wissinger et al. 1966; Lee and Kaplan 1974; Bourguignon 1981). The phalanges are the typical location for the lesion, but a case involving a metacarpal has been reported (Rubin and Steinberg 1996). The lesion usually occurs on the dorsal surface of the affected phalanx with only one case reported to date arising on the volar aspect (Mohanna et al. 2000).

A firm mass is usually palpable on clinical presentation, and there may be loss of function of the digit distal to the exostosis due to excursion of the extensor tendons (Mohanna et al. 2000). There is almost always an antecedent history of trauma usually in the form of a laceration. Radiographically, the earliest finding is soft tissue swelling. A poorly defined, fragmented collection of subperiosteal new bone may be seen up to about 4 months from the initial injury (James and Davies 2005). The mature lesion demonstrates a narrow body with a smooth dome and usually lies deep to the extensor apparatus (Fig. 19c). Most authors recommend a 6-month period between the episode of trauma and local excision of the lesion (Rubin and Steinberg 1996; Mohanna et al. 2000). Excision of the lesion before it has fully matured may result in recurrence. Serial radiographs and bone scan can be used to assess maturity of the lesion which is indicated by well-defined cortical margins on radiographs and decreasing activity on bone scintigraphy [Rubin].

2.5.4 Subungual Exostosis

Subungual exostosis is an uncommon benign condition arising in a distal phalanx beneath or adjacent to the nail bed. Though it most commonly occurs in the great toe, between 10 and 20% of cases are identified in the fingers (Landon et al. 1979; Carroll et al. 1992; Hoehn and Coletta 1992; Ippolito et al. 1987; Izuka et al. 1995). There is no preponderance for a particular digit in the hand. The incidence of subungual exostosis is 1.5 times higher in females than males (Izuka et al. 1995). Patients usually present in the second and third decades of life. Clinical presentation typically involves pain, swelling or surrounding ulceration of the nail bed. Secondary soft tissue infection may result. The aetiology remains unclear though trauma is felt by some authors to be the most likely precipitating factor (Landon et al. 1979; Resnick and Niwayama 1988).

The tumour is histologically characterized by mature trabecular bone and an overlying fibrocartilaginous cap. This feature distinguishes the tumour from osteochondroma which has a hyaline cartilage cap (Carroll et al. 1992). Radiographs demonstrate a mature trabecular bony excrescence arising from the dorsal aspect of the distal phalanx (Fig. 20). The fibrocartilage cap is radiolucent. The lesion may have a narrow or broad attachment, but there is no continuity with the underlying medulla, a distinguishing feature from osteochondroma. There should be no bony destruction (Landon et al. 1979). Occasionally, the lesion may be strictly more paraungual than subungual in location (Fig. 20). No cases of malignant change have been reported in the literature.

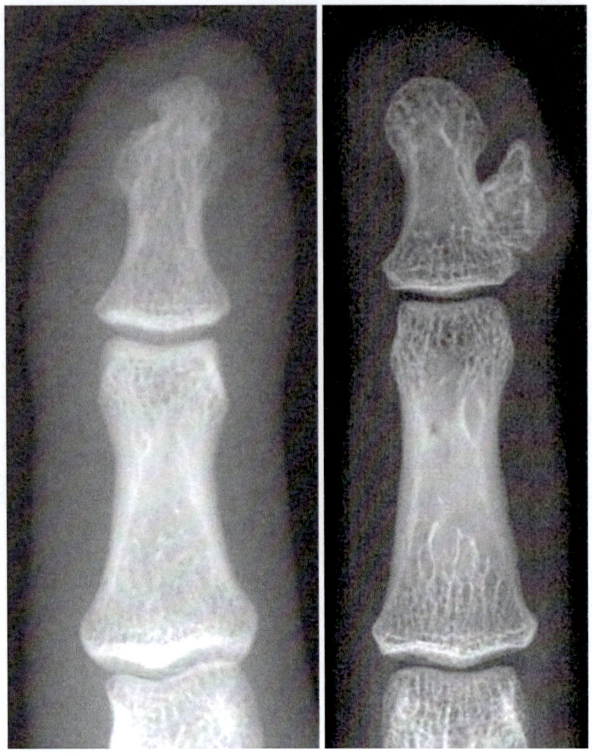

Fig. 20 Subungual and paraungual exostoses

2.5.5 Periostitis Ossificans

Myositis ossificans occurring in the hand is an extremely rare entity. When it occurs in a juxtacortical location, it is termed periostitis ossificans and may mimic BPOP or FRP (Fig. 21) (James and Davies 2005). It is usually seen in young adults. Patients may present with a rapid onset of pain, a palpable mass, oedema, joint contractures and decreased range of motion (Cushner and Morwessel 1992; De Smet and Vercauteren 1984; Ray and Basset 1984).

Initial radiographs may be normal or demonstrate a non-calcified soft tissue mass. The mass undergoes peripheral mineralization at 7–14 days, and adjacent periosteal reaction may also be observed (Fig. 21). By 6–8 weeks, a densely calcified periphery develops and a lucent centre is observed on radiographs. As the lesion matures, it undergoes ossification from the margins inwards. This 'zoning' phenomenon is the hallmark of myositis ossificans and helps differentiate it from parosteal osteosarcoma both radiologically and histologically (Fig. 21c).

2.6 Miscellaneous Benign Tumours

Chondroblastoma (CB) occurring in the hand and wrist is extremely rare and accounts for between 3 and 4% of all CB (Neviaser and Wilson 1972; Schajowicz and Gallardo 1970; Bloem and Mulder 1985). It typically occurs in an older age group to CB at other locations, most commonly presenting in the

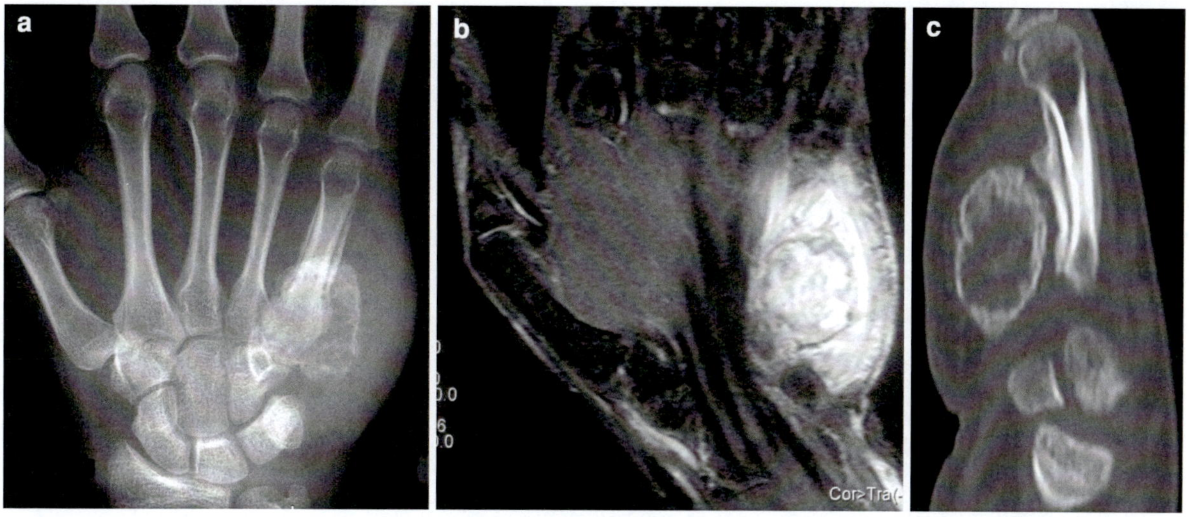

Fig. 21 Periostitis ossificans. **a** PA radiograph showing peripheral mineralization (zoning phenomenon) and reactive periosteal new bone. **b** Coronal STIR MR image showing the thin low signal intensity rim corresponding to the mineralization and a florid surrounding inflammatory response. **c** Sagittal CT reconstruction confirming the peripheral mineralization and periosteal reaction along the adjacent metacarpal

third decade of life (Davila et al. 2004; Bloem and Mulder 1985). Cases of CB occurring in the phalanges, metacarpals and carpal bones have been documented. The clinical presentation, as at other locations, almost always involves pain (Bloem and Mulder 1985). The typical radiographic appearance is of a lytic lesion with sclerotic margins, bony expansion, matrix mineralization and occasional septation (Dahlin and Unni 1986; Davila et al. 2004). At MRI, a secondary aneurysmal bone cyst component is frequently present and marrow oedema surrounding the lesion may be identified (Davila et al. 2004).

Osteoblastoma of the hand and wrist is also very rare and accounts for between 5 and 6% of all osteoblastomas (Adler 2000). On radiographs, osteoblastoma is typically eccentrically located and demonstrates a large focus of central osteolysis, between 4 and 10 cm in diameter, and a small area or peripheral sclerosis. In the short tubular bones, the lesions are much smaller, centrally located and expansile. They are well circumscribed and predominantly radiolucent (Adler 2000). Osteoblastoma has been reported in carpal, metacarpal and phalangeal bones (Wilner 1982). It is usually a solitary tumour however 3 cases of multifocal osteoblastoma involving the small bones of the hand and wrist have been reported (Adler 2000; Allieu et al. 1989; Muren et al. 1991).

Fibrous dysplasia of the hand and wrist is very uncommon. In a series of 225 cases of monostotic fibrous dysplasia, only 3 hand cases were reported (Schajowicz 1981). Of the cases described in the English speaking literature, the majority have been located in the metacarpal bone and have been of the polystotic form (Amillo et al. 1996; Gropper et al. 1985; Hayter and Becton 1984). An expansile, lytic lesion involving the shaft with a sclerotic border, trabeculations and a partially calcified matrix is described on radiographs in one of these cases (Fig. 22) (Gropper et al. 1985). Periosteal reaction and soft tissue extension as delineated on MRI has been reported (Amillo et al. 1996). Pathological fracture through an involved metacarpal was the presenting feature in another case (Hayter and Becton 1984).

Intraosseous epidermal cysts, or epidermal inclusion cysts, are squamous epithelial-lined benign cysts within bone. Peak incidence is within the 25–50 age group with a male to female ratio of 3:1 (Fisher et al. 1958). The most common site is the terminal phalanx of the left middle finger (Fisher et al. 1958). On radiographs, they usually appear as a well-defined, unilocular, osteolytic lesion with a sclerotic margin (Fig. 23) and may exhibit spotty calcifications (Musharrafieh et al. 2002; Patel et al. 2006). Enchondroma is the major differential diagnosis, but unlike intraosseous epidermal cysts, it is rarely symptomatic in the absence of a fracture.

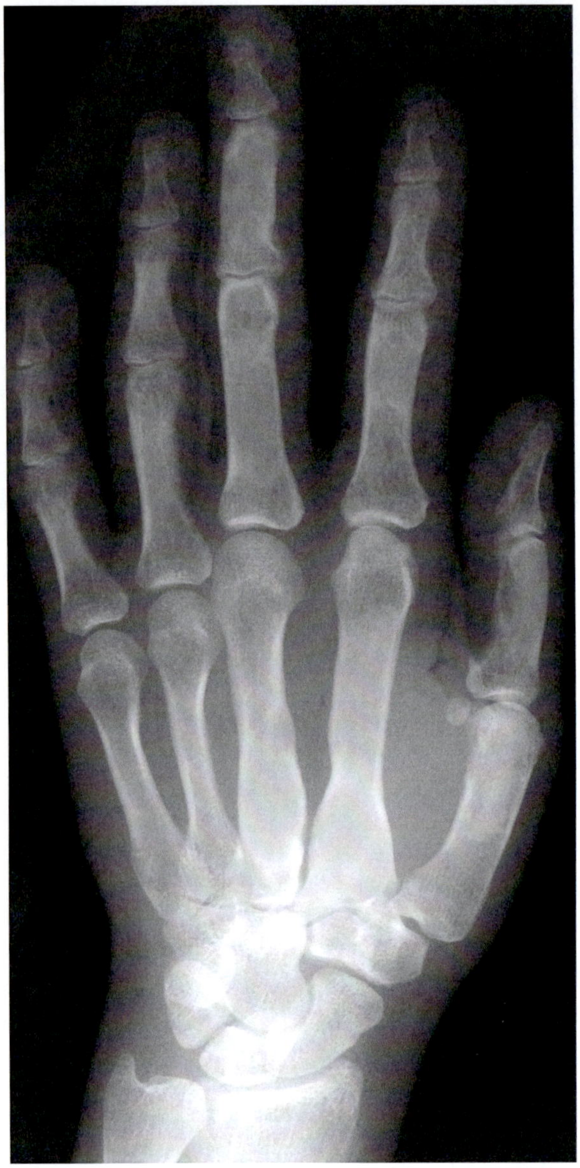

Fig. 22 Fibrous dysplasia. Polystotic involvement of the thumb, index and middle fingers. There is mild bony expansion with a ground glass matrix

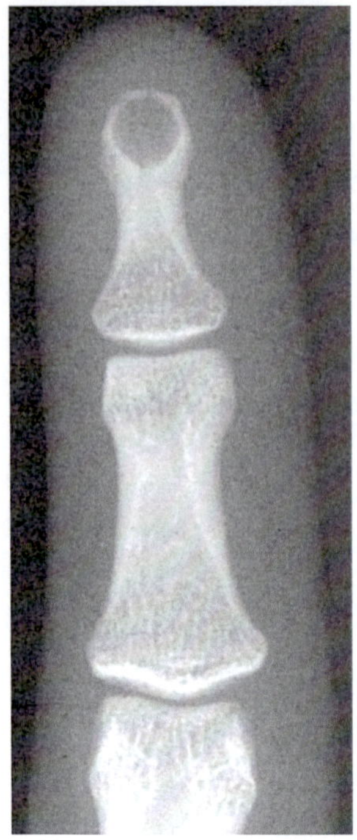

Fig. 23 Intraosseous epidermal cyst. Well-defined, rounded, lytic lesion in the tip of the terminal phalanx

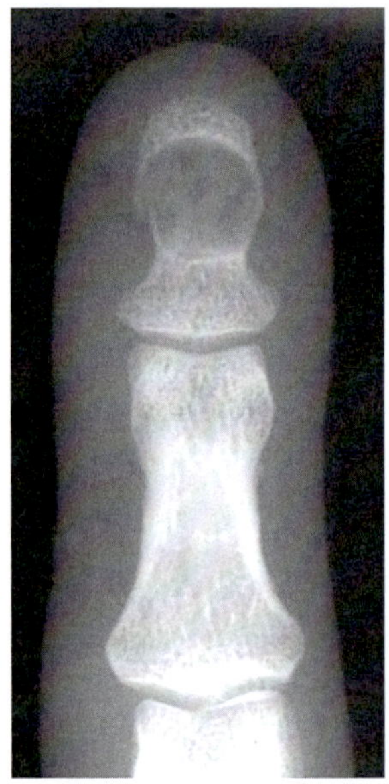

Fig. 24 Glomus tumour. Pathological fracture through well-defined lytic lesion in the terminal phalanx

Glomus tumours are benign hamartomas. They arise from the normal glomus apparatus within subcutaneous tissue. The tumours mainly occur in women and are most commonly located in the distal phalanx, usually in a subungual location (Fig. 24) (Dahlin et al. 2005). Intraosseous glomus tumours of the hand are extremely rare. Only ten had been reported in the literature by 1981 (Chan 1981). To our knowledge, only one further case has subsequently been described (Johnson et al. 1993). MRI has proved to be a valuable method of imaging glomus tumours (Theumann et al. 2002; Opdenakker et al. 1999). Most glomus tumours demonstrate high signal on spin echo T2-weighted sequences and avid enhancement post-gadolinium injection (Theumann et al. 2002). Cases have been reported where a tumour was present despite a negative MRI. On this basis, it has been

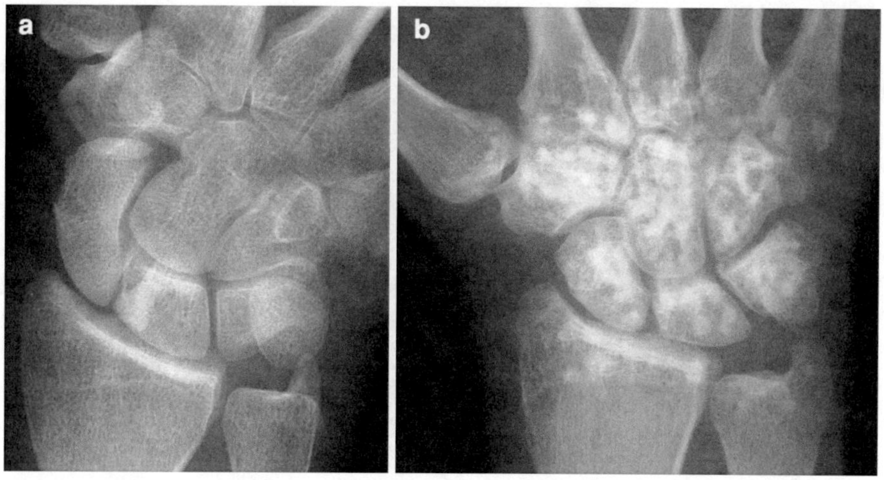

Fig. 25 Bone island. **a** Solitary sclerotic focus in the lunate, **b** Multiple small bone islands clustered around the bone ends (osteopoikilosis)

suggested that in the correct clinical context, surgical exploration should be considered even if MRI findings do not support the diagnosis (Dahlin et al. 2005).

Bone islands (enostosis) are relatively frequently encountered on routine imaging of the hand and wrist for other indications. They represent a focus of mature compact bone and are best considered a benign tumour-like lesion (Greenspan 1995). Radiographs demonstrate a sclerotic focus that often has a round or oval appearance which blends with the adjacent cancellous bone (Fig. 25a). CT shows a localized spiculate margin to the lesion and MRI will demonstrate the lesion to be low signal on all sequences. In the multiple form, osteopoikilosis, the bone islands are clustered around the bone ends (Fig. 25b).

There is a spectrum of vascular tumours that may arise in bone from benign haemangioma to malignant angiosarcoma. All are uncommon in the hand and wrist. Of particular note is that these lesions, including low-grade haemangioendothelioma, can be multicentric and so should be considered in the differential diagnosis when imaging reveals multiple lytic bony lesions (Fig. 26).

3 Malignant Bone Tumours of the Hand and Wrist

3.1 Chondrosarcoma

Chondrosarcoma of the hand accounts for 1.5% of all chondrosaromas (Unni 1996). From a Mayo Clinic series of 29 primary malignant tumours of the hand and wrist, 12 were chondrosarcomas (Unni 1996). A literature review by Damron et al. however identified only one case of chondrosarcoma from a total of 2,588 tumours of the hand (Damron et al. 1995). This may be explained by the fact that chondrosarcoma of the hand and wrist more commonly occurs from malignant degeneration of a pre-existing lesion than as primary chondrosarcoma (O'Connor and Bancroft 2004).

Chondrosarcoma of the hand and wrist occurs in an older age group than chondrosarcoma at other locations with presentation most commonly in the 6th and 7th decades of life (Saunders et al. 1997; Ogose et al. 1997). Females are slightly more commonly affected than males with a ratio of 1.3:1 (Saunders et al. 1997). Typical clinical features are of pain and swelling though not always in combination (Ogose et al. 1997; O'Connor and Bancroft 2004). Cawte et al. reported duration of symptoms between 1 month and 3 years before presentation (Cawte et al. 1998). Roberts and Price however noted a very long history in their older patients, averaging 19 years (Roberts and Price 1977).

As already discussed in this chapter, chondrosarcoma arising from pre-existing solitary enchondromas or osteochondromas or in conditions of enchondromatosis or multiple hereditary exostoses are well documented in the literature (Figs. 4 and 8). These "secondary" chondrosarcomas account for 27% of chondrosarcomas reported in the hand (Saunders et al. 1997). In all locations, 15–28% are secondary (Huvos and Marcove 1987; Salib 1967).

Chondrosarcoma of the hand is located at similar locations to enchondroma, originating near the site of

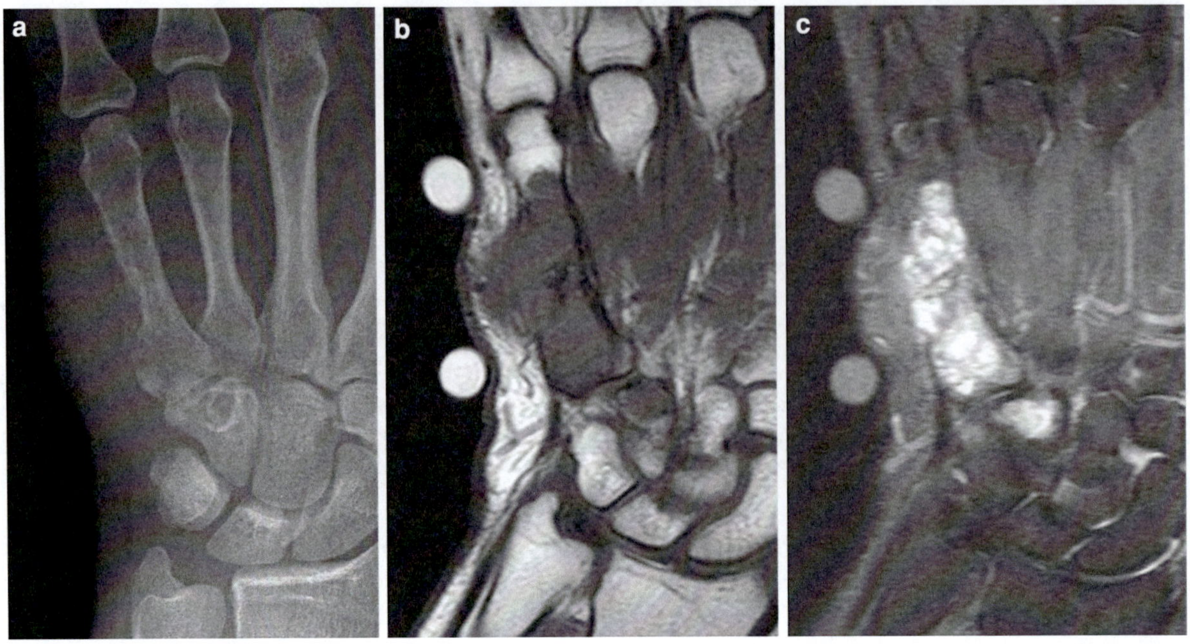

Fig. 26 Multifocal haemangioendothelioma. **a** PA radiograph, **b** Coronal T1-weighted and **c** STIR MR images showing extensive infiltration of the 5th metacarpal with a further focus of tumour in the hamate

the epiphyseal growth plate of the bone: proximally in the phalanx and distally in the metacarpal (Fig. 27) (Palmieri 1984; Roberts and Price 1977). The tumour most commonly occurs at the proximal phalanx (Saunders et al. 1997; Ogose et al. 1997; O'Connor and Bancroft 2004). Of a series of 88 chondrosarcomas of the hand reported by Ogose et al., the 5th digit was most commonly affected and the 4th was least commonly involved (Ogose et al. 1997). In the same series, the majority of chondrosarcomas located in the distal phalanx affected the thumb. Chondrosarcomas have been rarely described arising in the carpal bones (Dahlin and Salvador 1974; Granberry and Bryan 1978; Young et al. 1990; Ogose et al. 1997).

Chondrosarcoma of the hand can be difficult to differentiate radiographically from benign cartilaginous tumours particularly in the absence of clear extension through the cortex and an associated soft tissue mass (Cawte et al. 1998; Murphey et al. 2003). In a study of 160 cases of chondrosarcomas of the small bones of the hands and feet, endosteal erosion, cortical destruction and expansion were observed in 90% of the 111 cases where imaging was available (Ogose et al. 1997). Other features included an associated soft tissue mass (80%), poor margination (79%), mineralization (74%), a permeative lytic pattern (50%) and a periosteal reaction (14%) (Fig. 27). Extension of tumour across the joint in the hand has been described (Patil et al. 2003). In a study comparing the radiographic appearances of enchondroma and chondrosarcoma of the hands and feet, calcification of the chondroid matrix was observed in equal numbers (Cawte et al. 1998). Pathological fractures are observed in both enchondroma and chondrosarcoma. MRI better defines the extent of soft tissue involvement. Tumours classically demonstrate high signal on T2-weighted images and low signal on T1-weighted images, reflecting the hyaline cartilage content of the tumour (Fig. 27b, c).

The periosteal or juxtacortical type makes up an extremely rare subset of chondrosarcoma of the hand. Of 23 patients with chondrosarcoma of the small bones of the hand, Patil et al. identified one periosteal tumour (Patil et al. 2003). A further paper by Roberts and Price identified two patients out of 19 cases of chondrosarcoma of the hand that had a periosteal location. Review of the literature reveals a further two case reports (Wu et al. 1983; Jokl et al. 1971). A faintly radio-opaque mass with saucer-shaped erosion of the underlying phalanx was described in one case (Wu et al. 1983). Another description was of a radiolucent mass with stippling and calcification

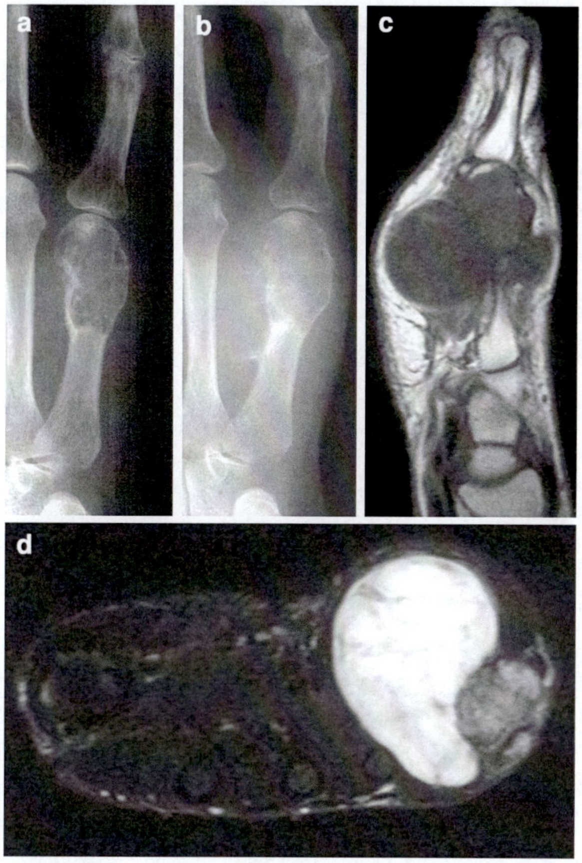

Fig. 27 Malignant transformation of enchondroma to chondrosarcoma. **a**, **b** PA radiographs obtained 18 months apart showing a significant increase in size of the lesion with cortical breaching. **c** Sagittal T1-weighted and **d** Axial T2-weighted fat saturated images showing the full extent of both intraosseous and extraosseous spread

around the middle phalanx (Jokl et al. 1971). Roberts and Price observed that the degree of cortical destruction and soft tissue tumour was less marked than in conventional chondrosarcoma (Roberts and Price 1977). It is probably for this reason that the distinction between periosteal chondroma and low-grade juxtacortical chondrosarcoma is sometimes difficult to make.

Most published series report no metastatic disease associated with chondrosarcoma of the hand (Patil et al. 2003; Palmieri 1984; Roberts and Price 1977) but in one study of patients with chondrosarcoma of the small bones of the hands and feet, Ogose et al. reported 12 distant metastatic lesions from the 70 patients where follow-up was available (Ogose et al. 1997). The risk of local recurrence after surgery necessitates long-term follow-up of these patients (O'Connor and Bancroft 2004).

3.2 Osteosarcoma

Osteosarcoma of the small bones of the hand is rare. Of 2,589 cases of skeletal osteosarcoma, Okada et al. found only 10 arising in the hand (Okada et al. 1993). A review of the English literature by Fowble et al. in 2005 found a total of 41 cases of osteosarcoma of the hand in 39 patients (Fowble et al. 2005). Since then a further 4 cases have been reported (Jones et al. 2006; Muir et al. 2008; Abe et al. 2007; Mathov et al. 2008).

Despite an age range of presentation between 13 months to 85 years (Sanchis-alfonso et al. 1994; D'antona 1934 quoted by Carroll 1957), osteosarcoma of the hand appears to affect an older age group than conventional osteosarcoma, the mean age being 42 years. Risk factors include Paget's disease, previous radiation treatment, trauma and metastasis from primary osteosarcoma located elsewhere in the skeleton (Fowble et al. 2005). Clinical presentation is typically pain and swelling (Okada et al. 1993). The long duration of symptoms, long interval before local recurrence and excellent response to treatment suggest that lesions in this location are less aggressive than conventional osteosarcomas (Okada et al. 1993).

Osteosarcoma of the hand shows a preferential distribution around the MCP joints, often sited within the metacarpal heads and bases of the proximal phalanges, with a slight predilection for the second and third digits (Fowble et al. 2005). These sites represent the fastest growing growth plates and the longest bones of the hand. Lesions of the carpus have only been reported twice, one in the scaphoid and the other in the trapezium (Marcuzzi et al. 1996; Bickerstaff et al. 1988). Two cases of bilateral osteosarcoma of the hand, both in patients with Paget's disease, have previously been reported (Drompp 1961; Friedman et al. 1982).

The radiographic findings are similar to the appearance of osteosarcoma at other sites with matrix mineralization, bone destruction and florid periosteal reaction (Fig. 28). The tumour is generally intramedullary in location with extension into the soft tissues (Fig. 28b). The presence of intramedullary involvement is helpful in distinguishing the lesion from benign entities such as BPOP and FRP that can otherwise

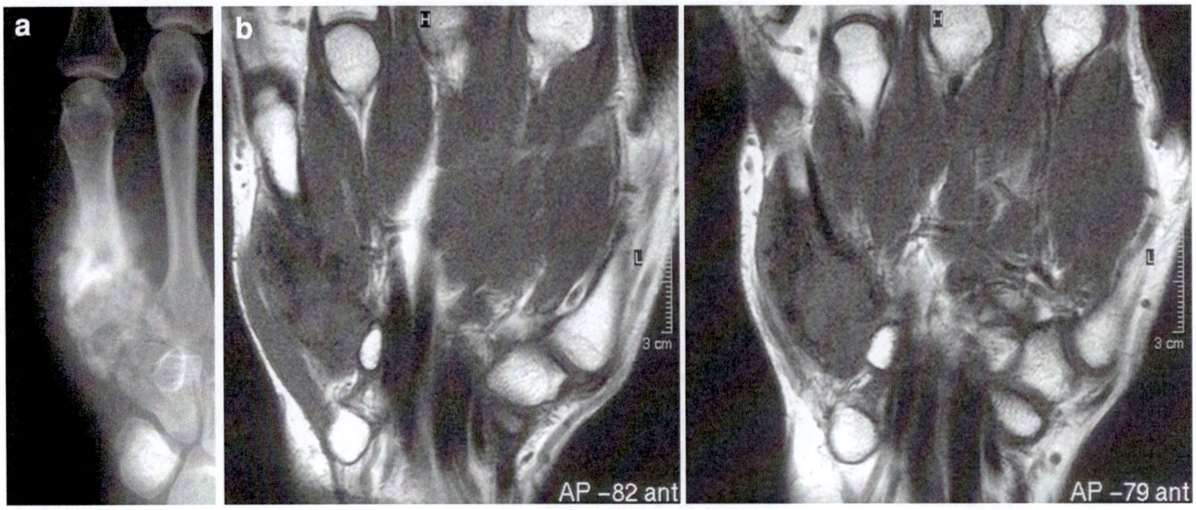

Fig. 28 Osteosarcoma. **a** Radiograph showing a mixed lytic and sclerotic lesion arising in the proximal half of the 5th metacarpal. **b** Coronal T1-weighted MR images showing the tumour infiltration and low signal intensity areas due to the malignant mineralization

appear similar on radiographs (Jones et al. 2006). The absence of zonal organization in osteosarcomas as characterized by peripheral density and central lucency can also help differentiate it from benign entities (Jones et al. 2006). MRI better assesses the soft tissue involvement and degree of intramedullary extension (Fig. 28b). The lesion may be isointense on T1-weighted imaging and of high-signal intensity on T2-weighted imaging (Honoki et al. 2001).

There appears to be a greater propensity for lesions to arise from the surface of the bone when compared to osteosarcoma at other sites. The majority of these surface tumours are parosteal with only two reported periosteal osteosarcomas of the hand (Okada et al. 1993; James and Davies 2005; Jones et al. 2006; Muir et al. 2008). Surface osteosarcomas often appear as a densely calcified mass adjacent to a metacarpal or phalanx on radiographs (Fig. 29) (Revell et al. 2000). They can be connected to bone by a stalk that may only be demonstrated on CT. These lesions may be difficult and sometimes impossible to differentiate from benign disorders on imaging (Okada et al. 1993). A rare variant of parosteal osteosarcoma is the osteochondroma-like parosteal osteosarcoma that has been reported in the hand (Fig. 30). On imaging, these lesions appear as a 'pasted on' ossified mass with an intact underlying cortex and no medullary involvement (Lin et al. 1998). Of the 6 cases of osteochondroma-like parosteal osteosarcoma reported by Lin et al., none of which occurred in the hand, all were misdiagnosed as benign entities on radiological and histological assessment.

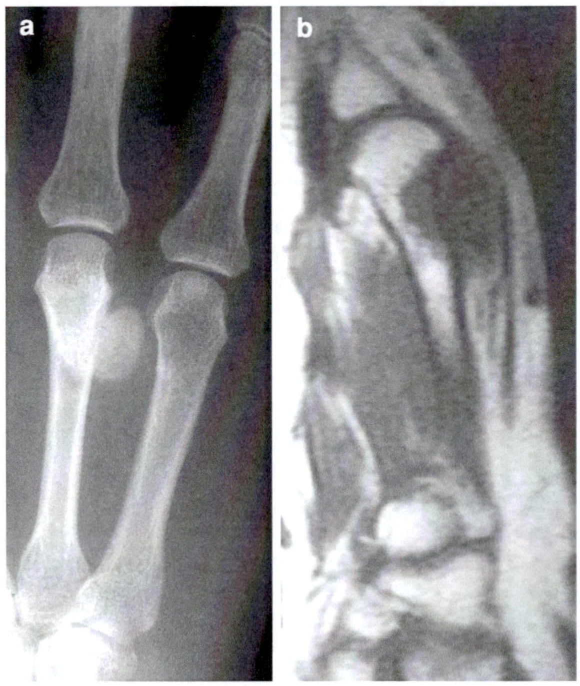

Fig. 29 Parosteal osteosarcoma. **a** The radiograph shows and ossified surface lesion arising from the 4th metacarpal. **b** Sagittal T1-weighted MR image showing the lesion is invading the underlying medulla

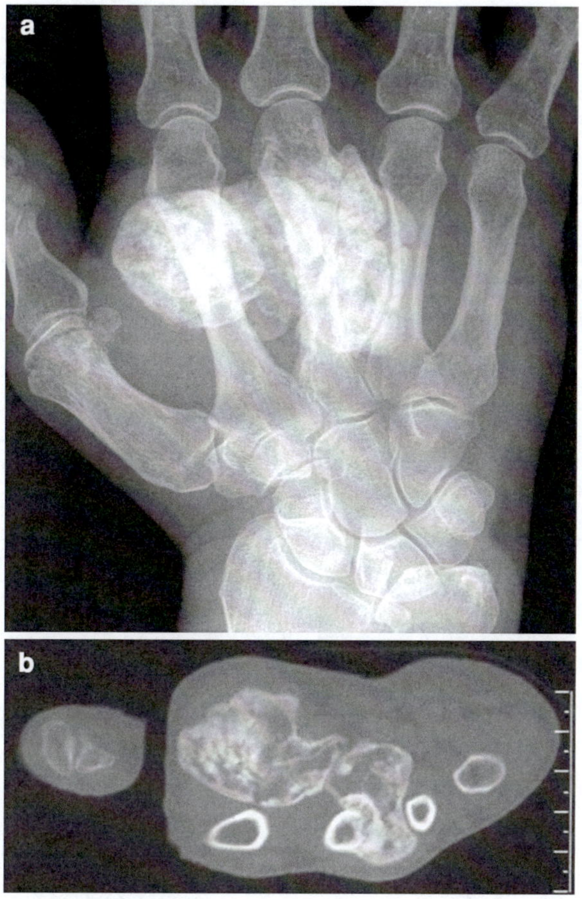

Fig. 30 Osteochondroma-like parosteal osteosarcoma. **a** The radiograph shows an ossifying mass overlying the metacarpals. **b** The CT shows it to be arising from the surface of the 3rd metacarpal but there is no trabecular continuity that would exclude the diagnosis of an osteochondroma

3.3 Ewing sarcoma

Ewing sarcoma (ES) of the hand has an incidence of between 0.3 and 1% of all ES of bone (Dahlin and Unni 1986; Kissane et al. 1983). Of 377 cases reported by the intergroup Ewing's sarcoma study, only two had lesions in the hand (Reinus et al. 1985). In Baraga's series of 43 cases of ES of the hand and feet, 11 involved the hands (Baraga et al. 2001). The demographics are similar to ES of bone at other sites with peak incidence in the second decade and males twice as commonly affected as females (Baraga et al. 2001). Typical clinical features are of pain and swelling and presentation may be acute or insidious. An antecedent history of trauma is uncommon (Dick et al. 1971; Dreyfuss et al. 1980).

ES of the hand is most likely to occur in the metacarpal bones (Lacey et al. 1987). In a literature review of ES of the phalanges, Yamaguchi et al. found that the proximal phalanx was most commonly involved (Yamaguchi et al. 1997). To the best of our knowledge, ES has never been reported in a carpal bone though it is known to occur in the tarsal bones of the feet. The tumour typically occurs in the meta-diaphyseal region of the short tubular bones of the hands and feet but may occupy the whole length of the bone (Baraga et al. 2001).

The classic radiographic findings of a permeative lytic lesion, with associated areas of sclerosis and a soft tissue mass, are almost as commonly seen in ES of the small bones of the hands and feet as at other locations (Fig. 31) (Reinus et al. 1985, Baraga et al. 2001). In the hand, it is less commonly a purely lytic lesion and more often demonstrates blastic or mixed change than at other sites (Baraga et al. 2001). Bone expansion is more commonly seen than elsewhere in the skeleton likely due to a smaller volume of bone (Reinus et al. 1985; Baraga et al. 2001). Reinus et al. originally reported a lower incidence of periosteal reaction in ES of the bones of the hands and feet than at other locations, but in Baraga et al. subsequent larger study, the rate was equal to ES at other sites (Reinus et al. 1985, Baraga et al. 2001). MRI can be used to accurately quantify the extent of the soft tissue mass both prior to and after chemotherapy (Ozaki et al. 1995). The main differential diagnosis for ES in the small bones of the hands is osteomyelitis, and misdiagnosis can lead to significant delay in treatment (Durbin et al. 1988).

A better prognosis than for ES arising at other sites has been reported (Daecke et al. 2005). This is thought to be due to less soft tissue in the extremities allowing for comparatively early presentation, diagnosis and excision with a wide margin (Yamaguchi et al. 1997). Smaller tumour volume and a lower incidence of metastasis at presentation are also thought to be important factors (Daecke et al. 2005). Akanwenze et al., in their series of 5 cases, have however reported a similar survival rate to ES at other sites (Anakwenze et al. 2009).

3.4 Metastasis

Metastasis to the hand is rare and accounts for approximately 0.1% of all metastatic bone lesions

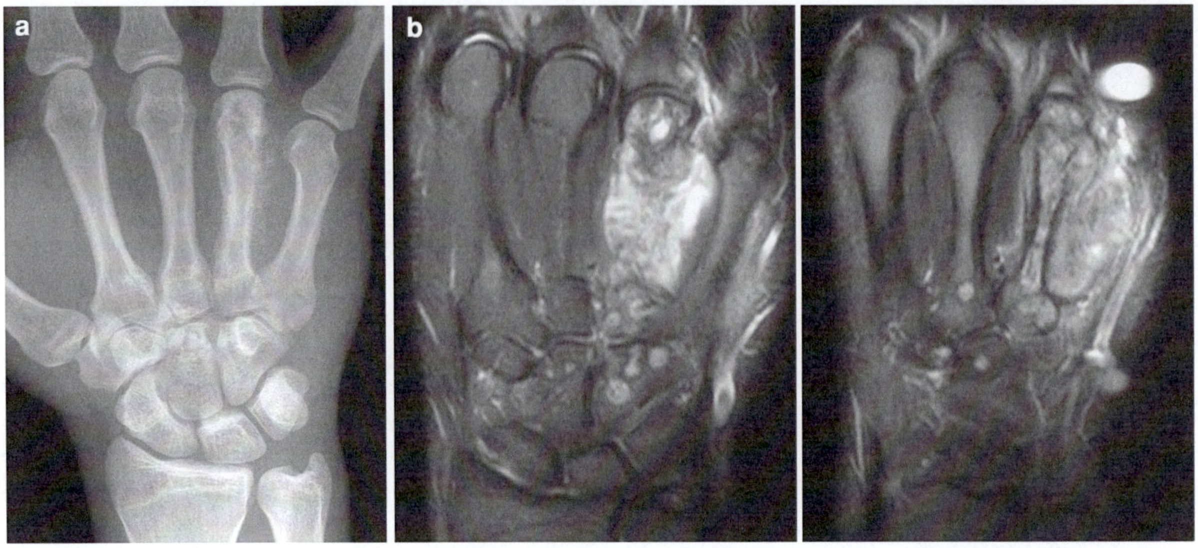

Fig. 31 Ewing sarcoma. **a** Radiograph showing typical features of an onion skin and spiculated periosteal reaction along the 4th metacarpal. **b** Two contiguous coronal STIR MR images showing extensive tumour infiltration of the metacarpal with soft tissue extension and multiple small skip metastases in the carpal bones and adjacent metacarpal

(Kerin 1983). In a series of approximately 75,000 patients diagnosed with a primary malignancy, 5 patients with metastasis to the bones of the hand and wrist were identified (Amadio and Lombadri 1987). Metastasis to the hand may rarely be the initial presentation of occult malignancy (Abrahams 1995). It is in this context in particular that acrometastasis can be misdiagnosed as other skeletal pathologies such as infection or inflammatory arthritis both clinically and radiologically.

Any bone in the hand and wrist can be involved, though the most commonly reported site is the terminal phalanx (Healey et al. 1986; Libson et al. 1987; Kerin 1983). This is probably because arterial flow is greatest in this area of the hand (Mulvey 1964). No one digit is preferentially involved (Wu and Guise 1978). The carpus is less commonly affected, being involved in only 10% of cases in two large studies of bone metastases to the hand and wrist (Healey et al. 1986; Kerin 1983; Libson et al. 1987). The majority of patients are in their fifth decade or older.

Of skeletal wrist and hand metastases, 40–50% are from primary bronchial carcinoma (Fig. 32) (Kerin 1983). This is thought to be due to the fact that primary tumours in the lung can shed cells directly into the systemic arterial circulation, whereas potential secondaries from other sites pass through the capillary bed of the lung or liver first. Wolff et al. (1966) reported

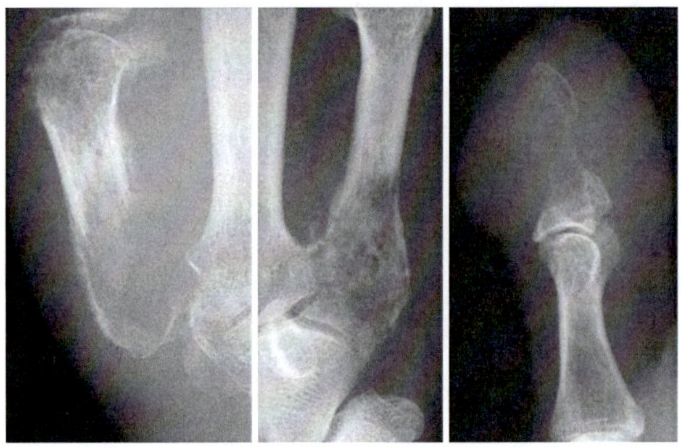

Fig. 32 Lytic metastases. Radiographs showing examples of bronchial metastases to the fingers in three different patients

metastases from the breast accounting for 25% of bone secondaries in the hand (cited by Amadio and Lombadri 1987). Renal cell carcinoma accounts for 10% of bone metastases to the hand and wrist (Ghert et al. 2001). Subdiaphragmatic tumours are generally more likely to metastasize to the feet, however in Kerin's review of the literature, metastatic hand lesions from the prostate, cervix and uterus were all noted (Kerin 1983). Sarcomatous metastases to the hand are much less frequent than metastases from carcinoma.

Clinically the patient may present with pain, swelling and loss of function. In the presence of widespread metastases at other locations, the

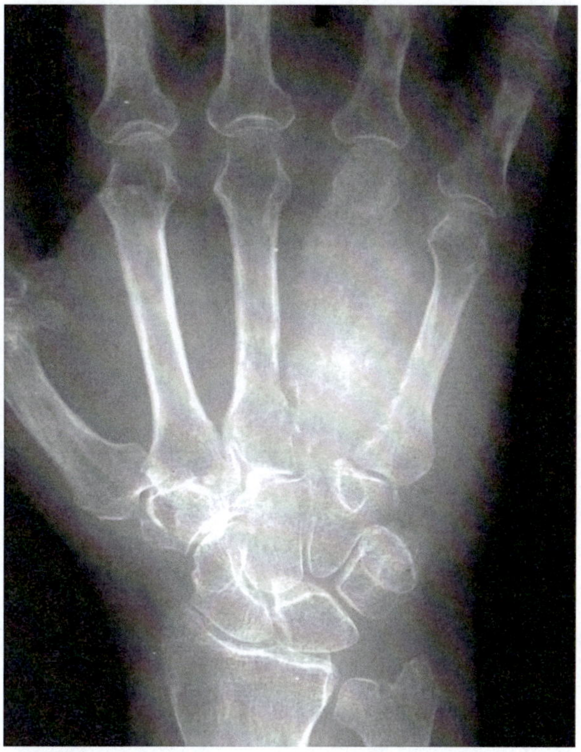

Fig. 33 Sclerotic metastasis. Radiograph showing a rare case in the 4th metacarpal from a primary mucinous adenocarcinoma of the colon

diagnosis may be straightforward. However in cases of occult malignancy, the lesion may clinically resemble osteomyelitis, septic arthritis or an acute monoarticular rheumatoid arthritis.

Metastases of the hand appear most frequently as nonspecific lytic, aggressive lesions (Fig. 32). The pattern of bone destruction varies but usually a thin rim of cortication is present around the lesion. The neoplasm may expand the cortical shell as it enlarges. Sclerotic forms have been described and are typical of metastatic osteosarcoma, but have also been seen with prostate and breast metastases (Fig. 33) (Abrahams 1995). Periosteal reaction is uncommon (Healey et al. 1986; Libson et al. 1987; Wu and Guise 1978; Chung 1983; Kerin 1958; Mulvey 1964). A soft tissue component is frequent (Libson et al. 1987). In juxta-articular lesions subchondral bone is usually spared and joint involvement is rare (Healey et al. 1986; Libson et al. 1987; Kerin 1958; Mulvey 1964).

The prognosis for patients with metastases to the hand and wrist is extremely poor with, in one series, 50% of patients dead within 6 months (Amadio and Lombadri 1987).

3.5 Lymphoma

Lymphoma involving bone usually occurs in the setting of widespread systemic disease. Non-hodgkins lymphoma however can arise primarily in bone. This is uncommon accounting for 3% of all extranodal lymphomas (Pinheiro et al. 2009). In a review of 82 cases of primary lymphoma of bone, Beal et al. found the femur to be the most common site of presentation, followed by the pelvis and tibia (Beal et al. 2006). In a Mayo clinic series of 422 cases of malignant lymphoma of bone, only 2 involved the small bones of the hand (Ostrowski et al. 1986). The authors do not state whether these were cases of primary lymphoma of bone or part of a multifocal disease. Only a few isolated case reports of primary lymphoma of bone occurring in the small bones of the hand have been published probably reflecting it's rarity (Davies et al. 1994; Archer et al. 2009; Baskar et al. 2009; Chua et al. 2009; Pinheiro et al. 2009). Of these in only one case, a solitary lesion involving the first metacarpal, was disease confined to the hands (Davies et al. 1994).

Primary lymphoma most commonly presents in adults with a median age in the 5th or 6th decades with males more frequently affected than females (Shoji and Miller 1971; Boston et al. 1974; Davies et al. 1994). Clinical presentation in the hand typically involves pain and swelling, often at an affected joint, and may mimic a rhematological disorder (Archer et al. 2009; Baskar et al. 2009). Constitutional 'B' symptoms are rare in primary bone lymphoma (Boston et al. 1974; Beal et al. 2006). Radiographs demonstrate a destructive lytic deposit with an associated soft tissue mass (Fig. 34). Despite the extensive destruction, pathological fractures are uncommon (6%) (Boston et al. 1974). MRI and CT may both demonstrate more extensive local disease than suggested on radiographs. A bone scan is required in all patients presenting with primary lymphoma of bone to assess for the presence of multifocal disease. Patients usually present with early stage disease and with modern curative modalities, the prognosis is excellent (Beal et al. 2006).

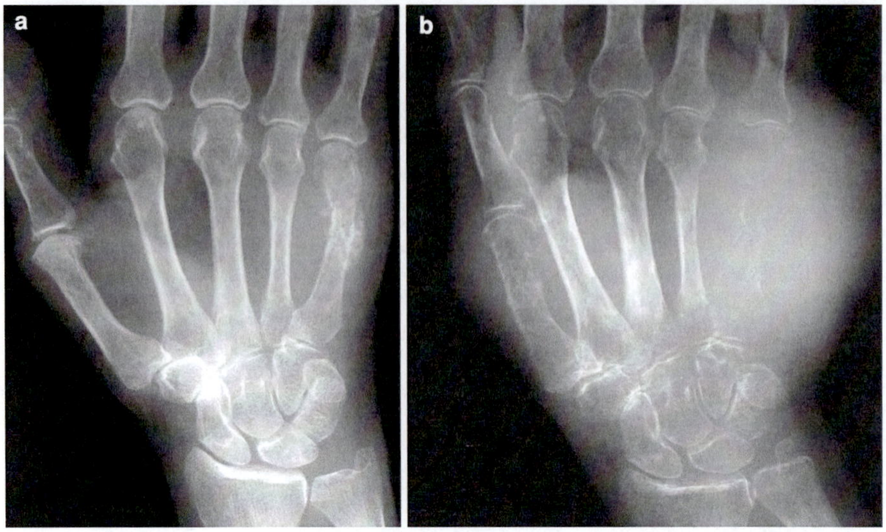

Fig. 34 Lymphoma. **a** Radiographs at presentation and **b** 4 months later. There is rapid progression of the permeative lytic lesion in the 5th metacarpal and on the latter film there is evidence of a further deposit in the 1st metacarpal

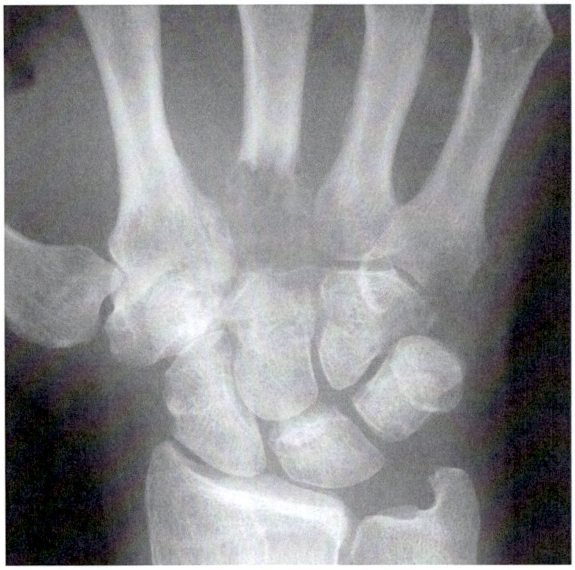

Fig. 35 Myeloma. There is a lytic lesion arising in the base of the 3rd metacarpal. The appearances are similar to both a metastasis and giant cell tumour

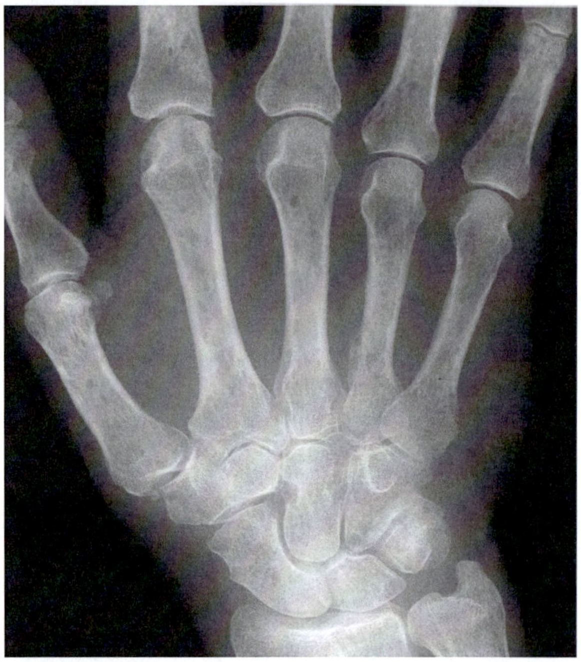

Fig. 36 Multiple myeloma. Multiple small cortical lucencies involving all the metacarpals

3.6 Multiple Myeloma

Multiple myeloma is the malignant proliferation of plasma cells involving more than 10% of bone marrow. Involvement of the extremities is rare and seen in less than 1% of all solitary bone plasmacytomas (Celik et al. 1996). Osteolytic lesions involving the small bones of the hand, either isolated or associated with multiple lytic lesions at other sites, have rarely been reported in multiple myeloma and plasma cell leukaemia (Fig. 35) (Farman and Degnan 1976; Ozguroglu et al. 1999; Dastgir et al. 1994, Antonijevic et al. 1994 Celik et al. 1996; Wandroo et al. 2005; Capalbo and Mascolo 2007). Lesions arising in the phalanges are most commonly described, but Capalbo and Moscolo have reported a case of multiple lesions involving the metacarpals and phalanges of both hands (Fig. 36). Antonijevic et al. have described multifocal lesions of both hands and feet presenting simultaneously (Antonijevic et al. 1994).

Typical radiographic features are that of an expansile lytic lesion with cortical erosion. Patients may present with a pathological fracture through a lytic lesion which could be initially mistaken for an enchondroma (Dastgir et al. 1994). Diagnosis is usually made by means of biopsy and routine haematological tests. A skeletal survey is mandatory once the diagnosis has been made to assess for synchronous lesions. Solitary bone plasmacytomas account for 5–7% of all bone plasmacytomas and generally have a good prognosis with a long duration of relapse free survival after local treatment. Celik et al. however have reported a case of solitary plamacytoma of the 5th phalanx that had a short duration of remission and aggressive type of clinical relapse (Celik et al. 1996).

4 Conclusion

Bone tumours of the hand and wrist are infrequently encountered in general clinical practice. The clinical history, physical findings and radiographic features are sufficient to make the diagnosis in the majority of cases. A wide variety of tumour and tumour-like lesions however can present in the hand and wrist. Due to their rare occurrence at this site, they present diagnostic challenges for both the radiologist and the clinician. Knowledge of the imaging characteristics specific to each lesion can facilitate more appropriate and timely management. The imaging findings should always be considered in conjunction with the demographics, clinical presentation and distribution for each individual case.

The superficial location leads to earlier presentation, allowing expeditious diagnosis and treatment of malignant neoplasms. This often results in a better clinical outcome when compared to the same tumours at other skeletal sites. Though rare, it is important to remember the possibility of a malignant neoplasm when encountering an aggressive bone lesion in the hand or wrist. It is also important to consider benign lesions that radiographically appear aggressive and may be misdiagnosed as malignant tumours. Thorough evaluation of the clinical history, imaging findings and any available histopathology should be made before arriving at a diagnosis in these cases.

5 Keypoints

- Though uncommon, a variety of tumour and tumour-like lesions may present in the bones of the hand and wrist
- The majority are benign
- Enchondroma is the commonest benign tumour
- Chondrosarcoma is the commonest malignant primary tumour
- A spectrum of benign proliferative disorders of the phalanges exists which may require close clinical and radiographic follow-up to avoid confusion with a malignant process
- Malignant tumours of the hand frequently have a better prognosis than at other skeletal sites due to earlier presentation
- The distribution of a lesion and demographic features of the patient should be considered in conjunction with the imaging findings when assessing bone lesions of the hand and wrist

References

Abe K, Kumagai K, Hayashi T et al (2007) High-grade surface osteosarcoma of the hand. Skeletal Radiol 36(9):869–873

Abrahams (1995) Occult malignancy presenting as metastatic disease to the hand and wrist. Skeletal Radiol 24:135–137

Adler C-P (2000) Multifocal osteoblastoma of the hand. Skeletal Radiol 29:601–604

Al-Harthy A, Rayan GM (2003) Phalangeal osteochondroma: a cause of childhood trigger finger. Br J Plast Surg 56(2):161–163

Allieu Y, Lussiez B, Benichou M et al (1989) A double nidus osteoid osteoma in a finger. J Hand Surg [Am] 14:538–541

Alnot JY, Badelon O, Grossin M et al (1983) Juxta-cortical aneurysmal cyst of the 3rd metacarpal bone. Apropos of a case. Ann Chir Main 2(4):358–361

Amadio P, Lombadri R (1987) Metastatic tumours of the hand. J Hand Surg 12A:311–316

Ambrosia JM, Wold LE, Amadio PC (1987) Osteoid osteoma of the hand and wrist. J Hand Surg 12A:794–800

Amillo S, Schweitzer D, San Julian M (1996) Monostotic fibrous dysplasia in the hand: a case report. J Hand Surg Am 21(2):290–292

Anakwenze OA, Parker WL, Wold LE et al (2009) Ewing's sarcoma of the hand. J Hand Surg [Eur] 34:35–39

Antonijević N, Radosević-Radojković N, Colović M et al (1994) Simultaneous occurrence of localized plasmacytoma in hand and feet bones. Srp Arh Celok Lek 122(9–10):294–296

Aoki J, Tanikawa H, Ishii K et al (1996) MR findings indicative of haemosiderin in giant-cell tumor of bone: frequency, cause, and diagnostic significance. Am J Roentgenol 166:145–148

Archer L, Wilson D, McCoubrie P (2009) Re: imaging features of primary extranodal lymphomas. Clin Radiol 64:948–950

Assoun J, Richardi G, Railhac J et al (1994) Osteoid osteoma: MRI versus CT. Radiology 191:217–223

Athanasian EA (2004) Aneurysmal bone cyst and giant cell tumor of bone of the hand and distal radius. Hand Clin 20:269–281

Athanasian EA, Wold LE, Amadio PC et al (1997) Giant cell tumors of the bones of the hands. J Hand Surg 22A:91–98

Averill RM, Smith RJ, Campbell CJ (1980) Giant cell tumors of the bones of the hand. J Hand Surg 5A:39–49

Baraga JJ, Amrami KK, Swee RG et al (2001) Radiographic features of Ewing's sarcoma of the bones of the hands and feet. Skeletal Radiol 30:121–126

Baskar S, Klocke R, Cushley M et al (2009) A killer Mocking bird. Rheumatology 48(8):882

Basu S, Basu P, Dowell JK (1999) Painless osteoid osteoma in a metacarpal. J Hand Surg [Br] 24(1):133–134

Beal K, Allen L, Yahalom J (2006) Primary bone lymphoma: treatment results and prognostic factors with long-term follow-up of 82 patients. Cancer 106:2652–2656

Bednar MS, McCormack RR Jr, Glasser D et al (1993) Osteoid Osteoma of the upper extremity. J Hand Surg Am 18(6): 1019–1025

Bednar M, Weiland A, Light T (1995) Osteoid osteoma of the upper extremity. Hand Clin 11:211–221

Bickerstaff DR, Harris SC, Kay NRM (1988) Osteosarcoma of the carpus. J Hand Surg [Br] 13(3):303–305

Biscaglia R, Bacchini P, Bertoni F (2000) Giant cell tumor of the bones of the hand and foot. Cancer 88:2022–2032

Bloem JL, Mulder JD (1985) Chondroblastoma: a clinical and radiological study of 104 cases. Skeletal Radiol 14:1–91

Boriani S, Bacchini P, Bertoni F et al (1983) Periosteal chondroma: a review of twenty cases. J Bone Joint Surg Am 65:205–212

Boston HC Jr, Dahlin DC, Ivins JC et al (1974) Malignant lymphoma (so-called reticulum cell sarcoma) of bone. Cancer 34:1131–1137

Bourguignon RL (1981) Recurrent turret exostoses—case report. J Hand Surg 6A:578–582

Callahan DJ, Walter NE, Okoye MI (1985) Florid reactive periostitis of the proximal phalanx: case report. J Bone J Surg 67A:968–970

Campanacci M, Giunti A, Olmi R (1979) Giant cell tumours of bone. A study of 209 cases with long term follow up in 130. Ital J Orthop Traumatol 1:249

Campbell DR, Millner PA, Dreghorn CR (1995) Primary bone tumours of the hand and wrist. J Hand Surg 20B(1):5–7

Capalbo S, Mascolo V (2007). Letter to the editor: phalangeal lytic lesions in multiple myeloma. Clin Lymphoma Multiple Myeloma 597

Carroll RE (1957) Osteogenic sarcoma in the hand. J Bone Joint Surg Am 39:325–331

Carroll RE, Chance JT, Inan Y (1992) Subungual exostosis in the hand. J Hand Surg [Br] 17(5):569–574

Cash S, Habermann E (1988) Chondrosarcoma of the small bones of the hand: case report and review of the literature. Orthop Rev 17:365–369

Cates HE, Burgess RC (1991) Incidence of brachydactyly and hand exostosis in hereditary multiple exostosis. J Hand Surg Am 16(1):127–132

Cawte TG, Steiner GC, Beltran J et al (1998) Chondrosarcoma of the short tubular bones of the hands and feet. Skeletal Radiol 27(11):625–632

Celik I, Baltali E, Barişta I et al (1996) Solitary phalanx plasmacytoma relapse with disseminated extramedullary plasmacytomas and myeloma after short duration of remission. Anticancer Res 16(2):959–962

Chalmers J (1981) Aneurysmal bone cyst of the phalanges: a report of three cases. The Hand 13(3):296–300

Chan CW (1981) Intraosseous glomus tumour: case report. J Hand Surg Am 6:368–369

Choi JH, Jin Gu M, Jin Kim M et al (2001) Fibrosarcoma in bizarre parosteal osteochondromatous proliferation. Skeletal Radiol 30:44–47

Chua SC, Rozalli FI, O'Connor SR (2009) Imaging features of primary extranodal lymphomas. Clin Radiol 64:574–588

Chung TS (1983) Metastatic malignancy to the bones of the hand. J Surg Oncol 24:99

Crandall BF, Field LL, Sparkes RS et al (1984) Hereditary multiple exostosis: report of a family. Clin Orthop 190.217

Crosby LA, Murphy RP (1988) Subperiosteal osteoid osteoma of the distal phalanx of the thumb. J Hand Surg [Am] 13(6):923–925

Culver J, Sweet D, McCue F (1975) Chondrosarcoma of the hand arising from a previously benign solitary enchondroma: case report and pathological description. Clin Orthop Rel Res 113:128–131

Cushner FD, Morwessel RM (1992) Myositis ossificans traumatica. Orthopaedic Review 21:1319–1326

Daecke W, Ahrens S, Juergens H et al (2005) Ewing's sarcoma and primitive neuroectodermal tumor of hand and forearm. Experience of the cooperative Ewing's sarcoma study group. J Cancer Res Clin Oncol 131:219–225

Dahlin DC (1995) Bone tumours, 3rd edn. General aspects and data on 6221 cases. Thomas, Springfield, Illinois

Dahlin DC, Salvador AH (1974) Chondrosarcomas of bones of the hands and feet: a study of 30 cases. Cancer 34:755–760

Dahlin DC, Unni KK (1986) Bone tumours, 3rd edn. Thomas, Springfield, Illinois

Dahlin LB, Besjakov J, Veress B (2005) A glomus tumor: classic signs without magnetic resonance imaging finding. Scand J Plast Reconstr Surg Hand Surg 39:123–125

Damron TA, Rock MG, Unni KK (1995) Subcutaneous involvement after a metacarpal chondrosarcoma. Case report and review of literature. Clin Orthop 316:189–194

Dastgir N, O'Dowd G, O'Rourke P (1994) Myeloma with predominant phalangeal involvement. Acta Orthop Belg 70:69–71

Davies AN, Salisbury JR, Dobbs HJ (1994) Primary Lymphoma of bone: report of an unusual case with review of the literature. Clin Oncol 6:411–412

Davila JA, Amrami KK, Sundaram M et al (2004) Chondroblastoma of the hands and feet. Skeletal Radiol 33:582–587

De Smet L (2004) Dysplasia epiphysealis hemimelica of the hand: two cases at the proximal interphalangeal joint. J Pediatr Orthop 13(5):323–325

De Smet L, Vercauteren M (1984) Fast-growing pseudomalignant osseous tumour (myositis ossificans) of the finger. A case report. J Hand Surg 9B:93–94

deSantos LA, Spjut HJ (1981) Periosteal chondroma: a radiographic spectrum. Skeletal Radiol 6:15–20

Dhondt E, Oudenhoven L, Khan S et al (2006) Nora's lesion, a distinct radiological entity? Skeletal Radiol 35:497–502

Dick KC, Francis HM, Johnston AD (1971) Ewing's sarcoma of the hand. J Bone Joint Surg 53A:345–348

Doyle LK, Ruby LK, Nalebuff EG et al (1985) Osteoid osteoma of the hand. J Hand Surg 10A:408–410

Dreyfuss UY, Auslander L, Bialik V et al (1980) Ewing's sarcoma of the hand following recurrent trauma: a case report. Hand 12:300–303

Drompp BW (1961) Bilateral osteosarcoma in the phalanges of the hand: a solitary case report. J Bone Joint Surg Am 43:199–204

Dupree WB, Enzinger FM (1986) Fibro-osseousopseudotumour of the digits. Cancer 58:2103–2109

Durbin M, Randall L, James M et al (1988) Ewing's sarcoma masquerading as osteomyelitis. Clin Orthop Relat Res 357:176–185

Ehara S, Nishida J, Abe M et al (1994) Magnetic resonance imaging of pseudomalignant osseous tumor of the hand. Skeletal Radiol 23:513–516

Farman J, Degnan TJ (1976) Multiple myeloma with small bone involvement. NY State J Med 76(6):990–992

Fisher R, Ruhn J, Skerrett P (1958) Epidermal cyst in bone. Cancer 11(3):643–648

Fowble VA, Pae R, Vitale A et al (2005) Osteosarcoma of the hand. Clin Orthop Rel Res 440:255–261

Friedman AC, Orcutt J, Madewell JE (1982) Paget disease of the hand: a radiographic spectrum. AJR 138:691–693

Fuhr SE, Hendron JH (1979) Aneurysmal bone cyst involving the hand. A review and report of two cases. J Hand Surg 4:152–159

Garcia J, Bianchi S (2001) Diagnostic imaging of tumors of the hand and wrist. Eur Radiol 11:1470–1482

Garrison RC, Unni KK, Mcleod RA et al (1982) Chondrosarcoma arising in osteochondroma. Cancer 49(9):1890–1897

Ghert MA, Harrelson JM, Scully SP (2001) Solitary renal cell carcinoma metastasis to the hand: the need for wide excision or amputation. J Hand Surg 26A:156–150

Gouin F, Grimaud E, Redini F et al (2003) Metatarsal giant cell tumor and giant cell reparative granuloma are similar entities. Clin Orthop 416:278–284

Granberry WM, Bryan W (1978) Chondrosarcoma of the trapezium: a case report. J Hand Surg [Am] 3:277–279

Greenspan A (1995) Bone island (enostosis): current concept—a review. Skeletal Radiol 24:111–115

Gropper PT, Mah JY, Gelfant BM et al (1985) Monostotic fibrous dysplasia of the hand. J Hand Surg Br 10(3):404–406

Harness NG, Mankin HJ (2004) Giant cell tumor of the distal forearm. J Hand Surg [Am] 29(2):188–193

Havulinna J, Parkkinen J, Laitinen M (2005) Aneurysmal bone cyst of the index sesamoid. J Hand Surg 30A:1091–1093

Hayter RG, Becton JL (1984) Fibrous dysplasia of a metacarpal. J Hand Surg Am 9(4):587–589

Healey JH, Turnbull ADM, Miedema B et al (1986) Acrometastases. J Bone Joint Surg Am 68:743

Heiple KG (1961) Carpal osteochondroma. J Bone Joint Surg 43A:861–864

Helliwell TR, O'Connor MA, Ritchie DA et al (2001) Bizarre parosteal osteochondromatous proliferation with cortical invasion. Skeletal Radiol 30:282–285

Hoehn JG, Coletta C (1992) Subungual exostosis of the fingers. J Hand Surg [Am] 17(3):468–471

Honoki K, Miyauchi Y, Yajima H et al (2001) Primary osteogenic sarcoma of a finger proximal phalanx: a case report and review of the literature. J Hand Surg [Am] 26(6):1151–1156

Howard RF, Slawski DP, Gilula LA (1996) Florid reactive periostitis of the digit with cortical erosion and review of the literature. J Hand Surg [Am] 21(3):501–505

Hutter RVP, Foote FW, Francis KC et al (1962) Parosteal fasciitis. Am J Surg 104:800–807

Huvos AG (1991) Aneurysmal bone cyst. In: Bone tumors: diagnosis, treatment, and prognosis, 2nd edn. W. B. Saunders, Philadelphia

Huvos A, Marcove R (1987) Chondrosarcoma in the young: a clinicopathologic analysis of 79 patients younger than 21 years of age. Am J Surg Pathol 11:930–942

Ippolito E, Falez F, Tudisco C et al (1987) Subungual exostosis. Histological and clinical considerations on 30 cases. Ital J Orthop Traumatol 13(1):81–87

Izuka T, Kinoshita Y, Fukumoto K (1995) Subungual exostosis of the finger. Ann Plast Surg 35(3):330–332

Jackson RP, Rackling FW, Mantz FA (1977) Osteoid osteoma and osteoblastoma. Similar histologic lesions with different natural histories. Clin Orthop Relat Res 128:303–311

Jaffe HL (1935) Osteoid osteoma: a benign osteoblastic tumour composed of osteoid and atypical bone. Arch Surg 31:709

Jaffe HL, Lichtenstein L, Portis RB (1940) Giant-cell tumour of bone: its pathological appearance, grading, supposed variants and treatment. Arch Pathol Lab Med 30:993–1031

Jambhekar NA, Desai SS, Puri A et al (2004) Florid reactive periostitis of the hands. Skelet Radiol 33:663–665

James SLJ, Davies AM (2005) Giant-cell tumours of the hand and wrist: a review of imaging findings and differential diagnoses. Eur Radiol 15:1855–1866

James SLJ, Davies AM (2006) Surface lesions of the bones of the hand. Eur Radiol 16:108–123

Johnson DL, Kuschner SH, Lane CS (1993) Intraosseous glomus tumour of the phalanx. A case report. J Hand Surg 18A:1026–1028

Jokl P, Albright JA, Goodman AH (1971) Juxtacortical chondrosarcoma of the hand. J Bone Joint Surg [Am] 53(7):1370–1376

Jones KB, Buckwalter A, McCarthy EF (2006) Parosteal osteosarcoma of the thumb metacarpal: a case report. Iowa Orthop J 26:134–137

Jongewood RH, Martel W, Louis D et al (1985) Care report 304. Skeletal Radiol 13:169–173

Justis E, Dart RC (1983) Chondrosarcoma of the hand with metastasis: a review of the literature and case report. J Hand Surg 8:320–324

Kamath BJ, Menezis R, Binu S et al (2007) Solitary osteochondroma of the metacarpal. J Hand Surg 32A(2):274–276

Karr MA, Aulicino PL, DuPuy TE et al. (1984) Osteochondromas of the hand in hereditary multiple exostosis: report of a case presenting as a blocked proximal interphalangeal joint. J Hand Surg [Am] 9(2):264–268

Kayser F, Resnick D, Haghighi P et al (1998) Evidence of the subperiosteal origin of osteoid osteomas in the tubular bones: analysis by CT and MR imaging. Am J Roentgenol 170(3):609–614

Kerin R (1958) Metastatic tumours of the hand. J Bone Joint Surg Am 40:263–277

Kerin R (1983) Metastatic tumors of the hand. J Bone Joint Surg Am 65:1331

Kissane JM, Askin FB, Foulkes M et al (1983) Ewing's sarcoma of bone: clinicopathologic aspects of 303 cases from the intergroup Ewing's sarcoma study. Hum Pathol 14:773–779

Koti M, Honakeri SP, Thomas A (2009) A Multilobed osteochondroma of the hamate: case report. J Hand Surg 34A:1515–1517

Kransdorf MJ, Sweet DE, Buetow PC et al (1992) Giant cell tumor in skeletally immature patients. Radiology 184(1): 233–237

Kreitner K-F, Löw R, Mayer A (1999) Unusual manifestation of an osteoid osteoma of the capitate. Eur Radiol 9:1098–1100

Kwittken J, Branche M (1969) Fasciitis ossificans. Am J Clin Pathol 51:251–255

Lacey SH, Danish EH, Thompson GH et al (1987) Ewing sarcoma of the proximal phalanx of a finger. J Bone Joint Surg Am 69:931–934

Landon GC, Johnson KA, Dahlin DC (1979) Subungual exostoses. J Bone Joint Surg [Am] 61(2):256–259

Landsman JC, Shall JF, Seitz Jr WH et al. (1990) Florid reactive periostitis of the digits. Orthop Rev 19(9):831–834

Lawrie TR, Alterman K, Sinclair AM (1970) Painless osteoid osteoma. A report of two cases. J Bone Joint Surg Am 52(7):1357–1363

Lee BS, Kaplan R (1974) Turret exostosis of the phalanges. Clin Orthop 100:186–189

Leeson MC, Lowry L, McCue RW (1988) Aneurysmal bone cyst of the distal thumb phalanx: a case report and review of the literature. Othopedics 11(4):601–604

Libson E, Bloom R, Husband JE et al. (1987) Metastatic tumors of the bones of the hands and foot. Skeletal Radiol 16:387

Lichtenstein L, Hall HE (1952) Periosteal chondroma. J Bone Joint Surg [Am] 34A:691–697

Lin J, Yoa L, Mirra JM et al (1998) Osteochondroma like parosteal osteosarcoma: a report of six cases of a new entity. Am J Roentgenol AJR 170:1571–1577

Liu J, Hudkins P, Swee R et al (1987) Bone sarcoma associated with Ollier's disease. Cancer 59:1376–1385

Logan SE, Gilula LA, Kyriakos M (1992) Bilateral scaphoid ganglion cysts in an adolescent. J Hand Surg Am 17:490–495

Lorente R, Moreno M, Quiles M (1992) Bilateral intraosseous ganglia of the lunate: a case report. J Hand Surg Am 17:1084–1085

Macdonald DF, Binhammer PA, Rubenstein JD et al (2003) Giant cell reparative granuloma: case report and review of giant cell lesions of the hands and feet. Can J Surg 46(6):471–473

Maiya S, Davies AM, Evans N et al (2002) Surface aneurysmal bone cysts: a pictorial review. Eur Radiol 12(1):99–108

Malhotra R, Maheshwari J, Dinda AK (1992) A solitary osteochondroma of the capitate bone: a case report. J Hand Surg 17A:1082–1083

Marcuzzi A, Maiorana A, Adani R et al (1996) Osteosarcoma of the scaphoid. A case report and review of the literature. J Bone Joint Surg [Br] 78-B:699–701

Marcuzzi A, Acciaro AL, Landi A (2002) Osteoid osteoma of the hand and wrist. J Hand Surg Br 27(5):440–443

Mathov SH, Bougie JD, Awad S (2008) Osteosarcoma of the hand: a rare case for radiographic appearance, location, and age. J Manipulative Physiol Ther 31:164–167

McDonald DJ, Sim FH, McLeod RA et al (1986) Giant-cell tumor of bone. J Bone Joint Surg Am 68(2):235–242

Meneses MF, Unni KK, Swee RG (1993) Bizarre parosteal osteochondromatous proliferation of bone (Nora's lesion). Am J Surg Pathol 17(7):691–697

Michelsen M, Abramovici L, Steiner G et al (2004) Bizarre parosteal osteochondromatous proliferation (Nora's Lesion) in the hand. J Hand Surg 29A:520–525

Minguella J (1982) Giant cell tumor of the metacarpal in a child of unusual age and site. Hand 14:93

Mohanna PN, Moiemen NS, Frame JD (2000) Turret exostosis of the thumb. Br J Plast Surg 53:629–631

Moore JR, Cutis RM, Wiglis EPS (1983) Osteocartilaginous lesions of the digits in children: an experience with 10 cases. J Hand Surg 8:309–315

Moser RP, Kransdorf MJ, Gilkey FW et al (1990) Giant cell tumor of the upper extremity. Radiographics 10:83–102

Muir TM, Lehman TP, Meyer WH (2008) Periosteal osteosarcoma in the hand of a paediatric patient: a case report. J Hand Surg 33A:266–268

Mulvey RB (1964) Peripheral bone metastases. Am J Roentgenol 91:155

Murase T, Moritomo H, Tada K et al (2002) Pseudomallet finger associated with exostoses of the phalanx: a report of two cases. J Hand Surg 27A:817–820

Muren C, Hoglund M, Engkvist O et al (1991) Osteoid osteomas of the hand: report of three cases and review of the literature. Acta Radiol 32:62–66

Murphey MD, Nomikos GC, Flemming DJ et al (2001) Imaging of giant cell tumor and giant cell reparative granuloma of bone: radiologic—pathologic correlation. Radiographics 21:1283–1309

Murphey MD, Walker A, Wilson JA et al (2003) From the archives of the AFIP imaging of primary chondrosarcoma: radiologic-pathologic correlation. Radiographics 23:1245–1278

Musharrafieh RS et al (2002) Epidermoid cyst of the thumb. Orthopedics 25(8):862–863

Nelson D, Abdul-Farim F, Carter J et al (1990) Chondrosarcoma of the small bone of the hand arising from an enchondroma. J Hand Surg 15A:655–659

Neviaser R, Wilson J (1972) Benign chondroblastoma in the finger. J Bone Joint Surg 54A:389

Nora FE, Dahlin DC, Beabout JW (1983) Bizarre parosteal osteochondromatous proliferations of the hands and feet. Am J Surg Pathol 7(3):245–250

O'Connor MI, Bancroft LW (2004) Benign and malignant cartilage tumors of the hand. Hand Clin 20:317–323

O'Donnell RJ, Springfield DS, Motwani HK et al (1994) Recurrence of giant cell tumor of long bones after curettage

and packing with cement. J Bone Joint Surg Am 6(12):1827–1833
Ogose A, Unni KK, Swee RG et al (1997) Chondrosarcoma of small bones of the hands and feet. Cancer 80(1):50–59
Okada K, Wold LE, Baebout JW et al (1993) Osteosarcoma of the hand. Cancer 72:719–725
Opdenakker G, Gelin G, Palmers Y (1999) MR imaging of a subungual glomus tumor. Am J Roentgenol 172:250–251
Orui H, Ishikawa A, Tsuchiya T et al. (2001) Magnetic resonance imaging characteristics of bizarre parosteal osteochondromatous proliferation of the hand: a case report. J Hand Surg 27A:1104–1108
Ostlere SJ, Gold RH, Mirra JM et al (1991) Chondrosarcoma of the proximal phalanx of the right fourth finger secondary to multiple hereditary exostoses (MHE). Skeletal Radiol 20(2):145–148
Ostrowski ML, Spjut HJ (1997) Lesions of the bones of the hands and feet. Am J Surg Pathol 21(6):676–690
Ostrowski ML, Unni KK, Banks PM et al (1986) Malignant lymphoma of bone. Cancer 58:2646–2655
Ozaki T, Hashizume H, Kawai A et al (1995) Ewings sarcoma of the hand: magnetic resonance images and treatment. J Hand Surg 20A:441–444
Ozguroglu M, Aki H, Demir G et al (1999) Unusual manifestation of B-cell disorders. J Clin Oncol 17:1083–1085
Palmieri TJ (1984) Chondrosarcoma of the hand. J Hand Surg [Am] 9(3):332–338
Patel, Desai SS, Gordon SL (1987) Management of skeletal giant cell tumors of the phalanges of the hand. J Hand Surg [Am] 12:70–77
Patel K, Bhuiya T, Chen S (2006) Epidermal inclusion cyst of the phalanx: a case report and literature review. Skeletal Radiol 35:861–863
Patil S, Silva MV, de Crossan J et al (2003) Chondrosarcoma of small bones of the hand. J Hand Surg Br 26(6):602–628
Peimer C, Schiller AL, Mankin HJ et al (1980) Multicentric giant cell tumor of bone. J Bone Joint Surg 62A:652–656
Pho RW (1981) Malignant giant cell tumour of the distal end of the radius treated by a free vascularized fibular transplant. J Bone Jt Surg, Am 63:877–884
Picci P, Manfrini M, Zucchi V et al (1983) Giant-cell tumor of bone in skeletally immature patients. J Bone Joint Surg Am 65:486
Pinheiro RF, Filho FDR, Lima GG et al (2009) Primary non-Hodgkin lymphoma of bone: an unusual presentation. J Can Res Ther 5:52–53
Platt AJ, Klugman DJ (1995) Aneurysmal bone cyst of the capitate. J Hand Surg Br 20B(1):8–11
Ratner V, Dorfman HD (1990) Giant-cell reparative granuloma of the hand and foot bones. Clin Orth Relat Res 260:251–258
Ray MJ, Basset RL (1984) Myositis ossificans. Orthopedics 7:532–535
Reinus WR, Gilula LA, Shirley SK et al (1985) Radiographic appearance of Ewing's sarcoma of the hands and feet: report from the intergroup Ewing sarcoma study. AJR 144:331–336
Resnick D, Niwayama G (1988) Diagnosis of bone and joint disorders, 2nd edn. WB Saunders, Philadelphia
Revell MP, Mulligan PJ, Grimer RJ (2000) Parosteal osteosarcoma of the ring finger metacarpal in a semi-professional pianist. J Hand Surg [Br] 25(3):314–316
Rex C, Jacobs L, Nur Z (1997) Painless osteoid osteoma of themmiddle phalanx. J Hand Surg [Br] 22(6):798–800
Robbin MR, Murphey MD (2000) Benign chondroid neoplasms of bone. Semin Musculoskel Radiol 4(1):45–58
Roberts PH, Price CH (1977) Chondrosarcoma of the bones of the hand. J Bone Joint Surg [Br] 59(2):213–221
Robinson P, White LM, Sundaram M et al (2001) Periosteal chondroid tumors: radiologic evaluation with pathologic correlation. Am J Roentgenol 177(5):1183–1188
Rock MG, Pritchard DJ, Unni KK (1984) Metastases from histologically benign giant-cell tumour of bone. J Bone Joint Surg Am 66:269–274
Rogers G, Brzeziensk M et al (1999) Florid reactive periostitis of the middle phalanx: a case report and review of the literature. J Hand Surg 24A:1014–1018
Rosborough A (1966) Osteoid osteoma: report of a lesion in the terminal phalanx of a finger. J Bone Joint Surg 48B:485–487
Rubin JA, Steinberg DR (1996) Turret exostosis of the metacarpal: a case report. J Hand Surg 21A:296–298
Rybak LD, Abramovici L, Kenan S et al (2007) Cortico-medullary continuity in bizarre parosteal osteochondromatous proliferation mimicking osteochondroma on imaging. Skeletal Radiol 36:829–834
Salib P (1967) Chondrosarcoma: a study of the cases treated at the Massachusetts General Hospital in 27 years (1937–1963). Am J Orthop 9:240–242
Sanchis-Alfonso V, Fernandez-Fernandez CI, Donat J (1994) Osteoblastic osteogenic sarcoma in a 13-month-old girl. Pathol Res Pract 190(2):207–210
Sanjay B, Raj G, Younge D (1996) Giant cell tumours of the hand. J Hand Surg Br 21(5):683–687
Saunders C, Szabo RM, Mora S (1997) Chondrosarcoma of the hand arising in a young patient with multiple hereditary exostoses. J Hand Surg Br 22(2):237–242
Sbarbaro J, Straub L (1960) Chondrosarcoma in a phalanx. Am J Surg 100:751–752
Schajowicz F (1981) Fibrous dysplasia. In: Schajowicz F (ed) Tumours and tumorlike lesions of bone and joints. Springer, Berlin, pp 478–490
Schajowicz F, Gallardo H (1970) Epiphyseal chondroblastoma of bone. J Bone Joint Surg 52B:205
Shankman S, Desai P, Beltran J (1997) Subperiosteal osteoid osteoma: radiographic and pathologic manifestations. Skeletal Radiol 26:457–462
Shigematsu K, Kobata Y, Yajima H et al (2006) Giant-cell tumors of the carpus. J Hand Surg 31A:1214–1219
Shoji H, Miller TR (1971) Primary reticulum cell sarcoma of bone: significance of clinical features upon the prognosis. Cancer 28:1234–1244
Solana J, Bosch M, Español I (2003) Florid reactive periostitis of the thumb: a case report and review of the literature. Chirurgie de la main 22:99–103
Solomon L (1967) Carpal and tarsal exostosis in hereditary multiple exostoses. Clin Radiol 18:412–416
Spjut HJ, Dorfman HD (1981) Florid reactive periostitis of the tubular bones of the hands and feet. Am J Surg Pathol 5:423–433
Sun T-C, Swee RG, Shives TC et al (1985) Chondrosarcoma in Maffucci's syndrome. J Bone Joint Surg [Am] 67:1214–1219
Sundaram M, Wang L, Rotman M et al (2001) Florid reactive periostitis and bizarre parosteal osteochondromatous

proliferation: pre-biopsy imaging evolution, treatment and outcome. Skeletal Radiol 30:192–198

Takagi T, Matsumura T, Shiraishi T (2005) Lunate osteochondroma: a case report. J Hand Surg 30A:693–695

Takigawa K (1971) Chondroma of the bones of the hand: a review of 110 cases. J Bone Joint Surg 53A:1591–1599

Taniguchi K (1995) A practical classification system for multiple cartilaginous exostosis in children. J Pediatr Orthop 15(5):585–591

Tannenbaum DA, Biermann JS (1997) Bizarre parosteal osteochondromatous proliferation of bone. Orthopedics 20:1186–1188

Theumann NH, Goettmann S, Leviet D et al (2002) Recurrent glomus tumors of the fingertips: MR imaging evaluation. Radiology 223:143–151

Tillman BP, Dahlin DC, Lipscomb PR et al (1968) Aneurysmal bone cyst: an analysis of ninety-five cases. Mayo Clin Proc 43:478–495

Torreggiani WC, Munk PL, Al-Ismail K et al (2001) MR imaging features of bizarre parosteal osteochondromatous proliferation of bone (Nora's lesion). Eur J Radiol 40:224–231

Trias A, Basna J, Sanchez G et al (1978) Chondrosarcoma of the hand. Clin Orthop Rel Res 134:297–301

Unni KK (1996) Dahlin's bone tumours: general aspects and data on 11087 cases, 5th edn. Lippincott-Raven, Philadelphia

van Alphen JC, te Slaa RL, Eulderink F et al (1996) Solitary osteochondroma of the scaphoid: a case report. J Hand Surg 21A:423–425

Vanhoenacker FM, Van Hul W, Wuyts W et al (2001) Hereditary multiple exostoses: from genetics to clinical syndrome and complications. Eur J Radiol 40(2001):208–217

Wandroo FA, Mahendra P, Khuroo RA et al (2005) Plasma cell leukaemia presenting with polyarthralgian and phalangeal lytic lesions. Clin Lab Hematol 27:203–205

Williams HJ, Davies AM, Allen G, Evans N, Mangham DC (2004) Imaging features of intraosseous ganglia: a report of 45 cases. Eur Radiol 14:1761–1769

Wilner D (1982) Radiology of bone tumors and allied disorders. Saunders, Philadelphia

Wiss DA, Reid BS (1983) Painless osteoid osteoma of the fingers: a report of three cases. J Hand Surg Am 8(6):914–917

Wissinger HA, McClain EJ, Boyes JH (1966) Turret exostosis: ossifying hematoma of the phalanges. J Bone Joint Surg 48A:105–110

Wold LE, Swee RG (1984) Giant cell tumor of the small bones of the hands and feet. Sem Diagn Pathol 1:173–184

Wold LE, Dobyns H, Swee RG et al (1986) Giant cell reaction (Giant cell reparative granuloma) of the small bones of the hands and feet. Am J Surg Pathol 10(6):491–496

Wu KK, Guise ER (1978) Metastatic tumors of the hand. a report of six cases. J Hand Surg 3:271

Wu K, Frost H, Guise E (1983) A chondrosarcoma of the hand arising from an asymptomatic benign solitary enchondroma of 40 years duration. J Hand surg 8:317–319

Yamaguchi T, Dorfman HD (2001) Giant cell reparative granuloma: a comparative clinicopathologic study of lesions in gnathic and extragnathic sites. Int J Surg Pathol 9:189–200

Yamaguchi T, Tamai K, Saotome K et al (1997) Ewings sarcoma of the thumb. Skeletal Radiol 27:725–728

Young CL, Sim FH, Unni KK et al (1990) Chondrosarcoma of bone in children. Cancer 66:1641–1648

Yuen M, Friedman L, Orr W et al (1992) Proliferative periosteal processes of phalanges: a unitary hypothesis. Skelet Radiol 21(5):301–303

Tumor and Tumor-Like Lesions of Soft Tissue

F. M. Vanhoenacker, P. Van Dyck, J. L. Gielen, and A. M. De Schepper

Contents

Abstract

Masses of the hand and wrist are a common clinical problem. Soft-tissue tumors of the hand and wrist are far more frequent than bone tumors. If clinical examination is equivocal, imaging is often requested. This chapter aims to present an overview of the imaging characteristics of the most frequent tumor and tumor-like soft-tissue lesions of the hand and wrist.

1 Introduction

Masses of the hand and wrist are a common clinical problem. Soft-tissue tumors of the hand and wrist are far more frequent than bone tumors (de La Kethulle de Ryhove et al. 2000; Capelastegui et al. 1999). If clinical examination is equivocal, imaging is often requested. This chapter aims to present an overview of the imaging characteristics of the most frequent tumor and tumor-like soft-tissue lesions of the hand and wrist.

F. M. Vanhoenacker · P. Van Dyck · J. L. Gielen · A. M. De Schepper
Department of Radiology, University Hospital Antwerp, Wilrijkstraat, 10, 2650 Edegem, Belgium

F. M. Vanhoenacker (✉)
General Hospital Sint-Maarten Duffel-Mechelen, Rooienberg 25, 2570 Duffel, Belgium
e-mail: filip.vanhoenacker@telenet.be

A. M. Davis et al. (eds.), *Imaging of the Hand and Wrist*, Medical Radiology. Diagnostic Imaging,
DOI: 10.1007/174_2010_113, © Springer-Verlag Berlin Heidelberg 2013

2 Benign Soft-Tissue Tumors

2.1 Synovial Cyst, Ganglion Cyst and Tendon Sheath Cyst

2.1.1 Definition and Nosological Classification

Cystic lesions are the most common mass lesions arising in the hand and wrist, accounting for 50–70% of all soft-tissue tumors of the hand and wrist (De Beuckeleer et al. 2001; Angeledes 1999). The terminology of cystic lesions is very confusing and depends on a combination of parameters such as topography, the presence or absence of joint communication, and the histologic composition.

The term *synovial cyst* describes a continuation or herniation of the synovial membrane through the joint capsule. In the French literature, the term "arthro-synovial" cyst is preferred, which refers to its intimate relationship with the adjacent joint. Indeed, there is always a communication with the adjacent joint, and the histologic composition is identical to those of the joint cavity. It consists of a collection of intraarticular fluid, lined by a continuous layer of "true" synovial cells. Usually associated joint diseases are present, like osteoarthrosis, inflammatory, and posttraumatic joint diseases. Thirty percent of the lesions are associated with underlying interosseous ligament injury (Lowden et al. 2005). The elevated intraarticular pressure, due to an accumulation of joint fluid in these diseases causes herniation of joint fluid and synovium through a "locus minoris resistentiae" within the joint capsule.

Ganglia contain also mucinous fluid, but their wall consists of a (discontinuous) layer of flattened pseudosynovial cells, surrounded by connective tissue (pseudocapsule).

A communication with the adjacent joint is not always present.

There remains much controversy in the literature, concerning the pathogenesis of ganglion cysts. Several theories have been proposed, including displacement of synovial tissue during embryogenesis, proliferation of pluripotential mesenchymal cells, degeneration of connective tissues after trauma, and migration of synovial fluid into the cyst (synovial herniation theory).

Based upon the similar appearance on imaging, surgery and similar wall composition of synovial cysts and ganglion cysts, we believe that the synovial herniation hypothesis is the most satisfactory. According to this theory, synovial cysts or ganglion cysts are formed by a herniation of synovium through a breach in the adjacent articulation.

Whereas a synovial cyst has a continuous synovial lining of true synovial cells, the wall composition of a ganglion cyst consists of a discontinuous layer of pseudosynovial cells.

A ganglion cyst may represent an advanced stage of a degenerated synovial cyst, in which the continuous synovial lining and the communication with the joint may be lost during the process of degeneration (Vanhoenacker et al. 2006b).

A tendon sheath cyst consists of a special subtype of a ganglion cyst located on the course of a tendon sheath.

2.1.2 Clinical Findings

Cystic lesions of the hand and wrist occur most frequently between 20 and 40 years of age, but may arise in the pediatric population and the elderly (Nahra and Bucchieri 2004; Wang and Hutchinson 2001). There is a female predominance (Nahra and Bucchieri 2004). Half of the patients are asymptomatic (Lowden et al. 2005), whereas the others may suffer from chronic wrist pain, tenderness or functional impairment (Peh et al. 1995).

The lesion may fluctuate in size, particularly during flexion of the wrist.

The majority of ganglion cysts are located at the dorsal aspect of the wrist adjacent to the scapholunate ligament (60–70%), whereas volar wrist cysts account for approximately 18–20%. Approximately two-thirds of anterior wrist ganglions arise from the radiocarpal joint and one third arise from the scaphotrapezial joint (Greendyke et al. 1992). Volar cysts may cause median and ulnar nerve palsies (Kobayashi et al. 2001; Christiaanse et al. 2010). Some cysts may adhere directly to the tendon sheath (Nahra and Bucchieri 2004). Rarely, cysts arise from the dorsal aspect of the interphalangeal joints, often secondary to Heberden osteoarthritis in elderly patients (Nahra and Bucchieri 2004).

2.1.3 Imaging Findings

The role of imaging is to define the cystic nature of those lesions and to demonstrate a possible communication with the joint. This is important for the surgeon, because the resection of the communicating stalk with the joint is essential to avoid post-surgical recurrence of the cyst.

2.1.4 Conventional Radiography

Standard radiography is non-specific and may reveal an ill-defined or rounded, non-calcified soft-tissue mass. Rarely gas, or calcified loose bodies may be seen within in a communicating cyst.

2.1.5 Ultrasound

On US, synovial cysts and ganglion cysts appear as anechoic masses (Fig. 1), and may have a visible communication with a joint (Fig. 1) or tendon sheath (Fig. 2a). The lesion may be multiseptated and may contain some fine internal septations. US is an accurate technique to define the cystic nature in superficial cysts around the wrist and the hand, but it has limited ability to visualize deeper lying structures and their relationship with the adjacent joint. Furthermore, cysts containing debris or hyperplastic synovium may simulate solid mass lesions on ultrasound examinations (Vanhoenacker et al. 2006b).

2.1.6 CT-Scan

Due to its low soft-tissue contrast, CT is of limited value in assessing soft-tissue lesions. Para-articular cysts are of lower attenuation than muscle and of higher attenuation than fat. Rim enhancement is seen after intravenous contrast administration (Steiner et al. 1996). A possible communication with the joint is sometimes difficult to define on axial images.

2.1.7 MRI

MR imaging demonstrates the exact location and extent of the cystic lesions, and its relationship to the joint and surrounding structures (Fig. 2b, c). The diagnosis of a cystic mass is usually straightforward by analysis of the signal intensities of the lesion. They are typically hypo- or iso-intense to muscle on T1-weighted images, and homogeneously hyperintense on T2-weighted images. However, there are some pitfalls. Atypical cyst content due to debris or hemorrhage may alter the imaging appearance of the cysts. Chronic inflammation may cause marked thickening of the synovial membrane and, therefore, mimic a solid soft-tissue mass. Cystic lesions are well circumscribed, but may be lobulated, or multicystic with internal septa. Ruptured cysts, due to an elevated pressure, are irregularly delineated and must be differentiated from other soft-tissue tumors and hemorrhagic or inflammatory lesions.

After gadolinium contrast administration, subtle rim enhancement of the peripheral fibrovascular tissue in the cyst wall is seen, but there is never central enhancement like in other well-delineated soft-tissue lesions with high signal intensity on T2-weighted images, such as myxoma, myxoid liposarcoma, hemangioma, synovial sarcoma, and mucinosis.

2.2 Epidermoid Cyst

2.2.1 Definition and Histopathology

Epidermoid cyst, also known as epidermal inclusion cyst or infundibular cyst, results from the proliferation of surface epidermal cells within the dermis. The lesion is typically located within the subcutaneous tissue and is often secondary to trauma. It is more frequently seen in men than in women (Nahra and Bucchieri 2004).

Macroscopically, the lesion is filled with keratin (Ergun et al. 2010). The walls of the cyst resemble follicular epithelium (Murphy and Elder 1991). The cyst wall may rupture with secondary foreign body-type reaction, granulomatous reaction, granulation tissue or abscess formation (Murphy and Elder 1991; Jin et al. 2008).

2.2.2 Imaging

On plain radiographs, epidermal cyst may be located in the subcutaneous tissue or within the bone (most frequently at the terminal phalanges of the fingers). Lesions located within the dermis may cause well-defined osteolysis on the adjacent bone (Fig. 3a)

Ultrasound is more sensitive than clinical examination for the diagnosis of a epidermoid cyst (after palpation, 93.5%; after ultrasonography, 99.3%) (Kuwano et al. 2009). The lesion is usually well defined. Echogenicity varies with the content of the cyst. The lesions are usually hypoechoic, with posterior acoustic enhancement. Large lesions may show intralesional hyperechoic debris or keratin clusters (Fig. 4) (Gielen et al. 2006). Rupture of the cysts may

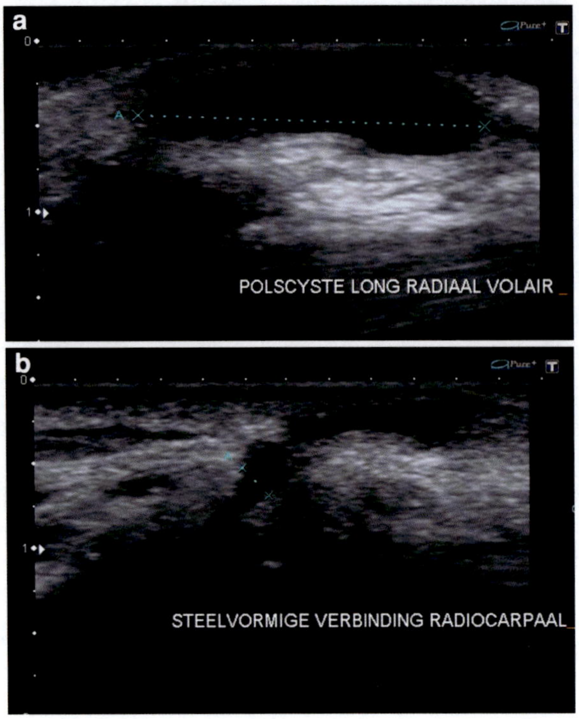

Fig. 1 Ganglion cyst. **a** Longitudinal ultrasound showing a well-defined anechoic structure at the palmar aspect of the carpus. **b** Longitudinal ultrasound shows a stalk-like connection with the adjacent radiocarpal joint

result in changes in shapes (either lobulations, protrusions or abscess pocket formations), pericystic changes, and increased vascularity on power Doppler ultrasound (Jin et al. 2008).

In the case of epidermoid inclusion cysts occurring in the fingertips, there may be bony involvement in which the cyst erodes into the bone causing a lytic lesion within the distal phalanx. Cortical destruction and osteolysis may mimic a malignant or infectious process (Nahra and Bucchieri 2004).

On CT and MRI, the lesion is well defined. MR features depend on the chemical composition of cholesterol and keratin content. Lesions with a high lipid content are hyperintense on both pulse sequences, whereas acrystalline form of cholesterol and the presence of keratin and microcalcifications may result in a low signal on T2-weighted images. After administration of intravenous gadolinium contrast, there is lack of contrast enhancement in non-complicated epidermoid cysts (Fig. 3b–d) (Ergun et al. 2010).

2.3 Lipoma

2.3.1 Definition

Lipomas are well-encapsulated masses composed of mature adipose cells. They are the most frequently encountered benign lipomatous lesions of the hand (Peh et al. 1995; Ergun et al. 2010).

2.3.2 Clinical Findings

Lipomas are most frequently located under the skin (superficial lipoma) but can also be seen in muscles (often within thenar or hypothenar muscles), bones, and tendons (deep seated lipoma) (Peh et al. 1995; Ergun et al. 2010). The lesions are usually asymptomatic, but may occasionally compress adjacent nerves, vessels, or tendons (Peh et al. 1995). Most frequently, lipoma affects patients in the fifth to sixth decade (De Beuckeleer et al. 2001)

2.3.3 Imaging

Radiographs are usually normal, but a low to intermediate density may be seen in larger lesions (Murphey et al. 2004).

On ultrasound, superficial lipomas have an elongated shape and are usually parallel to the skin. Intramuscular lesions are often more difficult to distinguish from the surrounding muscle fibers. The reflectivity is highly variable ranging from hypo- to hyper-reflective compared to subcutaneous fat.

CT shows a homogeneous mass with low density (−60 to −130 HU). Intramuscular lesions may contain thin fibromuscular septa. There is no significant contrast enhancement.

On MRI, the lesion has similar signal characteristics as subcutaneous fat on all pulse sequences. Fat-suppression techniques show homogeneous suppression. Minor (<2 mm) internal septa and a low signal intensity capsule may be seen. After administration of intravenous gadolinium contrast, there is no contrast enhancement, except for the peripheral fibrous capsule or the subtle internal septa (Fig. 5) (Ergun et al. 2010).

2.4 Lipomatosis of Nerve

2.4.1 Definition

Lipomatosis of nerve has also been designated in the past as fibrolipomatous hamartoma, fibrofatty overgrowth, lipomatous hamartoma, lipofibroma, neurolipoma,

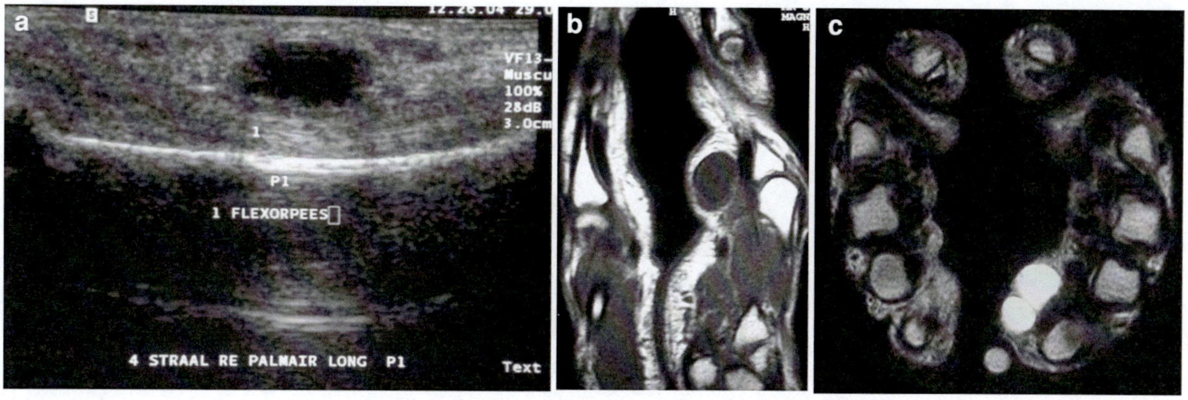

Fig. 2 Cyst of the tendon sheath. **a** Longitudinal ultrasound showing a well-delineated sonolucent structure on the course of the flexor tendon of right fourth finger. **b** Sagittal SE T1-weighted image. **c** Axial TSE T2-weighted image in another patient with a tendon sheath cyst of the flexor tendon. The lesion is isointense to muscle on T1-weighted images (**b**) and hyperintense on T2-weighted images (**c**)

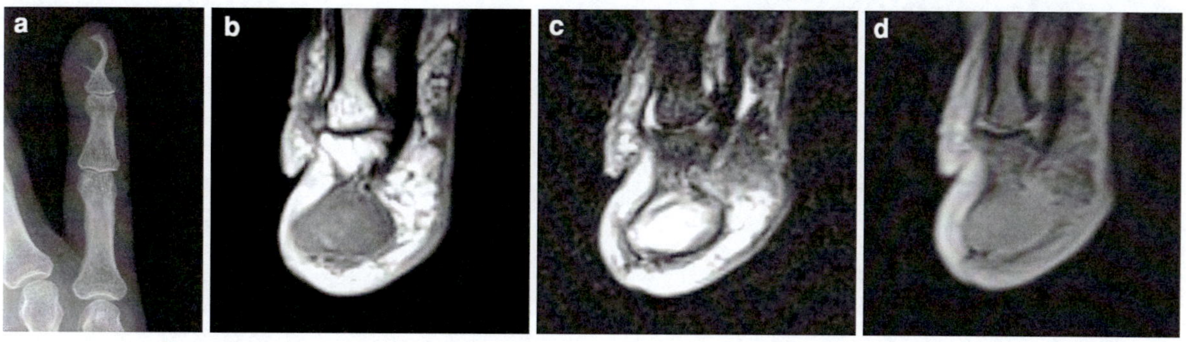

Fig. 3 Subcutaneous epidermoid cyst with involvement of the adjacent bone of the terminal phalanx of the right fifth finger. **a** Plain radiograph showing a well-defined osteolytic defect at the radial side of the distal phalanx. Note cortical destruction of the radial cortex. **b** Coronal SE T1-weighted image. The lesion is of intermediate signal intensity with some internal areas of relatively high signal. **c** Coronal TSE T2-weighted image. High signal intensity of the lesion. **d** Coronal SE T1-weighted image after intravenous injection of gadolinium contrast. There is only subtle peripheral enhancement of the lesion (Case courtesy of C. Kenis, Antwerp)

intraneural lipoma and fatty infiltration of the nerve and neural fibrolipoma. In 2002, the WHO adopted the designation of lipomatosis of nerve (Christopher et al. 2002). It is a very rare tumor, characterized by a proliferation of fatty and fibrous components that surrounds the thickened nerve bundles and infiltrates both the epineurium and the perineurium. Its cause is unknown, but some consider this condition as a congenital lesion, since it is occasionally present at birth whereas others believe to exist a relationship with a history of a prior trauma.

2.4.2 Clinical Findings

This tumor affects predominantly children or young adults. Males are affected more frequently than females

Lipomatosis of nerve occurs chiefly in the volar aspects of the hands, wrist, and forearm and usually involves the median nerve. A soft-tissue mass is frequently present several years before onset of symptoms. Lipomatosis of nerve usually gives rise to pain, paresthesia, or decreased sensation or muscle strength, in the area innervated by the affected nerves. It may be associated with bone overgrowth and macrodactyly of the fingers, a condition described as macrodystrophia lipomatosa (Fig. 6) (Vanhoenacker et al. 2005; Vanhoenacker et al. 2006a).

2.4.3 Imaging

On plain radiographs, lipomatosis of nerve may manifest by a soft-tissue mass or only be suspected by indirect signs such as the presence of macrodactyly, usually affecting the second and third digits of the hand. There is a soft-tissue and osseous

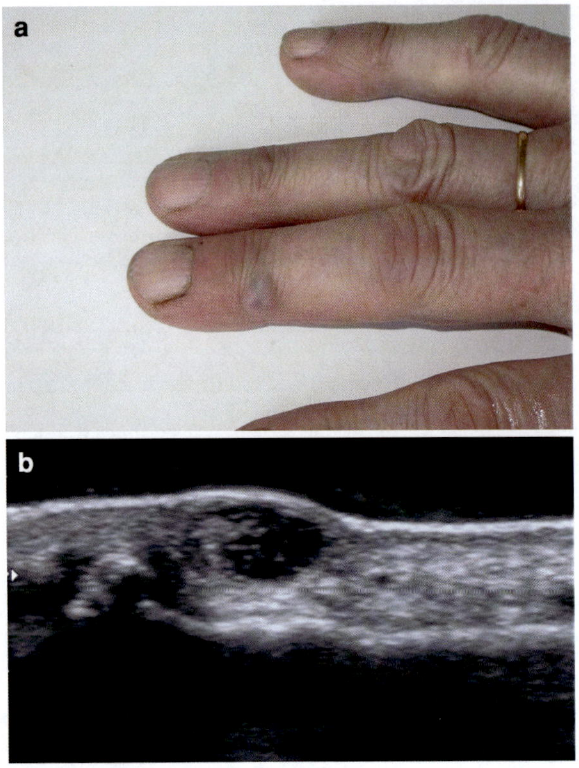

Fig. 4 Subcutaneous epidermoid cyst. **a** Clinical picture showing a small soft-tissue lesion with bluish skin discoloration at the third finger. **b** Longitudinal ultrasound showing a well-defined subcutaneous lesion with variable echogenicity (anechoic components and some internal hyperechoic debris)

hypertrophy including long, broad and splayed phalanges (Fig. 6).

CT and MRI can identify the nervous origin of the tumor due to the presence of tortuous tubular structures, corresponding to enlarged nerve bundles within a predominantly fatty mass (Fig. 7). These structures, clearly depicted on MRI, show low signal intensity on both T1- and T2-weighted images according to their fibrous content. The tumor has the tendency to spread along the branches of the nerve, with a significant variation in the distribution of fat along the nerves and their innervated muscle. The contrast between the low-signal nerve fascicles and surrounding high-signal fat results in a "cable-like" appearance of the tumor, when visualized on axial planes on T1-weighted MR images (Fig. 7) and a "spaghetti-like" appearance on coronal planes. The MR imaging findings of lipomatosis of nerve are very characteristic, obviating the need for biopsy (Marom and Helms 1999). Lipomatosis of nerve must be differentiated from a nerve sheath lipoma associated with altered sensibility along the course of some nerves. MRI allows differentiation between these two entities, since lipoma manifests as a focal mass separated from the nerve bundles.

2.5 Giant Cell Tumor of Tendon Sheath (GCTTS)

2.5.1 Definition

GCTTS are benign proliferative lesions of synovial origin and represent a localized extra-articular form of pigmented villonodular synovitis (Nguyon et al. 2004; Peh et al. 1995). In the hand and the wrist, this is the second most common soft-tissue lesion after a ganglion cyst. The pathogenesis remains unclear but is probably due to a reactive inflammatory process. GCTTS may arise from the tendon sheath, joint capsule, bursae, fascia or ligaments (Nguyon et al. 2004; Peh et al. 1995). Histologically, they are composed of histiocytes, macrophages, multinucleated giant cells and hemosiderin due to repeated hemorrhage (Nguyon et al. 2004; Peh et al. 1995; Wan et al. 2010).

2.5.2 Clinical Findings

The lesions are more common in the fingers than in the wrist and palm. The most affected site is the volar aspect of the first three digits (Ushijima et al. 1986). They are usually well-circumscribed firm masses that grow slowly and are typically painless. If located near a joint, they may cause decreased joint motion (Capelastegui et al. 1999).

2.5.3 Imaging

Standard radiography may be normal or display a well-circumscribed soft-tissue mass in about half of the patients. Pressure erosions at the underlying bone is present in about 20% of patients, while periosteal reaction, calcifications, or cystic changes are extremely unusual (De Beuckeleer and Vanhoenacker 2006; Wan et al. 2010; De Schepper et al. 2007).

Ultrasound shows a hypoechoic, solid mass with well-defined margins usually located near tendons

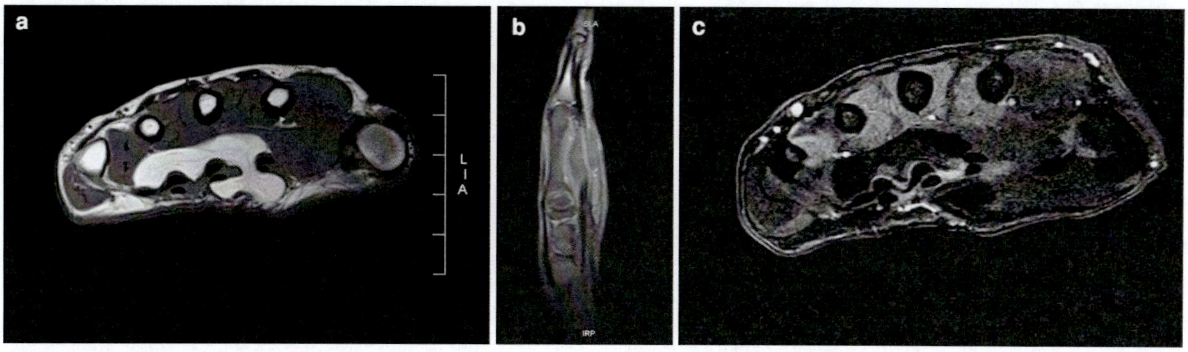

Fig. 5 Deep-seated lipoma of the hand in a 43-year-old women. **a** Axial SE T1-weighted image. Note the presence of a dumbbell shaped mass at the flexor compartment of the hand. The lesion is well defined and isointense to subcutaneous fat. **b** Sagittal fatsuppressed TSE T2-weighted image. There is homogeneus fat suppression of the lesion. **c** Axial fatsuppressed SE T1-weighted image after intravenous injection of gadolinium contrast. There is absence of enhancement of the lesion

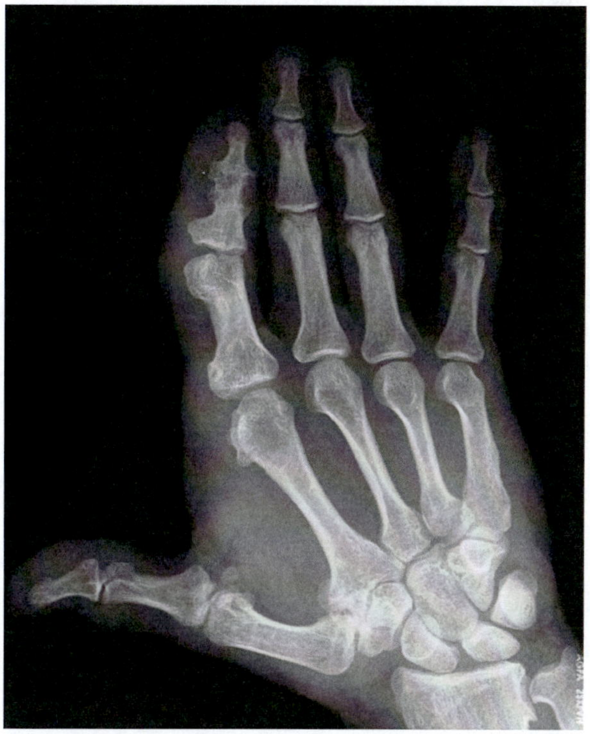

Fig. 6 Macrodystophia lipomatosa. Posterioanterior radiograph of the right hand. Note osseous and soft-tissue enlargement, affecting the second finger. (From Vanhoenacker et al. 2006a, with permission)

(Fig. 8). Bone erosions due to pressure of the tumor on the cortex may be demonstrated as well. The tendon usually exhibits normal shape and echogenicity. Contrary to ganglia, the giant cell tumor lacks posterior acoustic enhancement, presents always with internal echoes, and shows hypervascularity on color or power Doppler imaging (Wan et al. 2010).

MR images typically show a well-defined mass adjacent to or enveloping a tendon, with a signal intensity similar to or less than that of skeletal muscle on T1-weighted images. On T2-weighted images, the signal intensity is predominantly low, with a variable degree of heterogeneity. Blooming artifact is seen on gradient-echo sequences due to the presence of hemosiderin (Wan et al. 2010). GCTTS usually enhance after gadolinium contrast administration (Fig. 9).

Fibroma of the tendon sheath may have a similar presentation as GCTTS on MR imaging (Sect. 2.10), but it lacks giant cells (Nguyon et al. 2004)

2.6 Pigmented Villonodular Synovitis

2.6.1 Definition

The articular counterpart of giant cell tumors of the tendon sheath is also known as pigmented villonodular synovitis (PVNS).

PVNS is a rare monoarticular arthropathy that usually occurs between the ages of 20 and 50, with a peak incidence between the third and the fourth decades of life. There is no sex predilection.

It usually involves the knee (80%) or the hip, while the ankle, elbow, shoulder, and wrist are less frequent locations.

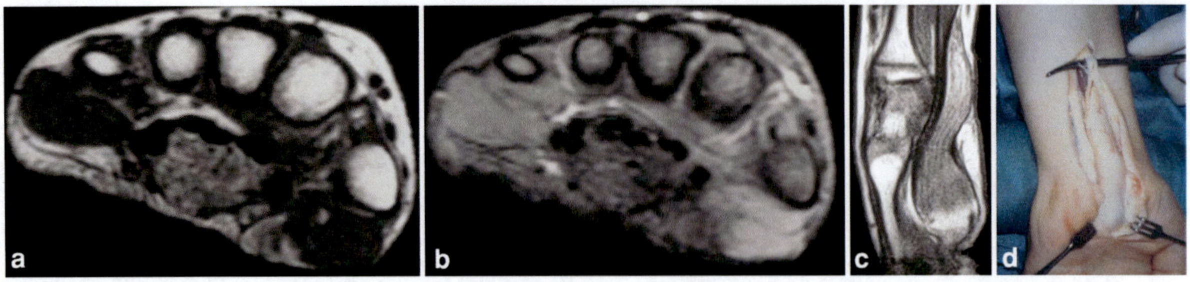

Fig. 7 Lipomatosis of nerve of the median nerve at the level of the carpal tunnel in a 40-year-old man. **a** Axial SE T1-weighted MR image. **b** Axial gradient echo T2*-weighted MR image. **c** Sagittal SE T1-weighted MR image and corresponding preoperative view (**d**) of the median nerve. A heterogeneous mass is seen within the carpal tunnel. There is a mixed SI of fatty components, fibrous components and neural fascicles (**a**, **b**, **c**, cable-like appearance). The signal intensity and localization are highly characteristic of lipomatosis of the median nerve. Note fusiform thickening of the median nerve (**d**). (From Vanhoenacker et al. 2006a, with permission)

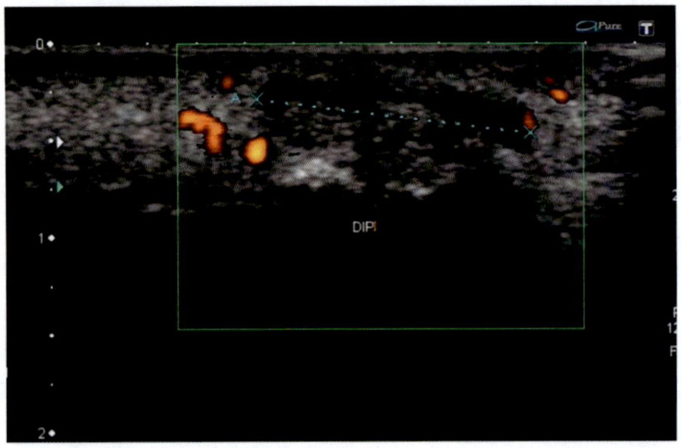

Fig. 8 Giant cell tumor of the tendon sheath. Longitudinal ultrasound showing a well-defined hypoechoic mass adjacent to the flexor tendon. There is increased Doppler signal at the periphery of the lesion

2.6.2 Clinical Findings

The clinical picture is characterized by the insidious onset of monoarticular swelling in young adults, stiffness, and progressive pain. Symptoms tend to be continuous, but exacerbations occur from time to time. Aspirated synovial fluid is typically xanthochromic or serosanguineous.

Microscopically, the lesions are composed of solid or finger-like masses of hyperplastic synovium with multinucleated giant cells, xanthoma cells, and intra- and extracellular hemosiderin, lying in a fibrous stroma. Long-standing lesions show fibrosis and hyalinization.

When the villi become matted together, clefts lined by synovial cells are seen and may give an appearance alarmingly similar to synovial sarcoma.

2.6.3 Imaging Findings

Conventional radiographs may be normal, or show a non-specific periarticular soft-tissue mass and associated joint effusion. Visible calcifications are extremely unusual. The presence of calcifications should suggest an alternative diagnosis such as synovial osteochondromatosis. Despite the absence of calcification in PVNS, high iron content may be present within the synovium, producing a higher radiodensity than adjacent joint effusion or soft tissue. Associated bone erosions (Fig. 10a) with sclerotic margins may be present on both sides of the affected joints, particularly in joints with a tight capsule, such as the wrist. These erosive changes are probably due to a pressure phenomenon resulting from entrapment of soft-tissue masses between articulating surfaces. These lesions are usually present in non-marginal locations and may be multiple. If solitary, they may mimic primary osteolytic bone neoplasms. The preservation of the articular space until late in the disease and the absence of peri-articular osteopenia are helpful in the differential diagnosis from an inflammatory synovitis.

Ultrasonography shows a heterogeneous mass lesion. Sometimes related enlarged or disconnected synovial cysts or bursae with internal septa are noted.

CT is able to sharply define lytic bone lesions associated with pigmented villonodular synovitis. Also associated intraosseous soft-tissue masses extending with a narrow pedicle to the synovium are easily visualized. Joint effusion is atypical, and the tumoral mass itself is also not as characteristic as on MR imaging. Sometimes a high attenuation tissue is

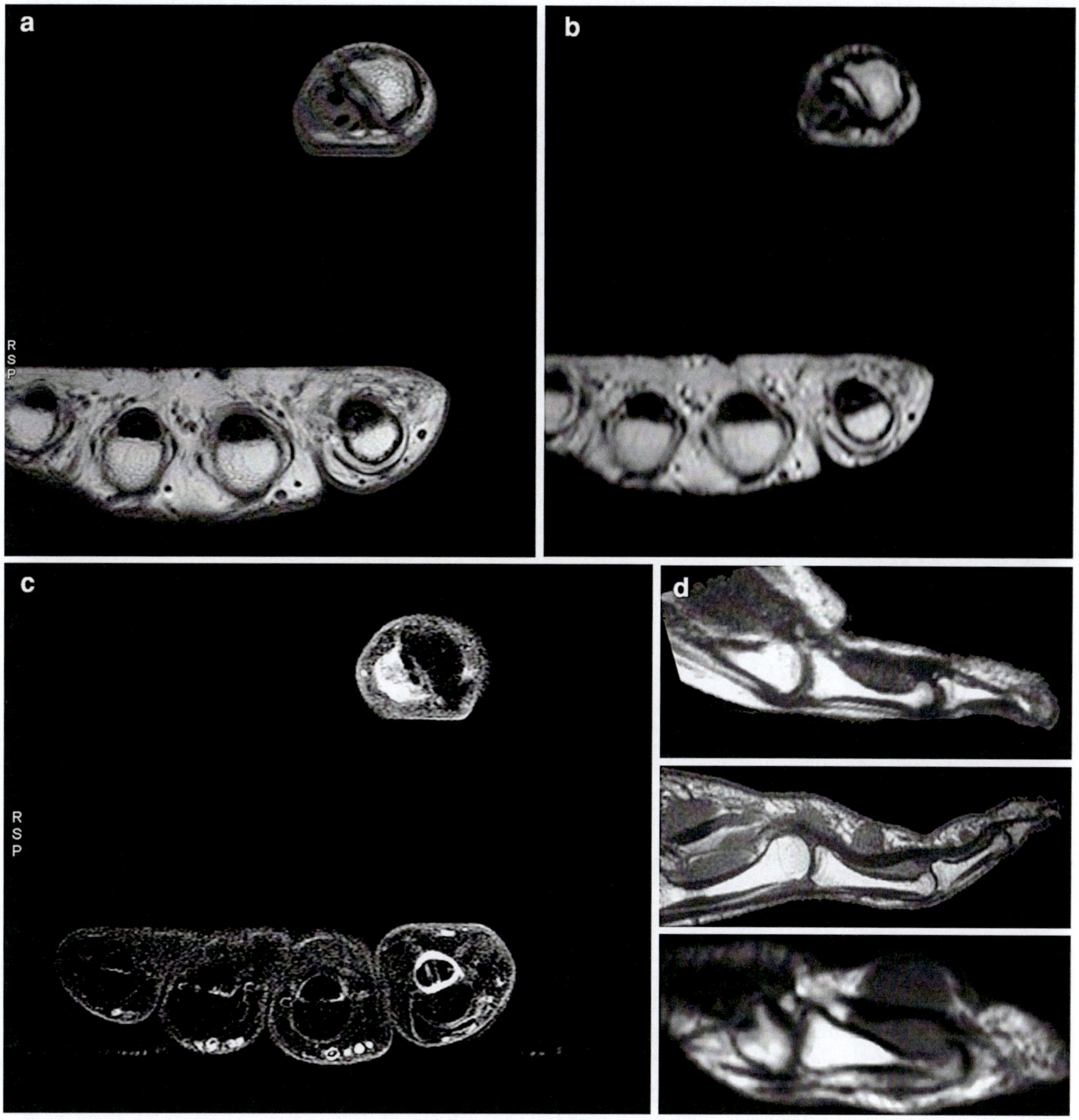

Fig. 9 Giant cell tumor of the tendon sheath. **a** Axial SE T1-weighted image. A hypointense structure is surrounding the flexor tendons of the thumb. **b** Axial TSE T2-weighted image. The lesion is of low signal intensity. **c** Axial SE T1-weighted image after intravenous injection of gadolinium contrast (subtraction image). There is marked inhomogeneous enhancement of the lesion. **d** Sagittal SE T1-weighted image in another patient with a giant cell tumor of tendon sheath. A hypointense structure is surrounding the flexor tendon, which is a typical location for a GCTTS

identified within the joint, due to the presence of hemosiderin. The differential diagnosis consists of iron deposition in the joint due to hemophilia or chronic bleeding and calcification. Enhancement after intravenous contrast administration appears to be the rule.

The MR appearance of pigmented villonodular synovitis as a rule is quite characteristic, due to the presence of hemosiderin within the synovial masses. A heterogeneous, hyperplastic synovial process with significant areas of low signal intensity on all

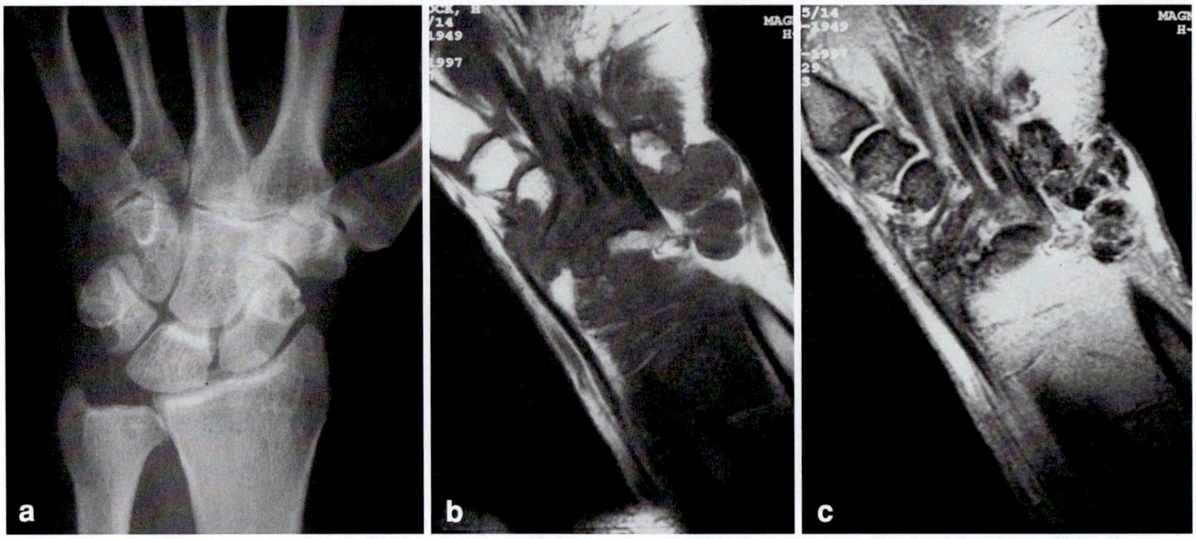

Fig. 10 Pigmented villonodular synovitis. **a** Plain radiograph of the left wrist. There are multiple erosions at the distal aspect of the scaphoid bone and at the proximal aspect of the triquetral bone. **b** Coronal SE T1-weighted image. The lesion is located intra-articularly within the wrist joint and is of low signal intensity (isointense to muscle). Note also erosions at the carpal bones. **c** Coronal gradient T2* image showing blooming artifact of the lesion

sequences, particularly T2-weighted images, is typical. The presence of hemosiderin causes local changes in susceptibility and therefore loss of MR signal. This is especially true for gradient-echo sequences and at high field strengths. This decreased signal intensity is most prominent in the periphery of the lesions (the so-called "blooming" artifact) (Fig. 10b, c). Occasionally, intralesional areas of high signal intensity on both pulse sequences may be present, due to fat, edema, or inflammation. Joint effusion appears as hyperintense areas entrapped between the low signal intensity areas on T2-weighted images.

After gadolinium contrast administration, homogeneous or septal enhancement may be observed. The differential diagnosis on MR imaging includes other causes of chronic hemarthrosis such as chronic trauma, hemophilia, synovial hemangioma and "burnt out" rheumatoid pannus and amyloid arthropathy. These disorders can be separated on the basis of clinical history, laboratory findings, and enhancement pattern. In hemophilia, there are usually diffuse changes in cartilage and bone, including cartilaginous and subchondral erosions, as well as joint space narrowing. Synovial chondromatosis could potentially simulate pigmented villonodular synovitis on MR, and in general this is true for all low signal intensity masses with calcified or ossified components. This should be no problem, since these areas are well recognized on plain films and CT. Tophaceous gout may also mimic PVNS, if there is a high concentration of calcium within the tophus. Finally, desmoid tumors, benign fibrous histiocytoma and sclerosing hemangioma could be mistaken for pigmented villonodular synovitis due to their low signal on MR imaging, which is due to their dense fibrous content. The lack of intraarticular changes should alert one to consider another diagnosis besides pigmented villonodular synovitis.

MR imaging is the imaging technique of choice to evaluate the possible extra-articular extension and areas of the joint, which are difficult to see arthroscopically.

2.7 Vascular Tumors and Lymphatic Tumors

2.7.1 Definition

Benign vascular tumors are common benign soft-tissue masses, which can be classified into localized hemangioma and diffuse angiomatosis. Klippel-Trénaunay syndrome is a separate entity in which hemangiomas are accompanied by unilateral hypertrophy of the

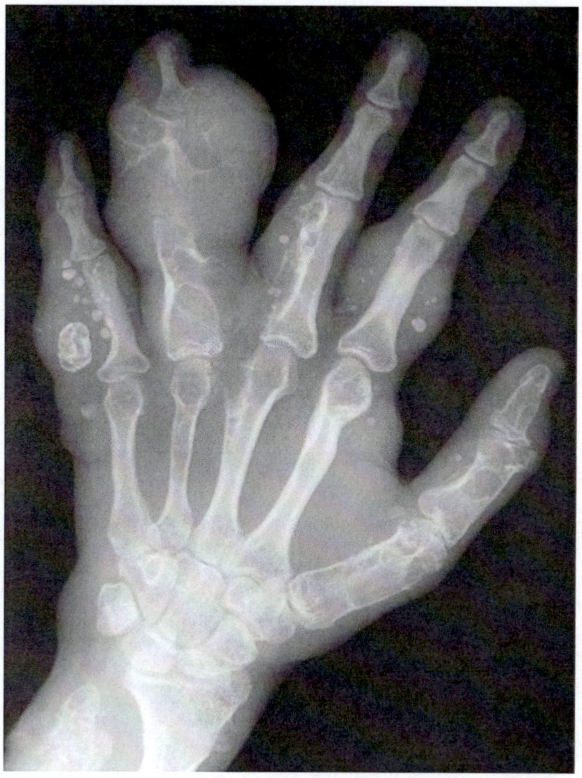

Fig. 11 Mafucci's syndrome. Plain radiograph of the left hand. Note multiple enchondromas and soft-tissue haemangiomas with intralesional phleboliths

extremity. Maffucci's syndrome consists of the combination of hemangiomas and enchondromatosis (Fig. 11). Semimalignant vascular tumors include hemangioendotheliomas (Nguyon et al. 2004; Peh et al. 1995; Ergun et al. 2010). Hemangiomas represent a broad spectrum of vascular tumors which may be classified by vessel size into capillary, cavernous, venous or arteriovenous malformations (Ergun et al. 2010). Apart from vessels, the lesions contain variable amounts of non-vascular elements including thrombus, fat, fibrous tissue, bone and muscular tissue (Nguyon et al. 2004; Schmitt 2008; Ergun et al. 2010).

Lymphangiomas of the hand are rare.

2.7.2 Clinical Findings

Most hemangiomas are asymptomatic, but they may present at an early age secondary to cosmetic deformity or pain. Women are more affected than men, and the incidence peaks in early adulthood. A familial disposition may occur (Schmitt 2008). The hand is frequently affected. The cutaneous and subcutaneous compartments are often involved, and there is frequently an overlying skin discoloration (Fig. 12a). Less often, the lesion is found in tendon sheaths (Fig. 12), muscles or the median nerve (Nguyon et al. 2004; Schmitt 2008).

Capillary hemangiomas are most frequent and are usually located in the skin and subcutaneous tissue. Clinically, they are characterized as port-wine spot lesions. Because of the superficial location, the diagnosis is often made clinically and imaging is rarely required.

Venous hemangiomas typically involve the deep structures (Ergun et al. 2010).

2.7.3 Imaging

Radiographs often provide little information (Fig. 12b). Phleboliths are sometimes seen (Fig. 11). Linear or arciform calcifications are less common (Nguyon et al. 2004; Schmitt 2008). Adjacent osseous remodeling can occur (Fig. 13a), including erosion, overgrowth, periosteal reaction, and osteoporosis (Nguyon et al. 2004).

On ultrasound, hemangiomas have a variable appearance, presenting as circumscribed or diffuse, homogeneous or inhomogeneous lesions. Doppler reveals blood flow within the lesion (Fig. 12c) (Nguyon et al. 2004).

On MRI, arteriovenous malformation often appears as an enlarged vascular channel without a discrete soft-tissue mass (Ergun et al. 2010).

Cavernous hemangiomas are well-circumscribed lobulated masses which are usually isointense to muscle on T1-weighted images, with variable areas of interspersed fat (Fig. 13b). On T2-weighted sequences, the lesion is heterogeneously hyperintense (Fig. 13c), as a result of the mixed amounts of fat and pooled blood in larger vessels. Thrombotic vessel segments have different signal intensities depending on the age of thrombosis (Fig. 12). Fast blood flow generally causes a flow void with a dark lumen, whereas a slow or stagnant flow in dilated or tortuous vessels can cause increased signal ("paradoxical enhancement"). Linear or serpiginous flow voids with round filing defects may be demonstrated on both pulse sequences, indicating the presence of high-flow vessels and phleboliths (Fig. 14). Smaller cavernous hemangiomas are more likely to have an atypical appearance (Nguyon et al. 2004).

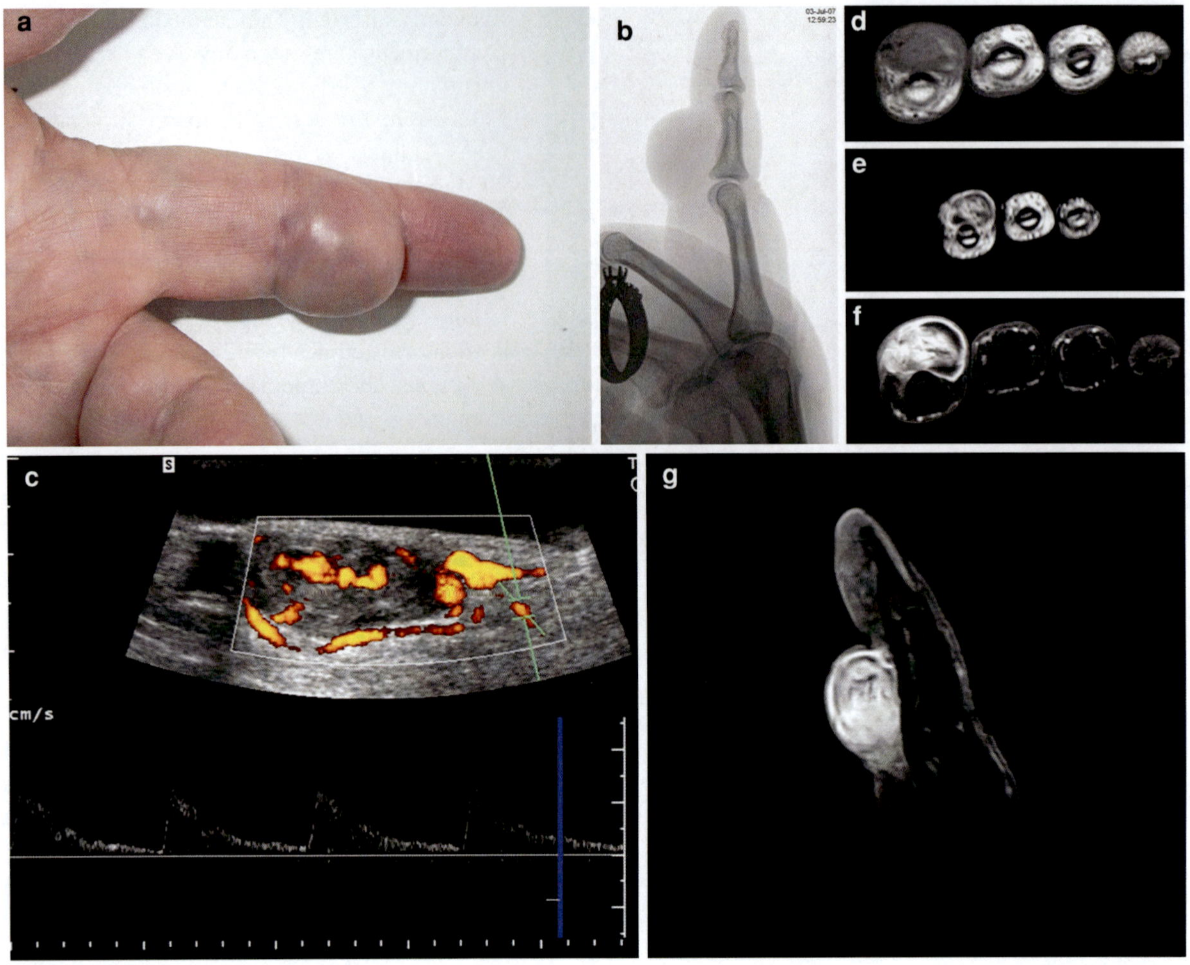

Fig. 12 Partially thrombosed arteriovenous malformation adjacent to the flexor tendon. **a** Clinical image showing a soft-tissue mass at the palmar aspect of the index. There is bluish discoloration of the overlying skin. **b** Plain radiograph (lateral view) demonstrates a non-specific soft-tissue mass at the palmar aspect of the index. **c** Longitudinal ultrasound showing an oval shaped hypoechoic structure with increased intralesional power Doppler signal and an arterial feeder at the proximal side of the lesion. **d** Axial T1-weighted images shows that the lesion is of heterogeneous signal intensity. Areas of high signal intensity may correspond to thrombosis. **e** Axial TSE T2-weighted image. The lesion is heterogeneous with areas of high and low signal intensity. **f**, **g** Axial and sagittal fatsuppressed T1-weighted images after intravenous injection of gadolinium contrast. There is heterogeneous enhancement of the lesion. Areas of non-enhancement may correspond to thrombosis of vascular structures

After intravenous injection of gadolinium contrast, occasionally the arterial feeders and draining veins may be seen both on CT- (Fig. 15) and MR Angiography. Delayed imaging after a few minutes allows evaluation of the precise extent of the tumor (Schmitt 2008) (Fig. 13d, e).

On CT, lymphangiomas usually have a negative density due to high lipid content of the lymphatic fluid.

On T1-weighted MR images, the lesion is of intermediate signal intensity, whereas it is typically hyperintense on T2-weighted images.

2.8 Benign Neurogenic Tumors

2.8.1 Definition

The most frequent subtypes of neurogenic tumors in the hand and wrist are neurinomas (schwannomas) and neurofibromas.

Schwannomas originate from the Schwann cells surrounding the peripheral nerves. The lesions are eccentric to the nerve of origin and are surrounded by a capsule of connective tissue. A schwannoma originates usually from the deeper and broader

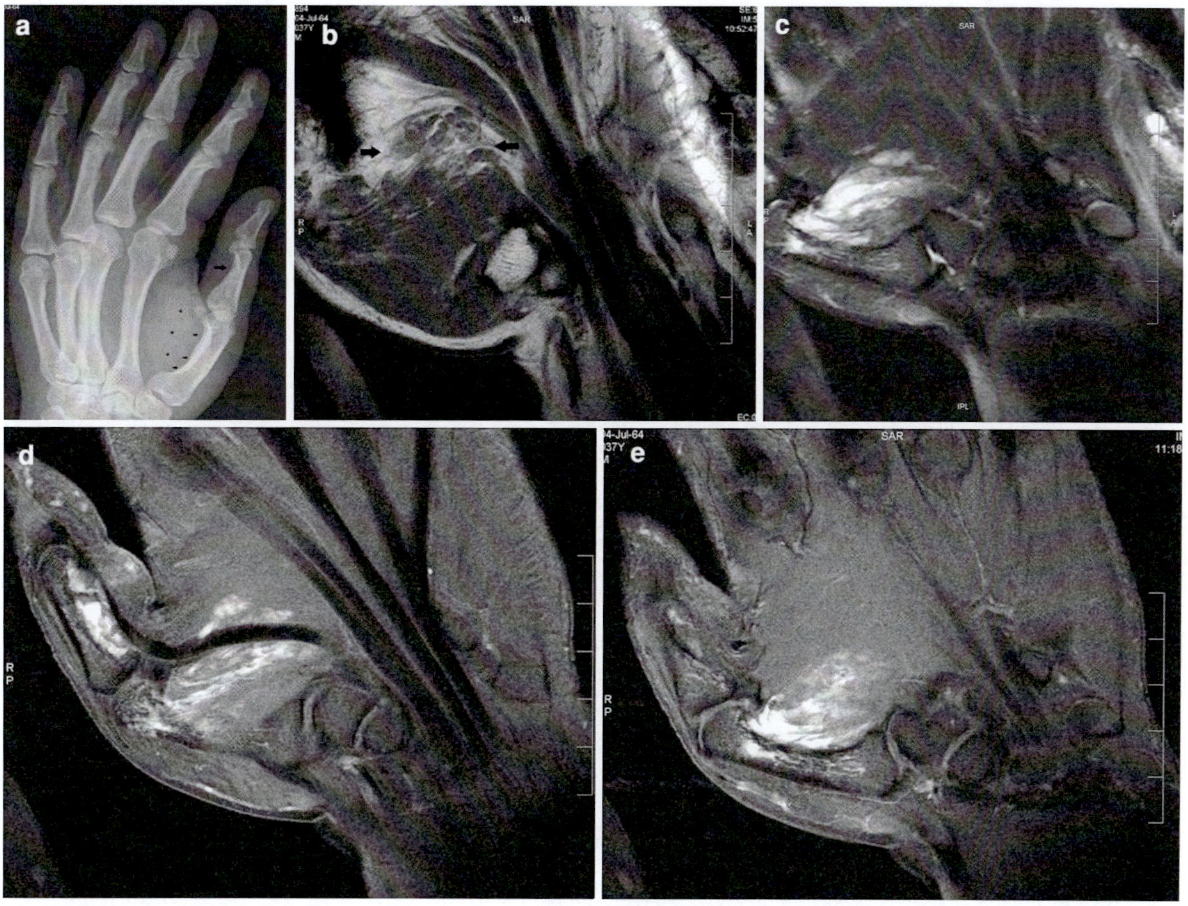

Fig. 13 Haemangioma of the thenar muscle. **a** Plain radiograph of the left hand. There is a non-specific soft-tissue mass (*asterisks*), containing some streaks of fat and causing pressure erosion of the ulnar side of the first metacarpal and proximal phalanx of the thumb (*arrows*). **b** Coronal SE T1-weighted image shows a well-defined lobulated mass in the thenar muscle (*arrows*) with areas of interspersed fat. **c** Coronal fatsuppressed TSE T2-weighted image. The lesion is located within the thenar muscle and has a heterogeneous high signal intensity. There is also osseous remodeling of the ulnar side of the cortex of metacarpal 1. Note some streaks of high signal within the medullary bone of metacarpal 1, due to intra-osseous extension in the metacarpal bone. **d**, **e** Coronal SE fatsuppressed T1-weighted images after intravenous injection of gadolinium contrast. There is marked serpiginous enhancement of the intramuscular and intraosseous component of the lesion (metacarpal 1 and proximal phalanx of the thumb)

nerves of the hand and wrist and is primarily located at the palmar side (Schmitt 2008; Ergun et al. 2010).

Neurofibromas cause diffuse thickening of the nerve sheath. The nerve fascicles run through the concentric tumor. The lesion involves the smaller cutaneous nerves and has no capsule. Neurofibromas occur as solitary lesions or in conjunction with von Recklinghausen disease (Neurofibromatosis type I). Multiple schwannomas as part of schwannomatosis is much more rare.

2.8.2 Clinical Findings

Patients present with a palpable mass (Fig. 16a) and rarely complain of pain. Pain may be elicited by percussion of the mass (Hoffmann-Tinel sign).

2.8.3 Imaging Findings

Plain radiographs are usually normal, but paraosseous neurogenic tumors can cause scalloping of the adjacent bone.

On ultrasound, neurinomas are located eccentric to the surrounding nerve, whereas neurofibromas are

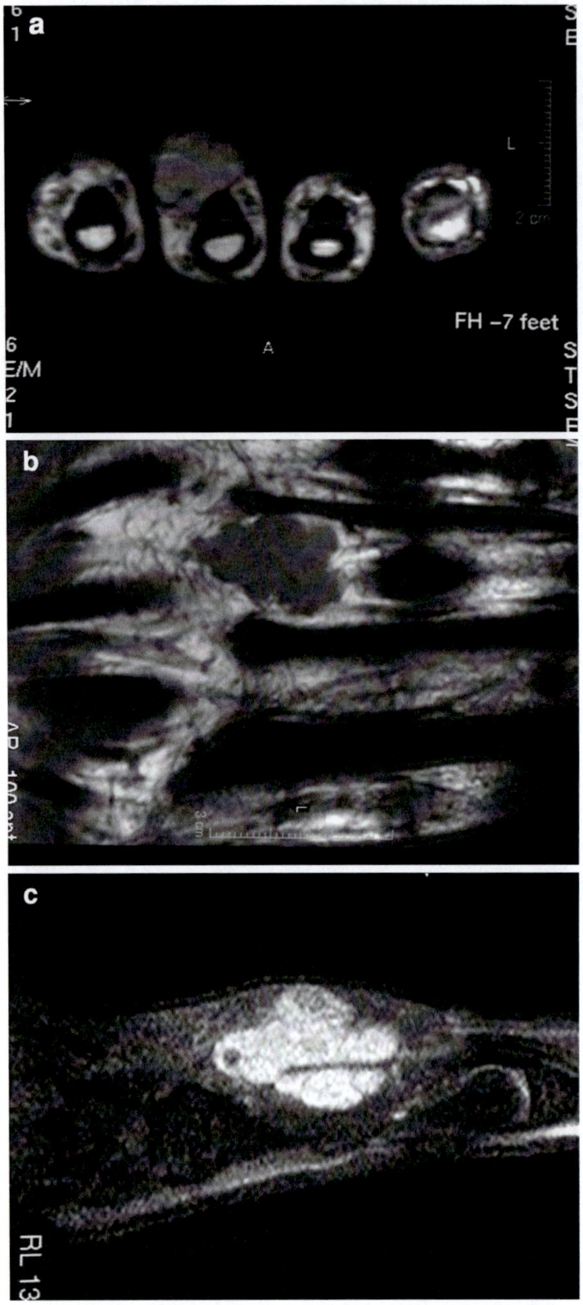

Fig. 14 Haemangioma of the finger. **a** Axial SE T1-weighted image and **b** coronal SE T1-weighted image shows a well-defined lobulated at the flexor side of the third finger. **c** Coronal fatsuppressed TSE T2-weighted image. The lesion is predominantly of high signal intensity. Note also some intralesional round areas of low signal intensity (phleboliths)

concentric in relation to the affected nerve. The Hoffman-Tinel sign can be provoked by sonographic palpation of the affected nerve.

On MRI, benign nerve sheath tumors are well-demarcated masses. The lesions are isointense or slightly hyperintense to muscle on T1-weighted images and heterogeneously hyperintense on T2-weighted images. A target sign consisting of a central low signal and a hyperintense periphery is highly suggestive for a neurogenic tumor (Fig. 16). Other morphological signs of neurogenic tumors are the split fat sign (displaced fat around the mass on the neurovascular bundle), the fascicular sign (nerve fascicles on the course of the tumor), and the presence of a fusiform mass on the course of the involved nerve (Schmitt 2008; Ergun et al. 2010).

2.9 Glomus Tumor

2.9.1 Definition

The glomus tumor is a neoplasm consisting of cells which closely resemble smooth muscle cells of the normal glomus body. The glomus body is an arteriovenous anastomosis that has an important role in thermoregulation. It is located in the subungual region, digits, and palms. The lesion shows both muscle fibers and epithelial-appearing glomus cells (Enzinger and Weiss 1995).

2.9.2 Clinical Findings

Glomus tumors are uncommon, with an equal frequency of occurrence in both sexes. The most common location is the subungual tissue at the tip of the finger. For this location however, there is a striking female predominance. Glomus tumors are also seen at the palm, wrist, forearm, and foot. Multiple lesions may be present, especially during childhood. Glomus tumors cause a radiating pain which is elicited by a change in temperature. Clinical examination usually reveals a characteristic blue-red nodule. Therapy aims at complete excision, still leaving a recurrence rate of 10% (Enzinger and Weiss 1995).

2.9.3 Imaging

Plain films may show a small mass at the dorsal aspect of the finger, associated with a small erosion of the adjacent bone. However, this sign is non-specific and is only found in 12–60% of glomus tumors (Drape et al. 2009) Ultrasound may detect

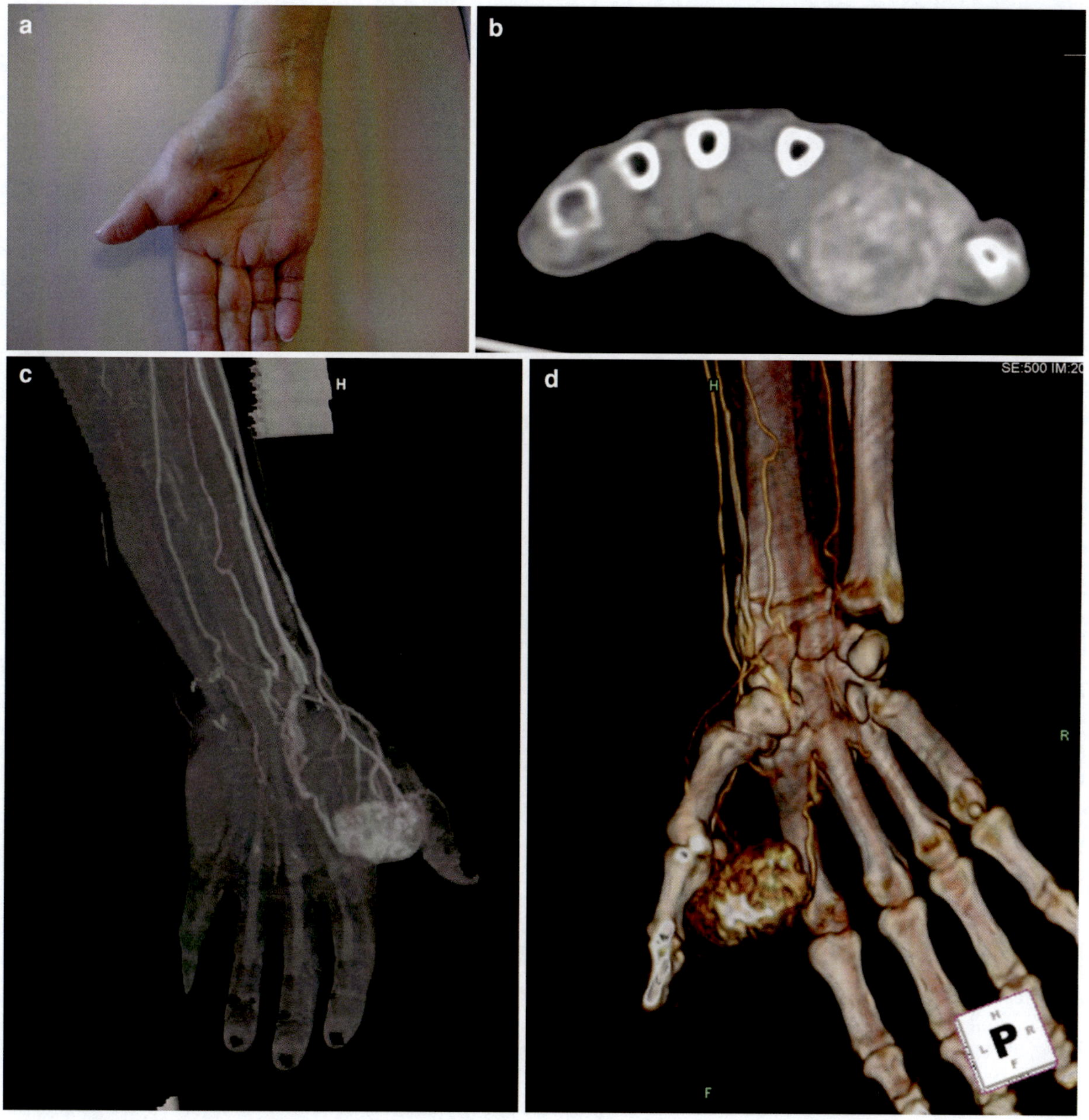

Fig. 15 Arteriovenous malformation of the thumb. **a** Clinical image showing a soft-tissue mass at the palmar aspect of the thumb. **b** Axial contrast-enhanced CT showing an intramuscular mass within the thenar with heterogeneous contrast enhancement. **c–d** CT-angiography (MIP and VRT image) showing the feeding arteries and draining veins

lesions as small as 2 mm (Drape et al. 2009; Matsunga et al. 2007). Ultrasound is more sensitive than plain films to detect cortical erosions at the dorsal aspect of the distal phalanx in up to 78% of cases (Drape et al. 2009). Ultrasound is able to detect 92% of glomus tumors (Drape et al. 2009; Marchadier et al. 2006). The lesion is usually rounded and the echogenicity may be variable (usually hypoechoic to the subungual region). Most glomus tumors are hypervascular on power Doppler (Fig. 17a, b), but 21% of the lesions may be hypovascular (Drape et al. 2009).

On MRI, glomus tumors are of low to intermediate signal intensity on T1-weighted images and of

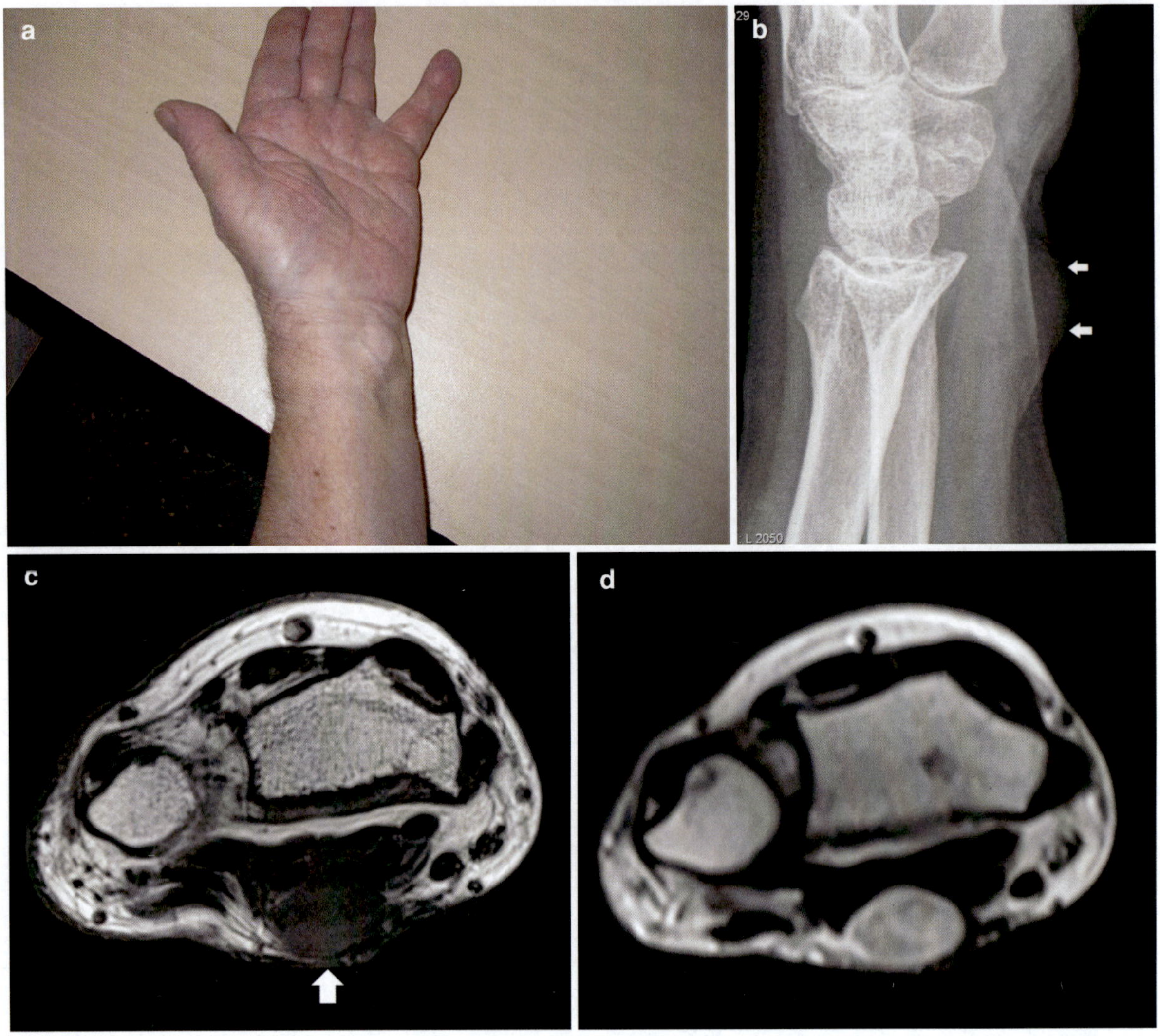

Fig. 16 Schwannoma of the median nerve. **a** Clinical image showing a soft-tissue mass at the palmar aspect of the wrist. **b** Plain radiograph. Non-specific soft-tissue mass at the palmar aspect of the wrist (*arrows*). **c** Axial SE T1-weighted image. Well-defined hypointense mass on the course of the median nerve (*arrow*). **d** Axial fatsuppressed TSE T2-weighted image. Target-like appearance consisting of a hyperintense periphery and central areas of relatively hypointense signal

high signal intensity on T2-weighted images. After intravenous administration of gadolinium contrast, moderate to strong enhancement is seen (Fig. 17c–f). MR angiography is a very useful technique to demonstrate the hypervascular nature of the lesion and an entangled arteriovenous anastomosis. Delayed imaging is sometimes required to demonstrate the hypervascular nature of some lesions (late interstitial diffusion of a minority of lesions) (Drape et al. 2009).

2.10 Fibroma of the Tendon Sheath

2.10.1 Definition

A fibroma of the tendon sheath is a circumscribed tumor, rarely larger than 2 cm in diameter, attached to the tendon sheath of the digits. The thumb is the most commonly involved digit (Nguyon et al. 2004; Plate et al. 2003). Histologically, the lesion is composed of scatters benign fibroblasts with dense collagen, but lack giants cells and xanthoma cells, in

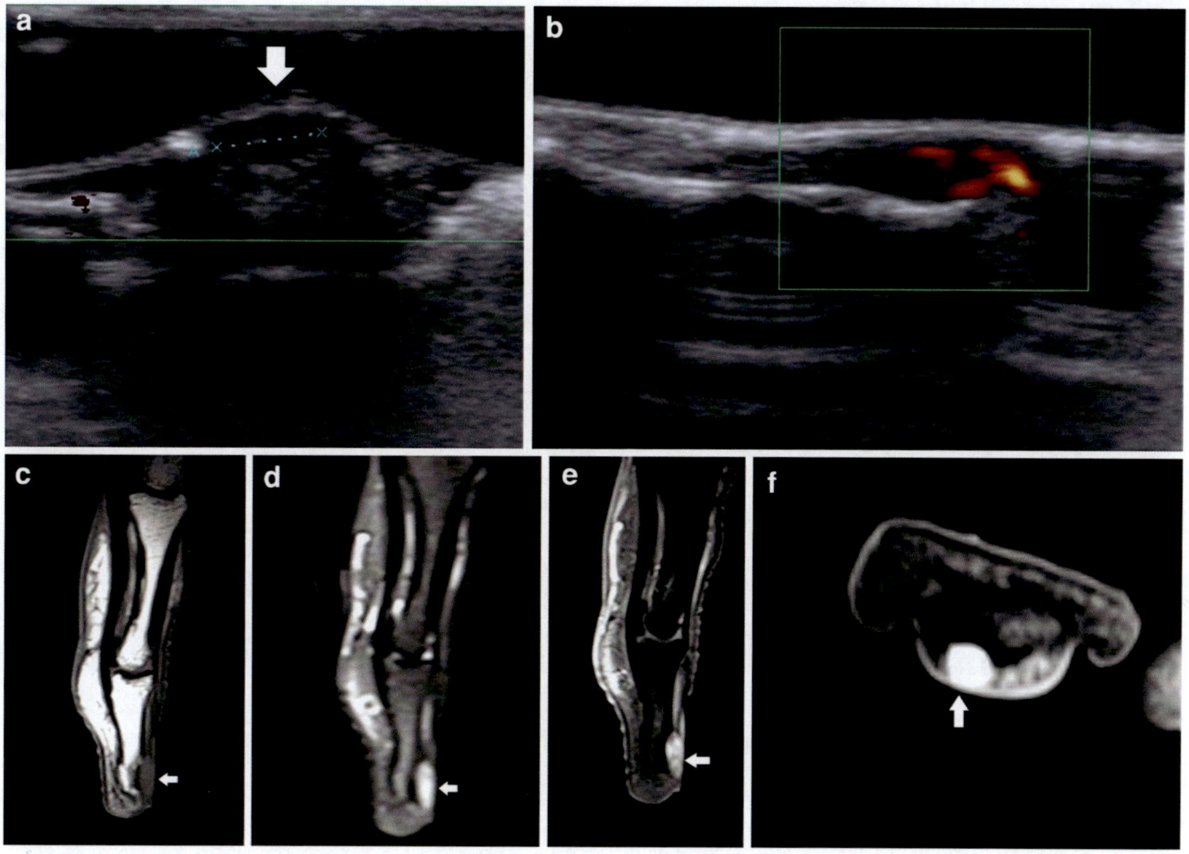

Fig. 17 Subungual glomus tumor. **a** Transverse ultrasound. Note a small hypoechoic subungual lesion causing cortical erosion of the dorsal aspect of the distal phalanx (*arrow*). **b** Longitudinal ultrasound showing increased intralesional power Doppler signal. **c** Sagittal SE T1-weighted image. There is a well-defined subungual hypointense lesion (*arrow*), causing cortical erosion of the distal phalanx. **d** Sagittal fatsuppressed TSE T2-weighted image. Hyperintense signal of the lesion (*arrow*). **e**, **f** Sagittal and axial SE fatsuppressed T1-weighted images after intravenous injection of gadolinium contrast. Marked enhancement of the tumor (*arrow*)

contradistinction to GCTTS (Nguyon et al. 2004; Peh et al. 1995; Wan et al. 2010).

2.10.2 Clinical Findings

They are less common than GCTTS and they often present as slow-growing, firm, and non-tender masses. The mean age of presentation is 42 years (Nguyon et al. 2004). Lesions are typically located on the flexor surfaces, occurring most often in men (75%) (Fox et al. 2003).

2.10.3 Imaging Findings

Pressure erosion of the underlying bone on plain films is very rare. Ultrasound shows a non-specific hypoechoic mass adjacent to the tendon sheath (Fig. 18a). The lesion is usually hypointense on MR sequences, and no or minimal enhancement is seen.

Increased capillary vascularity near the lesion surface may cause minor peripheral enhancement (Figs. 18, 19). The MR imaging findings vary when areas of increased cellularity or myxoid change occur within the lesion. Myxoid changes within the lesion may cause an intermediate to high signal intensity on T2-weighted images, whereas areas of increased cellularity may enhance (Ergun et al. 2010; Fox et al. 2003). In these instances, differentiation of fibroma of the tendon sheath from other tumors, such as giant cell tumor of the tendon sheath, is problematic (Fig. 18d).

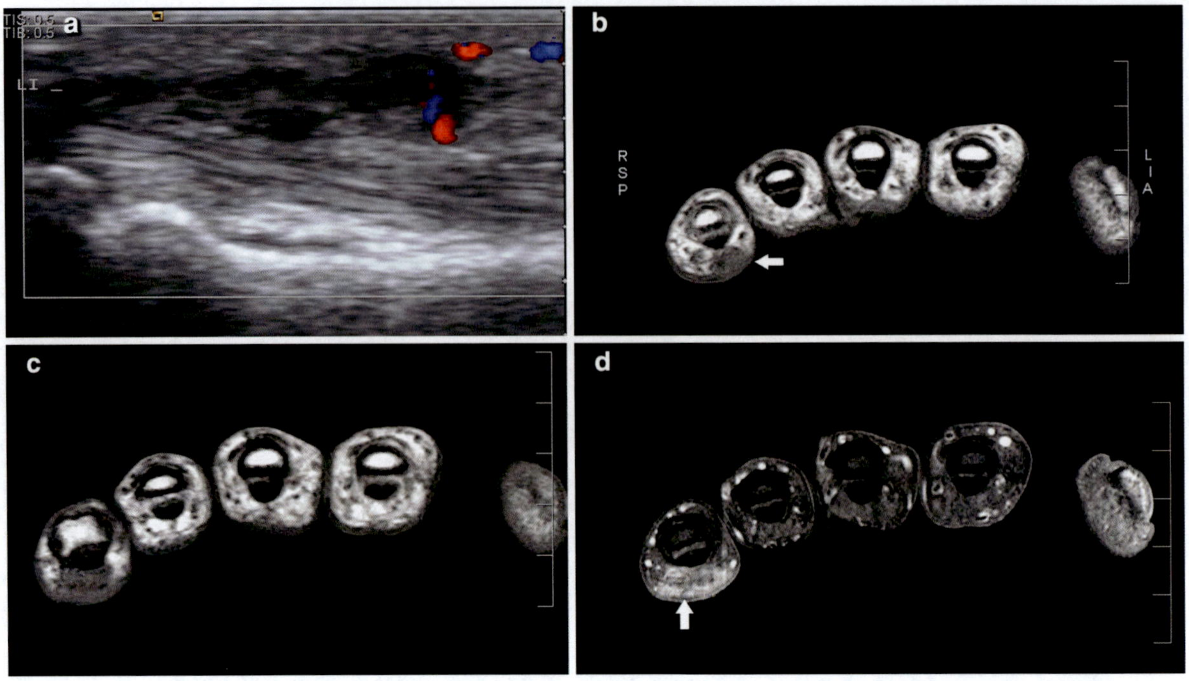

Fig. 18 Fibroma of the tendon sheath of the left fifth finger. **a** Longitudinal ultrasound. Polylobular hypoechoic lesion adjacent to the flexor tendons. Note some increased power Doppler signal at the proximal part of the lesion. **b** Axial SE T1-weighted image. The lesion is isointense to muscle (*arrow*). **c** Axial TSE T2-weighted image. The lesion remains of low signal intensity. **d** Axial SE fatsuppressed T1-weighted images after intravenous injection of gadolinium contrast. There is moderate enhancement of the lesion (*arrow*). In case of contrast enhancement, differentiation of a tendon sheath fibroma from a GCTTS may be difficult

2.11 Palmar Fibromatosis (Dupuytren Disease)

2.11.1 Definition

Palmar fibromatosis was originally described in 1831 by the French physician Dupuytren and is often referred to as Dupuytren disease or contracture. It is the most common of the superficial fibromatoses, affecting 1–2% of the general population. The disease is seen almost exclusively in Caucasians and is rare in populations of African or Asian descent.

The etiology of palmar fibromatosis is not completely understood, but it is thought to be multifactorial, including associations with trauma, microvascular injury, immunologic processes, and genetic factors (Murphey et al. 2009).

2.11.2 Clinical Features

The disease most commonly occurs in patients over 65 years of age, with a frequency of 20% in this age group. Men are three to four times more likely to be affected by the disease than women, and lesions are bilateral in 40–60% of patients. Patients present clinically with painless, subcutaneous nodules (Murphey et al. 2009). These nodules may progress slowly to fibrous cords or bands that attach to and cause traction on the underlying flexor tendons, resulting in flexion contractures of the digits. The fourth and fifth digits are most commonly involved. Patients commonly have related diseases such as plantar fibromatosis (5–20%), Peyronie disease, and knuckle pad fibromatosis. Other associated diseases include diabetes mellitus (20% of patients), epilepsy (50% of male patients and 25% of female patients), alcoholism (particularly liver disease related to alcoholism), and keloid (Murphey et al. 2009).

2.11.3 Imaging Findings

Plain radiographs are typically normal, other than the flexion contractures.

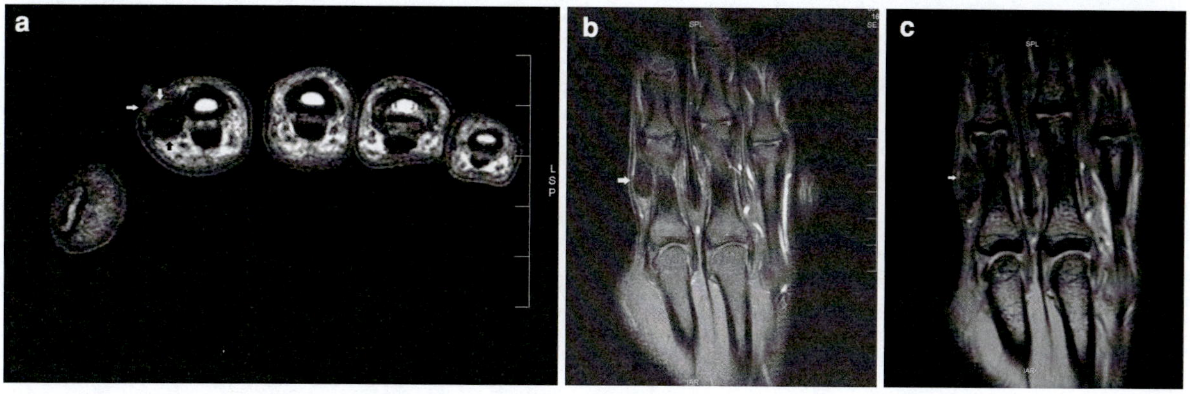

Fig. 19 Typical MR characteristics of a fibroma of the index. **a** Axial SE T1-weighted image. The lesion hypointense to muscle (*arrows*). **b** Coronal fatsuppressed TSE T2-weighted image. The lesion remains of low signal intensity (*arrow*). **c** Coronal gradient echo T2*-weighted image. There is absence of blooming artifact (*arrow*)

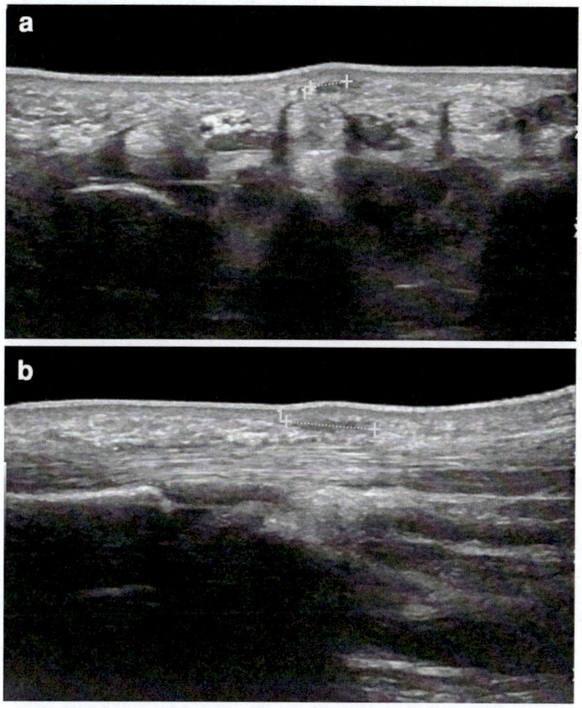

Fig. 20 Palmar fibromatosis. **a** Transverse ultrasound. **b** Longitudinal ultrasound. Hypoechoic nodule adjacent to the flexor tendon of the palm of the hand (third ray)

Ultrasound reveals hypervascular, hypoechoic nodules (Fig. 20) in the palmar subcutaneous tissues, superficial to the flexor tendons.

CT shows non-specific, nodular soft-tissue thickening.

At MR imaging, there are multiple nodular or cordlike, superficial soft-tissue masses that arise from the proximal palmar aponeurosis and extend superficially in parallel with the flexor tendons. Lesion length varies from 10 to 55 mm (2–10 mm in diameter), and lesions terminate in either a branching or nodular configuration at the level of the distal metacarpal.

The signal intensity of palmar fibromatosis is variable along with the cellularity and the collagen content of the lesion. Lesions of low signal intensity on all pulse sequences are relatively hypocellular and contain abundant dense collagen. In contradistinction, the lesions of intermediate signal intensity on both T1- and T2-weighted images are more cellular or mixed, with less abundant collagen (Murphey et al. 2009; Yacoe et al. 1993). Lesions with a higher cellular component have been shown to have a higher local recurrence rate following local excision. This information is important because preoperative MR imaging may assist the surgeon in determining the appropriate timing for excision (Yacoe et al. 1993; Robbin et al. 2001). After intravenous administration of gadolinium contrast, hypercellular lesions are enhancing more vividly than hypocellular lesions (Murphey et al. 2009).

2.12 Desmoid Tumors (Desmoid Type Fibromatosis)

2.12.1 Definition

Extra-abdominal desmoids are rare benign soft-tissue tumors arising from connective tissue of muscle, overlying fascia, or aponeurosis. They have been designated previously as desmoids tumor, aggressive fibromatosis, or musculoaponeurotic fibromatosis. The term "desmoid" means band-like or tendon-like lesion (De Schepper and Vandevenne 2006). Currently, the term desmoid type fibromatosis is used. The lesions can be regarded as deep seated fibromatosis in contradistinction to palmar fibromatosis which is a superficially located. Desmoid fibromas are infiltrative tumors, known for their frequent recurrences. Complete surgical excision is often difficult.

2.12.2 Clinical Features

The most commonly encountered locations are the upper arm (28%), chest wall and paraspinal area (17%), thigh (12%), neck (8%), knee (7%), pelvis or buttock (6%), lower leg (5%). The hand and forearm is rarely affected in up to 5% (Murphey et al. 2009; Berthe et al. 2003). Desmoids occur most frequently in patients in the second to fourth decades of life, with a peak incidence between the ages of 25 and 35 years (Murphey et al. 2009). The lesion is typically deeply seated and poorly circumscribed. Slow insidious growth is the rule, and most lesions are painless (Murphey et al. 2009).

2.12.3 Imaging Findings

Plain radiographs are often normal. A non-specific soft-tissue mass may be apparent in patients with larger lesions. Calcification is uncommon, although underlying pressure erosion or cortical scalloping may be seen.

The US appearance of desmoid-type fibromatosis has not been extensively described. Ultrasound may demonstrate a non-specific poorly defined, hypoechoic soft-tissue mass. Large lesions may demonstrate posterior acoustic shadowing. Increased vascularity is seen on Doppler-ultrasound (Murphey et al. 2009).

On CT, the lesion has a variable attenuation and enhancement (up to 110 HU). The attenuation is usually similar to that of skeletal muscle, but lesions with more prominent collagen content may reveal mildly higher attenuation. Low attenuation is rare and is associated with myxoid components. The margins are often indistinct (Murphey et al. 2009).

On MRI, the lesion may be well demarcated or ill defined. The signal intensity of desmoid-type fibromatosis is variable, dependent on the extent of collagen and degree of cellularity of the lesion. Low signal intensity areas on T2-weighted images correspond histologically to hypocellular and collagen-rich portions of the tumor, whereas more cellular areas with a large extracellular space are of high signal on T2-weighted images. In addition, high T2 signal may be seen in myxoid portions.

Postcontrast MR images typically reveal heterogeneous and often moderate to marked enhancement of these lesions. Hypocellular, collagenized bands do not enhance and therefore are often accentuated at postcontrast MR imaging (Fig. 21) (Murphey et al. 2009).

2.13 Synovial Chondromatosis

2.13.1 Definition

Primary synovial chondromatosis represents an uncommon benign neoplastic process with hyaline cartilage nodules in the subsynovial tissue of a joint, tendon sheath (Fig. 21), or bursa. The nodules may enlarge and detach from the synovium (Murphey et al. 2007). Synovial chondromatosis may be divided into primary and secondary forms. Secondary chondromatosis represents a non-tumoral condition associated with underlying degenerative, destructive or posttraumatic joint disease that causes intraarticular chondral bodies. On the contrary, primary synovial chondromatosis can be regarded as a true benign neoplastic disorder (Murphey et al. 2007; Buddingh et al. 2003).

2.13.2 Clinical Findings

Male adults are the most commonly involved patient population.

Primary chondromatosis involves usually large joints such as the knee and hip. The metacarpophalangeal, interphalangeal, and distal radioulnar joints

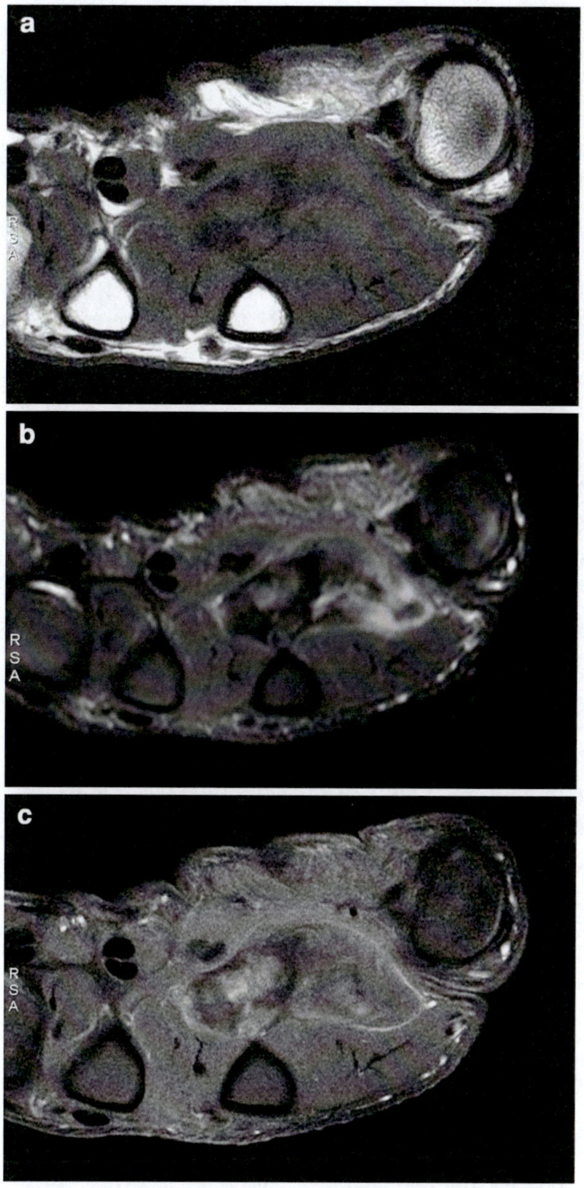

Fig. 21 Desmoid tumor. **a** Axial SE T1-weighted image. Ill-defined intramuscular lesion in the thenar muscle. The mass is of heterogeneous signal with isointense and hypointense areas compared to muscle. **b** Axial fatsuppressed TSE T2-weighted image. Heterogeneous signal intensity with areas of low and intermediate signal. The areas of low signal intensity on both pulse sequences correspond to areas of hypocellularity and collagenized areas. **c** Axial SE fatsuppressed T1-weighted images after intravenous injection of gadolinium contrast. Hypocellular, collagenized areas do not enhance

of the hand and wrist are less commonly involved (Murphey et al. 2007). Primary synovial chondromatosis can also involve extraarticular sites (Sect. 17.2.14). This subtype arises probably in synovium about the tendons or bursa and is frequently referred to as tenosynovial (Fig. 22) or bursal chondromatosis, respectively (Murphey et al. 2007).

2.13.3 Imaging

Radiologic findings are frequently pathognomonic. Radiographs reveal multiple intra-articular calcifications (70–95% of cases) of similar size and shape, distributed throughout the joint, with typical chondroid "ring-and-arc" pattern of mineralization. Extrinsic erosion of bone is seen in 20–50% of cases. The joint space is typically maintained, unless the disease is complicated by secondary osteoarthritis.

Ultrasound shows a heterogeneous mass containing foci of hyperechogenicity, representing either chondral fragments or fronds of synovium with underlying cartilage nodule formation. The nodules are usually multiple and have a lobular contour. If the lesion contains sufficient mineralization or enchondral ossification, posterior acoustic shadowing may be present (Murphey et al. 2007). Synovial chondromatosis is avascular on power Doppler (Roberts et al. 2004).

Computed tomography (CT) may depict calcified intra-articular fragments and more subtle extrinsic bone erosion.

Magnetic resonance (MR) imaging findings are more variable, depending on the degree of mineralization, although the most common pattern (77% of cases) reveals low to intermediate signal intensity with T1-weighting and very high signal intensity with T2-weighting with hypointense calcifications. These signal intensity characteristics on MR images and low attenuation of the non-mineralized regions on CT scans reflect the high water content of the cartilaginous lesions. CT and MR imaging depict the extent of the synovial disease (particularly surrounding soft-tissue involvement) and lobular growth. Following intravenous administration of contrast, peripheral or arc-like enhancement may be observed (Wittkop et al. 2002). With delayed imaging after intravenous

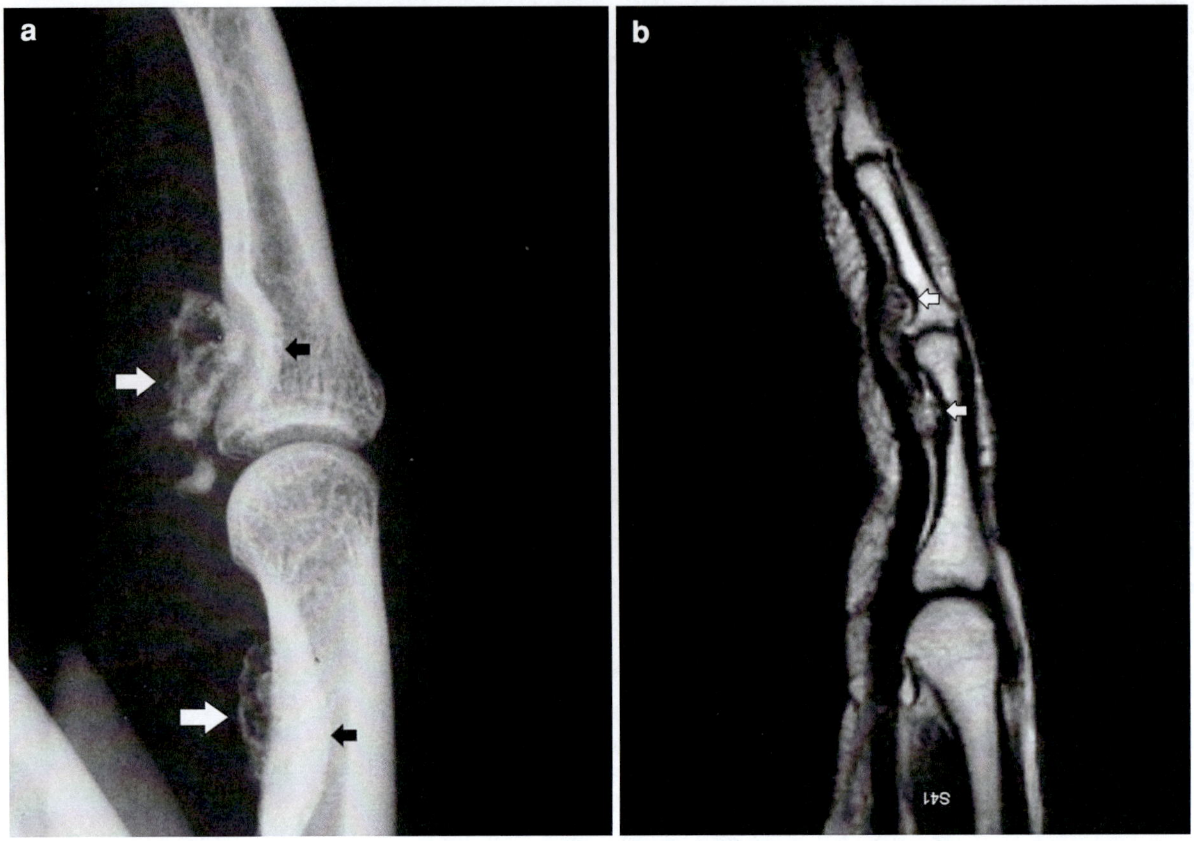

Fig. 22 Tenosynovial chondromatosis of the finger. **a** Plain radiograph. Chondroid-like calcifications adjacent to the flexor side of the proximal and middle phalanx (*white arrows*). There is scalloping of the adjacent cortical bone (*black arrows*). **b** Sagittal TSE T2-weighted image. The lesions are of variable signal intensity corresponding to calcified and non-calcified chondroid areas. Note the intimate relationship with the flexor tendons and the presence of cortical erosions (*arrows*)

contrast administration, an indirect MR arthrographic effect may be obtained, showing multiple intraarticular nodules within the joint cavity (Brassens and Cotten 2010).

Secondary synovial chondromatosis can be distinguished from primary disease both radiologically (underlying articular disease and fewer chondral bodies of variable size and shape) and pathologically (concentric rings of growth) (Murphey et al. 2007).

2.14 Soft-Tissue Chondroma (Tenosynovial Chondromatosis)

2.14.1 Definition

Soft-tissue chondroma, also known as extraskeletal chondroma or chondroma of soft-tissue parts is a rare soft-tissue tumor accounting for only 1.5% of benign soft-tissue tumors (Hondar Wu et al. 2006). The origin is not known but is assumed to be synovial, since the lesion is typically attached to the synovial capsule or tendon sheath (Ergun et al. 2010).

2.14.2 Clinical Features

Soft-tissue chondroma occurs at almost any age, but most commonly in 30–60-year-old patients. The tumor occurs most commonly in the hands and feet (Hondar Wu et al. 2006). Men are affected more often than women in the third decades of life. When the disease is diagnosed in older patients (after the fifth decade), there is a female predominance (Murphey et al. 2007). The patient presents most frequently with a painless mass or only mild tenderness upon palpation of the lesion. Duration of the symptoms ranges

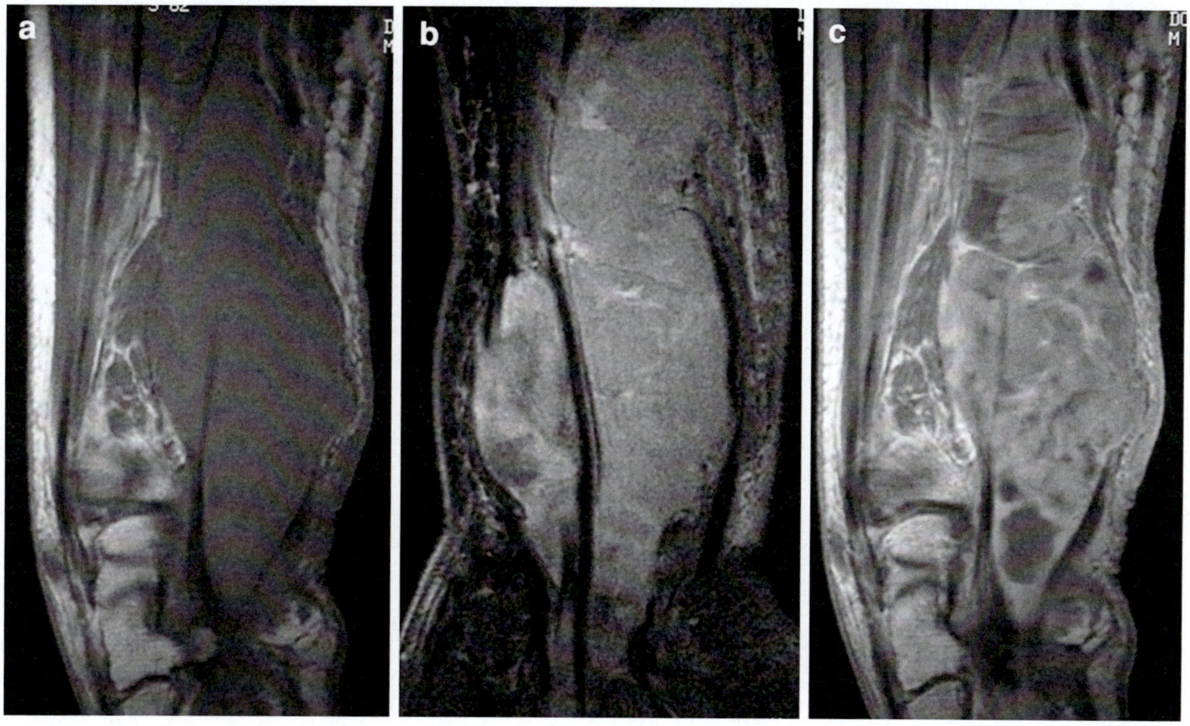

Fig. 23 Typical example of a malignant soft-tissue tumor of the wrist (highly malignant sarcoma NOS). **a** Sagittal SE T1-weighted image. **b** Sagittal fatsuppressed TSE T2-weighted image. **c** Sagittal fatsuppressed SE T1-weighted images after intravenous injection of gadolinium contrast. The lesion is large, inhomogeneous on T2-weighted images and shows marked and inhomogeneous enhancement

between 5 and 18 years with a median of 2 years (Fetsch et al. 2003).

2.14.3 Imaging Features

Plain films demonstrate calcifications in 33–80% of soft-tissue chondromas. The pattern of calcifications is variable, including curvilinear, punctate, mixed and dystrophic or focal dense pattern (Fig. 22) (Hondar Wu et al. 2006).

On MRI, the signal intensity varies along with the degree of calcified matrix within the lesion (Fig. 22). Highly calcified lesions are of low signal intensity on both pulse sequences, whereas non-calcified lesions are of intermediate signal intensity on T1-weighted images and of high signal on T2-weighted images. The high signal is due to a high water content of the mucopolysaccharide component or myxoid changes (Hondar Wu et al. 2006). Following intravenous administration of contrast, septal or peripheral enhancement may be observed, corresponding to fibrovascular tissue surrounding the avascular nodules (Ergun et al. 2010).

Table 1 MR Imaging features that may suggest malignancy (modified from De Schepper and Bloem 2007)

Large volume (any lesion exceeding 3 cm in H/W)
Ill defined margins
Inhomogeneity on all pulse sequences
Intralesional hemorrhage
Intralesional necrosis
Extensive and peripheral enhancement pattern (with papillary projections) on static contrast examination
Rapid enhancement with steep slope on dynamic contrast examination
Extracompartmental extension
Invasion of adjacent bones and neurovascular bundles.

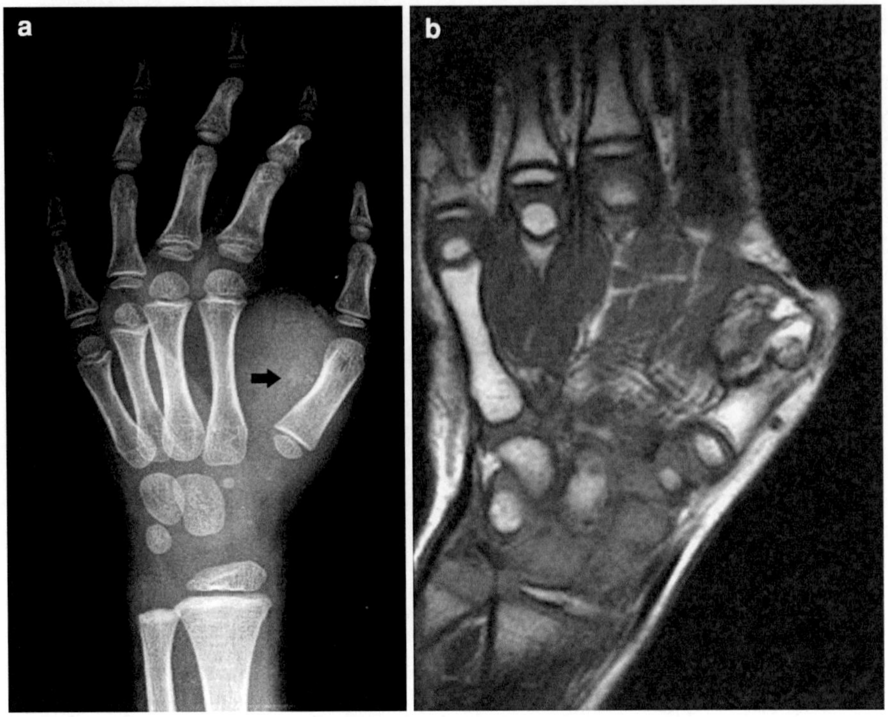

Fig. 24 Myositis of the thenar in a 7-year-old boy, presenting with pain and swelling at the thumb. **a** Plain radiograph. Note calcifications in the thenar (*arrow*). **b** Coronal SE T1-weighted image 9 month later shows an intramuscular ossified mass with central high signal intensity (fatty bone marrow) with peripheral and central areas of low signal (Courtesy of J. Vandevenne, Genk)

3 Malignant Soft-Tissue Tumors

Malignant soft-tissue tumors are much more rare than benign tumor and tumor-like conditions in the hand and wrist (de La Kethulle de Ryhove et al. 2000; Capelastegui et al. 1999).

Soft-tissue sarcomas of the hand may be found in young adults and clinical symptoms are usually non-specific, as most patients present with a painless mass without functional deficit.

Plain radiographs and CT are usually non-diagnostic. Amorphous (synovial sarcoma, extraskeletal osteosarcoma) or arc-like (extraskeletal chondrosarcoma) calcifications may be seen in certain malignant tumors. Destruction of the adjacent bone is very rare.

Most malignant soft-tissue tumors are hypoechoic on ultrasound and may show intralesional necrosis. The tumor extent cannot be reliably determined on ultrasound.

MRI is the imaging modality of choice for grading (differentiation between benign and malignant tumors and assessment of malignancy grade) and local staging of malignant soft-tissue tumors of the hand and wrist (H/W).

Important grading parameters which may suggest malignancy based on MR imaging (Fig. 23) are summarized in Table 1. There are some exceptions to these rules of thumb as some malignant tumors may have relatively well-defined margins and may demonstrate homogeneous enhancement (e.g. clear cell sarcoma). The value of each individual parameter being rather low, correct differentiation can be achieved by a combination of multiple parameters (Gielen et al. 2004; Van Rijswijk et al. 2004). Although a correct histologic diagnosis (tissue specific diagnosis) of malignant soft-tissue tumors cannot be reached based on imaging studies alone, the main task of the radiologist is to select any soft tissue that may be potentially malignant. These lesions should be further evaluated by incisional biopsy without jeopardizing definitive treatment options (Terek and Brien 1995).

The most common malignant soft-tissue tumors involving the hand are synovial sarcoma, liposarcomas, rhabdomyosarcoma, clear cell sarcoma, myxofibrosarcoma, malignant vascular tumors (angiosarcoma and Kaposi sarcoma), and malignant peripheral nerve sheath tumors. As the imaging features of these histologic subtypes are often non-

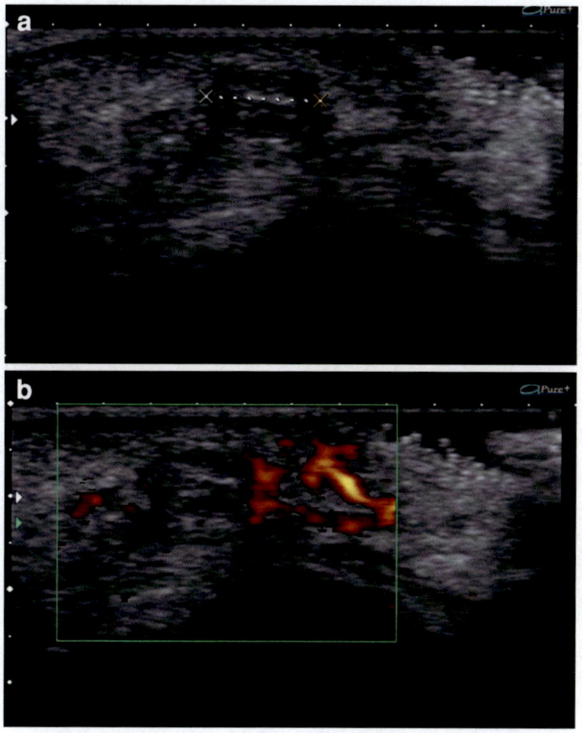

Fig. 25 Foreign body (wood). **a** Ultrasound shows a central hyperechoic wood fragment surrounded by a hypoechoic inflammatory reaction. **b** On power Doppler examination, there is increased signal at the periphery of the lesion

specific, further discussion is beyond the scope of this chapter.

4 Pseudotumoral Lesions

4.1 Myositis Ossificans

Myositis ossificans (MO) is a benign condition of heterotopic bone formation, which can mimic soft-tissue malignancies. It is rarely seen in the hand region (Chadha and Agarwal 2007; Van Zwieten et al. 2007). The ossification on plain films is centripetal (in contrast to the ossification in extraskeletal osteosarcoma).

Zonal pattern is the typical imaging characteristic (Fig. 24) (Ergun et al. 2010). Detailed discussion of the imaging features of MO is beyond the scope of this chapter.

4.2 Foreign-Body Granuloma

4.2.1 Definition

Foreign body granuloma is usually observed due to previous penetrating trauma, in which the foreign body is not properly retrieved.

4.2.2 Clinical Findings

Most patients will present with a palpable mass, pain, and discomfort.

4.2.3 Imaging Findings

Plain radiographs are only capable of demonstrating radio-opaque foreign bodies, where ultrasound is the imaging technique of choice to demonstrate non-radio-opaque foreign bodies and the surrounding inflammatory reaction (Fig. 25).

In the early course of the lesion, high T2-signal and contrast enhancement is seen surrounding the foreign body, while the granulation tissue may be of low T2-signal without contrast uptake in the chronic stage of the disease (Ergun et al. 2010).

4.3 Rheumatoid Nodule

4.3.1 Definition

Rheumatoid nodules may be rarely observed in cases of long-standing RA, or other rheumatic disease such as lupus, spondylarthropathy, agammaglobulinemia and rheumatic fever. Rarely, it may precede the articular manifestations of rheumatic disease. Histologically, the lesion consists of chronic inflammation, with or without central necrosis.

4.3.2 Clinical Findings

The lesions are usually located at the dorsal aspect of the hand within the subcutaneous tissue (particularly at sites of pressure or repetitive trauma), but bursae, joints, tendons and ligaments may be involved as well (Ergun et al. 2010).

4.3.3 Imaging Findings

Ultrasound is non-specific. MRI may demonstrate iso- to hypointense lesions compared to muscle on

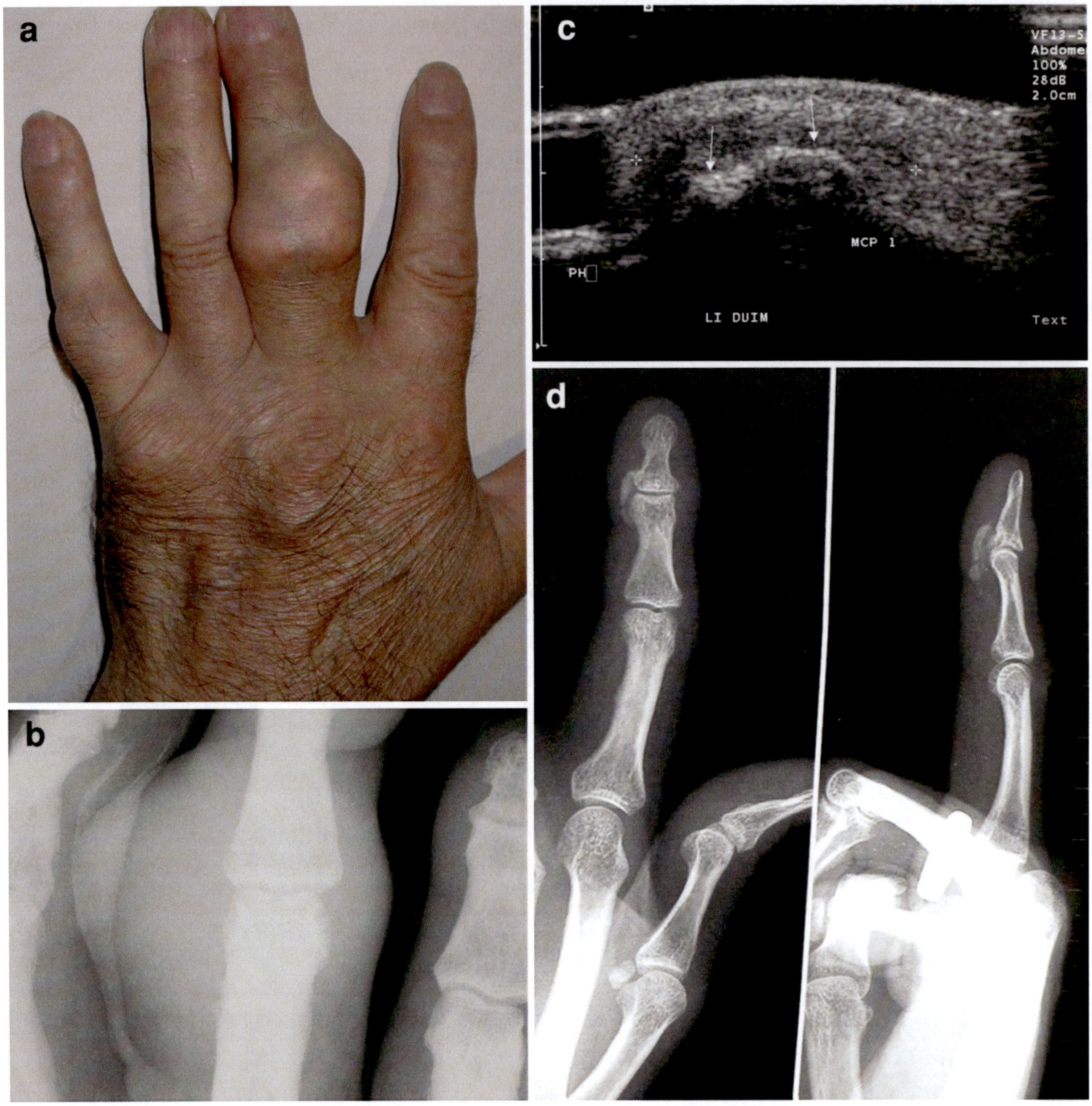

Fig. 26 Examples of pseudomasses due to metabolic diseases. **a** Clinical picture of tophaceous gout. Peri-articular soft-tissue swelling best seen at the proximal interphalangeal joint of the third finger. **b** Corresponding plain radiograph showing the soft-tissue swelling and adjacent periosteal new bone formation. **c** On ultrasound, there is a hypoechoic mass with intralesional reflections with retro-acoustic shadowing due to urate deposition. **d** Pseudogout (hydroxyapatite deposition disease) in another patient. Plain radiograph showing linear and amorphous calcifications at the joint capsule of the distal interphalangeal joint of the index

T1-weighted images. Solid lesions are hypointense on T2-weighted images, whereas cystic lesions are hyperintense. The enhancement pattern is variable ranging from marked in solid lesions to peripheral ring like in cystic lesions (Ergun et al. 2010).

4.4 Gout, Tophaceous Pseudogout, and Other Metabolic Disease

Crystal disease such as gout and pseudogout (hydroxyapatite and calcium pyrophosphate dehydrate

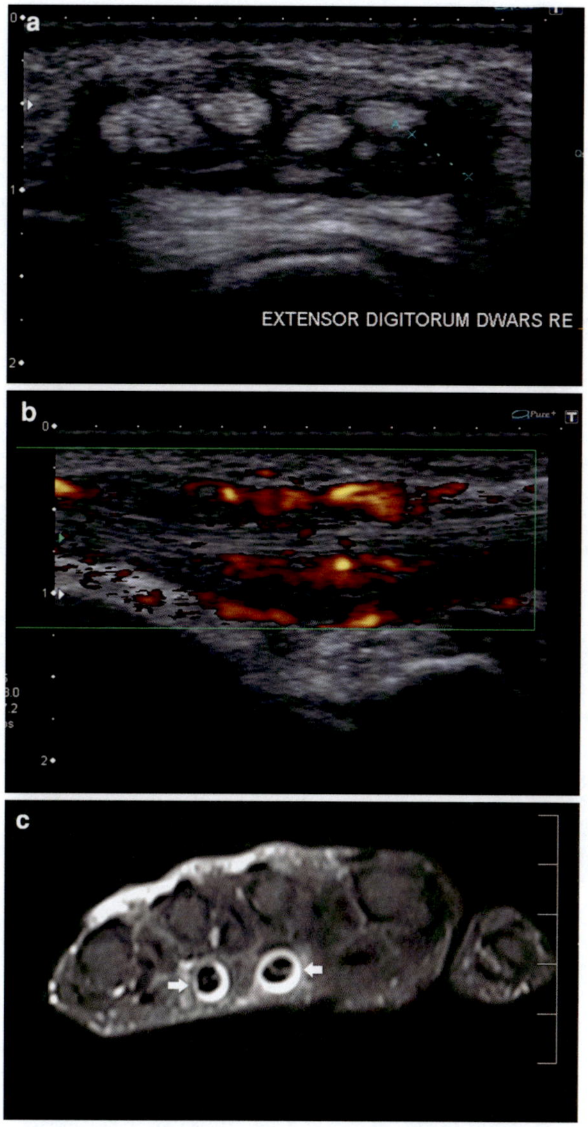

Fig. 27 Tenosynovitis. **a** Transverse ultrasound of the extensor tendons of the wrist showing fluid surrounding the extensor tendons of compartment 4. **b** Longitudinal power Doppler examination shows increased signal within the tendon sheath and tendons. **c** Axial fatsuppressed TSE T2-weighted image showing increased fluid around the flexor tendons of the third and fourth finger (*arrows*) in another patient with known rheumatoid arthritis

deposition disease) and amyloid deposition may occasionally present as peri-articular soft-tissue masses (Fig. 26). Imaging findings are discussed in another chapter of this book.

4.5 Tenosynovitis and Soft-Tissue Abscess

Tenosynovitis consists of inflammation of the tendon sheath. The etiology may include acute and chronic trauma, infection or inflammatory or metabolic disease (Fig. 27).

Infection of the hand and wrist can rapidly spread along the numerous tendon sheath, fascial planes, and lymphatics of the hand. Imaging findings are discussed elsewhere in this book.

4.6 Anomalous and Accessory Muscles

4.6.1 Definition

Accessory muscles are congenital anatomic variants that may clinically simulate mass lesions. The most encountered accessory muscles of the hand and wrist are the accessory palmaris longus muscle, the extensor digitorum brevis muscle, the accessory abductor pollicis minimi muscle, and the anomalies of the flexor digitorum muscles.

4.6.2 Clinical Findings

The lesion may present as a wrist mass. Palmaris longus and accessory flexor digitorum superficialis muscle may be associated with median or ulnar nerve entrapment.

4.6.3 Imaging Findings

Ultrasound shows a hypoechoic structure with a typical striated appearance of muscle. Dynamic ultrasound will show changes in the shape of the mass with active muscle contraction. Accessory muscles are isointense to muscles on all MR pulse sequences.

4.7 Anomalous Osseous Structures

Accessory osseous structures such as a carpal boss may sometimes simulate soft-tissue masses clinically. A carpal boss consists of a firm osseous prominence on the dorsum of the hand at the base of the second or third metacarpal and adjacent to the capitate and trapezoid bone (Fig. 28). On MRI, there may be reactive bone

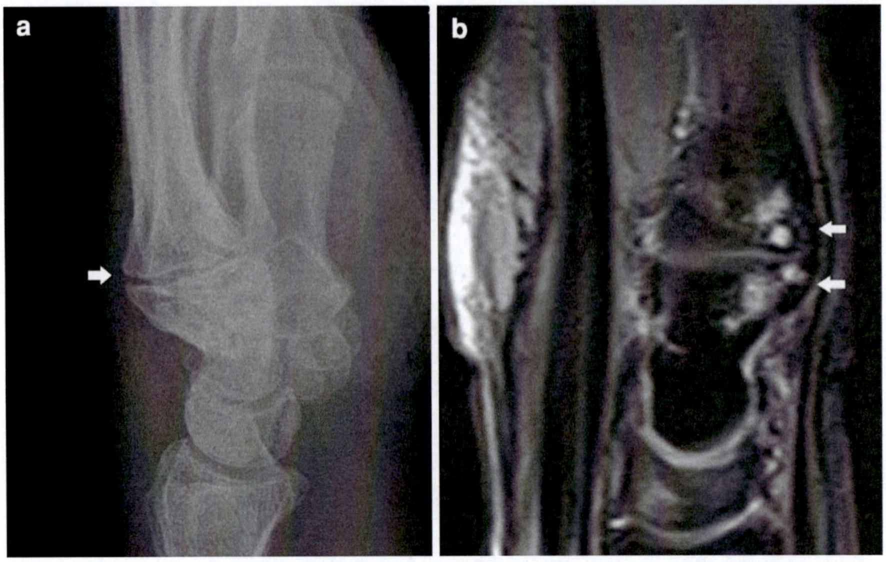

Fig. 28 Carpal boss. **a** Plain radiograph (*lateral view*) showing a bony prominence at the dorsal aspect of the carpometacarpal joint (*arrow*). **b** Sagittal fatsuppressed TSE T2-weighted image. Note bone marrow edema and subchondral cyst formation at the carpo-metacarpal joint (*arrows*)

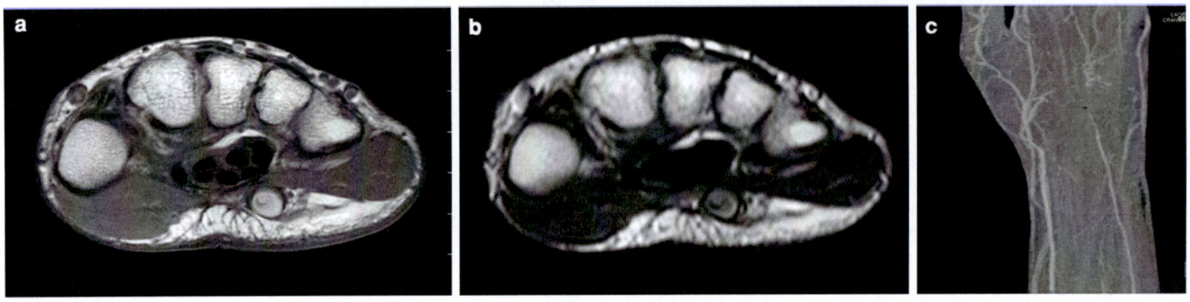

Fig. 29 Hypothenar hammer syndrome. **a** Axial SE T1-weighted image shows a well defined oval mass superficial to the flexor tendons and immediately distal to the hamulus of the hamate. The lesion is of high signal with central area of lower signal intensity. **b** Axial TSE T2-weighted image shows comparable signal intensities, consistent with thrombosis. **c** CT-angiography shows occlusion of the ulnar artery (*arrow*)

marrow edema and associated joint effusion at the carpo-metacarpal joint (Nguyon et al. 2004).

4.8 Bizarre Parosteal Osteochondromatous Proliferation (BPOP)

This reactive lesion and other surface lesions of bone are discussed in Tumours and Tumour-like Lesions of Bone.

4.9 Knuckle Pads

Knuckle pads are caused by focal fibrous thickening dorsally at the proximal interphalangeal (PIP) or metacarpophalangeal (MCP) joint may precede the development of palmar fibromatosis. They are usually asymptomatic. Imaging features are non-specific. On MRI, a nodular thickening is seen at the dorsal aspect of the PIP or MCP joint, with intermediate signal intensity compared to muscle on both pulse sequences and moderate enhancement (Murphey et al. 2009).

4.10 Subcutaneous Granuloma Annulare

Subcutaneous granuloma annulare is a rare inflammatory dermatosis that may be encountered in children, usually located in the pretibial area or the scalp. The lesion presents as an ill-demarcated fast-growing painless subcutaneous lesion, with variable signal intensity and contrast enhancement.

4.11 Hypothenar Hammer Syndrome

A posttraumatic partially thrombosed palmar aneurysm resulting from repeated trauma to the wrist (hypothenar hammer syndrome) may mimic a soft-tissue tumor (Van Zwieten et al. 2007).

The typical location of the lesion on the distal part of the ulnar artery distal to the hamulus of the hamate, the history of repeated trauma, the signal intensity of the lesion (indicative of thrombosis), and direct demonstration of occlusion of the ulnar artery on different imaging modalities (Doppler-ultrasound, MR and CT-angiography) may allow a correct diagnosis (Fig. 29).

5 Conclusion

Most benign soft-tissue tumors or tumor-like conditions of the hand have a predilection for certain location in the hand or wrist or may present with characteristic imaging features. This applies particularly for ganglion cysts, epidermoid inclusion cysts, lipoma, haemangiomas, glomus tumors, and nerve sheath tumors. These lesions can be confidently characterized by imaging. On the contrary, malignant tumors and certain locally aggressive tumors such as desmoid tumor present with non-specific imaging features. Further histologic confirmation is mandatory in order to allow proper management of these lesions.

6 Key Points

- Soft-tissue tumors of the hand and wrist (H&W) are more frequent than bone tumors.
- Benign tumors largely outnumber their malignant counterparts.
- There are some tumors having the H&W as a preferential location, i.e. ganglion cysts, GCTTS, lipomatosis of nerve…
- Benign tumors mostly have distinctive features on MRI, i.e. cysts, GCTTS, hemangiomas, lipomas, neurogenic tumors…
- Ultrasound is the initial technique for evaluation of superficial cystic lesions and may have role in the evaluation of small glomus tumors
- MRI is the preferred technique that contributes substantially in detection, staging, grading, and characterization of soft-tissue tumors. There is only a limited role for plain radiography or CT scan.
- The goal of MRI is to characterize as much as benign tumors and to advocate a biopsy in MRI-non-specific lesions.

References

Angeledes AC (1999) Ganglions of the hand and wrist. In: Green DP, Hotchkiss RN, Pederson WC (eds) Operative hand surgery. Churchill Livingstone, New York, pp 2171–2183

Berthe JV, Loréa P, De Prez C, De Mey A (2003) A case report of desmoid tumor of the finger. Chir Main 22(6):312–314

Brassens H, Cotten A (2010) Chondromatose synoviale. In: Cotten A, Malghem J (eds) 10èmes mises au point en imagerie ostéo-articulaire. Bruxelles Lille, pp 111–125

Buddingh EP, Krallman P, Neff JR, Nelson M, Liu J, Bridge JA (2003) Chromosome 6 abnormalities are recurrent in synovial chondromatosis. Cancer Genet Cytogenet 1:18–22

Capelastegui A, Astigarraga E, Fernandez-Canton G et al (1999) Masses and pseudomasses of the hand and wrist: MR findings in 134 cases. Skeletal Radiol 28:498–507

Chadha M, Agarwal A (2007) Myositis ossificans traumatica of the hand. Can J Surg 50(6):E21–E22

Christiaanse ECY, Jager T, Vanhoenacker FM, Van Hedent E, Van Damme R (2010) Piso-Hamate hiatus syndrome. JBR-BTR 93:34

Christopher D, Unni K, Mertens F (2002) Adipocytic tumors. WHO Classification of tumors. Pathology and genetics: tumors of soft tissue and bone. IARC, Lyon, pp 19–46

De Beuckeleer LHL, Vanhoenacker FM (2006) Lipomatous tumors. In: De Schepper AM, Vanhoenacker F, Parizel PM, Gielen J (eds) Imaging of soft tissue tumors. Springer, Berlin, Heidelberg, New York, pp 203–226

De Beuckeleer LH, De Schepper AM, de La Kethulle de Ryhove D, Nishimura H (2001) Imaging of soft tissue tumors of the hand and wrist. In: Guglielmi G, Van Kuijk C, Genant HK (eds) Fundamentals of hand and wrist imaging. Springer, Berlin, Heidelberg, New York, pp 331–363

de La Kethulle de Ryhove D, De Beuckeleer L, De Schepper A (2000) Magnetic resonance imaging of soft tissue tumors of the hand and wrist. J Radiol 81(5):493–507

De Schepper AM, Bloem JL (2007) Soft tissue tumors: grading, staging, and tissue-specific diagnosis. Top Magn Reson Imaging 18(6):431–444

De Schepper AM, Vandevenne JE (2006) Tumors of connective tissue. In: De Schepper AM, Vanhoenacker F, Parizel PM, Gielen J (eds) Imaging of soft tissue tumors. Springer, Berlin, Heidelberg, New York, pp 167–202

De Schepper AM, Hogendoorn PC, Bloem JL (2007) Giant cell tumors of the tendon sheath may present radiologically as intrinsic osseous lesions. Eur Radiol 17(2):499–502

Drape JL, Rousseau J, Guerini H, Feydy A, Chevrot A (2009) Tumeurs glomiques sous-ungéales: confrontations echo-

IRM. In: Drape JL et al (eds) Poignet et main. SIMS, Sauramps Medical, Montpellier, pp 327–332
Enzinger FM, Weis SW (1995) Perivascular tumors. In: Enzinger FM, Weis SW (eds) Soft tissue tumors, 3rd edn. Mosby, St Louis, pp 701–755
Ergun TE, Lakadamyali H, Derincek A, Tarhan NC, Ozturk A (2010) Magnetic resonance imaging in the visualization of benign tumors and tumor-like lesions of hand and wrist. Curr Probl Diagn Radiol 1–16
Fetsch JF, Vinh TN, Remotti F, Walker EA, Murphey MD, Sweet DE (2003) Tenosynovial (extraarticular) chondromatosis: an analysis of 37 cases of an underrecognized clinicopathologic entity with a strong predilection for the hands and feet and a high local recurrence rate. Am J Surg Pathol 27:1260–1268
Fox MG, Kransdorf MJ, Bancroft LW, Peterson JJ, Flemming DJ (2003) MR imaging of fibroma of the tendon sheath. AJR Am J Roentgenol 180:1449–1453
Gielen JL, De Schepper AM, Vanhoenacker F, Parizel PM, Wang XL, Sciot R, Weyler J (2004) Accuracy of MRI in characterization of soft tissue tumors and tumor-like lesions. A prospective study in 548 patients. Eur Radiol 14(12): 2320–2330
Gielen J, Ceulemans R, van Holsbeeck M (2006) Ultrasound of soft tissue tumors. In: De Schepper AM, Vanhoenacker F, Parizel PM, Gielen J (eds) Imaging of soft tissue tumors. Springer, Berlin, Heidelberg, New York, pp 3–18
Greendyke SD, Wilson M, Shepier TR (1992) Anterior wrist ganglia from the from the scaphotrapezial joint. J Hand Surg Am 17(3):487–490
Hondar Wu HT, Chen W, Lee O, Chang CY (2006) Imaging and pathological correlation of soft-tissue chondroma: a serial five-case study and literature review. Clin Imaging 30(1):32–36
Jin W, Ryu KN, Kim GY, Kim HC, Lee JH, Park JS (2008) Sonographic findings of ruptured epidermal inclusion cysts in superficial soft tissue: emphasis on shapes, pericystic changes, and pericystic vascularity. J Ultrasound Med 27(2):171–176 quiz 177–178
Kobayashi N, Koshino T, Nakazawa A, Saito T (2001) Neuropathy of motor branch of median or ulnar nerve induced by midpalm ganglion. J Hand Surg (Am) 26: 474
Kuwano Y, Ishizaki K, Watanabe R, Nanko H (2009) Efficacy of diagnostic ultrasonography of lipomas, epidermal cysts, and ganglions. Arch Dermatol 145(7):761–764
Lowden CM, Attiah M, Gravin G, Macdermid JC, Osman S, Farber KJ (2005) The prevalence of wrist ganglia in a asymptomatic population: magnetic resonance evaluation. J Hand Surg (Br) 30B(3):302–306
Marchadier A, Cohen M, Legre R (2006) Subungual glomus tumors of the fingers: ultrasound diagnosis. Chir Main 25:16–21
Marom EM, Helms CA (1999) Fibrolipomatous hamartoma: pathognomonic on MR imaging. Skeletal Radiol 28:260–264
Matsunga A, Ochiai t, Abe I et al (2007) Subungual glomus tumour: evaluation of ultrasound imaging in preoperative assessment. Eur J Dermatol 17:67–69
Murphey MD, Carroll JF, Flemming DJ, Pope TL, Gannon FH, Kransdorf MJ (2004) From the archives of the AFIP. Benign musculoskeletal lipomatous lesions. Radiographics 24:1433–1466
Murphey MD, Vidal JA, Fanburg-Smith Gajewski DA (2007) From the archives of the AFIP. Imaging of synovial chondromatosis with radiologic-pathologic correlation. Radiographics 27:1465–1488
Murphey MD, Ruble CM, Tyszko SM, Zbojniewicz AM, Potter BK, Miettinen M (2009) From the archives of the AFIP: musculoskeletal fibromatoses: radiologic-pathologic correlation. Radiographics 29(7):2143–2173
Murphy GE, Elder DE (1991) Atlas of tumor pathology: nonmelanotic tumors of the skin. Armed Forces Institute of Pathology, Washington
Nahra ME, Bucchieri JS (2004) Ganglion cysts and other tumor related conditions of the hand and wrist. Hand Clin 20:249–260
Nguyon V, Choi J, Davis KW (2004) Imaging of Wrist masses. Curr Probl Diagn Radiol 147–160
Peh WCG, Truong NP, Totty WG, Gilula LA (1995) Pictorial review: magnetic resonance imaging of benign soft tissue masses of the hand and wrist 50:519–525
Plate AM, Lee SJ, Steiner G, Posner M (2003) Tumorlike lesions and benign tumors of the hand and wrist. J Am Acad Orthop Surg 11:129–141
Robbin MR, Murphey MD, Temple HT, Kransdorf MJ, Choi JJ (2001) Imaging of musculoskeletal fibromatosis. Radiographics 21(3):585–600
Roberts D, Miller TT, Erlanger SM (2004) Sonographic appearance of primary synovial chondromatosis of the knee. J Ultrasound Med 23:707–709
Schmitt R (2008) Soft-tissue tumors. In: Schmitt R, Lanz U (eds) Diagnostic imaging of the hand. Georg Thieme Verlag, Stuttgart, pp 502–521
Steiner E, Steinbach LS, Schnarkowski P, Tirman PF, Genant HK (1996) Ganglia and cysts around joints. Radiol Clin North Am 34:395–425
Terek RM, Brien EW (1995) Soft-tissue sarcomas of the hand and wrist. Hand Clin 11(2):287–305
Ushijima M, Hashimoto H, Tsuneyoshi M et al (1986) Giant cell tumor of the tendon sheath (nodular tenosynovitis). A study of 207 cases to compare the large joint group with the common digit group. Cancer 15:875–884
van Rijswijk CS, Geirnaerdt MJ, Hogendoorn PC, Taminiau AH, van Coevorden F, Zwinderman AH, Pope TL, Bloem JL (2004) Soft-tissue tumors: value of static and dynamic gadopentetate dimeglumine-enhanced MR imaging in prediction of malignancy. Radiology 233(2):493–502
Van Zwieten KJ, Brys P, Van Rietvelde F et al (2007) Imaging of the hand, techniques and pathology: a pictorial essay. JBR-BTR 90(5):395–455
Vanhoenacker FM, De Schepper AM, Gielen JL, Parizel PM (2005) MR imaging in the diagnosis and management of inheritable musculoskeletal disorders. Clin Radiol 60: 160–170
Vanhoenacker FM, Marques MC, Garcia H (2006a) Lipomatous tumors. In: De Schepper AM, Vanhoenacker F, Parizel PM, Gielen J (eds) Imaging of soft tissue tumors. Springer, Berlin, Heidelberg, New York, pp 227–261
Vanhoenacker FM, Van Goethem JWM, Vandevenne JE, Shahabpour M (2006b) Synovial tumors. In: De Schepper AM, Vanhoenacker F, Parizel PM, Gielen J (eds) Imaging

of soft tissue tumors. Springer, Berlin, Heidelberg, New York, pp 311–324

Wan JM, Magarelli N, Peh WC, Guglielmi G, Shek TW (2010) Imaging of giant cell tumour of the tendon sheath. Radiol Med 115:141–151

Wang AA, Hutchinson DT (2001) Longitudinal observation of pediatric hand and wrist ganglia. J Hand Surg (Am) 26:599–602

Wittkop AM, Davies AM, Mangham DC (2002) Primary synovial chondromatosis and synovial chondrosarcoma. Eur Radiol 12:2112–2219

Yacoe ME, Bergman AG, Ladd AL, Hellman BH (1993) Dupuytren's contracture: MR imaging findings and correlation between MR signal intensity and cellularity of lesions. AJR Am J Roentgenol 160(4):813–817

Miscellaneous Conditions with Manifestations in the Hand and Wrist

Vikram S. Sandhu, A. Mark Davies, and Steven L. James

Contents

V. S. Sandhu
Imaging Department, Royal Orthopaedic Hospital, Bristol Road South, Birmingham, B31 2AP, UK
e-mail: viksandhu@doctors.org.uk

A. M. Davies (✉) · S. L. James
Department of Radiology, Royal Orthopaedic Hospital, Birmingham, B31 2AP, UK
e-mail: wendy.turner1@nhs.net

Abstract

In any textbook dealing with conditions affecting a particular anatomical site, there will be some which do not fit conveniently under the standard chapter headings. The purpose of this chapter is to review these miscellaneous localised and systemic disorders that may affect the hand and wrist.

1 Introduction

In any textbook dealing with conditions affecting a particular anatomical site, there will be some which do not fit conveniently under the standard chapter headings. The purpose of this chapter is to review these miscellaneous localised and systemic disorders that may affect the hand and wrist.

2 Paget's Disease

Paget's disease of bone is a benign disorder affecting 3–4% of the population over 40 years of age predominantly in Caucasian races (Smith et al. 2002). There is recent evidence of decreasing prevalence (Cundy 2006). The abnormality in Paget's disease is excessive and abnormal remodelling of bone. Three pathologic phases have been described: the lytic phase, the mixed phase and the blastic phase. Initially there is osteolysis, followed by trabecular and cortical thickening and enlargement in the mixed phase of the disease, followed by sclerosis in the blastic phase. Paget's disease is usually polyostotic and asymmetric.

A. M. Davis et al. (eds.), *Imaging of the Hand and Wrist*, Medical Radiology. Diagnostic Imaging,
DOI: 10.1007/174_2010_114, © Springer-Verlag Berlin Heidelberg 2013

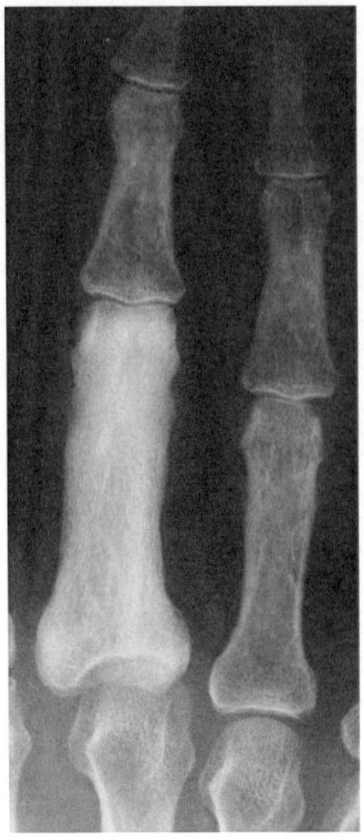

Fig. 1 Paget's disease. There is bony sclerosis and expansion of the proximal phalanx of the middle finger

Polyostotic disease (65–90%) is more frequent than monostotic disease.

Involvement in the hand and wrist has been reported infrequently, although bone scintigraphy studies reveal hand localisation varying from 6.4 to 11.6% (Friedman et al. 1982). Clinically, Paget's disease in the hands is usually asymptomatic; however, several cases with pain in the hands have been reported (Friedman et al. 1982). When Paget's disease occurs in the hand, there is usually a polyostotic involvement (Haverbush et al. 1972). Monostotic localisation in the hand is less frequent (De Smet et al. 1994; Rodriguez-Peralto et al. 1994; Calif et al. 2007). It typically affects the phalanges and metacarpals, with carpal involvement rare and distal phalangeal involvement almost unknown. The most common radiographic pattern of disease in the hand is sclerosis (Fig. 1; Haverbush et al. 1972) and is seen in 45% of cases (Friedman et al. 1982). However, all patterns as found elsewhere in the body (cortical destruction, bone expansion, coarsened trabeculae and bone sclerosis) may be seen in the hand (Friedman et al. 1982). Sarcomatous transformation is the most sinister complication of Paget's disease and is rarely seen in the hand. A review by Lopez et al. (2003) looked at 340 cases of Paget's sarcoma in the literature and identified no cases in the hand and wrist. Isolated cases of malignant transformation have, however, been recorded (Friedman et al. 1982). The MR imaging appearances of Pagetic marrow can be variable (Smith et al. 2002) but a useful diagnostic sign is the preservation of the hyperintense marrow signal on T1-weighted images (Fig. 2; Boutin et al. 1998; Kaufmann et al. 1991; Sundaram et al. 2001; Vande Berg et al. 2001).

3 Sarcoid

Sarcoidosis is a granulomatous disorder of unknown cause that affects multiple organ systems. It is characterised by the presence of multiple non-caseating granulomas, most commonly seen in the lungs, lymph nodes, skin and eyes. The diagnosis is made by a combination of clinical, radiological and histological features.

Skeletal involvement has been reported in 1–13% of patients with the disease. Radiographic evaluation is often limited to the hands or feet, which demonstrate predominantly osteolytic lesions. The hand is the commonest site of skeletal sarcoidosis. The lesions may be unilateral or bilateral, but symmetrical involvement is unusual. Lesions in the hand are most commonly seen in the middle and distal phalanges, and less often in the proximal phalanges and metacarpals (Van Linthoudt and Ott 1986). There are several types of lesion that are seen. The characteristic lesion is the alteration of the trabecular lattice resulting in a honeycomb lytic appearance (Fig. 3). Cystic lesions may also occur leading to a punched-out appearance that may be located centrally or eccentrically (Fig. 3). Osseous destruction may appear rapidly if these lesions are associated with cortical erosion, which can lead to pathological fracture (Neville et al. 1976, 1977). Periosteal new bone formation is uncommon.

Acro-osteolysis (terminal phalangeal resorption) has been reported in sarcoid involvement of the hands (Fig. 4). The finding is non-specific. In both the hand and the wrist, tenosynovitis is a recognised complication of sarcoidosis (Katzman et al. 1997; Moore 2003). Other soft tissue changes can be seen on MR imaging. These include focal and diffuse muscle lesions, soft tissue infiltration and masses (Moore 2003). MR imaging may also be useful in the

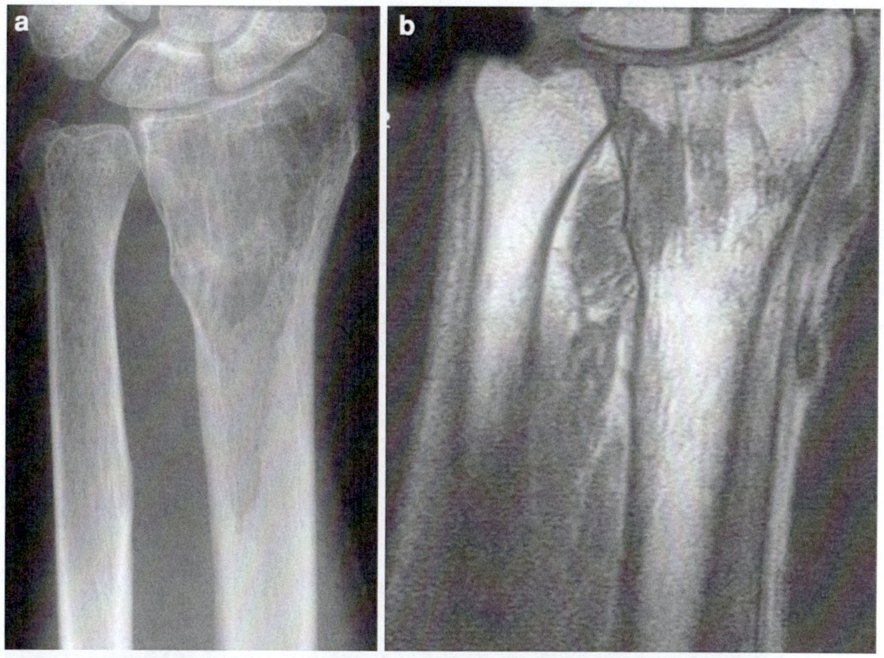

Fig. 2 **a** Radiograph and **b** coronal T1-weighted MR imaging of Paget's disease of the distal radius. The radiograph was initially misinterpreted as showing a giant cell tumour but the preservation of the hyperintense marrow signal in **b** is highly suggestive of Paget's disease

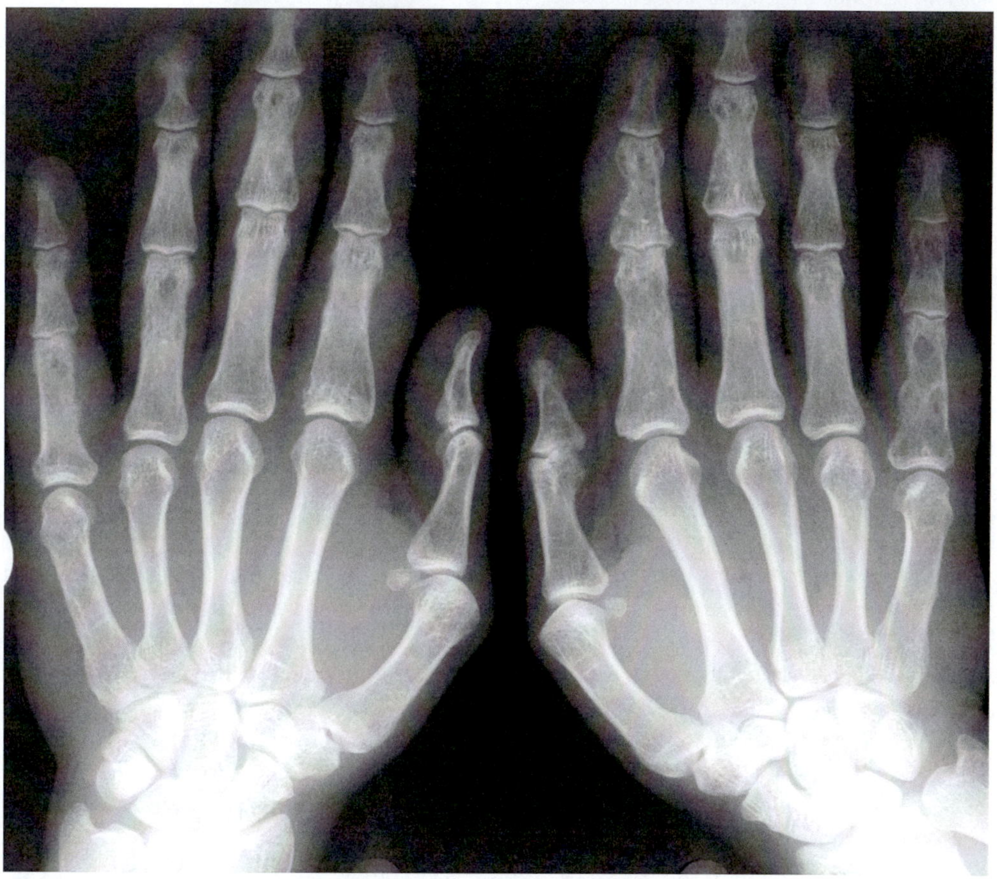

Fig. 3 Sarcoidosis. There is involvement of the proximal and middle phalanges of both hands. The appearances are more punched-out on the *left* with honeycomb osteolysis on the *right*

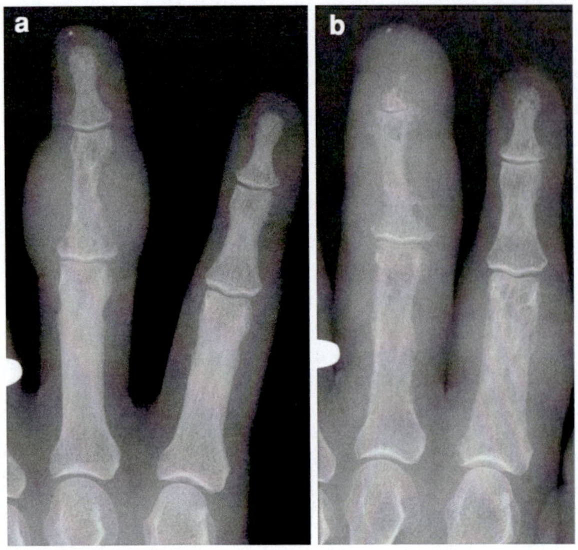

Fig. 4 Sarcoidosis. At presentation, **a** showing eccentric soft tissue swelling and lacy osteolysis of the middle phalanx of the middle finger; 14 years later, **b** showing soft tissue swelling of both index and middle fingers and progression of disease with terminal phalangeal resorption and further destruction of the middle phalanx of the middle finger. There is now also involvement of the proximal phalanges of both fingers

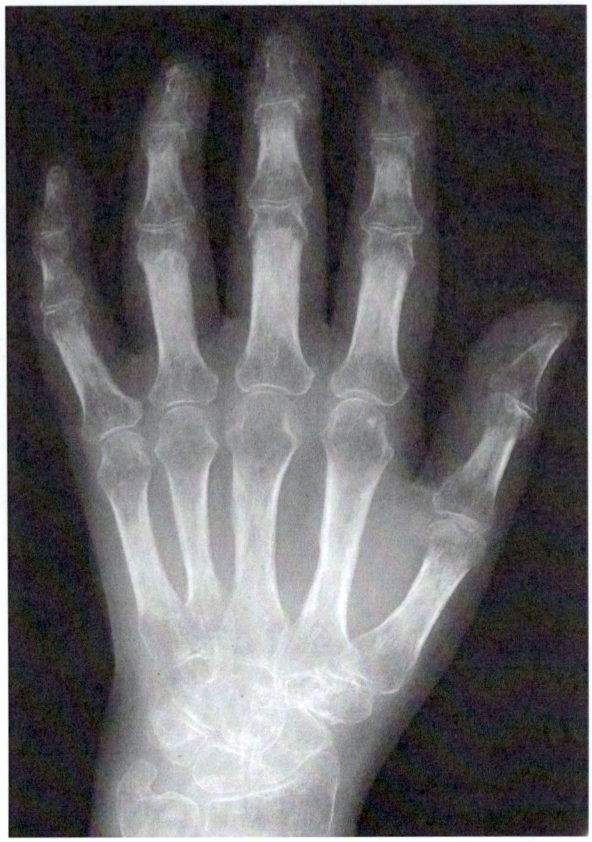

Fig. 5 Reflex sympathetic dystrophy. There is intense juxta-articular osteopenia mimicking an acute inflammatory arthropathy

differential diagnosis, for example in the evaluation of soft tissue nodules distinguishing gout from sarcoidosis. Intermediate-weighted MR images typically show tophi as hypointense, whereas sarcoid nodules will usually be hyperintense.

Lofgren syndrome is a well-recognised manifestation of sarcoidosis, with patients exhibiting arthralgias, erythema nodosum and bilateral hilar lymphadenopathy. Polyarthritis involving the interphalangeal joints, wrists, elbows, knees or ankles is common. Monoarthritis and effusion are uncommon. Ten to thirty-five percentage of sarcoidosis patients will also experience joint symptoms due to granulomatous arthritis with a chronic transient or relapsing arthropathy. Sausage-like dactylitis of the fingers can also occur (Fig. 4). Pain is usually not severe. The uptake of FDG in PET scanning from sarcoid tissue is non-specific. However, Brudin et al. (1994) have described how the degree of FDG uptake correlates with disease activity, and although FDG PET is not useful for initial diagnosis, it could be used for evaluating the extent of active disease and monitoring response to therapy (Love et al. 2005).

4 Reflex Sympathetic Dystrophy

Reflex sympathetic dystrophy (RSD) is a distinct condition that occurs in a variety of clinical situations. There are several terms that are used to describe the same condition including: causalgia, algodystrophy, Sudeck's atrophy, post-traumatic osteoporosis and complex regional pain syndrome. Although the cause is often idiopathic, many visceral, musculoskeletal, neurological and vascular conditions can cause RSD with trauma the most common. The most frequent site for RSD is in the hand. Clinical symptoms include stiffness, pain, tenderness and weakness. Radiographic changes range from soft tissue swelling with juxta-articular osteopenia (Fig. 5) to a more generalised osteopenia (Fig. 6). The former can mimic the

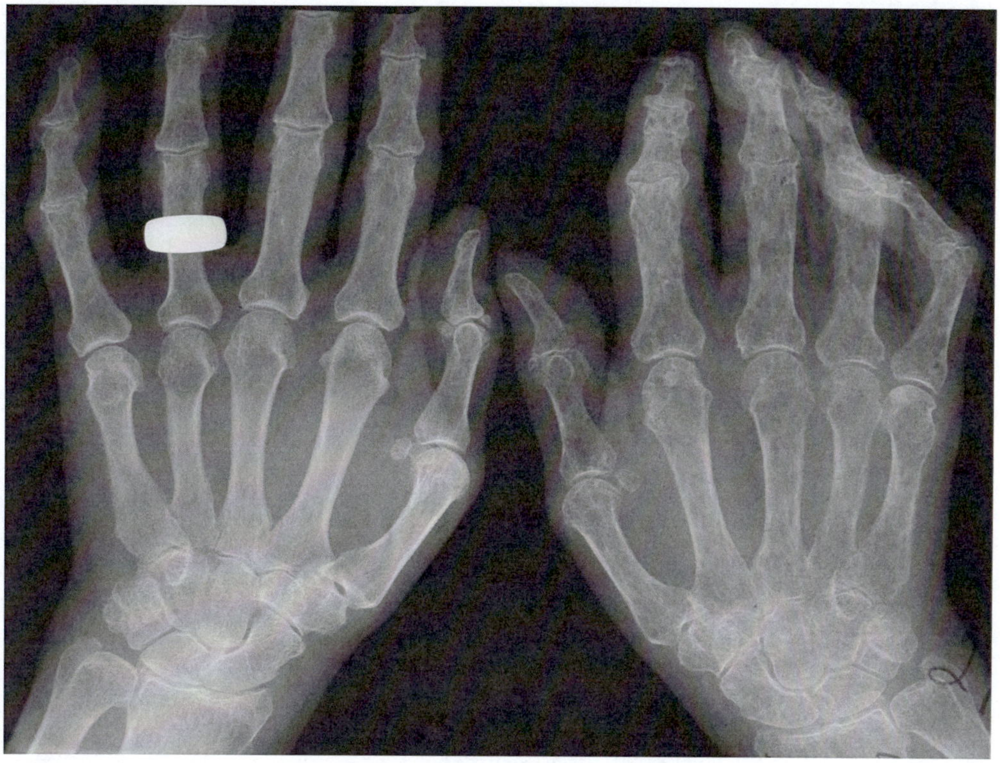

Fig. 6 Reflex sympathetic dystrophy. In this chronic case affecting the right hand, there is intense generalised osteopenia with multiple intracortical lucencies. Note the normal bone density of the unaffected left hand

presentation of an acute inflammatory arthropathy but in RSD there is no joint space narrowing or erosions. Both three-phase bone scintigraphy and MR imaging can be used to assess the "activity" of this disorder over time (Park et al. 2009).

5 Haematological and Marrow Disorders

This section covers the imaging manifestations in the hand and wrist of haematological and marrow disorders including haemophilia, sickle cell anaemia and thalassaemia.

5.1 Haemophilia

Haemophilia and related bleeding disorders are a group of conditions that are characterised by abnormality in blood coagulation caused by deficiency in certain plasma clotting factors. The two most common types associated with intraosseous and intraarticular bleeding are haemophilia A (deficiency in clotting factor VIII) and haemophilia B (deficiency in clotting factor IX). Haemarthrosis occurs in 75–90% of people with haemophilia and in time leads to a haemophilic arthropathy. This begins between the ages of 2–3 years and increases in frequency till the ages of 8–13 years. The joints most commonly affected include the knee, elbow, ankle, hip and shoulder. Usually, a single joint is involved in each episode, though eventually multiple joints become affected in this disease. Intraarticular bleeding is rare in the hand and wrist. A well-recognised but rare complication occurring in approximately 2% of patients with severe haemophilia is the so-called haemophilic pseudotumour. These result from chronic recurrent haemorrhage that may be intraosseous, subperiosteal or arise in the soft tissues. The bones most frequently involved, in order of decreasing frequency, are the femur, pelvis, tibia and the small bones of the hand

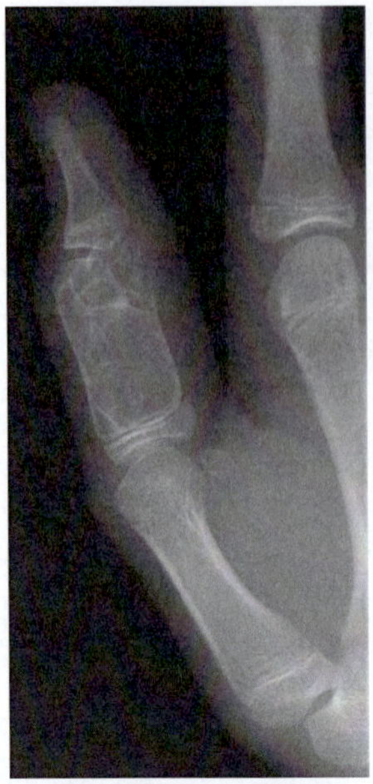

Fig. 7 Haemophilic pseudotumour proximal phalanx of the thumb. The age of the patient and the radiographic appearances mimic an aneurysmal bone cyst

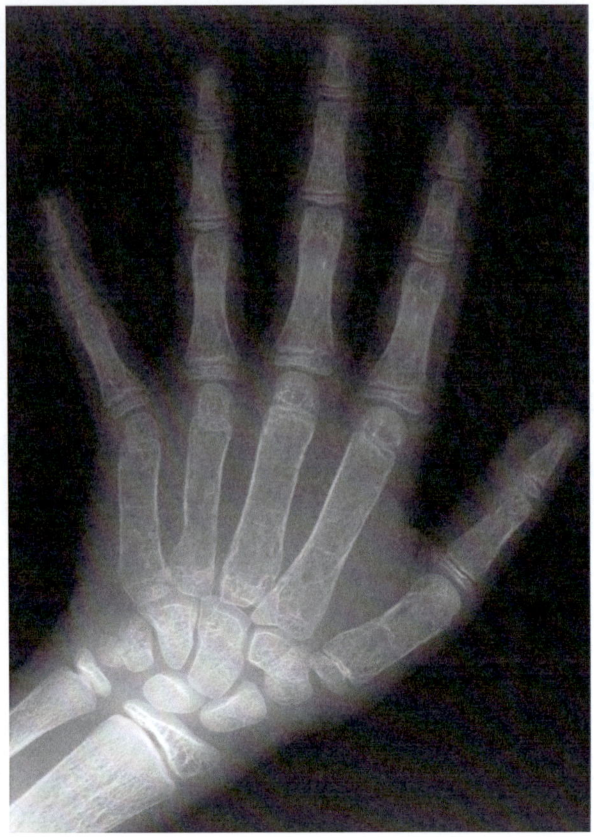

Fig. 9 Thalassaemia. The marrow hyperplasia is causing severe generalised osteopenia, trabeculation and minor expansion of the long bones

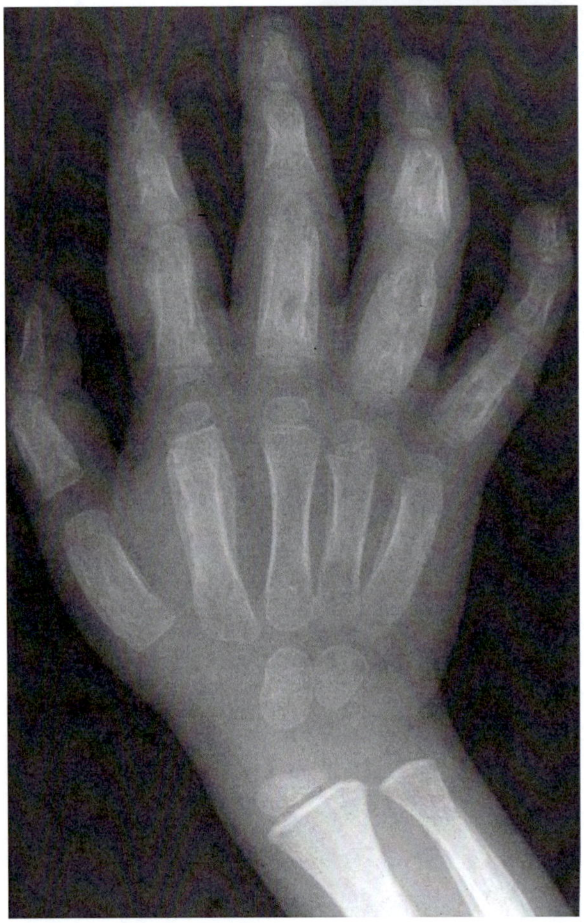

Fig. 8 Sickle cell disease. A young child with severe hand–foot syndrome showing medullary lucencies and periosteal new bone formation involving all the long bones of the hand and the distal ulna. The visible mineralised carpal bones are not involved

(Park and Ryu 2004). Cases have also been reported affecting the distal forearm bones (Ahlberg 1975; Shaheen and Alasha 2005). Cases involving the hand and wrist are usually of intraosseous origin, whereas pseudotumours arising in the lower limbs and pelvis tend to be extraosseous with secondary pressure erosion of adjacent bones. In the long bones of the hand, intraosseous haemophilic pseudotumour shows an expansile benign-appearing lytic lesion mimicking amongst other pathologies an aneurysmal bone cyst (Fig. 7; Shaw and Wilson 1993).

5.2 Sickle Cell Disease

Sickle cell disease is one of the hereditary haemoglobinopathies characterised by an abnormal haemoglobin chain (HbS). Clinical manifestations of the disease include painful crises affecting the bones and joints of the extremities. In children with sickle cell anaemia, 30% will present with hand–foot syndrome

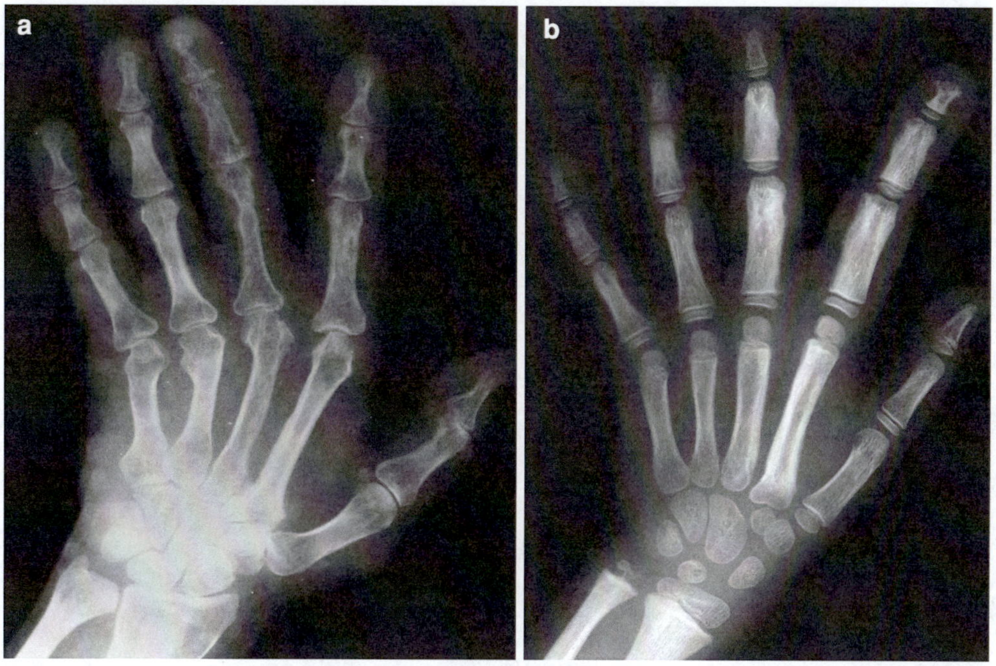

Fig. 10 Two different cases of neurofibromatosis. **a** Multiple soft tissue lumps due to subcutaneous neurofibromas and bone erosions in the index and middle fingers. **b** There is focal gigantism and sclerosis of the index and middle metacarpals and fingers

between the ages of 6–24 months with pain and swelling of the hands due to marrow infarction (Watson et al. 1963). The radiographic changes are those of a dactylitis with osteolysis and periosteal new bone formation (Fig. 8; Bohrer 1970). Hand–foot syndrome is rare after 6 years of age because the red marrow recedes from the distal tubular bones of the hand and is replaced by yellow marrow with reduced oxygen requirements. Severe dactylitis may cause premature growth plate fusion thereby causing relative shortening of one or more long bones of the hand (Cockshott 1963). Ischaemic changes in the carpal bones are uncommon (Lanzer et al. 1984).

5.3 Thalassaemia

Thalassaemia is a hereditary haemoglobinopathy with an abnormality in the globin chain production of the red blood cell. This can involve a deficiency in alpha-globin chain synthesis or beta-globin chain synthesis. In severe untreated cases, there is generalised osteopenia and the tubular bones of the hand are expanded secondary to marrow hyperplasia (Fig. 9; Caffey 1957; Middlemiss and Raper 1966). There is also cortical thinning with a coarse, trabeculated appearance. When MR imaging is used in the assessment of the tubular bones of the hand, the findings may include an indistinct physeal–metaphyseal junction, altered signal intensity in the metaphysis, physeal widening and metadiaphyseal and epiphyseal lesions. Severe radiographic changes are not often seen in the developed world these days as most cases are treated from early infancy with repeated blood transfusions thereby reducing the marrow hyperplasia.

5.4 Other Marrow Disorders

The radiographic appearances in the hands of other marrow and deposition disorders such as Gaucher's disease and Niemann-Pick disease are relatively minor when compared with changes elsewhere in the skeleton. The authors have reported a single case of Erdheim–Chester disease presenting with a lytic lesion in a metacarpal mimicking a giant cell tumour or metastasis (Davies et al. 2010). Marrow malignancies are covered in chapter "Tumours and Tumour-like Leisions of Bone".

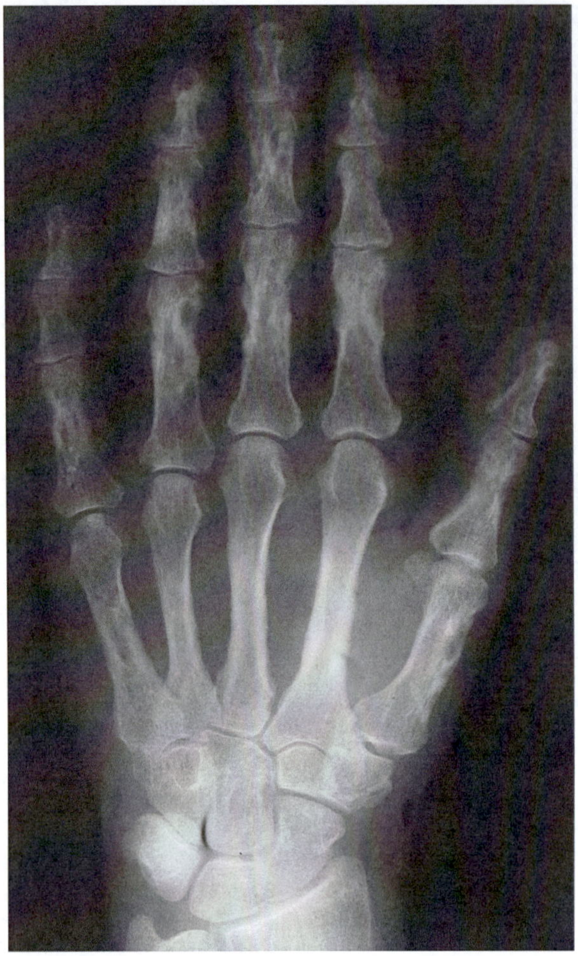

Fig. 11 Tuberous sclerosis. Multiple cyst-like radiolucencies involving the first and fifth metacarpals and all the fingers

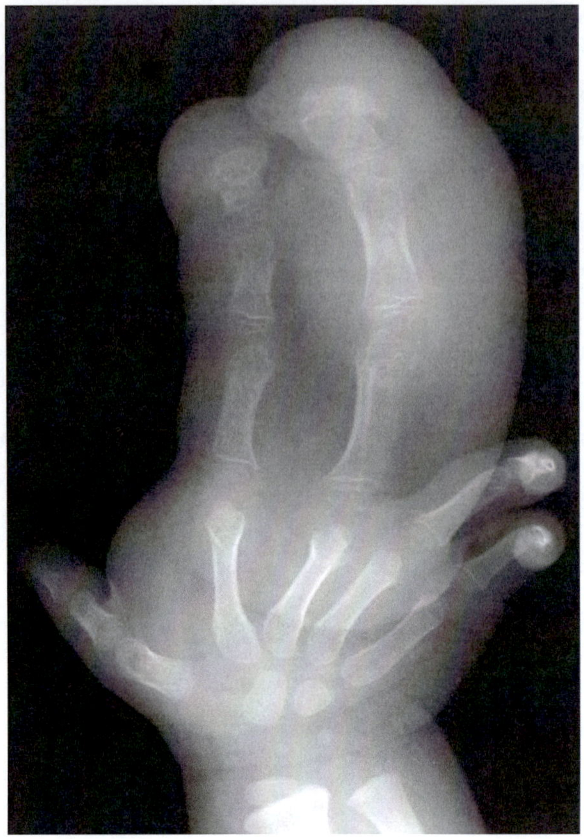

Fig. 12 Macrodystrophia lipomatosa in a child. Focal gigantism of the index and middle fingers with bony overgrowth and soft tissue syndactyly

6 Amyloidosis

Amyloidosis is the deposition of abnormal insoluble proteins in soft tissues and bone. It is not a single disease entity with to-date over 20 variants identified. The World Health Organization has proposed a classification based on the precursor fibril protein (Westermark et al. 2002). This includes primary systemic, secondary systemic, familial, dialysis-related, etc. Soft tissue amyloid deposition produces nodules that are often prominent over the joints of the hand and wrist. Similar deposits in the carpal canal may lead to carpal tunnel syndrome. Ten to thirty percentage of patients with primary amyloidosis have carpal tunnel syndrome. Typically, a bilateral distribution is seen, and signs and symptoms related to carpal tunnel syndrome often precede other manifestations of the disease. Amyloid deposition has also been documented in the wrists of patients on dialysis for chronic renal failure with carpal tunnel syndrome. The radiographic findings of amyloidosis in the hand and wrist include asymmetric soft tissue masses, periarticular osteoporosis, widening of the articular spaces and subchondral cysts and erosions. The appearance differs from rheumatoid disease of the hands and wrist as there is preservation of the joint space with soft tissue nodular masses. Extensive joint destruction is occasionally encountered in amyloidosis resulting from neuropathic arthropathy or osteonecrosis of the epiphyseal surfaces. On MR imaging, the amyloid deposits tend to be iso- or slightly hypointense with respect to muscle (Cobby et al. 1991; Kiss et al. 2005).

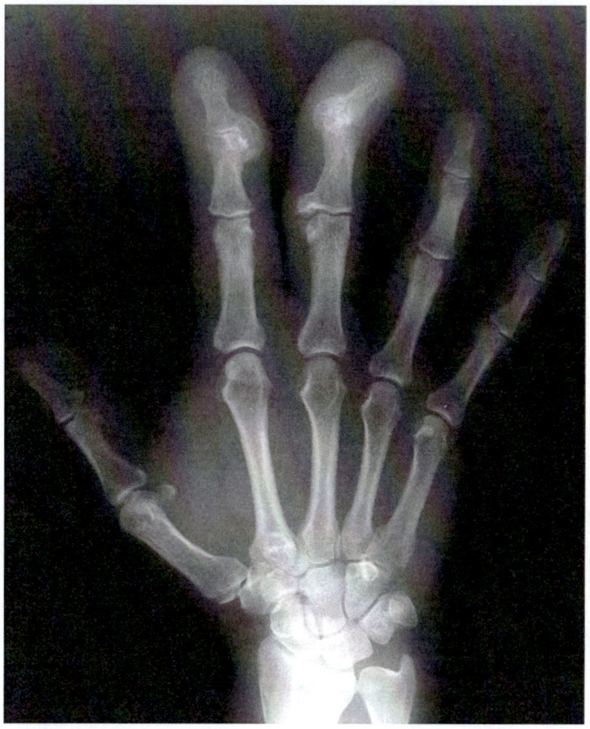

Fig. 13 Macrodystrophia lipomatosa in an adult: focal gigantism of the index and middle fingers with periarticular exostoses

Table 1 Diseases associated with hypertrophic osteoarthropathy (modified from Gibson et al. 2008)

Pulmonary
Bronchogenic carcinoma
Metastases
Mesothelioma
Pulmonary abscess
Tuberculosis
Bronchiectasis
Cystic Fibrosis
Cardiac
Cyanotic heart disease
Bacterial endocarditis
Gastrointestinal
Inflammatory bowel disease
Biliary atresia
Cirrhosis
Miscellaneous
Nasopharyngeal carcinoma
Hodgkin's lymphoma
AIDS

7 Haemochromatosis

Haemochromatosis results from excessive iron storage in the soft tissues. It may be primary, inherited as an autosomal recessive disorder, or secondary to chronic anaemias with multiple transfusions and dietary iron overload. In the hand and wrist, calcium pyrophosphate dihydrate (CPPD) crystal deposition causes chondrocalcinosis of the triangular fibrocartilage in up to 60% cases. In chronic cases, particularly the primary form, a structural arthropathy develops with a predilection for the second and third metacarpo-phalangeal joints with joint space narrowing and hook-like exostoses on the radial aspect of the metacarpal heads (Schumacher 1964).

8 Phakomatoses

The phakamatoses are a group of neurocutaneous syndromes typified by the development of benign tumours and malformations, especially in organs of ectodermal origin. The two such conditions that may manifest in the hands are neurofibromatosis and tuberous sclerosis. In neurofibromatosis, this includes soft tissue masses, bone erosion from adjacent neurofibromas and localised gigantism (macrodactyly; Fig. 10). In tuberous sclerosis, there may be multiple cyst-like radiolucencies, periosteal thickening and localised gigantism (Fig. 11; Bernauer 2001).

9 Macrodystrophia Lipomatosa

This is a rare congenital form of localised gigantism due to overgrowth of the mesenchymal tissues particularly hypertrophy of adipose tissue. This results in enlargement of one or more adjacent digits (Fig. 12; Hildebrandt et al. 1993). Most of the reported lesions are present at birth and are associated with a high incidence of local anomalies including syndactyly, polydactyly and clinodactyly. In the adult, the bony hypertrophy can be associated with periarticular exostoses (Fig. 13). The condition may also be associated with carpal tunnel syndrome (Ranawat et al. 1968).

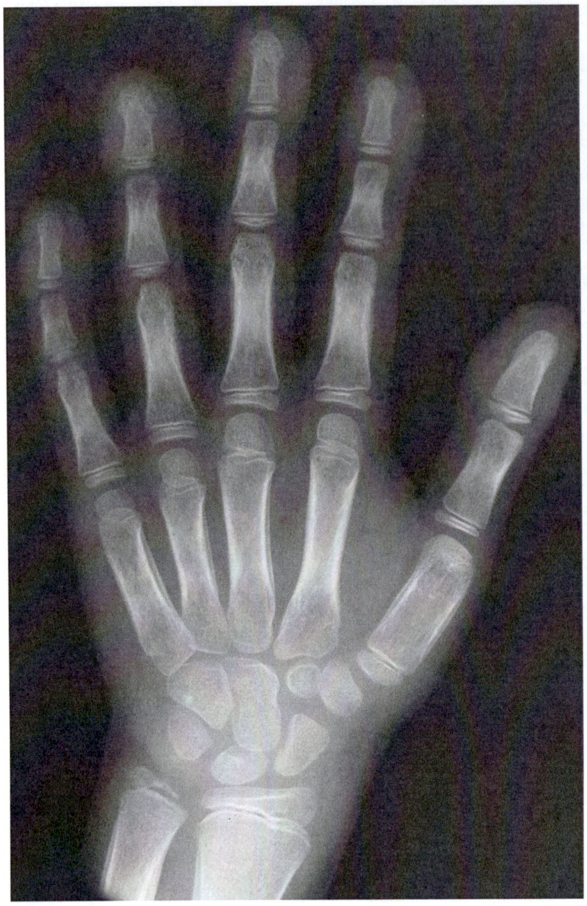

Fig. 14 Hypertrophic osteoarthropathy. Child with long-standing, untreated cyanotic heart disease. There is a single-layer lamellar periosteal reaction along the distal radius and ulna, the metacarpals and to a lesser extent the phalanges. There is also evidence of digital clubbing

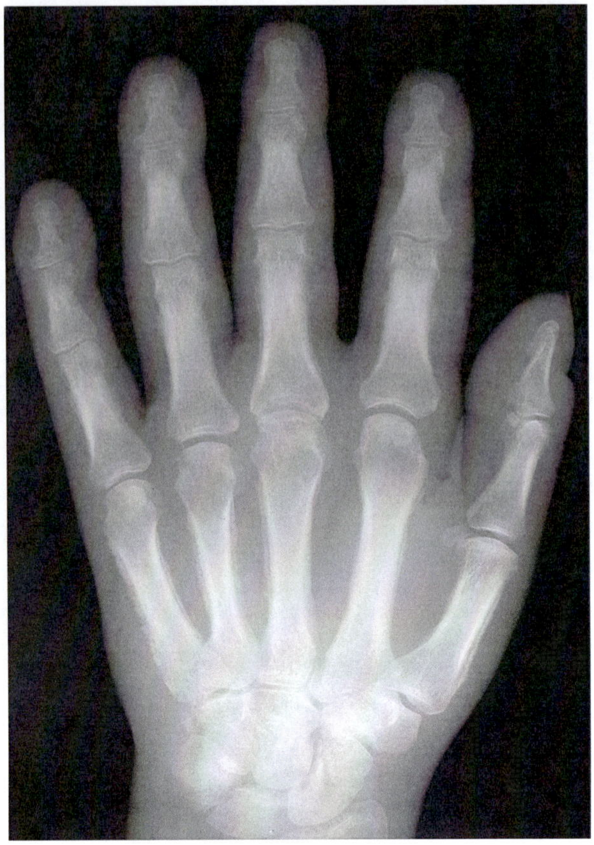

Fig. 15 Hypertrophic osteoarthropathy. Adult with known bronchogenic carcinoma. There is symmetrical coarse periosteal new bone formation along all the metacarpals and to a lesser extent the phalanges

10 Hypertrophic Osteoarthropathy

Originally called hypertrophic pulmonary osteoarthropathy, this condition was first described in the French literature at the end of the nineteenth century (Marie 1890). Clinical presentation is with pain and tenderness of the extremities with digital clubbing. Although most commonly associated with lung diseases, classically bronchogenic carcinoma, the term pulmonary has been dropped in recognition of the non-pulmonary associations (Table 1). The typical radiographic appearance is symmetrical periosteal new bone formation along the tubular bones. This occurs in the diaphyses of the radius and ulna, and less frequently in the metacarpals and phalanges. The severity can vary from simple elevation of the periosteum (Fig. 14), to a lamellated "onion-skin" appearance, to irregular periosteal "cloaking" with an undulating contour (Fig. 15; Ali et al. 1980; Pineda et al. 1987). The differential diagnosis for hypertrophic pulmonary osteoarthropathy includes pachydermoperiostitis sometimes referred to as primary hypertrophic osteoarthropathy. This is a rare, often familial, lesion predominantly of males with a predisposition for Afro-Caribbean populations. Clinically, there is clubbing of the fingers, thickening of the skin and hyperhydrosis. Compared with hypertrophic pulmonary osteoarthropathy, it is relatively pain free. The bones most commonly affected are the radius and ulna, followed by the tubular bones of the hands. The periosteal reaction is similar to hypertrophic pulmonary osteoarthropathy but is more solid and spiculated and also involves the epiphyses to produce outgrowths around joints (Fig. 16).

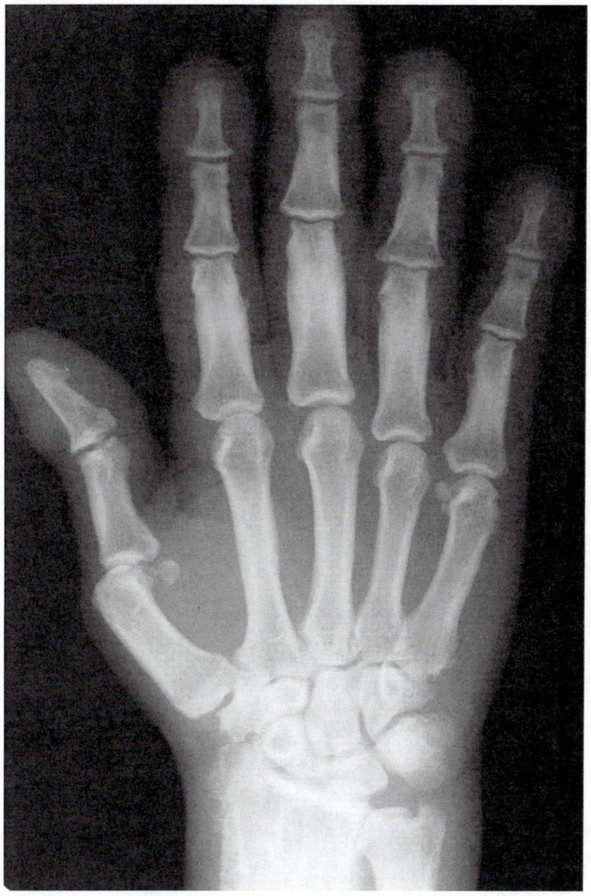

Fig. 16 Pachydermoperiostosis in an adult of Afro-Caribbean ethnic origin. Digital clubbing with coarse periosteal new bone formation along the distal radius and proximal phalanges

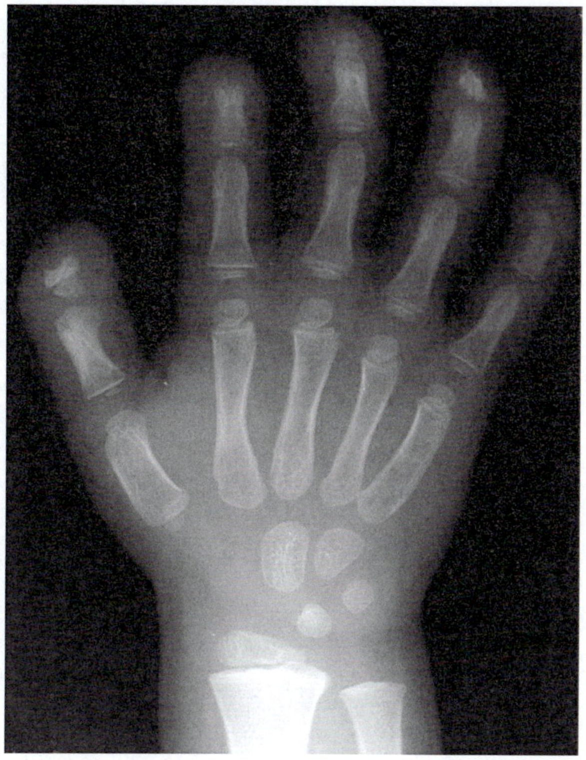

Fig. 17 Congenital insensitivity to pain. There is extensive terminal phalangeal resorption (acro-osteolysis) secondary to the underlying neuropathy. The appearances are non-specific and may be seen in other causes of neuropathy such as leprosy or following "trauma" such as frostbite

11 Congenital Insensitivity to Pain

Congenital insensitivity to pain, first described in 1932 (Dearbon 1932), is a rare hereditary sensory and autonomic neuropathy characterised by the congenital inability to register pain or temperature changes (Rahalkar et al. 2008; Reilly 2009). The principal orthopaedic manifestations are recurrent fractures, neuropathic joints and osteomyelitis (Silverman and Gilden 1959; Siegelman et al. 1966; Karmani et al. 2001). The changes in the hand include acro-osteolysis, amputations and secondary osteomyelitis (Fig. 17; Gwathmey and House 1984). In children, epiphyseal separation and growth plate fragmentation may occur at the wrist.

12 Toxic Agents and Pharmacological Agents

Toxic effects manifested in the hand may be localised or systemic. An example of a localised toxic effect is soft tissue necrosis and contractures secondary to snake bite venom (Huang et al. 1978). Snake and scorpion venom have also both been reported as causing acro-osteolysis (Qteishat et al. 1985). Osteolysis resulting from secondary infections due to animal bites is well recognised. The animals include domestic pets, rodents, exotic animals such as camels (Al-Boukai et al. 1989) and of course humans (Resnick et al. 1985).

Systemic toxic effects include lead poisoning seen in the past in children who had ingested lead-based paints. Radiographs show a radiodense line paralleling the growth plates in the metaphyses of

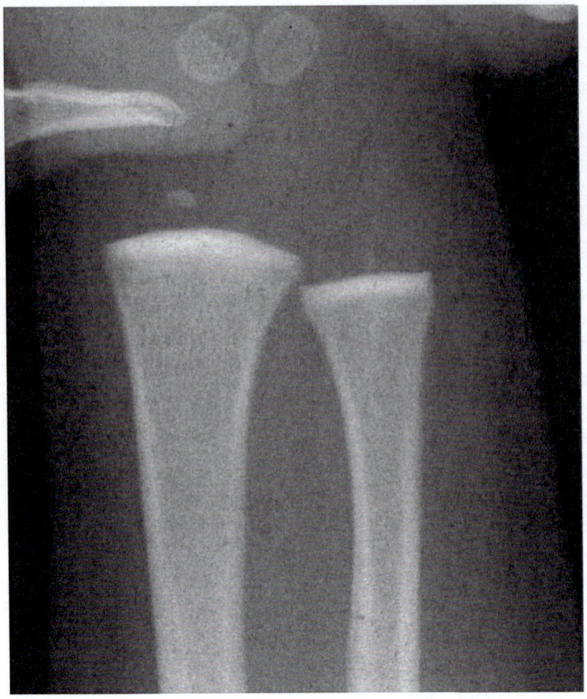

Fig. 18 Lead poisoning. An infant with a radiodense "lead line" in the distal radial and ulnar metaphyses

the distal radius and small tubular bones of the hand (Fig. 18; Leone 1968; Sachs 1981). Multiple lead lines may be seen if the exposure to the lead has been repeated. The differential diagnosis of radiodense lines in the distal radial metaphysis include other forms of heavy metal poisoning (e.g. bismuth and phosphorus) and the healing phase of rickets and scurvy and treated leukaemia. A toxic cause of more generalised bony sclerosis is fluorosis that is endemic in certain areas of India. In children, this may be associated with rickets-like changes (Christie 1980). An unusual form of occupational acro-osteolysis has been described in polyvinylchloride (PVC) poisoning (Gama and Meira 1978). The typical radiographic feature is a band of osteolysis through the terminal phalanges (Fig. 19a). With removal of exposure to the PVC manufacturing process, there is healing of the defects with shortening and widening of the terminal phalanges (Fig. 19b). A similar appearance may be seen with familial acro-osteolysis (Hajdu–Cheney syndrome) and has also been reported in a guitarist (Destouet and Murphy 1981).

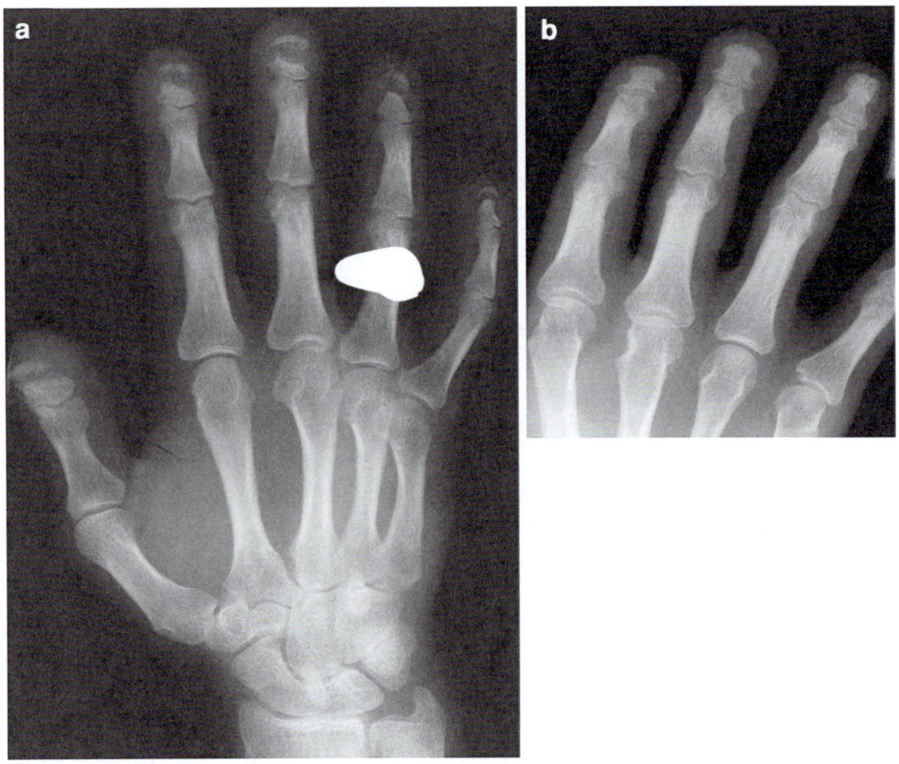

Fig. 19 Polyvinylchloride (PVC) poisoning. **a** Typical band-like acro-osteolysis across the terminal phalanges. **b** On removal from exposure to the PVC manufacturing process, there has been healing of the defects with shortening and widening of the terminal phalanges

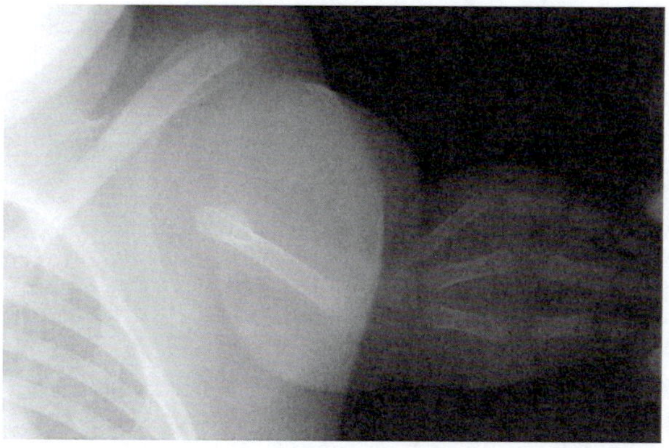

Fig. 20 Teratogenic effects of thalidomide therapy during pregnancy. The child has been born with proximal phocomelia and severe skeletal abnormalities of the hand

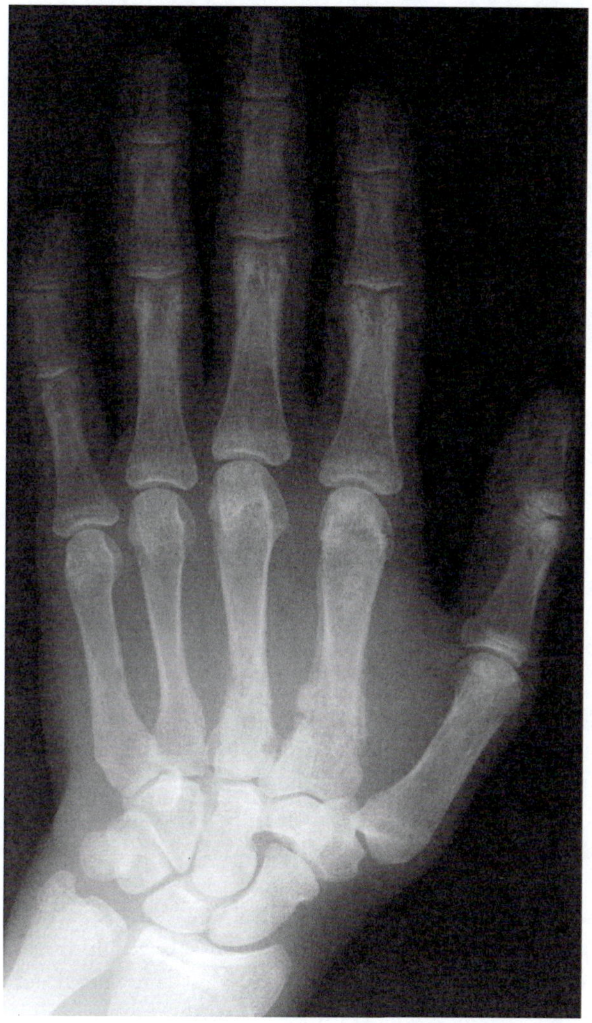

Fig. 21 Dialysis-related aluminium bone disease. Osteomalacic pattern with Looser's zone in the 2nd and 3rd metacarpals

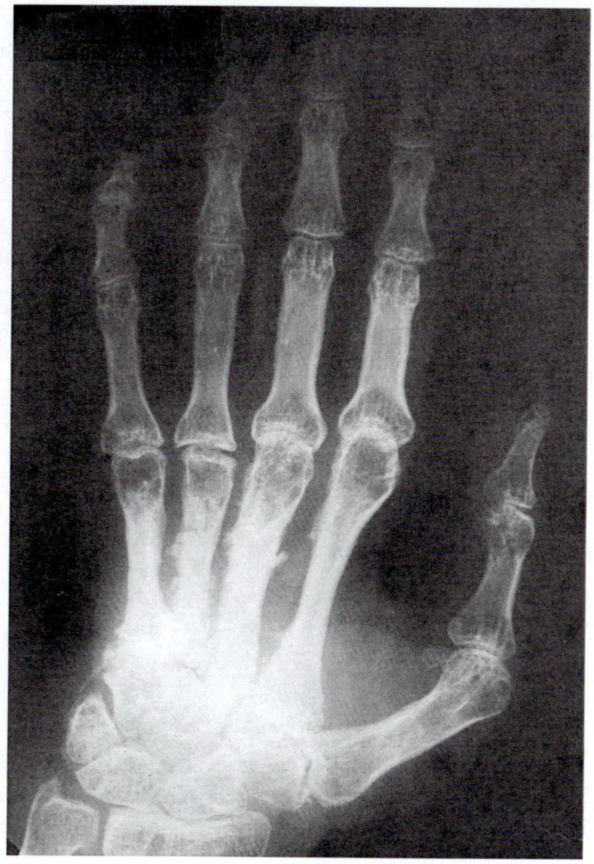

Fig. 22 Radionecrosis. Historical case of a seamstress who underwent protracted fluoroscopy for the removal of a sewing needle embedded in the soft tissues. This caused skin ulceration and contractures and radionecrosis of the metacarpals (from the collection of Dr Philip Jacobs—deceased)

Prolonged and excessive exposure to numerous pharmacological agents may cause skeletal abnormalities identifiable on radiographs of the hand. These range from the devastating teratogenic effects of thalidomide (Fig. 20) to the rickets-like or osteomalacia pattern associated with phenytoin, phenobarbital, deferoxamine, diphosphonates and dialysis-related aluminium toxicity (Fig. 21). Hypervitaminosis A can cause generalised periosteal reactions (Caffey 1951) and hypervitaminosis D sclerotic metaphyseal bands (De Wind 1961).

13 Radiation Changes

It was not long after the discovery of X-rays in 1895 by Wilhelm Roentgen that the deleterious effects were being reported. An eminent British Radiologist,

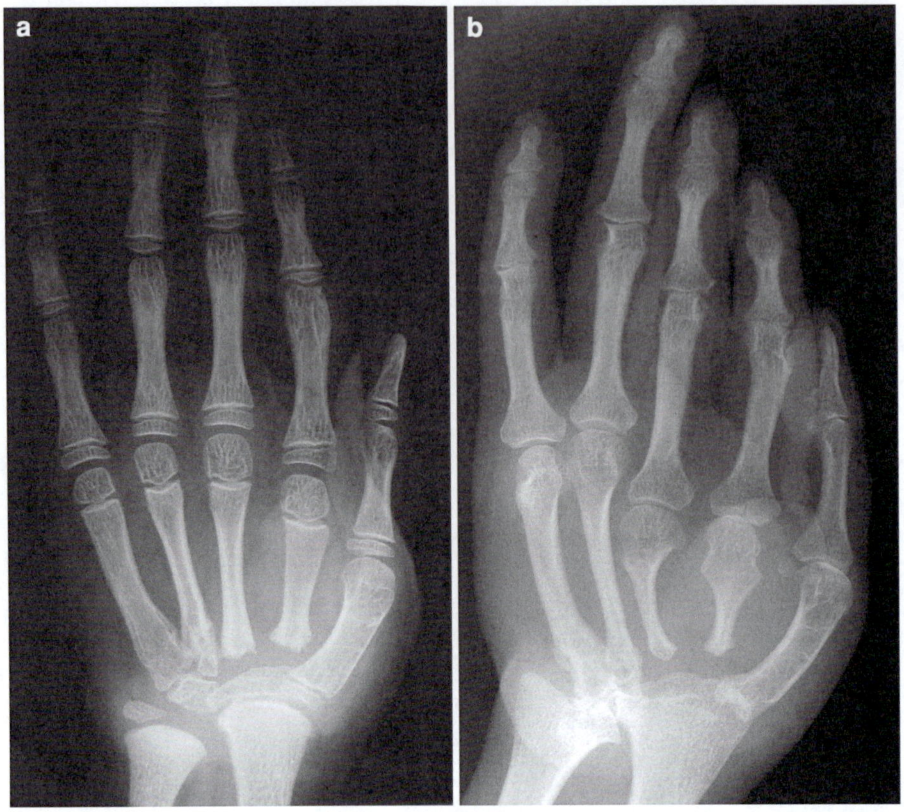

Fig. 23 Idiopathic Multicentric Osteolysis (Carpal-Tarsal Osteolysis). **a** Child showing marked resorption of the carpal bones with involvement of the bases of the 2nd and 3rd metacarpals. **b** Same case as an adult showing disease progression with further involvement of the metacarpals

John Hall-Edwards, working at the General Hospital in Birmingham was one of the first to give a comprehensive description of the adverse effects of X-rays on the bones of the hand—using his own hands for case material (Hall-Edwards 1908). Complications include radiation-induced dermatitis with an increased risk of malignant transformation, growth plate damage in children and radionecrosis of the bones (Fig. 22; Hartwell et al. 1964; De Smet et al. 1976). Radiation-induced damage to the hands from diagnostic X-rays is mercifully rare in this day and age but modern radiologists do need to be aware of the potential increase in radiation dose to the hands when undertaking interventional procedures under either fluoroscopic or CT control. Radiation-induced tumours of the hand following radiotherapy are rare (Libshitz and Cohen 1982). It is possible that the incidence of radiation-induced osteochondromas in the hands may rise due to the increasing use of whole-body irradiation in children as part of the preparative regimen for haematopoietic stem cell (bone marrow) transplantation.

14 Massive Osteolysis

Bone destruction is a non-specific feature of numerous different bone conditions. There is a rare group of idiopathic disorders causing significant bone destruction that can be categorised under the title of primary osteolysis syndromes (Resnick 2002). The commonest is known as Gorham's disease or Massive Osteolysis characterised by uncontrolled, destructive proliferation of vascular or lymphatic vessels within bone and the surrounding soft tissues (Gorham and Stout 1955). Radiographs show dramatic, progressive resorption of bone that can cross joints and involve adjacent bones. The shoulder and the pelvis are the most common sites of involvement but cases have been reported in the hand (Patel 2005). Another rarer form of primary osteolysis is Idiopathic Multicentric Osteolysis also known as Carpal-Tarsal Osteolysis. Radiographs show progressive carpal bone resorption with in time involvement of the metacarpals (Fig. 23). Cases may be associated with a nephropathy (Warady et al. 1991).

15 Key Points

- the hand is the commonest site of bone involvement with sarcoid.
- the hand is the commonest site for reflex sympathetic dystrophy (complex regional pain syndrome).
- dactylitis may be seen in numerous diseases including sarcoidosis and sickle cell anaemia.
- hypertrophic osteoarthropathy may be associated with both pulmonary and non-pulmonary disorders.

References

Ahlberg AK (1975) On the natural history of hemophilic pseudotumor. J Bone Joint Surg Am 57A:1133–1136

Al-Boukai AA, Hawass NE, Patel PJ, Kolawole TM (1989) Camel bites: report of severe osteolysis as late bone complications. Postgrad Med J 65:900–904

Ali A, Tetalman MR, Fordham EW et al (1980) Distribution of hypertrophic pulmonary osteoarthropathy. AJR Am J Roentgenol 134:771–780

Bernauer TA, Mirowski GW, Caldemeyer KS (2001) Tuberous sclerosis: II. Musculoskeletal and visceral findings. J Am Acad Dermatol 45:450–452

Bohrer SP (1970) Acute long bone diaphyseal infarcts in sickle cell disease. Br J Radiol 43:685–697

Boutin RD, Spitz DJ, Newman JS, Lenchik L, Steinbach LS (1998) Complications in Paget disease at MR imaging. Radiology 209:641–651

Brudin L, Valind S, Rhodes C et al (1994) Fluorine-18 deoxyglucose uptake in sarcoidosis measured with positron emission tomography. Eur J Nucl Med 21:297–305

Caffey J (1951) Chronic poisoning due to excess vitamin A. AJR Am J Roentgenol 65:12–26

Caffey J (1957) Cooley's anemia: a review of the roentgenographic findings in the skeleton. Hickey Lecture. AJR Am J Roentgenol 78:381–391

Calif E, Vlodavsky E, Stahl S (2007) Ivory fingers: monostotic Paget's disease of the phalanges. J Clin Endocrinol Metabolism 92:1590–1591

Christie DP (1980) The spectrum of radiographic bone changes in children with fluorosis. Radiology 136:85–90

Cobby MJ, Adler RS, Swartz R, Martel W (1991) Dialysis-related amyloid arthropathy: MR findings in four patients. AJR Am J Roentgenol 157:1023–1027

Cockshott WP (1963) Dactylitis and growth disorders. Br J Radiol 36:19–26

Cundy T (2006) Is Paget's disease of bone disappearing. Skeletal Radiol 35:350–351

Davies AM, Colley SP, James SLJ, Sumathi VP, Grimer RJ (2010) Erdheim–Chester disease presenting with destruction of a metacarpal. Clin Radiol 65:250–253

De Smet AA, Kuhns LR, Fayos JV, Holt JF (1976) Effects of radiation therapy on growing long bones. AJR Am J Roentgenol 127:935–939

De Smet L, Roosen P, Zachee B et al (1994) Monostotic localization of Paget disease in the hand. Acta Orthop Belg 60:184–186

De Wind LT (1961) Hypervitaminosis D with osteosclerosis. Arch Dis Child 36:373–380

Dearbon GV (1932) A case of congenital general pure analgesia. J Nerv Ment Dis 75:612

Destouet JM, Murphy WA (1981) Guitar player acro-osteolysis. Skeletal Radiol 6:275–277

Friedman A, Orcutt J, Madewell J (1982) Paget disease of the hand: radiographic spectrum. Am J Roentgenol 138(4): 691–693

Gama C, Meira JB (1978) Occupational acro-osteolysis. J Bone Joint Surg Am 60A:86–90

Gibson MS, Jennings BT, Murphey MD (2008) Hypertrophic osteoarthropathy. In: Pope TL Jr, Bloem HL, Beltran J, Morrison WB, Wilson DJ (eds) Imaging of the musculoskeletal system, vol 2. Saunders Elsevier, Philadelphia, p 1612

Gorham LW, Stout AP (1955) Massive osteolysis (acute spontaneous absorption of bone, phantom bone, disappearing bone): its relation to haemangiomatosis. J Bone Joint Surg Am 37A:985–1004

Gwathmey FW, House JH (1984) Clinical manifestations of congenital insensitivity of the hand and classification of syndromes. J Hand Surg [Am] 9A:863–869

Hall-Edwards J (1908) The effects upon bone due to prolonged exposure to X-rays. Arch Roentgen Ray 13:44

Hartwell SW Jr, Huger W Jr, Pickrell K (1964) Radiation dermatitis and radiogenic neoplasms of the hands. Ann Surg 160:828–834

Haverbush T, Wilde A, Phalen G (1972) The hand in Paget's disease of bone: report of two cases. J Bone Joint Surg Am 54A:173–175

Hildebrandt JW, Olson P, Paratainen H, Griffiths H (1993) Macrodystrophia lipomatosa. Orthopedics 16:1075–1077

Huang TT, Blackwell SJ, Lewis SR (1978) Hand deformities in patients with snake bite. Plast Reconstr Surg 62:32–36

Karmani S, Shedden R, De Sousa C (2001) Orthopaedic manifestations of congenital insensitivity to pain. J R Soc Med 94:139–140

Katzman BM, Caligiuri DA, Klein DM, Perrier G, Dauterman PA (1997) Sarcoid flexor tenosynovitis of the wrist: a case report. J Hand Surg Am 22:336–337

Kaufmann GA, Sundaram M, McDonald DJ (1991) MR imaging in symptomatic Paget's disease. Skeletal Radiol 20:413–418

Kiss E, Keusch G, Zanetti M, Jung T, Schwarz A, Schocke M, Jaschke W, Czermak BV (2005) Dialysis-related amyloidosis revisited. AJR Am J Roentgenol 185: 1460–1470

Lanzer W, Szabo R, Gelberman R (1984) Avascular necrosis of the lunate and sickle cell anemia: a case report. Clin Orthop Relat Res 187:168–171

Leone AJ Jr (1968) On lead lines. AJR Am J Roentgenol 103:165–167

Libshitz HI, Cohen MA (1982) Radiation-induced osteochondromas. Radiology 142:643–647

Lopez C, Thomas DV, Davies AM (2003) Neoplastic transformation and tumour-like lesions in Paget's disease of bone: a pictorial review. Eur Radiol 13:L151–L163

Love C, Tomas M, Tronco G et al (2005) FDG PET of infection and inflammation. Radiographics 25:1357–1368

Marie P (1890) De l'osteoarthropathie hypertrophiante pneumonique. Rev Med (Paris) 10:1–36

Middlemiss JH, Raper AB (1966) Skeletal changes in the haemoglobinopathies. J Bone Joint Surg Br 48B:693–701

Moore S (2003) Musculoskeletal sarcoidosis: spectrum of appearances at MR imaging. Radiographics 23:1389–1399

Neville E, Carstairs LS, James DG (1976) Bone sarcoidosis. Ann N Y Acad Sci 278:475–487

Neville EW, Carstairs LS, James DG (1977) Sarcoidosis of bone. Q J Med 46:215–217

Park JS, Ryu KN (2004) Hemophilic pseudotumor involving the musculoskeletal system: spectrum of radiologic findings. AJR Am J Roentgenol 183:55–61

Park SA, Yang CY, Shin YI, Oh GJ, Lee M (2009) Patterns of three-phase bone scintigraphy according to the time course of complex regional pain syndrome type 1 after a stroke or traumatic brain injury. Clin Nucl Med 34:773–776

Patel DV (2005) Gorham's disease or massive osteolysis. Clin Med Res 3:65–74

Pineda CJ, Martinez-Lavin M, Goodbar JE et al (1987) Periostitis in hypertrophic osteoarthropathy: relationship to disease duration. AJR Am J Roentgenol 148:773–778

Qteishat WA, Whitehouse GH, Hawass N (1985) Acroosteolysis following snake and scorpion envenomisation. Br J Radiol 58:1035–1039

Rahalkar MD, Rahalkar AM, Joshi SK (2008) Case series: congenital insensitivity to pain and anhidrosis. Indian J Radiol Imaging 18:132–134

Ranawat CS, Arora MM, Singh RG (1968) Macrodystrophia lipomatosa with carpal tunnel syndrome: a case report. J Bone Joint Surg Am 50A:1242–1244

Reilly MM (2009) Classification and diagnosis of inherited neuropathies. Ann Indian Acad Neurol 12:80–88

Resnick D (2002) Osteolysis and chondrolysis. In: Resnick D (ed) Diagnosis of bone and joint disorders, 4th edn. WB Saunders Co., Philadelphia, pp 4920–4944

Resnick D, Pineda CJ, Weisman HM, Kerr R (1985) Osteomyelitis and septic arthritis of the hand following human bites. Skeletal Radiol 14:263–266

Rodriguez-Peralto J, Ro J, McCabe K et al (1994) Case report 806: monostotic Paget's disease of the hand. Skeletal Radiol 23:55–57

Sachs H (1981) The evolution of the radiologic lead line. Radiology 139:81–85

Schumacher HR Jr (1964) Hemochromotosis and arthritis. Arthritis Rheum 7:41–50

Shaheen S, Alasha E (2005) Hemophilic pseudotumor of the distal parts of the radius and ulna: a case report. J Bone Joint Surg Am 87A:2546–2549

Shaw JA, Wilson SC (1993) Multiple hemophilic bone cysts in the hand. J Hand Surg Am 18:262–264

Siegelman SS, Heimann WG, Manin MC (1966) Congenital indifference to pain. AJR Am J Roentgenol 97:242–247

Silverman FN, Gilden JJ (1959) Congenital insensitivity to pain: a neurologic syndrome with bizarre skeletal lesions. Radiology 72:176–190

Smith S, Murphey M, Motamedi K et al (2002) Radiologic spectrum of Paget's disease of bone and its complications with pathologic correlation. Radiographics 22: 1191–1216

Sundaram M, Khanna G, El-Khoury GY (2001) T1-weighteds MR imaging for distinguishing large osteolysis of Paget's disease from sarcomatous degeneration. Skeletal Radiol 30:378–383

Van Linthoudt D, Ott H (1986) An unusual case of sarcoid dactylitis. Br J Rheumatol 25:222–224

Vande Berg B, Malghem J, Lecouvet F et al (2001) Magnetic resonance appearance of uncomplicated Paget's disease of bone. Semin Musculoskelet Radiol 1:69–77

Warady BA, Haug SJ, Lindsley CB (1991) Multicentric osteolysis: an infrequently recognized renal-rheumatologic syndrome. J Rheumatol 18:142–145

Watson RJ, Burko H, Megas H, Robinson M (1963) The hand–foot syndrome in sickle cell disease in young children. Pediatrics 31:975–982

Westermark P, Benson MD, Buxbaum JN et al (2002) Amyloid fibril protein nomenclature. Amyloid J Protein Folding Disord 9:197–200

Imaging the Post-Operative Wrist and Hand

R. S. D. Campbell and D. A. Campbell

Contents

R. S. D. Campbell (✉)
Department of Radiology, Consultant Musculoskeletal Radiologist, Royal Liverpool University Hospital, Liverpool, L7 8XP, UK
e-mail: Rob.Campbell@rlbuht.nhs.uk

D. A. Campbell
Consultant Hand and Wrist Surgeon, Leeds General Infirmary, Leeds, LS1 3EX, UK

Abstract

Orthopaedic procedures of the hand and wrist are performed for a wide variety of pathologic conditions. Acute fracture fixation and treatment of fracture complications account for the majority of surgical interventions. Other indications for surgery include management of chronic arthropathy, ligament or tendon injury, soft tissue and bone tumours and infection.

1 Introduction

Orthopaedic procedures of the hand and wrist are performed for a wide variety of pathologic conditions. Acute fracture fixation and treatment of fracture complications account for the majority of surgical interventions. Other indications for surgery include management of chronic arthropathy, ligament or tendon injury, soft tissue and bone tumours and infection.

It is important for the radiologist to understand the primary aims of surgical treatment in order to accurately assess the post-operative imaging to identify potential complications. The aims of surgery include:

- Restoration of normal anatomy
- Pain management

A. M. Davis et al. (eds.), *Imaging of the Hand and Wrist*, Medical Radiology. Diagnostic Imaging,
DOI: 10.1007/174_2010_140, © Springer-Verlag Berlin Heidelberg 2013

- Restoration of function
- Treatment of cosmetic disfigurement
- Prevention of secondary osteoarthritis (OA)

There are a large number of fixation devices and prostheses available to the orthopaedic surgeon, and radiologists should be familiar with the most commonly used devices. It is important to distinguish between acceptable and unacceptable alignment of the bony structures and metalware, and to recognise when poorly positioned devices may lead to complications. In soft tissue reconstruction, it is necessary to know when normal structures have been utilised to achieve the repair (e.g. tendon harvesting), in order to be able to recognise the anatomy on cross-sectional imaging.

Common complications include non-union and mal-union of fractures, poor operative correction of bone and joint deformity and mal-positioned orthopaedic hardware. Non-union of joint arthrodesis, implant failure and infection may also be encountered.

Radiographs are the primary imaging modality used to supplement clinical examination in the post-operative period. Cross-sectional imaging may be required when complications arise. The choice of image modality is guided by clinical findings, and may depend on the presence of orthopaedic metalware which limits the use of MRI in particular.

CT is excellent for documenting bony detail and is useful for assessment of fracture healing and some hardware complications. US is a useful alternative to MRI for assessment of the soft tissues. Nuclear medicine studies are rarely required, but white cell scans may occasionally be useful for evaluation of infected implants.

2 Fracture Fixation

2.1 Indications

Fixation of hand or wrist fractures is indicated when the fracture fragments lie in an unacceptable position, or the fracture pattern is unstable and redisplacement likely.

Fixation of a hand or wrist fracture would also be considered in certain circumstances where the patient's personal circumstances or characteristics would make such treatment more appropriate. These relative indications include:

- Co-existent skeletal injuries where mobility will be assisted by crutches or load bearing through the wrist
- Bilateral hand or wrist fractures
- Co-existent soft tissue injuries which require early treatment, physiotherapy or rehabilitation out of plaster cast
- Patient request (e.g. professional sportsman/woman)

2.2 Implant Choice

A variety of implants are used to stabilise fractures in the hand and wrist. These are either applied to directly stabilise the fracture fragments (Kirschner wires, or internal fixation materials), or applied indirectly to stabilise the fracture fragments from a distance (external fixators).

2.2.1 Kirschner Wires

These are small, thin pins made of stainless steel or titanium. They come in a variety of diameters, typically 1.0–1.6 mm in diameter. They have a sharp tip at one end or both ends ("double-ended"). K-wires with a threaded tip are designed for use as guide wires for cannulated devices and should never be left in situ, since removal is extremely difficult without adequate anaesthesia.

When inserted, the K-wires should engage both cortices to be mechanically effective. They cannot compress fracture fragments, and will only maintain a reduction achieved by other means. Most often, they are inserted percutaneously after a closed reduction, but may occasionally be used following open reduction. K-wires may need to cross joints to be mechanically effective in some circumstances, and this provides a potential route for spread of infection (Fig. 1).

2.2.2 Internal Fixation Materials

Internal fixation may be achieved by the use of compression screws, plate and screw devices or bone anchors.

The best known screw, the Herbert screw, was designed for use in the scaphoid. The pitch varies along the length of the screw, so that differential longitudinal movement occurs in the fracture fragments at each end of the screw as it is tightened, bringing the fragments closer together resulting in fracture compression. The 'Headless Compression Screw' (HCS), which provides significantly greater

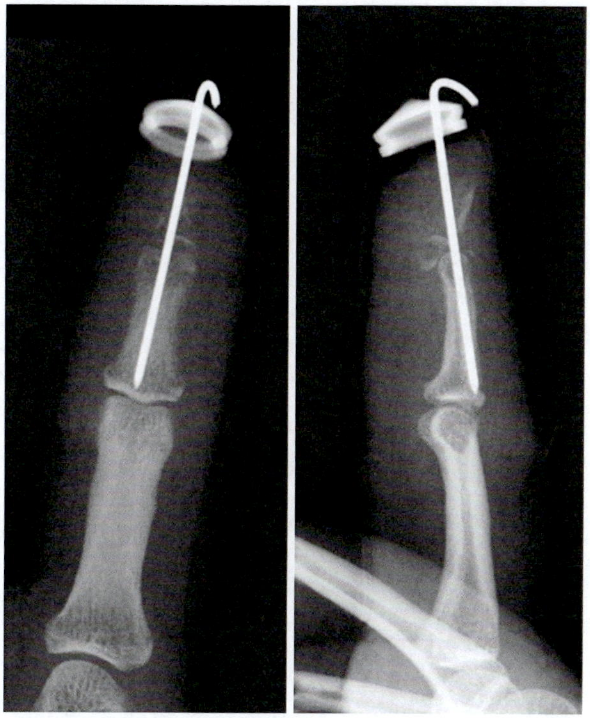

Fig. 1 AP and lateral radiographs acquired a few weeks following K-wire fixation of an open fracture of the distal phalanx due to a dog bite. There is osteomyelitis of the distal phalanx with marked lytic bony destruction. In addition, the presence of the K-wire has allowed spread of infection across the DIP joint into the middle phalanx, with diffuse osteopaenia and periosteal reaction

fracture compression and stability, has now largely replaced the Herbert screw. It is sometimes possible to fix fractures percutaneously by utilising cannulated screws, which have a central channel through which a thin guide wire can be inserted under image guidance across the fracture allowing the screw to be introduced over the temporary guide wire (Fig. 2).

Traditional 'plate and screw' implants for the hand and wrist have undergone a revolution in design in recent years. These changes have involved three separate developments:

- Angular stability
- Anatomic implants
- Indirect reduction technique (in distal radius fractures)

Anatomic implants such as the volar plate are commonly used in distal radial fractures. Modified contoured implants traditionally used by craniomaxillofacial (CMF) surgeons in the maxilla, mandible and facial bones have been adapted for use in the small bones of the fingers.

Bone anchors are small metallic or absorbable implants which are inserted into a small drill hole made in bone. Pre-threaded with suture material, they allow soft tissues to be reattached to the bone when this interface has been disrupted by injury. The most common use of these implants in the hand and wrist, is in the treatment of ulnar collateral ligament (UCL) injuries in the metacarpophalangeal (MCP) joint of the thumb (skiers thumb).

2.2.3 External Fixation

This technique involves the application of two or more threaded pins into the bone on each side of the fracture. These pins are then connected by means of an externally applied rigid bar, which may be radiolucent to help in assessment of radiographs. The pins must engage the cortex on both surfaces to withstand the forces attempting to redisplace the fracture.

When the distal fragment is large and not comminuted, two pins can be placed in the distal fragment, so that the fixator does not cross the adjacent joint (non-bridging fixator), and does not prevent joint movement. However, if one fracture fragment is small, and unable to securely hold two threaded pins, the pins must be placed in a bone beyond the adjacent joint.

2.3 Distal Radial Fractures

Traditionally, K-wires were used to treat extra-articular and simple-articular fractures in the elderly, although evidence has suggested that they may be significantly less effective in maintaining reduction in osteoporotic bone (Greatting and Bishop 1993). For this reason, internal fixation is increasingly employed in the elderly wrist fracture, although K-wires are still utilised for unstable epiphyseal fractures in children (Fig. 3). Radiographs are utilised to ensure K-wire and fracture alignment is maintained until fracture healing is achieved and the wires can be removed.

Implants placed on the dorsal surface of the distal radius were commonly complicated by attrition rupture of the extensor tendons, and are now less frequently utilised.

Current implants are 'anatomic' and designed to fit flush to the volar surface of the distal radius. The plate

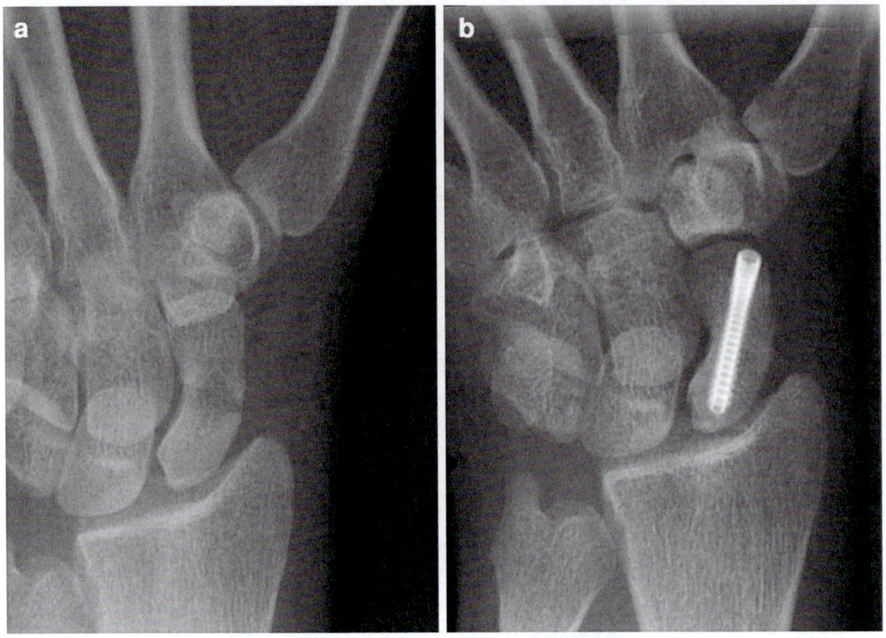

Fig. 2 Oblique PA radiograph (**a**) demonstrating an un-united waist of scaphoid fracture at 6 weeks. The fracture has been stabilised by a cannulated screw (**b**), and has now fully united. Note that the pitch of the screw is wider distally than proximally. NB: the screw is inserted distal to proximal, so the tip of the screw is in the proximal scaphoid

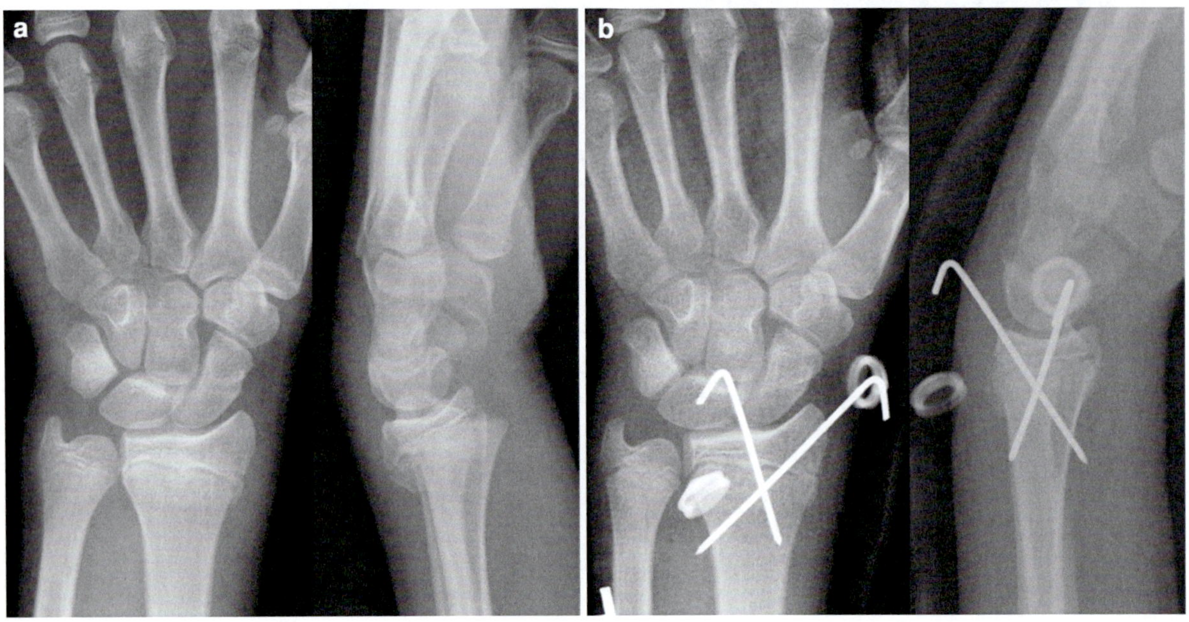

Fig. 3 PA and lateral radiographs (**a**) of a teenager with an unstable Salter–Harris type II fracture. The PA and lateral radiographs (**b**) acquired following K-wire fixation demonstrate good fracture reduction. Each K-wire traverses two bony cortices, ensuring mechanical stability

forces the distal fragments to re-align in a perfect position with multiple sub-chondral angularly stable screws (Fig. 4). This technique is known as 'indirect reduction' and is widely used in all types of distal radius fractures. It has the added advantage of automatically correcting any malrotation of the distal fragment. There are over 40 different designs of volar locking plates for the distal radius currently available.

A variety of neurovascular, soft tissue and osseous complications may arise as a result of volar plate

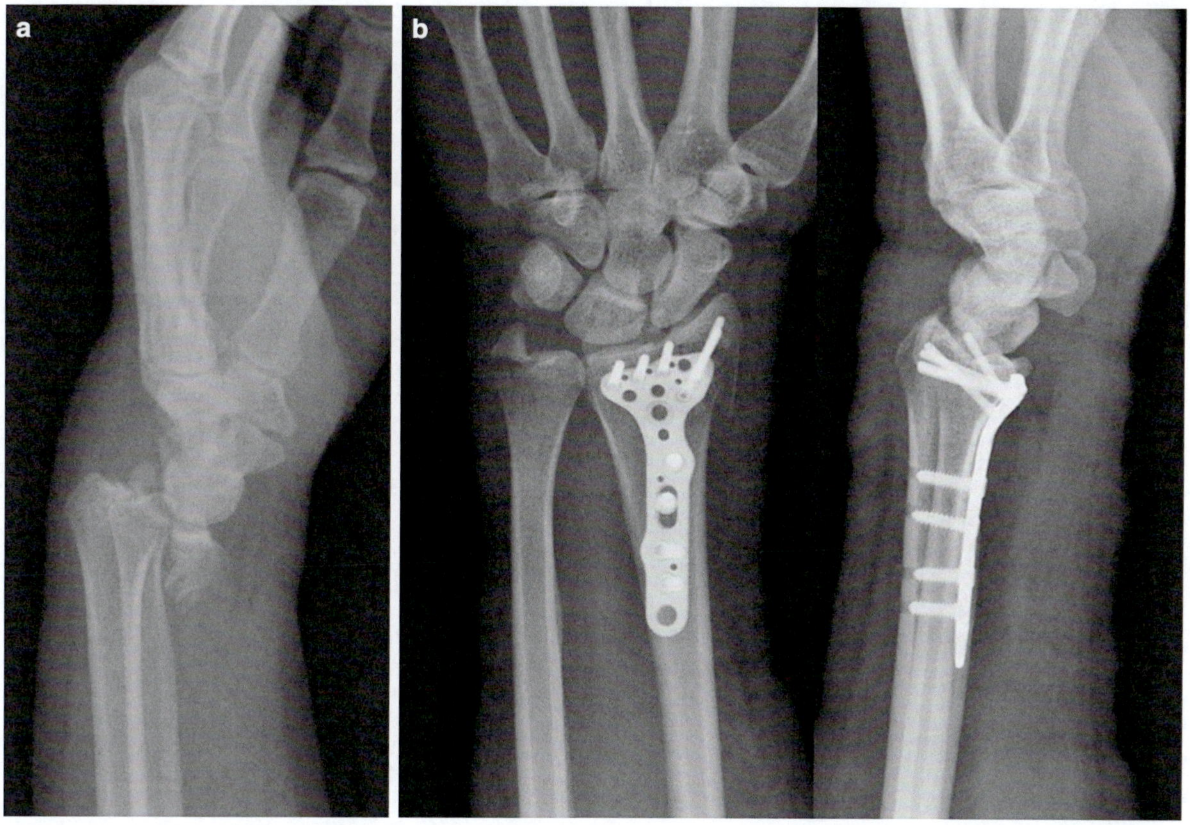

Fig. 4 Lateral radiograph (**a**) of a displaced volar shearing, comminuted and intra-articular fracture of the distal radius. PA and lateral radiographs (**b**) acquired following volar plate fixation demonstrate good restoration of anatomical alignment, with the articular fragments maintained by the sub-chondral screws. The screws in the proximal plate do not engage the dorsal cortex of the distal radial metaphysis, consequently they do not protrude into the soft tissues, but the resulting lack of bicortical fixation may be prone to early redisplacement. Note also the minimally displaced fracture at the base of the ulnar styloid

fixation (Berglund 2009). Flexor pollicis longus tendinopathy and rupture may be associated with a distally mal-positioned volar plate and plate 'lift-off'. Fracture mal-reduction may also contribute to tendon rupture. Extensor tendon ruptures may be seen with overlong or mal-positioned screws (Fig. 5). Intra-articular screw placement within the radio-carpal joint may also be encountered, and pre-dispose to accelerated secondary OA change. Other complications include carpal tunnel syndrome, complex regional pain syndrome and delayed union (Arora et al. 2007).

Patients' with pain or crepitus over the flexor or extensor tendons may be assessed by US to identify tendon impingement with the volar plate and exclude tendinopathy, and tendon rupture. The relationship of mal-placed screws to tendons can also be assessed. Significant tendon disease may necessitate removal of the volar plate once bony union is achieved.

External fixation is usually reserved for open or excessively comminuted fractures, although this mode of fixation is the preferential choice for some surgeons. Pins are placed in the radial shaft and the shaft of the index (second) metacarpal. The pins must engage the cortex on both surfaces to withstand the forces attempting to redisplace the fracture, and it is important to obtain consistent positioning of serial post-operative radiographs to ensure there is no metalware failure, and the pins remain fixed in the bone cortices.

2.4 Scaphoid Fractures

Internal fixation is indicated in the treatment of displaced waist of scaphoid fractures and undisplaced proximal pole scaphoid fractures. It is most frequently employed in the treatment of non-union of scaphoid

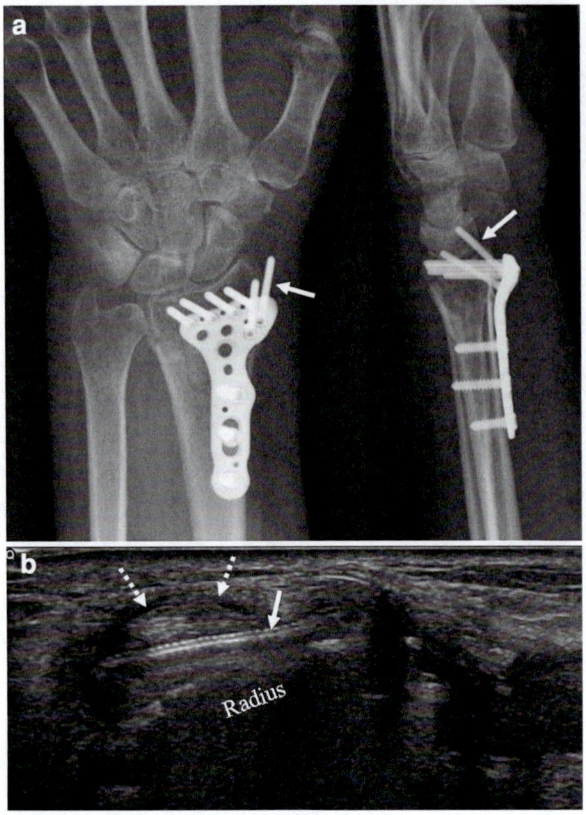

Fig. 5 PA and lateral radiographs (**a**) of a distal radial fracture fixated with a volar plate. The plate is positioned too far distally, and is not aligned with the centre of the shaft of the distal radius. One of the radial styloid screws is extra-osseous (*white arrows*). An oblique transverse US image (**b**) shows the screw (*white arrow*) extending into the extensor group I tendons (*broken white arrows*)

fractures in order to improve the chances of bony union. Cannulated screws are most commonly used and stabilise both the fracture fragments and interposed bone graft.

Grafting and fixation of scaphoid non-union is not indicated if there is established OA, and other salvage procedures such as denervation, proximal row carpectomy or wrist arthrodesis may be required. Radiographs are notoriously inaccurate in demonstrating avascular necrosis of the proximal pole (Downing et al. 2002). Pre-operative MR imaging is more accurate in assessing the vascularity of the proximal fragment.

Fracture non-union and hardware failure occurs in up to 8% of patients undergoing dorsal percutaneous cannulated screw fixation of undisplaced scaphoid fractures (Bushnell et al. 2007). Fracture healing on serial radiographs is normally expected by 12 weeks

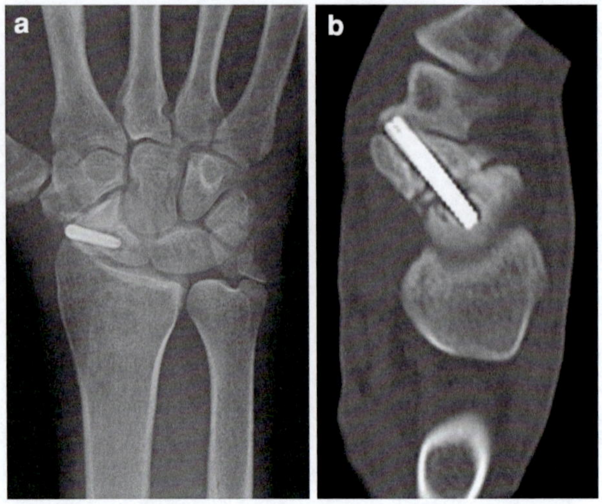

Fig. 6 PA radiograph (**a**) of a fractured scaphoid stabilised by a cannulated compression screw. It is difficult to assess fracture union on this examination, although there is clear evidence of lysis around the screw, suggesting loosening due to non-union. Sagittal oblique CT (**b**) confirms the presence of fracture non-union. In addition the proximal end of the screw impinges within the scapho-trapezial joint

post-fixation, and a persistent fracture line indicates delayed or non-union. Persistent non-union is more frequent in patients undergoing fixation of chronic non-union, even with bone grafting, and occurs in up to one-third of cases (Megerle et al. 2008). If radiographs are equivocal, CT is a reliable method of evaluating the status of fracture healing (Fig. 6). Progressive lucency around the screw is indicative of screw loosening. Avascular necrosis of the proximal pole segment is manifest by sclerosis, sub-chondral flattening and fragmentation. Screw fracture is rarely encountered.

2.5 Hamate Fractures

The treatment for non-displaced hamate fractures is usually conservative. However, the majority of displaced fractures are treated by either fixation with pins or screws (Fig. 7), or by excision of the fragment (Walsh and Bishop 2000) if a symptomatic non-union of the hook of the hamate is present. Non-union is common in displaced fractures managed non-operatively, although long-term outcome may be no worse than those treated operatively (Scheufler et al. 2005). Compression screw fixation generally achieves better fracture stability than fixation with Kirschner wires, although this does not necessarily correlate with outcome scores (Wharton et al. 2010).

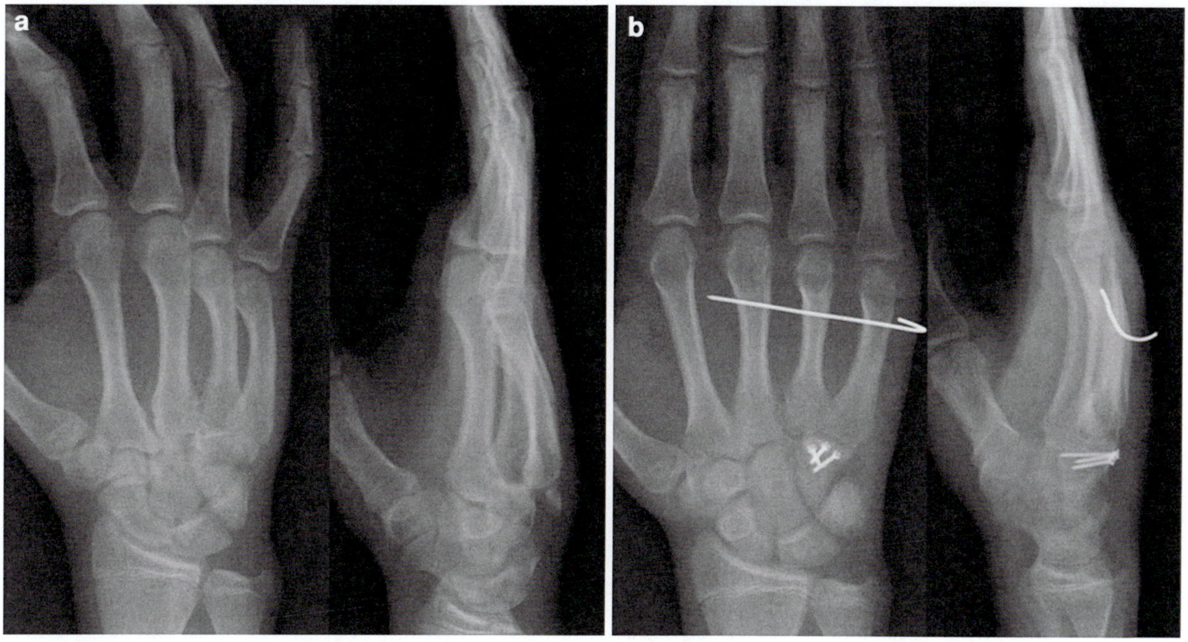

Fig. 7 Oblique PA and lateral radiographs (**a**) of a displaced dorsal hamate fracture associated with dislocation of the fourth and fifth metacarpal bases. The post-operative PA and lateral radiographs (**b**) demonstrate good anatomical alignment of the fracture fragment maintained by three cortical screws. The metacarpal dislocation has been reduced, and the K-wire transfixing from third to fifth metacarpals helps maintain stability during ligamentous healing

CT imaging of hamate fractures is utilised to detect occult fractures (Welling et al. 2008), to aid surgical planning of complex fractures, or to diagnose fracture non-union. Serial radiographs are required post-operatively to assess progression of bony union and exclude hardware failure. The PA and oblique views may be supplemented with a lateral view in cases with associated carpo-metacarpal dislocation, to assess adequacy of reduction. CT is rarely required in the post-operative period but may be helpful where bony union is equivocal.

2.6 Other Carpal Bones

Carpal fractures at other sites occur much less frequently. The peculiar anatomy of each carpal bone (irregular shape and significant surface area coverage by articular cartilage) does not lend itself to an easy solution when designing an internal fixation implant. However, the usually dense cancellous bone in this region, allows intraosseous devices to be designed, which will stabilise each carpal bone fracture appropriately.

When carpal bones dislocate, they are usually held in a reduced position by multiple K-wires inserted percutaneously. These are an excellent implant choice because compression is not required between bones as the ligaments heal. K-wires used for these indications will normally remain in place for approximately 8 weeks.

2.7 Metacarpal and Phalangeal Fractures

K-wires remain popular in the management of metacarpal fractures because of the high cortex:cancellous ratio of these bones. A combination of PA, oblique and true lateral post-operative radiographs, dependant on fracture location, may be required to assess fracture alignment. Good fracture reduction is especially important for intra-articular fractures to maintain function and prevent long-term secondary OA.

Internal fixation using plates and screws is indicated in unstable, irreducible and open fractures. They are employed in cases where early skeletal stabilisation will facilitate earlier movement and rehabilitation.

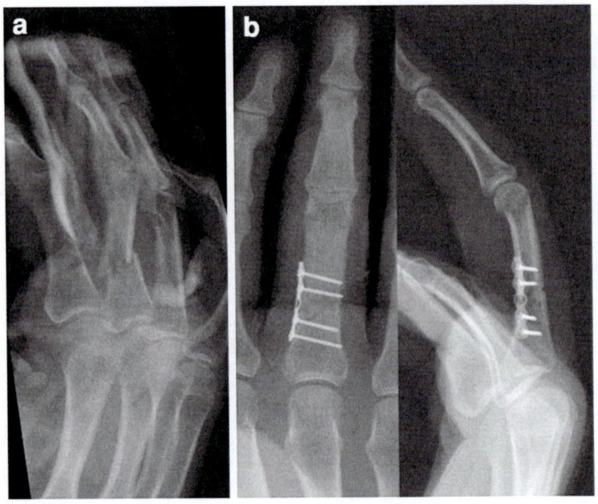

Fig. 8 Oblique radiograph (**a**) of an angulated, transverse fracture of the proximal phalanx of the middle finger. The PA and lateral radiographs (**b**) demonstrates anatomical fracture reduction and fixation with a CMF type implant. Note that the screws transfix the opposite cortex. The limited thickness and small size of the implant, combined with the lateral placement of the plate, suggest that this fixation is at significant risk of early redisplacement and failure. Larger implants situated on the dorsal surface of the bone (to resist the force of the flexor tendon) have a greater chance of success

Scaled down versions of standard long bone implants are too bulky for the confined areas adjacent to the bones of the hand, and often cause adhesion of the soft tissues in contact with the implant, requiring plate removal and division of peritendinous adhesions (tenolysis), as a second surgical procedure in up to 75% of cases (Buchler and Fischer 1987). Hand fracture implants now closely match the original CMF implants rather than orthopaedic implants. A whole new generation of anatomic implants for use in certain pre-defined areas of the hand has evolved (Fig. 8), such that external fixators are now rarely used in the hand (Fig. 9).

Radiographs are evaluated for fracture or displacement of either the plate or screws.

3 Prosthetic Joint Replacement

3.1 Indications

Joint prostheses are rarely indicated in the management of hand and wrist conditions. Finger joints require flexibility and mobility to be useful. Implants can rarely provide this since the surgical approach itself will result in stiffness. The function of the wrist joint demands both stability and flexibility, both of which are difficult to create and match in a prosthetic joint.

The commonest indication for arthroplasty in the hand and wrist is rheumatoid arthritis. Prosthetic joint replacement is indicated when an individual's personal needs or lifestyle are such that arthrodesis would be unsuitable. In some instances, this may be unilateral, with an arthrodesis preferred in the opposite wrist to provide maximum stability and strength.

Osteoarthritis is more common than rheumatoid arthritis, but OA patients have very different demands of hand and wrist function, and prosthetic replacement is usually unsuitable because of their greater functional needs. Prosthetic replacement may be considered for secondary OA of a single interphalangeal joint, when the remaining interphalangeal joints are unlikely to develop similar changes, but their function can be significantly downgraded by the arthritic changes present in the affected joint.

3.2 Implant Choice

3.2.1 Wrist

There are a number of different implants available, although none have proved overwhelmingly successful. Most have two parts, one for each side of the wrist 'joint'. They are made of metal, although a high density plastic insert is situated between the components in most implants.

Prostheses can either be described as 'constrained' or 'unconstrained', depending on the design characteristics and the relative freedom of movement between the components, or as 'cemented' or 'uncemented'. Newer designs try to mimic the natural movements of the wrist and carpal bones/ligaments.

Serial radiographs should be assessed for prosthesis alignment and migration, and bony osteolysis (Fig. 10). Early designs were subject to distal component loosening, although this is less frequently encountered with newer implants. Proximal subsidence may be identified but is often non-progressive and asymptomatic (Adams 2004). However, outcome measures for wrist arthroplasty are comparable or slightly worse than wrist fusion (Cavaliere and Chung 2008), and surgical options need to be carefully assessed.

Prosthetic surgery in the distal radioulnar joint (DRUJ) is more frequently indicated than in the

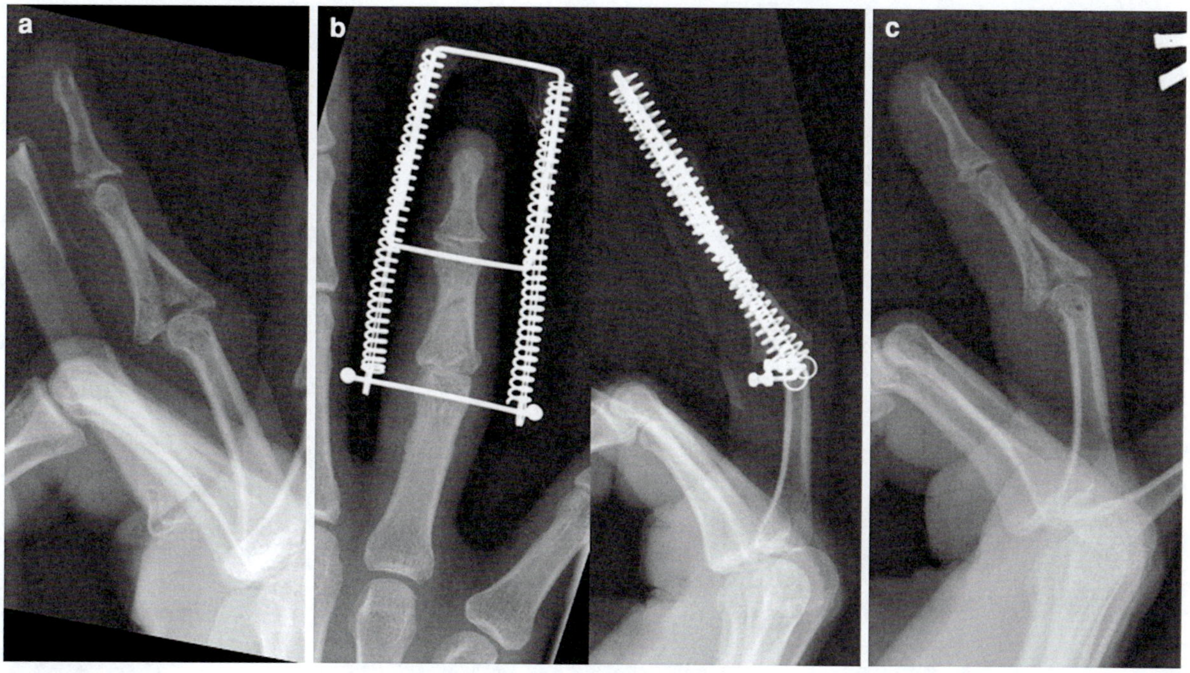

Fig. 9 Lateral radiograph (**a**) of a longitudinal, coronal plane fracture of the base of the middle phalanx, with separation and depression of the intra-articular fragments. The fracture has been stabilised with an external fixator (**b**), although fracture reduction is difficult to assess on the lateral view due to the presence of the fixator. The PA view demonstrates persistent displacement of an articular fragment on the ulnar side of the base of the phalanx. Following removal of the fixator, the lateral radiograph (**c**) demonstrates incomplete fracture reduction and incomplete bony union

radiocarpal joint (Kopylov and Tagil 2007). This type of surgery is most frequently performed to stabilise the unstable distal ulnar stump after excision (Darrach's procedure). Prosthetic surgery is also indicated in degenerative disease of the DRUJ and after unreconstructible fracture of the ulnar head. Prostheses either replace the distal ulna alone (distal ulnar prosthesis) (Fig. 11), or both the distal ulna and sigmoid notch of the distal radius (DRUJ prosthesis). They are usually uncemented.

3.2.2 Hand

Interphalangeal or metacarpophalangeal replacements are either made of:

- Silicon
- Metal and plastic
- Pyrocarbon

Silicon implants are commonly used for multiple MCP joint replacements in rheumatoid arthritis. Long-term outcomes for silicone implants are good with 63% survivorship at 17-year follow up (Trail et al. 2004), and have better outcomes than non-surgical groups (Chung et al. 2009). Metal and plastic implants mimic other large joint prostheses in other areas of the body but are almost always inserted without the use of cement. Pyrocarbon implants are radiopaque and are always inserted cementless.

Post-operative radiographs are assessed for the position of each implant, and joint alignment. At long-term follow up, loosening, bony osteolysis and prosthetic deformity and fracture may occur (Fig. 12). Fracture of silicone prostheses eventually occurs in up to two-thirds of cases, although clinical outcomes may not be adversely affected (Trail et al. 2004). Amyloid- and silicone-induced synovitis is a well documented complication of silicone implants and is also referred to as giant cell arthritis. Patients present with pain and swelling localised to the affected joint. Onset of symptoms can vary from 6 months to 9 years. Radiographs may show nodular soft tissue swelling, well defined sub-chondral lytic defects and erosions. The bony changes evolve over time and must be distinguished from pre-existing arthropathy which necessitates review of previous radiographs. MRI demonstrates effusions with peri-articular low signal intensity silicone particles and fibrosis in

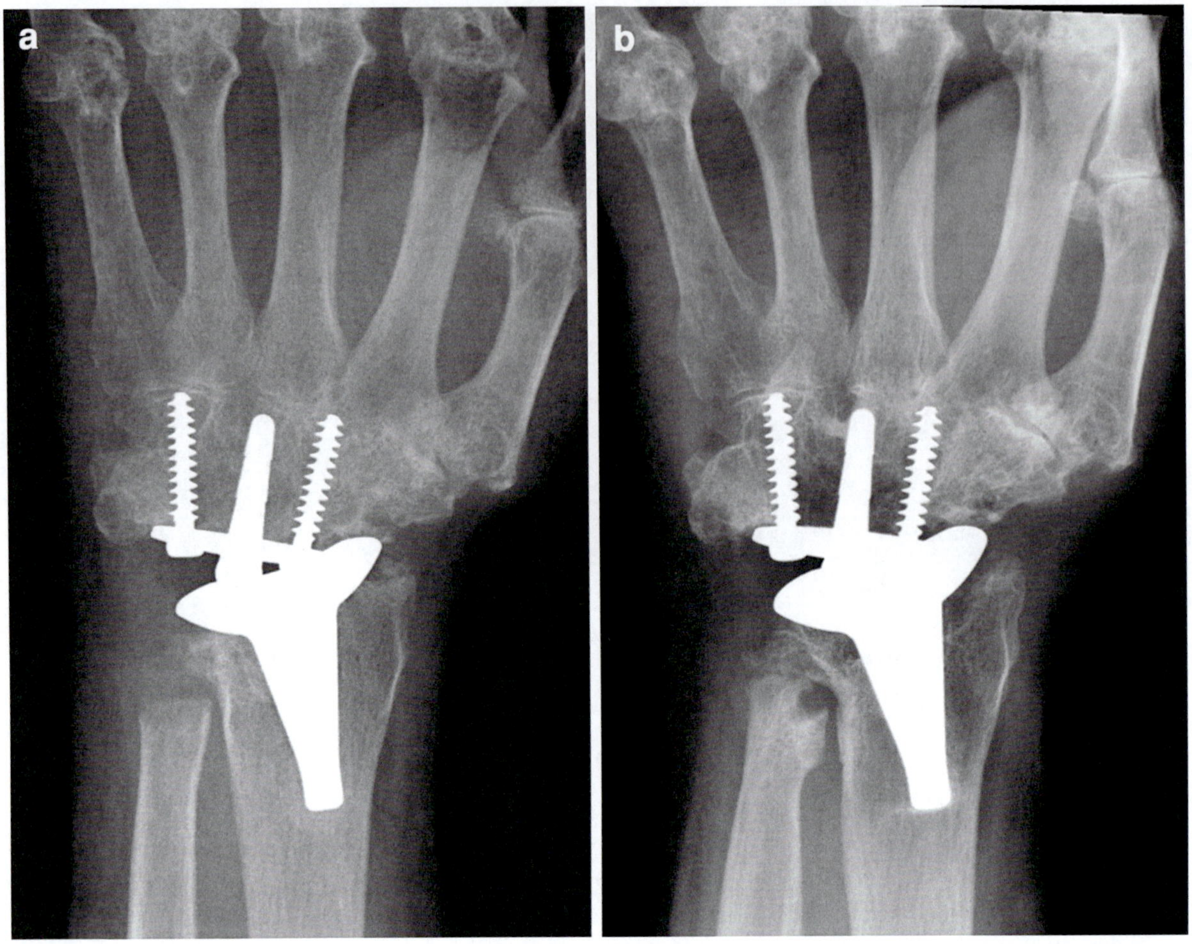

Fig. 10 PA radiograph (**a**) of a 'Re-Motion' wrist prosthesis, in a patient with severe rheumatoid arthritis. The prosthesis is angulated and there is reasonable bone density around the wrist. Although there is no subsidence or change in position of the prosthesis, a follow up radiograph (**b**) acquired 3 years later, demonstrates progressive bony lysis around both proximal and distal components, due to either infection or sterile loosening caused by repetitive loading on the radial border of the prosthesis secondary to malposition

addition to prosthetic deformity and fracture. The sub-chondral lucencies are lower signal intensity on T2W images than typical sub-chondral cysts (Chan et al. 1998). However, most diagnoses can be made on conventional radiographs.

4 Arthrodesis

4.1 Indications

Arthrodesis (surgical fusion) is performed to stabilise a joint by permanently removing its movement in order to remove pain or improve the position of a stiff joint. Surgical removal of the remaining cortical bone is performed on each side of the joint, so that a healthy, vascular bed of cancellous bone is exposed. Opposing cancellous surfaces are brought together and an implant is used to stabilise them whilst osseous healing occurs. Following successful fusion, the implant may be removed in a second surgical procedure if there are soft tissue complications.

Arthrodesis of the wrist may be total or partial. A total wrist arthrodesis involves the radiolunate, radioscaphoid, scapholunate, scaphocapitate and capitolunate joints. The third CMC joint is not always surgically prepared for fusion, but is often left untouched with the intention of removing the stabilising

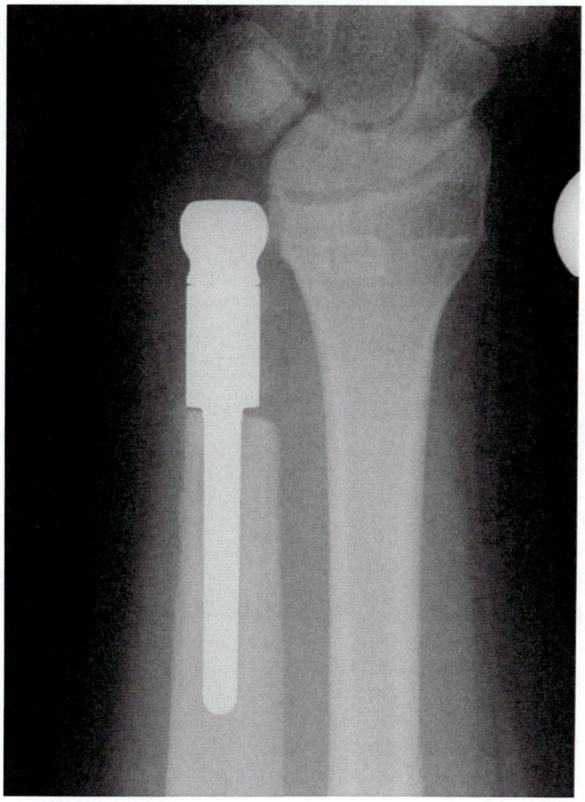

Fig. 11 PA radiograph of an uncemented distal ulnar prosthesis inserted to treat instability of the distal ulnar stump after excision of the ulnar head (Darrach's procedure)

implant at a later date once fusion is sound. This preserves an important movement in the hand, allowing 'cupping' of the fingers and improved dexterity.

A 'partial' wrist arthrodesis is otherwise known as 'intercarpal arthrodesis'. Adjacent carpal bones are arthrodesed to produce a specific anatomical fusion depending on the primary condition (rheumatoid arthritis, OA or carpal instability). Radiolunate arthrodesis is indicated in rheumatoid arthritis to prevent ulnar drift of the hand from the radius. Scaphotrapeziotrapezoid joint arthrodesis is indicated for OA, and when preservation of carpal height is required.

OA of the first CMC joint is very common and a wide range of surgical options are available including arthrodesis. In the hand, the most commonly fused joint is the MCP joint of the thumb. Instability and pain may produce loss of power and precision grip. The terminal joints of the thumb and the fingers are usually fused for patients with OA to restore the effective length of the digit, and improve stability, pain, dexterity and fine movements.

4.2 Implant Choice

4.2.1 Wrist

4.2.1.1 Total Wrist Arthrodesis

Total wrist arthrodesis can be difficult to achieve in patients with OA, and requires specifically designed implants which are strong, but which do not cause irritation of the overlying gliding tendons. These implants come with two different pre-set angles, so that the wrist is arthrodesed in either 20° of extension (commonly utilised) (Fig. 13) or in neutral flexion/extension. One of each type may be used in bilateral arthrodesis to give different abilities with each wrist. The newer versions of these implants include locking screw options to provide angular stability when used in osteoporotic bone.

Rheumatoid patients often have a thin dermis and a potential for poor wound healing. Successful bony fusion can be achieved by the use of an intramedullary stainless steel pin (usually of 3 or 4 mm diameter), without the risks of a substantial metal implant. This is introduced through the head of the middle metacarpal (or occasionally in the second intermetacarpal space) and passed across the carpus and into the medullary canal of the radius (Fig. 14). No rotational stability is provided by this implant, but healing is usually so rapid that this is not a functional problem.

4.2.1.2 Partial Wrist Arthrodesis

Four corner fusion of the lunate, triquetrum, hamate and capitate using a circular plate device was introduced in 1999. It is usually performed in combination with total excision of the scaphoid, as a salvage procedure for scapholunate advanced collapse (SLAC), and scaphoid non-union advanced collapse (SNAC), and has largely replaced traditional fusion procedures using wires, staples and compression screws (Fig. 15). Scaphoidectomy alone would result in inevitable carpal collapse, and a 'four corner arthrodesis' prevents this complication.

Early studies demonstrated higher complications rates than with conventional methods of fusion. Radiographic non-union (26%) and dorsal hardware

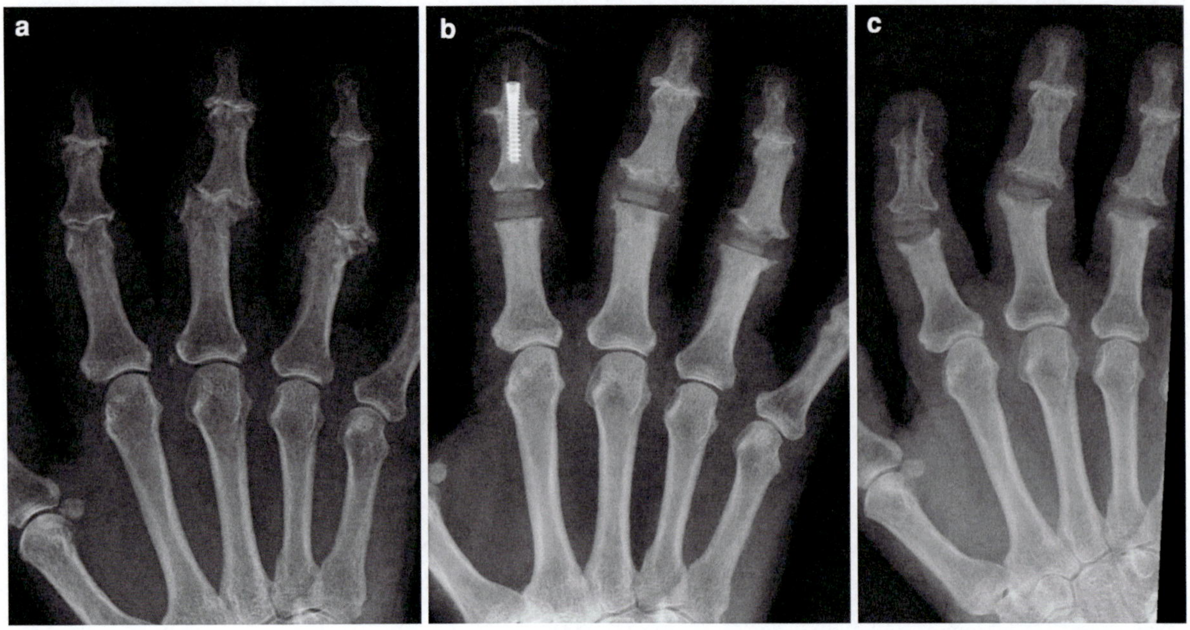

Fig. 12 PA radiograph (**a**) of a patient with severe interpalangeal (IP) joint erosive OA with joint deformity and subluxation. The post-operative radiograph (**b**) illustrates the silastic implants from the second to fourth PIP joints, with restoration of normal joint alignment. There has also been an arthrodesis of the DIP joint of the index finger. A follow up film (**c**) 2 years later (after removal of the arthrodesis screw) shows early deformation of the implants, with early bony resorption of the cut ends of the proximal phalanges. There is recurrent ulnar drift particularly affecting the middle finger. There is no fracture of the implants, and no soft tissue swelling

impingement (22%) are most frequently encountered (Vance et al. 2005). Other complications include implant breakage or back-out, and carpal tunnel syndrome (Bedford and Yang 2010). However, a recent study has shown a much higher rate of radiographic union, achieved over a mean follow up period of 22 months, with very few other complications observed (Bedford and Yang 2010).

Serial radiographs are used to assess the progress of bony union and identify hardware failure. Cross-sectional imaging is rarely required, but US may have a role when dorsal impingement or protruding screw tips through the carpal tunnel floor are suspected clinically.

4.2.2 Hand

Arthrodesis of the first CMC joint with screw and plate fixation may be complicated by plate failure and non-union (Fig. 16). However, there is no evidence that other surgical options such as trapeziectomy and ligament reconstruction offer any significant advantage (Wajon et al. 2009). Complications include tendon adhesion or rupture and complex regional pain syndrome (type I). These occur in up to 10–22% of patients.

Crossed K-wires or small intraosseous screws (such as mini-Herbert screws or HCSs) are used to arthrodesis finger joints (Fig. 17). If the finger joint is larger in cross-sectional area, a dorsal tension band wiring system may be used which gives the advantage of allowing early movement. The tension band wiring system consists of two parallel K-wires crossing the fusion site obliquely, with a dorsal ‘figure-of-8’ wire loop (Fig. 18).

Screw fixation results in bony fusion in 85–100% over 7–10 weeks (Leibovic 2007). Complications include screw migration, breakage and infection (Fig. 19). K-wire fixation allows fusion in 5–10% of flexion which improves dexterity, but is associated with higher rates of non-union and other complications.

5 Osteotomy

5.1 Indications

Osteotomy is indicated when the shape of a bone requires modification. In the wrist, this is most commonly required for fracture malunion of the distal

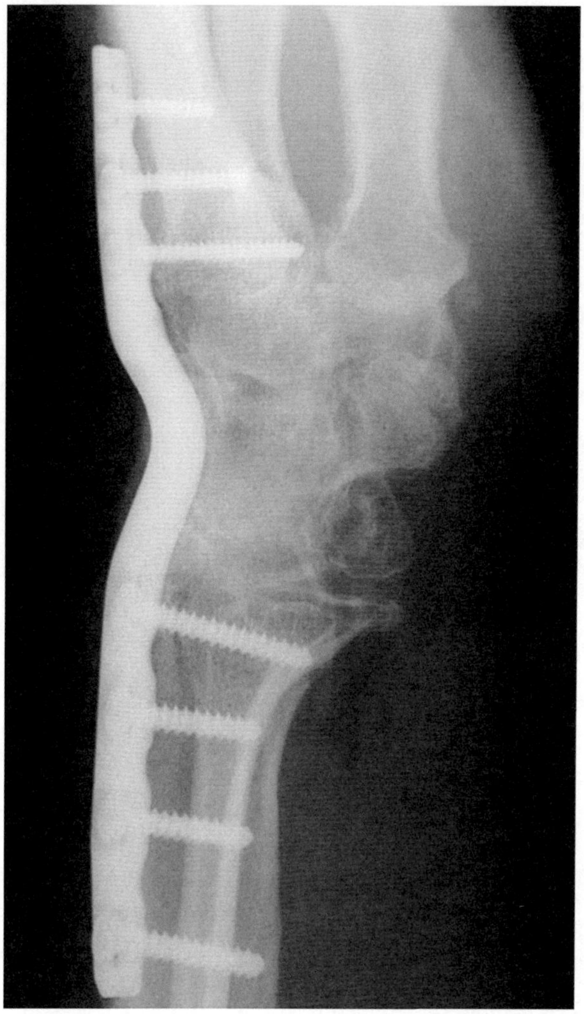

Fig. 13 Lateral radiograph of total wrist arthrodesis using a wrist fusion plate. The arthrodesis has been performed with the wrist in slight extension to allow improved power grip

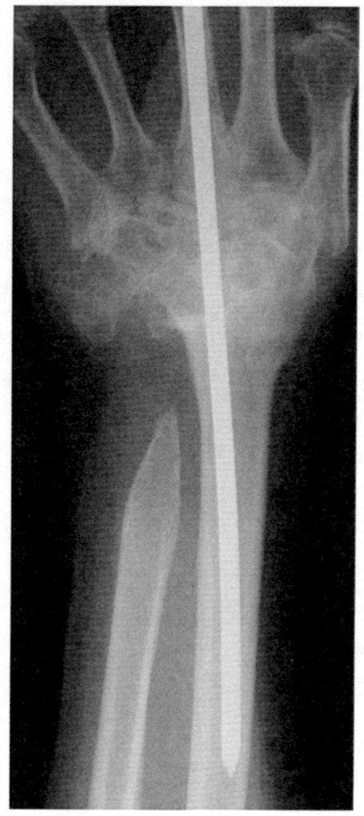

Fig. 14 Wrist arthrodesis in a rheumatoid patient achieved using a single longitudinal Steinman pin

radius, usually for an extra-articular deformity, but occasionally for more complex intra-articular deformity. The relative shortening of the radius caused by fracture is usually a 3D deformity which requires radial osteotomy and bone grafting to correct it. However, in unusual circumstances, if the radial deformity is simply one of shortening, an ulnar shortening osteotomy alone will realign the DRUJ surfaces (Fig. 20).

Osteotomy is also sometimes indicated for malunion of the scaphoid, when the classical 'hump back' deformity of a flexed scaphoid has resulted in secondary carpal instability, or in finger fractures which have healed with rotation. This produces a significant functional problem as the fingers 'cross over' each other as they bend into a fist.

Other indications for osteotomy relate to altering the pattern of load transfer across the joint. This used to be frequently performed for early OA, but is now reserved for conditions such as Kienbocks disease (where the radius is usually shortened at the metaphyseal level), and ulnar abutment (where the distal ulnar shaft is shortened to reduce the force across the degenerate or damaged TFCC).

5.2 Implants

Standard internal fixation implants are used for stabilisation of osteotomies around the wrist. For the distal radius, these are usually angularly stable implants, because indirect reduction techniques are used to correct the misshaped bone (Fig. 21).

Increasingly, surgeons are using 'anatomic' implants (shaped like the bone they are trying to correct) in radial osteotomy. These are usually applied on the volar surface of the distal radius. This did present problems in placing a large piece of cortico-cancellous bone graft into the defect when the 'natural' access for the graft was from the larger gap

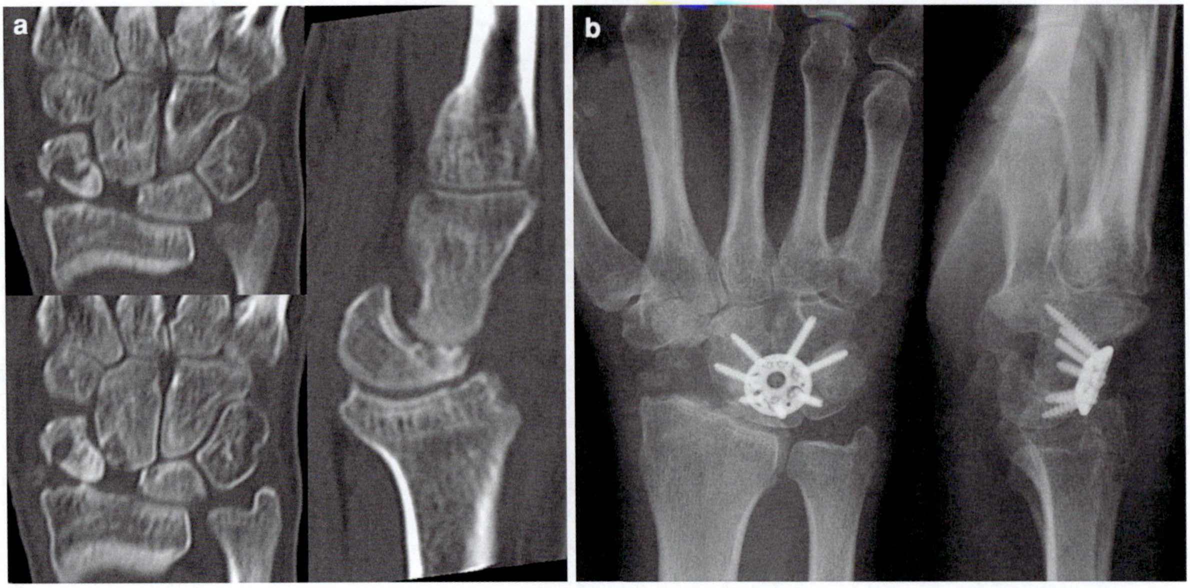

Fig. 15 Coronal and sagittal CT images (**a**) of a patient with a SNAC wrist. There is scaphoid non-union, scapholunate diastasis, DISI deformity and carpal collapse with secondary OA in the mid-carpal joint. There is also an un-united fracture of the radial styloid. A PA radiograph of the hand (**b**) shows the post-operative appearances following scaphoidectomy and a four corner fusion. The screws are well-sited in the capitate, hamate, lunate and triquetrum. However, there is residual dorsal angulation of the lunate with minor volar subluxation due to insufficient seating of the plate

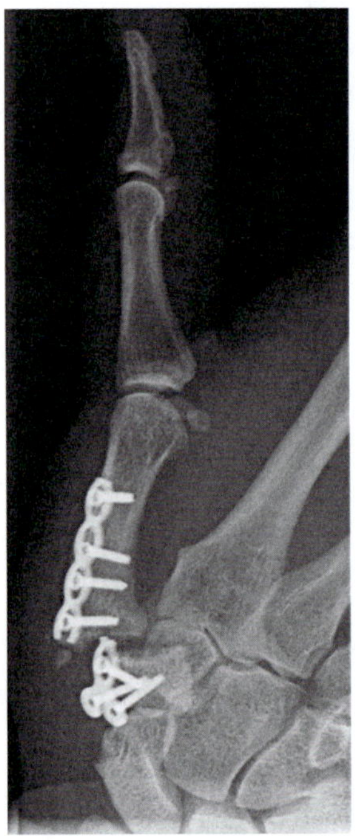

Fig. 16 Lateral radiograph of the thumb following arthrodesis of the first CMC joint with a mini fragment screw and plate fixation. The plate has fractured due to non-union of the arthrodesis with recurrent subluxation of the CMC joint

on the dorsal bone surface. However, the significant mechanical strength and stability provided by modern locking plates allows morselised cancellous bone or bone substitute to be packed into the defect through a small aperture.

Radial and ulnar osteotomies are generally very successful procedures. Complications are usually technique-related such as incomplete correction of deformity, implant-related issues (incorrect screw length, malposition of the implant) or delayed/non-union of the osteotomy. Similar complications exist in osteotomy of the scaphoid and fingers, but non-union is a more significant risk in scaphoid osteotomy than wrist or finger osteotomy.

6 Curettage and Bone Graft

6.1 Indications

Bone cysts are not uncommon in the phalanges, but are rare in the wrist. Occasionally, benign bone cysts and tumours, such as enchondromata, will require curettage and bone grafting.

Bone grafting is used more frequently to promote healing in conditions such as scaphoid non-union or after radial osteotomy.

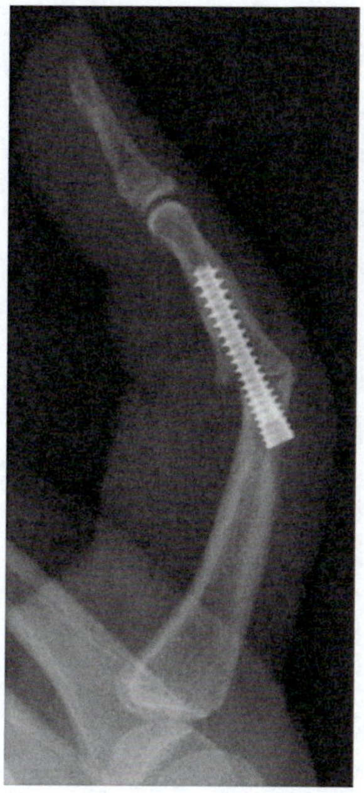

Fig. 17 Lateral radiograph showing satisfactory alignment of an IP joint arthrodesis with a compression screw. The joint is fixed in approximately 45° of flexion to help preserve function

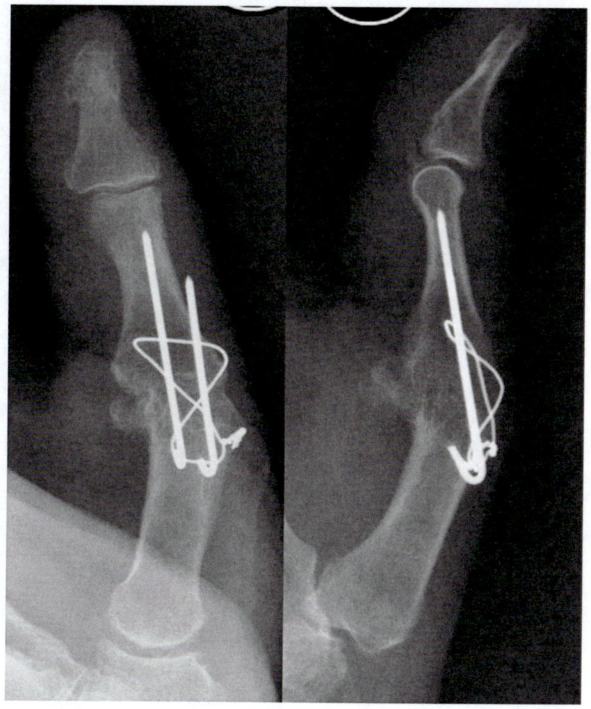

Fig. 18 PA and lateral radiographs of a first MCP arthrodesis performed for an unstable joint with secondary OA. The joint has been stabilised with K-wire and dorsal tension band wiring. Sound bony union has been achieved with the joint in flexion, although ideally the wires should penetrate the palmar cortex

6.2 Implant Choice

A structural bone graft is important in certain circumstances, and this will usually be harvested from the iliac crest (non-vascularised) or the distal radius on a vascular pedicle (vascularised). If the area to be grafted is stabilised by an appropriate strong implant (such as in corrective osteotomy for distal radius malunion), cancellous autograft or, increasingly, bone substitute will be indicated. Cancellous autograft can be harvested from the ipsilateral distal radius or the olecranon. Bone substitutes are either osteogenic (such as those containing bone morphogenic proteins (BMP) or hydroxyapatite) or inert stimulators of new bone growth (such as calcium sulfate). The former are more likely to be radiologically visible for months or even years after implantation, whilst the latter are usually only visible radiologically for a few weeks.

Radiographs are usually sufficient for follow up evaluation. MRI is indicated in cases where tumour recurrence is suspected (Fig. 22). The increasing use of bone substitutes has developed in response to the complications associated with harvesting of bone graft—particularly from the iliac crest. Haematoma, meralgia paraesthetica (injury to the lateral cutaneous nerve of the thigh) and scar tenderness may be encountered.

7 Tendon Repair

7.1 Indications

Tendon repair is indicated after traumatic division, attrition rupture or avulsion of the tendon insertion.

7.2 Implant Choice

No implants are used in primary tendon repair, which is achieved by intratendinous suturing of the tendon ends using non-absorbable suture material. Secondary reconstruction is performed when primary repair is not possible due to delayed presentation, infection, poor skin cover or other associated injuries. This usually involves two separate surgical procedures. The first stage is a re-creation of the tunnel for the tendon graft, which is necessary because of scarring and adhesions within the tendon sheath. It is achieved by the anatomical placement of a silastic rod (usually 2 mm

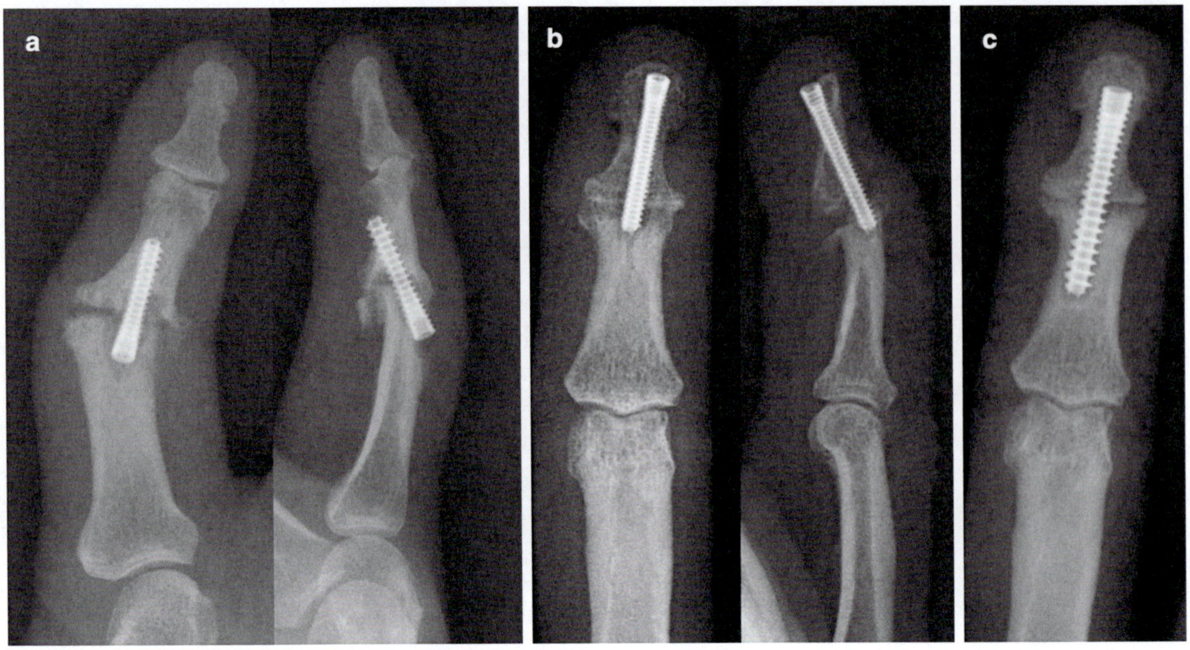

Fig. 19 Two examples of screw complications. In a PIP joint arthrodesis (**a**), the screw is placed too close to the dorsum of the cortex in the proximal phalanx, leading to loosening and bony lysis around the screw with non-union of the arthrodesis and recurrent joint malalignment. In the DIP joint arthrodesis (**b**), the screw is not sufficiently engaged within the middle phalanx. This arthrodesis will almost certainly fail, so a repeat arthrodesis was performed (**c**) which showed good screw alignment, but with some lysis around the screw indicating early loosening

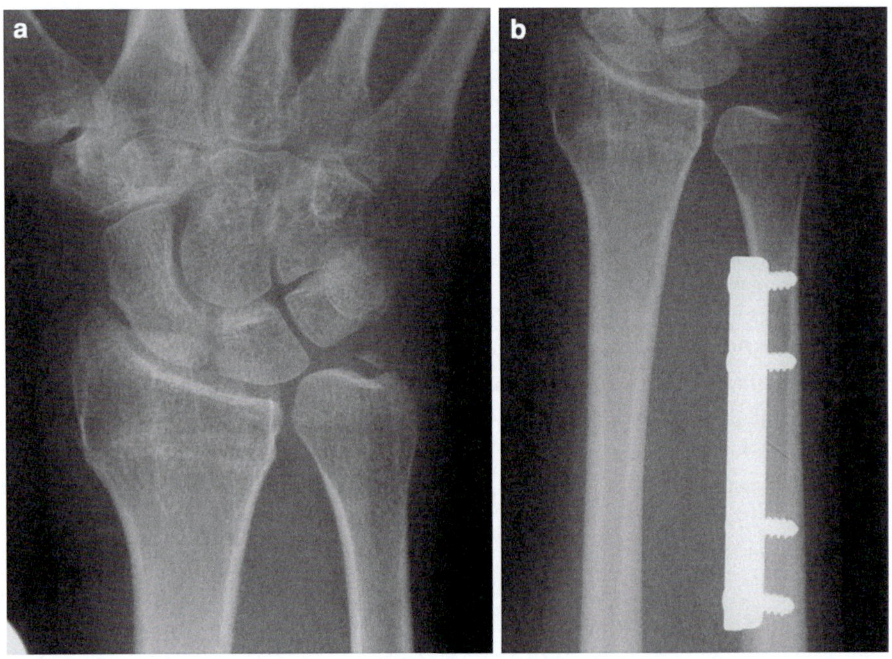

Fig. 20 PA radiograph (**a**) demonstrating uniplanar radial malunion with resultant length discrepancy between the radius and ulna, and abutment of the distal ulna onto the lunate and triquetrum. The post-operative radiograph (**b**) following shortening osteotomy of the ulna using a compression plate shows restoration of radioulnar alignment

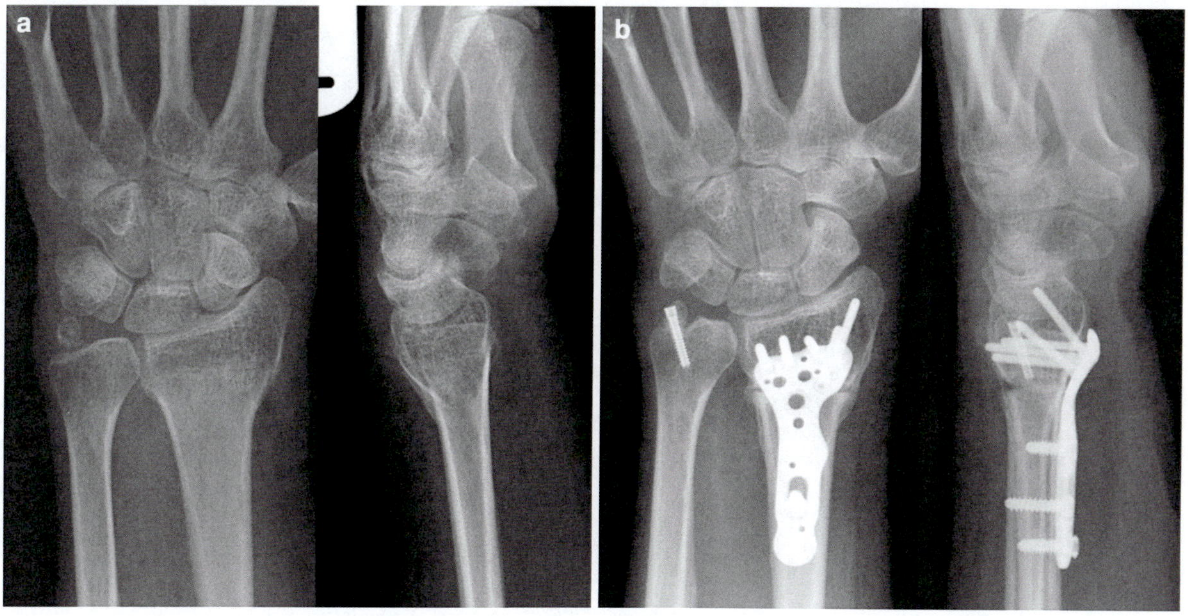

Fig. 21 PA and lateral radiographs (**a**) of a young adult with malunion of a distal radial fracture with residual dorsal angulation. There is also non-union of the ulnar styloid, and the DRUJ was clinically unstable. The post-operative radiographs (**b**) demonstrate bony union across the radial osteotomy which has been maintained in anatomic alignment with a volar plate. The ulnar styloid fracture has been stabilised with a compression screw to attempt to stabillise the DRUJ

diameter) along the whole length of the tendon sheath, around which a smooth lining forms over a number of months. It is replaced (in a second operation) with a tendon graft, which can now glide smoothly. This technique is most frequently performed on the flexor surface, but can also be used in extensor tendon defects.

Adhesion formation within the tendon sheath is common following tendon repair. Other complications include tendon re-rupture, pulley failure (or failure to recognise pulley injury at the time of repair), joint contracture and triggering (Lilly and Messer 2006). Breakdown of the repair requires further surgical repair, but clinical differentiation from adhesion formation may be difficult.

US can reliably assess the tendon repair, although access may be limited by finger flexion. Small headed 'hockeystick' probes allow improved visualisation. The repaired tendon is thickened and hyopechoic, and is surrounded by low reflective granulation tissue. Suture material is echogenic. Dynamic US evaluation of the tendon during gentle passive and active flexion/extension demonstrates paradoxical movement of the tendon ends when there is breakdown at the repair site.

8 Ligament Repair

8.1 Indications

Intrinsic ligament repair of the wrist is usually restricted to the ligaments of the proximal carpal row (the scapholunate and lunotriquetral ligaments). Surgical repair can be performed in the acute situation (usually within 3–4 weeks of injury) when the procedure is a true 'repair'. A high index of suspicion is essential to make an early diagnosis. Late presentation is more common and requires reconstruction rather than repair because of the irreversible shrinkage that occurs in the torn ligament surfaces over time.

Ligament injury secondary to joint dislocation is common in the thumb and fingers, although surgical repair is rarely necessary. Radiological monitoring of joint congruity will be necessary for 3–4 weeks after injury. Tears of the UCL of the thumb are caused by forced hyperextension and abduction. The ligament may either be partially or totally ruptured. Displaced UCL tears with the ligament remnant overlying the adductor aponeurosis (Stener lesion) will not heal and

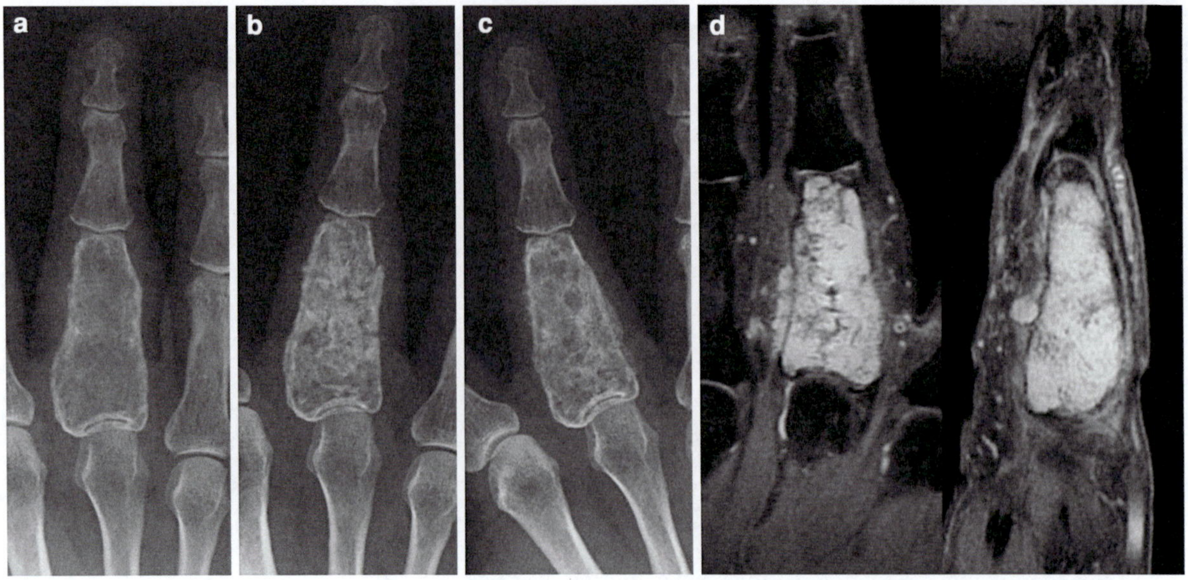

Fig. 22 PA radiograph (**a**) of a benign enchondroma within the proximal phalanx. The lesion has been treated by curettage and non-vascularised bone graft (**b**). However, several years later the patient represented with recurrent swelling and pain, and repeat radiograph (**c**) shows resorption of the bone graft material with internal lucency, cortical breakthrough and periosteal reaction. The coronal and sagittal T2FS MRI images (**d**) show high SI cartilage matrix. The appearances are strongly suggestive of chondrosarcoma transformation, which was confirmed following ray amputation

requires surgical repair or reattachment using a bone anchor.

8.2 Implant Choice

8.2.1 Wrist

Acute intrinsic ligament repairs must be stabilised until healing has occurred. This is either performed with multiple K-wires between the adjacent carpal bones, or with a small intraosseous screw, placed so as to hold the two adjacent bones tightly together. In both situations, the implants are always removed.

Reconstruction of an intrinsic ligament requires the same post-operative internal stabilisation as acute repair. Reconstruction of the scapholunate ligament is achieved by the use of a tendon graft, most usually from the flexor carpi radialis (FCR), passed through a substantial hole made in the scaphoid (up to 3 mm in diameter), and anchored to the lunate with a small bone anchor. This is termed as a Brunelli procedure, although other modifications are described (Brunelli and Brunelli 1995; Van Den Abbeele et al. 1998) (Fig. 23). The majority of patients experience improvement in pain and grip strength, although there is no long-term evidence to confirm that this will reduce the risk of development of OA.

A similar ligament reconstruction using tendon grafts is occasionally undertaken for instability of the first CMC joint of the thumb (Fig. 24). The procedure was described by Eaton and Littler using the FCR tendon, although other tendon grafts can be used (Brunelli et al. 1989; Eaton and Littler 1973). Long-term follow up has demonstrated good outcomes in the majority of patients, with prevention of secondary OA in those patients without pre-existing arthropathy (Eaton et al. 1984).

Post-operative radiographs demonstrate the location of drill holes and bone anchors, and the alteration in radiological measurements of instability. The radiographic appearances of scapholunate diastasis may persist post-operatively. Failure of reconstruction may be indicated by anchor migration. MRI can visualise the ligament reconstruction, but integrity throughout the whole of the tendon graft may be difficult due to magic angle effects. Interpretation of MRI will depend on knowledge of the exact procedure.

8.2.2 Hand

Stabilisation of an unstable finger dislocation is performed with a trans-articular K-wire, usually left in situ for 3 weeks.

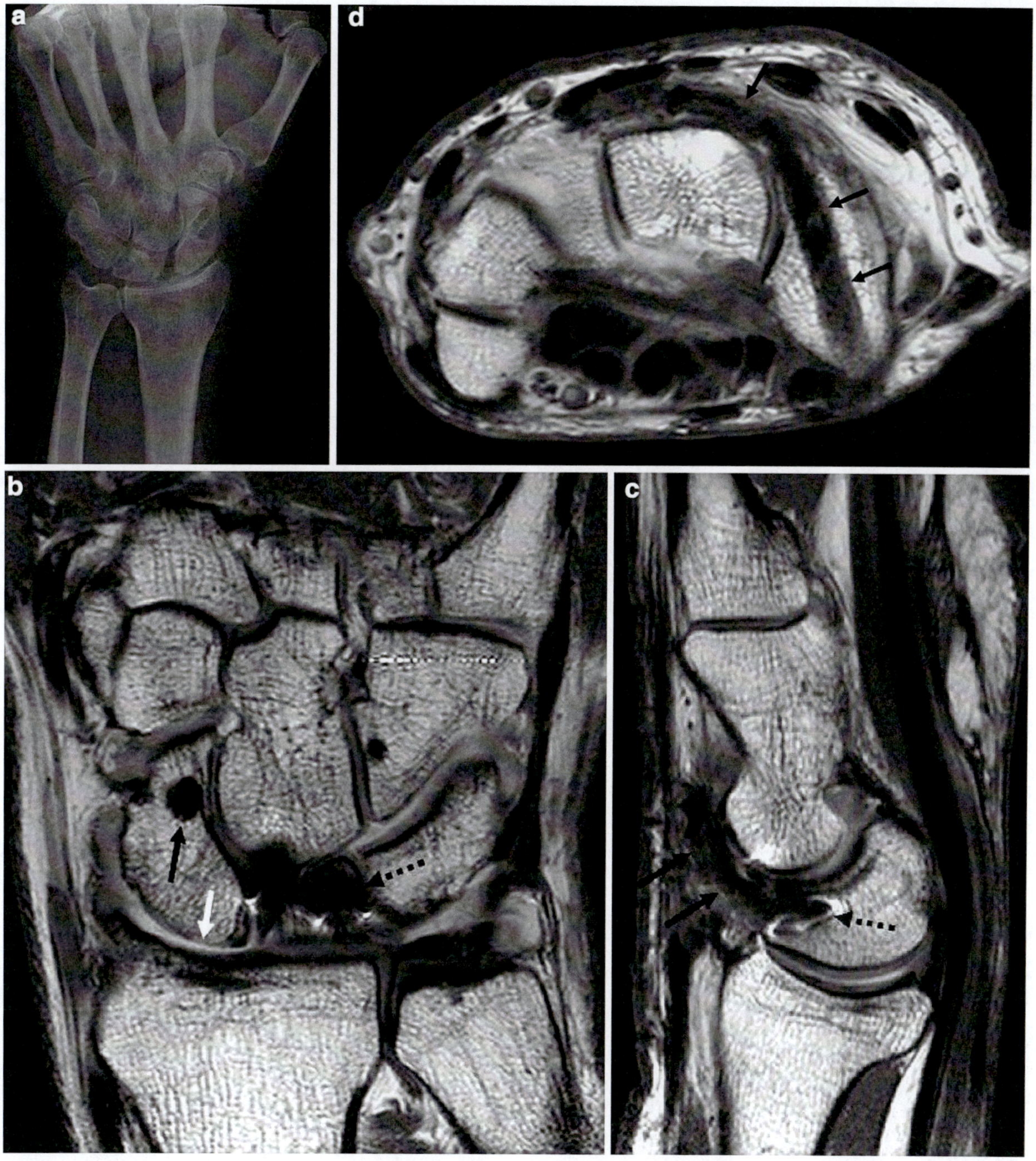

Fig. 23 PA radiograph (**a**) acquired following a Brunelli procedure for reconstruction of the scapholunate ligament. The tunnel within the scaphoid is clearly evident, and there is persistent scaholunate diastasis. The coronal (**b**), sagittal (**c**) and axial (**d**) T1W MR images also clearly show the scaphoid tunnel and ligament graft as low-signal intensity (*black arrows*). There is susceptibility artefact from the resorbable bone anchor in the dorsal aspect of the lunate (*broken arrow*). The graft appears intact. However, there is early articular cartilage loss on the proximal scaphoid (*white arrow*), which was not present on the pre-operative imaging, and there is residual dorsal tilt of the lunate

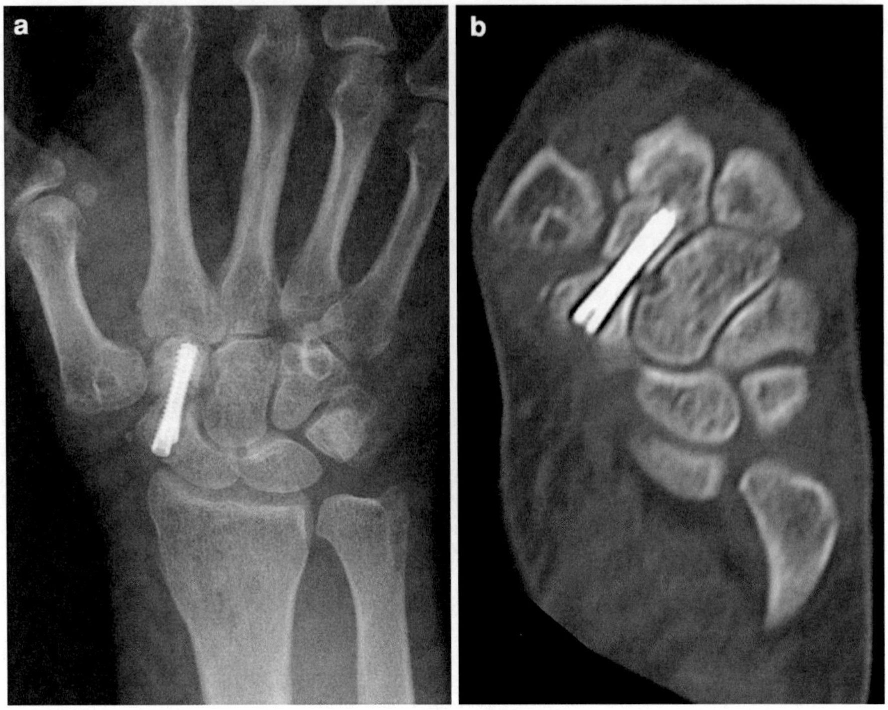

Fig. 24 PA radiograph (**a**) of a patient following trapeziectomy and arthrodesis of the scaphotrapezoid joint, and ligament reconstruction of the first CMC joint performed to treat pain and instability secondary to OA. The osseous tunnel, created for ligament reconstruction, is seen in the base of the first MC which remains subluxed. The screw has an area of lysis around it, suggesting loosening and persistent non-union. A coronal oblique CT image (**b**) confirms non-union of the arthrodesis and demonstrates the osseous tunnel within the first MC

Reattachment of an avulsion of the UCL of the thumb is usually performed with a small bone anchor. US may be utilised to identify failed ligament reconstruction. The ligament will be thickened and hypoechoic, and dynamic evaluation with radial stress helps identify abnormal joint widening. Adhesions between the repaired UCL and the adductor aponeurosis may cause pain and limitation of movement of the aponeurosis, which may be seen on US during flexion and extension of the MCP joint. Treatment is with physiotherapy.

Avulsion of the palmar (volar) plate is a common injury caused by hyperextension of, usually, the proximal interphalangeal joint. A small fleck of avulsed bone can often be seen adjacent to the palmar surface of the middle phalangeal base, or more subtle changes of erosion or blunting of the edge of the middle phalanx may also be noted. Avulsion of a fragment of bone which comprises more than one-third of the total articular surface will lead to inevitable instability of the joint and must be very carefully monitored. Subtle radiological evidence of dorsal subluxation of the affected joint must be sought in the first few weeks after injury, or in cases where functional recovery is delayed. If persistent subluxation or frank instability of the joint is identified, surgical reattachment of the volar plate to the base of the middle phalanx is indicated.

9 TFCC Repair

9.1 Indications

The triangular fibrocartilage complex (TFCC) stabilises the ulnar side of the wrist and the DRUJ. It is often injured during a fall onto the outstretched hand, and is associated with distal radius fractures. Injury to the ulnar styloid can be associated with a TFCC tear—especially if the ulnar styloid is fractured at its base. Repair of the TFCC is indicated if there is instability of the ulnocarpal joint or the DRUJ.

It is important to stress that not all abnormalities of the TFCC are true tears secondary to physical injury. Defects are commonly seen in the TFCC as either a congenital finding or a degenerative feature and the term 'TFCC *tear*' should be used with discretion, as this implies a traumatic aetiology. It may be prudent to describe these findings as 'TFCC *defects*'—where their aetiology is uncertain or yet to be determined.

9.2 Implant Choice

Repair is either performed through an open approach or arthroscopically. Whichever method is chosen, a

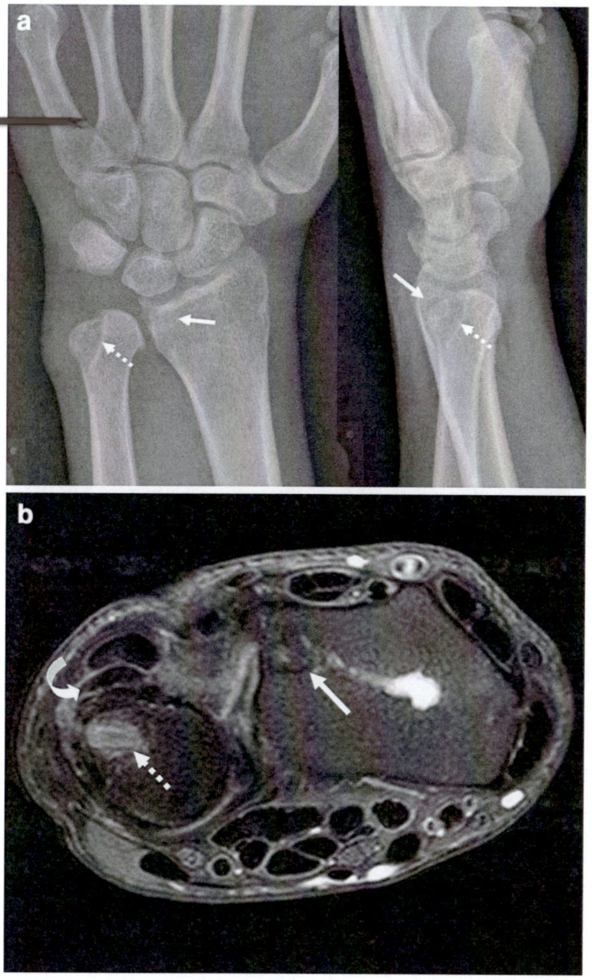

Fig. 25 PA and lateral radiographs (**a**) of the wrist following a ligamentous reconstruction of the DRUJ. Osseous tunnels can be seen in the distal radius (*white arrows*) and ulna (*broken white arrows*). The patient had persistent symptoms of pain and instability, and there is separation of the radius and ulna at the DRUJ. An axial T2WFS MR image (**b**) demonstrates a part of the tendon graft (*curved white arrow*) deep to the ECU tendon. However, the graft did not appear continuous and no graft is seen entering either the radial (*white arrow*) or ulnar (*broken white arrow*) tunnels. There is also marked recurrence of volar DRUJ instability indicating failure of the graft reconstruction

series of strong nylon sutures are passed through the cartilage disc to secure it to the external joint capsule. If the TFCC is irreparable, then a DRUJ ligament reconstruction may be indicated. The Adams procedure utilises a palmaris longus tendon graft to stabilise the DRUJ with drill holes placed through the distal radius and ulna (Adams and Berger 2002) (Fig. 25). Instability of the DRUJ in the presence of skeletal deformity, should first be addressed by correction of the skeletal deformity, which may be sufficient to restore complete stability (Lawler and Adams 2007). Recovery of strength and motion after repair, is seen in 85% of patients with chronic DRUJ instability (Adams and Lawler 2007).

If symptoms persist following TFCC repair, imaging may be required to exclude other causes of ulnar sided wrist pain, including ECU tendonitis or tendon subluxation, ulnar impaction, pisotriqutral chondromalacia or OA, and secondary OA of the DRUJ. In recurrent injury repeat MR arthrography may be required. Complications of DRUJ stabilisation include recurrent pain and instability. Radiographs document the location of the drill holes and the alignment of the DRUJ.

10 Conclusions

Radiological interpretation of the post-operative hand and wrist requires a thorough knowledge of the objectives of treatment in order to distinguish between acceptable findings and genuine complications on post-operative radiographs. Radiologists should be aware when cross-sectional imaging is indicated to provide diagnostic information that can help determine management protocols.

The range of orthopaedic implants and techniques of soft tissue reconstruction continue to evolve, and it is important to engage with the hand surgeon to be conversant with new techniques and procedures that are introduced in order to be able to correctly interpret radiological investigations.

References

Adams BD (2004) Total wrist arthroplasty. Tech Hand Up Extrem Surg 8(3):130–137

Adams BD, Berger RA (2002) An anatomic reconstruction of the distal radioulnar ligaments for posttraumatic distal radioulnar joint instability. J Hand Surg Am 27(2):243–251

Adams BD, Lawler E (2007) Chronic instability of the distal radioulnar joint. J Am Acad Orthop Surg 15(9):571–575

Arora R, Lutz M, Hennerbichler A, Krappinger D, Espen D, Gabl M (2007) Complications following internal fixation of unstable distal radius fracture with a palmar locking-plate. J Orthop Trauma 21(5):316–322

Bedford B, Yang SS (2010) High fusion rates with circular plate fixation for four-corner arthrodesis of the wrist. Clin Orthop Relat Res 468(1):163–168

Berglund LM, Messer TM (2009) Complications of volar plate fixation for managing distal radius fractures. J Am Acad Orthop Surg 17(6):369–377

Brunelli GA, Brunelli GR (1995) A new technique to correct carpal instability with scaphoid rotary subluxation: a preliminary report. J Hand Surg Am 20(3 Pt 2):S82–S85

Brunelli G, Monini L, Brunelli F (1989) Stabilisation of the trapezio-metacarpal joint. J Hand Surg Br 14(2):209–212

Buchler U, Fischer T (1987) Use of a minicondylar plate for metacarpal and phalangeal periarticular injuries. Clin Orthop Relat Res 214:53–58

Bushnell BD, McWilliams AD, Messer TM (2007) Complications in dorsal percutaneous cannulated screw fixation of nondisplaced scaphoid waist fractures. J Hand Surg Am 32(6):827–833

Cavaliere CM, Chung KC (2008) A systematic review of total wrist arthroplasty compared with total wrist arthrodesis for rheumatoid arthritis. Plast Reconstr Surg 122(3):813–825

Chan M, Chowchuen P, Workman T, Eilenberg S, Schweitzer M, Resnick D (1998) Silicone synovitis: MR imaging in five patients. Skeletal Radiol 27(1):13–17

Chung KC, Burns PB, Wilgis EF, Burke FD, Regan M, Kim HM et al (2009) A multicenter clinical trial in rheumatoid arthritis comparing silicone metacarpophalangeal joint arthroplasty with medical treatment. J Hand Surg Am 34(5):815–823

Downing ND, Oni JA, Davis TR, Vu TQ, Dawson JS, Martel AL (2002) The relationship between proximal pole blood flow and the subjective assessment of increased density of the proximal pole in acute scaphoid fractures. J Hand Surg Am 27(3):402–408

Eaton RG, Littler JW (1973) Ligament reconstruction for the painful thumb carpometacarpal joint. J Bone Joint Surg Am 55(8):1655–1666

Eaton RG, Lane LB, Littler JW, Keyser JJ (1984) Ligament reconstruction for the painful thumb carpometacarpal joint: a long-term assessment. J Hand Surg Am 9(5):692–699

Greatting MD, Bishop AT (1993) Intrafocal (Kapandji) pinning of unstable fractures of the distal radius. Orthop Clin North Am 24(2):301–307

Kopylov P, Tagil M (2007) Distal radioulnar joint replacement. Tech Hand Up Extrem Surg 11(1):109–114

Lawler E, Adams BD (2007) Reconstruction for DRUJ instability. Hand (N Y) 2(3):123–126

Leibovic SJ (2007) Instructional course lecture. Arthrodesis of the interphalangeal joints with headless compression screws. J Hand Surg Am 32(7):1113–1119

Lilly SI, Messer TM (2006) Complications after treatment of flexor tendon injuries. J Am Acad Orthop Surg 14(7): 387–396

Megerle K, Keutgen X, Muller M, Germann G, Sauerbier M (2008) Treatment of scaphoid non-unions of the proximal third with conventional bone grafting and mini-Herbert screws: an analysis of clinical and radiological results. J Hand Surg Eur Vol 33(2):179–185

Scheufler O, Andresen R, Radmer S, Erdmann D, Exner K, Germann G (2005) Hook of hamate fractures: critical evaluation of different therapeutic procedures. Plast Reconstr Surg 115(2):488–497

Trail IA, Martin JA, Nuttall D, Stanley JK (2004) Seventeen-year survivorship analysis of silastic metacarpophalangeal joint replacement. J Bone Joint Surg Br 86(7):1002–1006

Van Den Abbeele KL, Loh YC, Stanley JK, Trail IA (1998) Early results of a modified Brunelli procedure for scapholunate instability. J Hand Surg Br 23(2):258–261

Vance MC, Hernandez JD, Didonna ML, Stern PJ (2005) Complications and outcome of four-corner arthrodesis: circular plate fixation versus traditional techniques. J Hand Surg Am 30(6):1122–1127

Wajon A, Carr E, Edmunds I, Ada L (2009) Surgery for thumb (trapeziometacarpal joint) osteoarthritis. Cochrane Database Syst Rev (4): CD004631

Walsh JJ 4th, Bishop AT (2000) Diagnosis and management of hamate hook fractures. Hand Clin 16(3):397–403, viii

Welling RD, Jacobson JA, Jamadar DA, Chong S, Caoili EM, Jebson PJ (2008) MDCT and radiography of wrist fractures: radiographic sensitivity and fracture patterns. AJR Am J Roentgenol 190(1):10–16

Wharton DM, Casaletto JA, Choa R, Brown DJ (2010) Outcome following coronal fractures of the hamate. J Hand Surg Eur Vol 35(2):146–149

FSC
www.fsc.org
MIX
Papier | Fördert gute Waldnutzung
FSC® C083411

Kolibri 360 GmbH
Ferdinand-Jühlke-Straße 7
99095 Erfurt, Deutschland
produktsicherheit@kolibri360.de

Independent Review for Banks
The Complete BSA/AML Workbook

ISBN-13: **978-0-6152-3790-9**

Published By
ImpactAML–INX3 Financial Press
Las Vegas, Nevada

Other Books by the Authors:

SAR Investigations – The Complete BSA/AML Desktop Reference
Enhanced Due Diligence –The Complete BSA/AML Desktop Reference
Independent Review for MSBs –The Complete BSA/AML Audit Workbook
AML Risk Assessment for Tribal Casinos –The Complete BSA/AML Audit Workbook

Forward

Since passing the Bank Secrecy Act (BSA) decades ago, Congress and various non-governmental organizations, such as the Financial Action Task Force, have continued to add laws, regulations, guidance, and best practices to the regulatory landscape. After 2001, anti-money laundering regulatory enforcement became much more severe, and the burden on financial institutions to implement compliant anti-money laundering (AML) programs grew enormously. In response, the Federal Financial Institutions Examination Council (FFIEC) issued an examinations manual to bring clarity to the compliance and examination processes. While the FFIEC manual is an excellent resource guide for developing an AML compliance program, it has not made the auditing of such compliance programs much easier. Even since the publication of the FFIEC manual, more than a few financial institutions have found themselves facing regulatory enforcement actions and multi-million dollar fines!

It is almost impossible to simply read a several-hundred page manual on AML programs and then use that same manual for audit purposes. When you get on an airplane, you can be sure that the pilots have read the operating manual for the type of airplane being flown (which, for a typical airliner, makes the FFIEC manual look like a small pamphlet!). Yet the pilots will operate the flight using *checklists*. Checklists for downloading the weight and balance data, checklists for starting the engines, checklists for takeoff, climb, level-off, descent, landing and shutting the plane down at the destination gate. The checklists are developed by parsing the information in the airplane's manual such that is useful. The checklists allow the pilots an efficient method to make sure that all the i's are dotted and all the t's crossed for the successful conduct of their flight. This book accomplishes the same thing for the pilots of BSA compliance, i.e., BSA officers and auditors. We've taken the FFIEC manual and its voluminous information and parsed it into categories and questions such that its information becomes useful for audit purposes.

One of the four major pillars of the USA PATRIOT Act (Section 352) requires that financial institutions have an independent review conducted of their AML programs. Further, the person conducting the review cannot be the Bank Secrecy Act/AML compliance officer. In effect, this requirement forces a non-BSA specialist to try and digest all the information covered in the FFIEC manual and pass judgment. If you are a BSA auditor, you are already aware that increased regulatory complexity has made your job difficult and fraught with risk. As a non-BSA specialist, it is essential that you have the correct tools to navigate the vast regulatory requirements. This Workbook is such a tool.

The audience for this book is both BSA auditors *and* compliance officers. The latter can utilize the Workbook to design a comprehensive AML program. The former can use this Workbook to check their firm's BSA program status and carry out their duty to keep senior management informed.

In our remediation project work, we have seen deficiencies noted by regulators that do not seem to be obviously related to the BSA and do not appear anywhere in the FFIEC manual. Such items are generally noted in confidential documentation such as exit meeting minutes or memorandums. This Workbook adds additional value for the auditor by having these items included. Many BSA officers and inside counsel who have never performed BSA remediation work are often surprised that these items can actually be in scope for examination, but they most definitely are!

On the old hit television show, *Hill Street Blues*, at the beginning of each episode, Sergeant Phil Esterhaus would end his morning briefing to the patrol officers with the admonition: "Hey! Let's be careful out there!" Along with the functionality we try to provide you via this Workbook, I echo the good sergeant's counsel.

Howard Steiner

Table of Contents

Introduction

Each of the questions in this Workbook need to be answered in order to perform a complete and thorough review sufficient in the eyes of your regulator. Some questions may seem to be redundant across categories. This is so because each category is independent. So, when answering questions that you may think you've come across before, try answering them with regard to the specific requirements of the *category* of BSA compliance.

At the beginning of each section, there is guidance regarding the category's topic. The provided information is an amalgam of information from numerous public sources along with best practices added by the authors. Each question should be answered and an explanation or qualifying statement should be added. Use the guidance provided as a check to make sure you have covered the topic thoroughly in your answer

You should use the *Follow-up* section of each question to make notes of actions you plan to take in the future –if need be– to address the comments you have recorded.

AML Program

A written anti-money laundering program is one of the four main pillars of AML compliance as prescribed by Section 352 of the USA PATRIOT Act. (The other three are: the appointment of a BSA compliance officer; conducting an independent review; and providing training for appropriate personnel.) The questions in this category may seem very broad, but they will be drilled down upon in subsequent sections.

For purposes of compliance with the broad requirement of having a written AML program, FFIEC examiners are instructed to ensure that a financial institution's AML program addresses topics both generally and specifically. Topics that should be discussed generally in your BSA compliance manual include: basic AML information, descriptive information regarding the nature of your BSA program, reference to governing laws and regulations, money laundering risks, the implementation of policies, procedures and internal controls, board of directors approval of the compliance program, testing and independent reviews, and the existence of a customer information program.

Your AML program must also be written so as to address the risks that are associated with the nature of your bank's product/service offerings, customers, geographic footprint, and transaction types. The written program must address the fact that a risk assessment of your institution regarding exposure to these risks has been performed, and is periodically re-performed.

1. Do your anti-money laundering policies specifically define and state the risks presented by money laundering in its different forms (e.g., placement, layering, integration)?

☐ *Yes*

☐ *No*

Comments:

Follow-up:

2. Do your anti-money laundering policies address compliance with BSA and related anti-money laundering laws and regulations?

☐ ***Yes***

☐ ***No***

Comments:

Follow-up:

3. Does your AML program specifically address and identify high risk activities, businesses, and foreign countries commonly associated with money laundering?

☐ ***Yes***

☐ ***No***

Comments:

Follow-up:

4. Is your BSA/AML compliance program approved by your board of directors and noted in writing in the Board's minutes?

- ☐ *Yes*
- ☐ *No*

Comments:

Follow-up:

5. Is your bank's BSA/AML compliance program commensurate with its respective BSA/AML risk profile?

- ☐ *Yes*
- ☐ *No*

Comments:

Follow-up:

6. Does your BSA program provide a documented system of internal controls to ensure ongoing compliance?

☐ ***Yes***

☐ ***No***

Comments:

Follow-up:

7. Does your BSA program designate an individual or individuals responsible for managing BSA compliance (BSA compliance officer)? (A bank must designate one or more persons to coordinate and monitor day-to-day compliance. This requirement is detailed in the federal banking agencies' BSA compliance program regulations)

☐ ***Yes***

☐ ***No***

Comments:

Follow-up:

8. Does your BSA compliance program call for training of appropriate personnel? (Training is a mandatory component of Section 352 of the PATRIOT Act)

☐ *Yes*

☐ *No*

Comments:

Follow-up:

9. Does your BSA compliance program include a formal customer identification program (CIP)?

☐ *Yes*

☐ *No*

Comments:

Follow-up:

10. Does evidence exist to support the requirement that your bank's board of directors and management have created a culture of compliance to ensure staff adherence to your bank's BSA/AML policies, procedures, and processes?

☐ ***Yes***

☐ ***No***

Comments:

Follow-up:

11. Does your BSA program provide for independent testing of BSA/AML compliance by qualified personnel?

☐ ***Yes***

☐ ***No***

Comments:

Follow-up:

12. Is your firm's BSA compliance program fully implemented across all business units?

☐ *Yes*

☐ *No*

Comments:

Follow-up:

13. Is the level of sophistication of your bank's internal controls commensurate with the size, structure, risks and complexity of your bank (products, services, geography, etc.)?

☐ *Yes*

☐ *No*

Comments:

Follow-up:

14. If your bank is a large, complex financial institution, does your internal control structure address risks and compliance requirements unique to particular lines of business or departments?

☐ *Yes*

☐ *No*

Comments:

Follow-up:

15. Does your bank's AML program identify banking operations with respect to products, services, customers, and geographic locations that:

a. Are more vulnerable to abuse by money launderers and criminals;
b. Provide for periodic updates to the bank's risk profile; and,
c. Provide elements tailored to manage those risks?

☐ *Yes*

☐ *No*

Comments:

Follow-up:

16. Does your compliance process provide for informing the bank's board of directors (or a committee thereof) and senior management of:

☐ *Yes*

☐ *No*

Comments:

Follow-up:

Cash Intensive Businesses

Cash-intensive businesses and entities cover various industry sectors. Most of these businesses are conducting legitimate business; however, some aspects of these businesses may be susceptible to money laundering or terrorist financing. Common examples noted in FFIEC guidance include, but are not limited to, the following:

- Convenience stores.
- Restaurants.
- Retail stores.
- Liquor stores.
- Cigarette distributors.
- Privately-owned automated teller machines (ATMs).
- Vending machine operators.
- Parking garages.

Bank AML programs must include policies, procedures and controls for establishing and maintaining relationships with cash-intensive businesses, to include:

- The identification of high-risk relationships;
- The assessment of ML risks
- The performance of due diligence at account opening *and* periodically throughout the relationship; and,
- Application of sufficient monitoring for unusual or suspicious activity.

The AML program must address assignment of resources and/or efforts for conducting initial and ongoing risk assessments of cash-intensive businesses, with the preponderance of resources directed at accounts that pose the greatest risk of money laundering or terrorist financing.

1. When establishing and maintaining relationships with cash-intensive businesses, does your bank have policies, procedures, and processes to identify high-risk relationships; assess AML risks; complete due diligence at account opening and periodically throughout the relationship; and include such relationships in appropriate monitoring for unusual or suspicious activity?

☐ *Yes*

☐ *No*

Comments:

Follow-up:

2. At the time of account opening, does your bank have an understanding of the customer's:

a. Business type;
b. Operations;
c. Intended use of the account, including anticipated transaction volume, products, and services used; and,
d. The geographic locations involved in the relationship?

☐ *Yes*

☐ *No*

Comments:

Follow-up:

3. Does your AML program detail all of the following factors to be considered when identifying the risks associated with a cash intensive customer:

a. The purpose of the account;
b. The volume, frequency, and nature of currency transactions;
c. Customer history (e.g., length of relationship, Currency Transaction Report (CTR) filings,
d. Suspicious Activity Report (SAR) filings);
e. The primary business activity, products, and services offered *by* and *to* the customer;
f. The corporate or business structure;
g. The geographic locations and jurisdictions of the customer's operations.

☐ *Yes*

☐ *No*

Comments:

Follow-up:

4. For those customers deemed to be of particularly high risk, has bank management implemented sound practices such as periodic on-site visits, interviews with the businesses' management, or closer reviews of transactional activity?

☐ *Yes*

☐ *No*

Comments:

Follow-up:

CDD & EDD

The objective of CDD procedures should be to enable the bank to predict with relative certainty the types of transactions in which a customer is likely to engage. These procedures assist the bank in determining when transactions are potentially suspicious. The concept of CDD begins with verifying the customer's identity and assessing the risks associated with that customer. Procedures should also include enhanced CDD for high risk customers and ongoing due diligence of the customer base.

Effective CDD policies, procedures, and processes provide the critical framework that enables the bank to comply with regulatory requirements and to report suspicious activity. An illustration of this concept is provided in the FFIEC Examination Manual, Appendix K ("Customer Risk Versus Due Diligence and Suspicious Activity Monitoring").

BSA/AML policies, procedures, and processes should include CDD guidelines that:

- Are commensurate with the bank's BSA/AML risk profile, paying particular attention to high-risk customers.
- Contain a clear statement of management's overall expectations and establish specific staff responsibilities, including who is responsible for reviewing or approving changes to a customer's risk rating or profile, as applicable.
- Ensure that the bank possesses sufficient customer information to implement an effective suspicious activity monitoring system.
- Provide guidance for documenting analysis associated with the due diligence process, including guidance for resolving issues when insufficient or inaccurate information is obtained.
- Ensure the bank maintains current customer information.

Customer Risk

Management should have a thorough understanding of the money laundering or terrorist financing risks of the bank's customer base. Under this approach, the bank will obtain information at account opening sufficient to develop an understanding of normal and expected activity for the customer's occupation or business operations. Much of the CDD information can be confirmed through an information-reporting agency, banking references (for larger accounts), correspondence and telephone conversations with the customer, and visits to the customer's place of business. Additional steps may include obtaining third-party references or researching public information (e.g., on the Internet or commercial databases). CDD procedures should include periodic monitoring of the customer relationship to determine whether there are substantive changes to the original CDD information (e.g., change in employment or business operations).

Enhanced Due Diligence

Enhanced due diligence is defined and prescribed for foreign correspondent banking accounts and for private banking accounts carried for senior foreign political figures. The 312 guidance also uses the term "increased due diligence" for cases where the statutory triggers for EDD are not present.

Best practices and regulatory expectations, however, suggest that a risk based approach to BSA compliance be flexible to require, when appropriate, greater levels of due diligence across a range of high risk customer types.

Generally speaking then, enhanced/special due diligence (EDD) can be defined for practical purposes as:

Procedures established by a bank for higher-risk accounts, whom for risk mitigation purposes, require the bank to:

- Obtain a more detailed understanding of a customer's activities;
- Perform more frequent monitoring of transactions and account information; and
- More thoroughly investigate the backgrounds of these customers and affiliated individuals/businesses.

Regulatory guidance also requires that banks have a policy and procedures to be followed in circumstances where it cannot perform appropriate due diligence with respect to a private banking account, including when the covered financial institution should refuse to open the account, suspend transaction activity, file a suspicious activity report, or close the account.

1. Do your bank's policies and procedures address BSA objectives requiring banks to predict –with relative certainty– the types of transactions in which a customer is likely to engage?

☐ *Yes*

☐ *No*

Comments:

Follow-up:

2. Do your bank's CDD policies and procedures effectively address the assessment of the risks associated with each particular customer?

☐ *Yes*

☐ *No*

Comments:

Follow-up:

3. Do your bank's BSA/AML policies, procedures, and processes include CDD guidelines that:

a. Are commensurate with the bank's BSA/AML risk profile, paying particular attention to high-risk customers?
b. Contain a clear statement of management's overall expectations and establish specific staff responsibilities, including who is responsible for reviewing or approving changes to a customer's risk rating or profile, as applicable?
c. Ensure that the bank possesses sufficient customer information to implement an effective suspicious activity monitoring system?
d. Provide guidance for documenting analysis associated with the due diligence process, including such for resolving issues when insufficient or inaccurate information is obtained?
e. Ensure the bank maintains current customer information?

☐ *Yes*

☐ *No*

Comments:

Follow-up:

4. Does your bank obtain information at account opening sufficient to develop an understanding of *usual and expected* activity for a customer's occupation or business operations?

☐ *Yes*

☐ *No*

Comments:

Follow-up:

5. Do your bank's CDD procedures include periodic monitoring of customers' information and business relationships in order to determine whether there have been substantive changes to the original CDD information (e.g., change in employment or business operations)?

☐ *Yes*

☐ *No*

Comments:

Follow-up:

6. Do your bank's policies and procedures include provisions for more thorough review of high-risk customers and their transactions at account opening and more frequently throughout the term of their relationship with the bank?

☐ *Yes*

☐ *No*

Comments:

Follow-up:

7. For accounts that your bank determines as being of high risk, is the following information recorded:

a. Purpose of the account?
b. Source of funds and wealth?
c. Beneficial owners of the accounts, if applicable?
d. Customer's (or beneficial owners') occupation or type of business?
e. Financial statements?
f. Banking references?
g. Domicile (i.e., where the business is incorporated)?
h. Proximity of the customer's residence, place of employment, or place of business to the bank?
i. Description of the customer's primary trade area and whether international transactions are expected to be routine?
j. Description of the business operations, the anticipated volume of currency and total sales, and a list of major customers and suppliers.
k. Explanations for changes in account activity

☐ *Yes*

☐ *No*

Comments:

Follow-up:

8. Does your bank's management have a thorough understanding of the money laundering or terrorist financing risks of the bank's customer base, and is there documented proof to that effect?

☐ ***Yes***

☐ ***No***

Comments:

Follow-up:

9. Does your bank's determination of whom or what customer types constitute a high risk take into consideration:

a. Customers' business activity?
b. Ownership structure?
c. The anticipated or actual volume and types of transactions, including those transactions involving high-risk jurisdictions?

☐ ***Yes***

☐ ***No***

Comments:

Follow-up:

10. Does your bank consider the following examples of situations in which enhanced due diligence may be appropriate:

a. The bank is entering into a relationship with a *new* customer?
b. The customer's principals or beneficiaries reside in a foreign jurisdiction, or a *trust* or its funding mechanisms are established offshore?
c. Assets or transactions are *atypical* for the type and character of the customer?
d. The account type, size, assets, or transactions are *atypical* for the bank?
e. International funds transfers are conducted, particularly through offshore funding sources?
f. Accounts are funded with easily transportable assets such as gemstones, precious metals, coins, artwork, rare stamps, or negotiable instruments?
g. Accounts or relationships are maintained in which the identities of the principals, or beneficiaries, or sources of funds are unknown or cannot easily be determined?
h. Accounts benefit charitable organizations or other non-governmental organizations (NGOs) that may be used as a conduit for illegal activities?
i. Interest on lawyers' trust accounts (IOLTA) (e.g., holding and processing significant dollar amounts)?
j. Account assets which include PICs?
k. Senior Foreign Political Figures are parties to any accounts or transactions?

☐ *Yes*

☐ *No*

Comments:

Follow-up:

Concentration Accounts

OVERVIEW

Concentration accounts are internal accounts established to facilitate the processing and settlement of multiple or individual customer transactions within a bank, usually on the same day. These accounts may also be known as special-use, omnibus, suspense, settlement, intraday, sweep, or collection accounts. Concentration accounts are frequently used to facilitate transactions for private banking, trust and custody accounts, funds transfers, and international affiliates.

RISK FACTORS

Money laundering risk can arise in concentration accounts if the customer-identifying information, such as name, transaction amount, and account number, is separated from the financial transaction. If separation occurs, the audit trail is lost, and accounts may be misused or administered improperly. Banks that use concentration accounts should implement adequate policies, procedures, and processes covering the operation and record-keeping for these accounts. Policies should establish guidelines to identify, measure, monitor, and control the risks.

RISK MITIGATION

Because of the risks involved, management should be familiar with the nature of their customers' business and with the transactions flowing through the bank's concentration accounts. Additionally, the monitoring of concentration account transactions is necessary to identify and report unusual or suspicious transactions. Internal controls are necessary to ensure that processed transactions include the identifying customer information. Retaining complete information is crucial for compliance with regulatory requirements as well as ensuring adequate transaction monitoring. Adequate internal controls may include:

- ✓ Maintaining a comprehensive system that identifies, bank-wide, the general ledger accounts used as Concentration accounts, as well as the departments and individuals authorized to use those accounts.
- ✓ Requiring dual signatures on general ledger tickets.
- ✓ Prohibiting direct customer access to concentration acounts.
- ✓ Capturing customer transactions in the customer's account statements.
- ✓ Prohibiting customer's knowledge of concentration accounts or their ability to direct employees to conduct transactions through the accounts.
- ✓ Retaining appropriate transaction and customer identifying information.
- ✓ Frequent reconciling of the accounts by an individual who is independent from the transactions.
- ✓ Establishing timely discrepancy resolution process.
- ✓ Identifying recurring customer names.

1. Has your bank implemented adequate policies, procedures, and processes covering the operation and recordkeeping for concentration accounts, including establishment of guidelines to identify, measure, monitor, and control the risks?

☐ *Yes*

☐ *No*

Comments:

Follow-up:

2. Has your bank established adequate internal controls for mitigating concentration account risks that take into account the following:

a. Maintaining a comprehensive system that identifies, bank-wide, the general ledger accounts used as concentration accounts, as well as the departments and individuals authorized to use those accounts?
b. Requiring dual signatures on general ledger tickets?
c. Prohibiting direct customer access to concentration accounts?
d. Capturing customer transactions in the customer's account statements?
e. Prohibiting customers' knowledge of concentration accounts or their ability to direct employees to conduct transactions through the accounts?
f. Retaining appropriate transaction and customer identifying information?
g. Frequent reconciling of the accounts by an individual who is independent from the transactions?
h. Establishing timely discrepancy resolution process?
i. Identifying recurring customer names?

☐ *Yes*

☐ *No*

Comments:

Follow-up:

Business Entities

The term *business entities* refers to a variety of company formations that may be used for many purposes, such as tax and estate planning. Business entities are relatively easy to establish. Individuals, partnerships, and existing corporations establish business entities for legitimate reasons, but the entities may be abused for money laundering and terrorist financing.

Domestic Business

All states have statutes governing the organization and operation of business entities, including limited liability companies, corporations, general partnerships, limited partnerships, and trusts. Shell companies registered in the United States are a type of domestic[1] business entity that may pose heightened risks. Shell companies can be used for money laundering and other crimes because they are easy and inexpensive to form and operate. In addition, ownership and transactional information can be concealed from regulatory agencies and law enforcement, in large part because most state laws require minimal disclosures of such information during the formation process. According to a report by the U.S. Government Accountability Office (GAO), law enforcement officials are concerned that criminals are increasingly using U.S. shell companies to conceal their identity and illicit activities.[2]

Shell[3] companies can be publicly traded or privately held. Although publicly traded shell companies can be used for illicit purposes, the vulnerability of the shell company is compounded when it is privately held and beneficial ownership can more easily be obscured or hidden. Lack of transparency of beneficial ownership can be a desirable characteristic for some legitimate uses of shell companies, but it is also a serious vulnerability that can make some shell companies ideal vehicles for money laundering and other illicit financial activity. In some state jurisdictions, only minimal information is required to register articles of incorporation and maintain *good standing* for business entities — increasing the potential for their abuse by criminal and terrorist organizations.

Foreign Business

Frequently used foreign entities include trusts, investment funds, and insurance companies. Two foreign entities that can pose particular money laundering risk are:

- International business corporations (IBCs) and Private Investment Companies (PICs) opened in offshore financial centers (OFCs).[4] Many OFCs have limited organizational disclosure and record-keeping requirements for establishing foreign business entities, creating an opportune environment for money laundering;
- International Business Corporations.

IBCs are entities formed outside of a person's country of residence which can be used to maintain confidentially or hide assets. IBC ownership can, based on jurisdiction, be conveyed through registered or bearer shares. There are a variety of advantages to using an IBC which include, but are not limited to, the following:

- Asset protection
- Estate planning
- Privacy and confidentiality
- Reduction of tax liability

Through an IBC, an individual is able to conduct the following:

- Open and hold bank accounts;
- Hold and transfer funds;
- Engage in international business and other related transactions;
- Hold and manage offshore investments (e.g., stocks, bonds, mutual funds, and certificates of deposit), many of which may not be available to individuals, depending on their location of residence.);
- Hold corporate debit and credit cards, thereby allowing convenient access to funds.

Private Investment Companies

PICs are separate legal entities. They are essentially subsets of IBCs. Determining whether a foreign corporation is a PIC is based on identifying the purpose and use of the legal vehicle. PICs are typically used to hold individual funds and investments, and ownership can be vested through bearer shares or registered shares. Like other IBCs, PICs can offer confidentiality of ownership, hold assets centrally, and may provide intermediaries between private banking customers and the potential beneficiaries of the PICs. Shares of a PIC may be held by a trust, which further obscures beneficial ownership of the underlying assets. IBCs, including PICs, are incorporated frequently in secrecy havens.

Nominee Incorporation Services

Intermediaries, called nominee incorporation services (NIS), establish U.S. shell companies and bank accounts on behalf of foreign clients. NIS may be located in the United States or offshore. Corporate lawyers in the United States often use NIS to organize companies on behalf of their domestic and foreign clients because such services can efficiently organize legal entities in any state. NIS must comply with applicable state and federal procedures as well as any specific bank requirements. Those laws and procedures dictate what information NIS must share about the owners of a legal entity. Money launderers have also utilized NIS to hide their identities. By hiring a firm to serve as an intermediary between themselves, the licensing jurisdiction, and the bank, a company's beneficial owners may avoid disclosing their identities in state corporate filings and in corporate bank account opening documentation.

An NIS has the capability to form business entities, open full-service bank accounts for those entities, and act as the registered agent to accept service of legal process on behalf of those entities in a jurisdiction in which the entities have no physical presence. Furthermore, an NIS can perform these services without ever having to identify beneficial ownership on company formation, registration, or bank account documents.

Several international NIS firms have formed partnerships or marketing alliances with U.S. banks to offer financial services such as Internet banking and funds transfer capabilities to shell companies and non-U.S. citizens. U.S. banks participating in these marketing alliances by opening accounts through intermediaries without requiring the actual account-holder's physical presence, accepting by mail copies of passport photos, utility bills, and other identifying information may be assuming increased levels of BSA/AML risk.[5]

Risk Factors

Money laundering and terrorist financing risks arise because business entities can hide the true owner of assets or property derived from or associated with criminal activity[6]. The privacy and confidentiality surrounding some business entities may be exploited by criminals, money launderers, and terrorists. Verifying the grantors and beneficial owner(s) of some business entities may be extremely difficult, as the characteristics of these entities shield the legal identity of the owner. Few public records will disclose true ownership. Overall, the lack of ownership transparency; minimal or no record-keeping requirements, financial disclosures, and supervision; and the range of permissible activities all increase money laundering risk.

While business entities can be established in most international jurisdictions, the majority are incorporated in OFCs that provide ownership privacy and impose few or no tax obligations. To maintain anonymity, many business entities are formed with nominee directors, officeholders, and shareholders. In certain jurisdictions, business entities can also be established using bearer shares; ownership records are not maintained, rather ownership is based on physical possession of the stock certificates. Revocable trusts are another method used to insulate the grantor and beneficial owner and can be designed to own and manage the business entity, presenting significant barriers to law enforcement.

While the majority of U.S.-based shell companies serve legitimate purposes, some shell companies have been used as conduits for money laundering, to hide overseas transactions, or to layer domestic or foreign business entity structures[7]. For example, regulators have identified shell companies registered in the United States conducting suspicious transactions with foreign-based counter-parties. These transactions, primarily funds transfers circling in and out of the U.S. banking system, evidenced no apparent business purpose. Domestic business entities with bank-like names, but without regulatory authority to conduct banking, should be particularly suspect.[8]

The following indicators of potentially suspicious activity may be commonly associated with shell company activity:

- Insufficient or no information available to positively identify originators or beneficiaries of funds transfers (using Internet, commercial database searches, or direct inquiries to a respondent bank);
- Payments have no stated purpose, do not reference goods or services, or identify only a contract or invoice number;
- Goods or services, if identified, do not match profile of company provided by respondent bank or character of the financial activity;
- A company references remarkably dissimilar goods and services in related funds transfers;
- Explanation given by foreign respondent bank is inconsistent with observed funds transfer activity;
- Transacting businesses share the same address, provide only a registered agent's address, or other address inconsistencies;
- Many or all of the funds transfers are sent in large, round dollar, hundred dollar, or thousand dollar amounts;
- Unusually large number and variety of beneficiaries receiving funds transfers from one company;
- A foreign correspondent bank exceeds the expected volume in its client profile for funds transfers, or an individual company exhibits a high volume and pattern of funds transfers that is inconsistent with its normal business activity.
- Frequent involvement of multiple jurisdictions or beneficiaries located in high-risk offshore financial centers
- Use of nested correspondent banking situations;
- Multiple high-value payments or transfers between shell companies with no apparent legitimate business purpose;
- Purpose of the shell company is unknown or unclear.

Risk Mitigation

Management should develop policies, procedures, and processes that enable the bank to identify account relationships, in particular deposit accounts, with business entities, and monitor the risks associated with these accounts in all the bank's departments. Business entity customers may open accounts within the private banking department, within the trust department, or at local branches. Management should establish appropriate due diligence at account opening and during the life of the relationship to manage risk in these accounts. The bank should gather sufficient information on the business entities and their beneficial owners to understand and assess the risks of the account relationship. Important information for determining the valid use of these entities includes the type of business, the purpose of the account, the source of funds, and the source of wealth of the owner or beneficial owner.

The bank's Customer Identification Program (CIP) should detail the identification requirements for opening an account for a business entity. When opening an account for a customer that is not an individual, banks are permitted by 31 CFR 103.121 to obtain information about the individuals who have authority and control over such accounts in order to verify the customer's identity (the customer being the business entity). Required account opening information may include articles of incorporation, a corporate resolution by the directors authorizing the opening of the account, or the appointment of a person to act as a signatory for the entity on the account. Particular attention should be paid to articles of association that allow for nominee shareholders, board members, and bearer shares.

If a bank, through its trust or private banking departments, is facilitating the establishment of a business entity for a new or existing customer, the money laundering risk to the bank is typically mitigated. Since the bank is aware of the parties (e.g., grantors, beneficiaries, and shareholders) involved in the business entity, initial due diligence and verification is easier to obtain. Furthermore, in such cases, the bank frequently has ongoing relationships with the customers initiating the establishment of a business entity.

Risk assessments may include a review of the domestic or international jurisdiction where the business entity was established, the type of account (or accounts) and expected versus actual transaction activities, the types of products that will be used, and whether the business entity was created in-house or externally. If ownership is held in bearer share form, banks should assess the risks these relationships pose and determine the appropriate controls. For example, banks may choose to maintain (or have an independent third party maintain) bearer shares for new clients, or those without well-established relationships with the institution. For well-known, established customers, banks may find that periodically recertifying beneficial ownership is effective. The bank's risk assessment of a business entity customer becomes more important in complex corporate formations. For example, a foreign IBC may establish a layered series of business entities, with each entity naming its parent as its beneficiary.

Ongoing account monitoring is critical to ensure that the accounts are reviewed for unusual and suspicious activity. The bank should be aware of high-risk transactions in these accounts, such as activity that has no business or apparent lawful purpose, funds transfer activity to and from high-risk jurisdictions, currency intensive transactions, and frequent changes in the ownership or control of the nonpublic business entity.

---

[1] The term "domestic" refers to entities formed or organized in the United States. These entities may have no other connection to the United States, and ownership and management of the entities may reside abroad. [2] See GAO, Company Formations — Minimal Ownership Information is Collected and Available, GAO06-376, April 2006, at www.gao.gov. For additional information, refer to Failure to Identify Company Owners Impedes Law Enforcement, Senate Hearing 109-845, held on November 14, 2006 , and Tax Haven Abuses: The Enablers, The Tools & Secrecy, Senate Hearing 109-797, held on August 1, 2006, (particularly the Joint Report of the Majority and Minority Staffs of the Permanent Subcommittee on Investigations).

[3] The term "shell company" generally refers to an entity without a physical presence in any country. FinCEN has issued guidance alerting financial institutions to the potential risks associated with providing financial services to shell companies and reminding them of the importance of managing those risks. See FIN-2006-G014, Potential Money Laundering Risks Related to Shell Companies, November 2006, at www.fincen.gov.

[4] While some OFCs are well regulated, the primary attraction of the offshore sector remains the frequent existence of legal frameworks designed to obscure the identity of beneficial owners, to promote regulatory and supervisory arbitrage, and to provide mitigation or evasion of home-country tax regimes.

[5] Money Laundering Threat Assessment Working Group, *U.S. Money Laundering Threat Assessment*, December 2005.

[6] For a general discussion of the risk factors associated with the misuse of business entities, refer to the Financial Action Task Force's The Misuse of Corporate Vehicles, Including Trust and Company Service Providers, October 13, 2006, at www.fatf-gafi.org.

[7] 238 Failure to Identify Company Owners Impedes Law Enforcement. See Senate Hearing 109-845 held on November 14, 2006.

[8] The federal banking agencies notify banks and the public about entities engaged in unauthorized banking activities, both offshore and domestic. These notifications can be found on the federal banking agency's web sites.

1. Does your bank gather sufficient information on corporate entities (IBC's, PIC's and OBC's) and their beneficial owners to understand and assess the risks of the account relationship? (This information should include the type of business, the purpose of the account, the source of funds, and the source of wealth of the beneficiary.)

☐ *Yes*

☐ *No*

Comments:

Follow-up:

2. Does your bank pay particular attention in the CIP and due diligence process to articles of association that allow for nominee shareholders, board members, and bearer shares?

☐ *Yes*

☐ *No*

Comments:

Follow-up:

3. For ownership of corporations held in bearer share form, do bank policies provide for maintaining the physical control of the bearer shares either in-house or with a trusted third party to ensure that the ownership of the corporate entity does not change without the bank's knowledge?

☐ *Yes*

☐ *No*

Comments:

Follow-up:

4. Is your bank aware of high-risk transactions in these accounts, such as activity that have no business or apparent lawful purpose, funds transfer activity to and from high-risk jurisdictions, currency intensive transactions, and frequent changes in the ownership or control of an account for a nonpublic corporate entity?

☐ *Yes*

☐ *No*

Comments:

Follow-up:

Correspondent Accounts (Domestic)

Correspondent bank accounts are accounts banks maintain with each other on their own behalf in their own names. Correspondent bank account relationships are maintained between domestic banks and between domestic and foreign banks.

1. If your bank offers correspondent banking services to other domestic banks (the latter being known as respondent banks) are specific policies, procedures, and processes in place to manage the BSA/AML risks involved in these correspondent relationships and to detect and report suspicious activities? (**Note:** The level of risk varies depending on the respondent bank's BSA/AML compliance program, products, services, customers, and geographic locations. Each bank should monitor transactions related to domestic correspondent accounts.)

☐ *Yes*

☐ *No*

Comments:

Follow-up:

2. Are transactions related to domestic correspondent accounts specifically monitored?

☐ *Yes*

☐ *No*

Comments:

Follow-up:

Correspondent Accounts (Foreign)

Banks use international correspondent bank accounts for a variety of legitimate business purposes. Many are used to facilitate international trade and investment activities. Others are used for settlement purposes for funds transfer activity and clearing of foreign items. These accounts are designed to move legitimate funds and assets swiftly and securely around the world. International correspondent bank accounts may pose increased risk of potential illicit activities, including money laundering. Three of the more common types of activity found in international correspondent bank accounts that should receive heightened scrutiny are funds (wire) transfer, correspondent accounts used as "payable through accounts" and "pouch/cash letter activity." This heightened risk underscores the need for effective and comprehensive systems and controls particular to these types of accounts.

A bank must exercise caution and due diligence in determining the level of risk associated with each of its correspondent accounts. Information should be gathered to understand fully the nature of the correspondent's business. Factors to consider include the purpose of the account, whether the correspondent bank is located in a bank secrecy or money laundering haven (if so, the nature of the bank license, i.e., shell/offshore bank, fully licensed bank, or an affiliate/subsidiary of a major financial institution), the level of the correspondent's money laundering prevention and detection efforts, and the condition of bank regulation and supervision in the correspondent's country. The level of perceived risk in each account relationship, including the availability of the account to third parties, should dictate the nature of risk management. Banks must comply with 12 CFR 21.11 and 21.21 and 31 CFR 103.18 and report transactions that have no apparent lawful purpose or are not the sort in which a particular customer would normally be expected to engage.

With respect to audits of corresponding banking activities, examiners will review:

- Employee roles and responsibilities.
- Training and experience.
- Specific products and services offered by the bank.
- Violations cited.
- Concerns noted during prior audits or examinations.

For foreign correspondent banking activities, the auditors will:

1. Select a sample of high-risk foreign correspondent accounts and obtain account agreements, account-opening information, and account statements for a three-month period.
2. Evaluate the adequacy of the account approval process and consider information obtained on the sampled accounts, such as the foreign bank's anti-money laundering programs; licensing information; third-party access to the account; and the expected frequency, type, and volume of account activity, and other relevant information.
3. Review the account statements sampled to determine whether the transactions in the account are consistent with expectations. Examiners may need to request additional supporting documentation on the transactions to understand account activity fully (e.g., copies of checks, debit and credit tickets, and/or wire advices).
4. Evaluate the bank's system to identify suspicious activity in foreign correspondent accounts.

Te Patriot Act prohibits accounts with foreign shell banks. Foreign correspondent accounts, as noted in past U.S. Senate investigative reports,[1] are a gateway into the U.S. financial system. This section of the manual covers the regulatory requirements established by sections 312, 313, and 319(b) of the Patriot Act and by the implementing regulations at 31 CFR 103.177, 103.181, and 103.185. Additional discussions and procedures regarding specific money laundering risks for foreign correspondent banking activities, such as pouch activity, cash letters, U.S. dollar drafts, and payable through accounts, are included in the expanded sections.

FOREIGN SHELL BANK PROHIBITION AND FOREIGN CORRESPONDENT ACCOUNT RECORDKEEPING

On October 28, 2002, final regulations (31 CFR 103.177 and 103.185) implementing sections 313 and 319(b) of the Patriot Act became effective. The regulations implemented new provisions of the BSA that relate to foreign correspondent accounts.[2] Under 31 CFR 103.177 a bank is prohibited from establishing, maintaining, administering, or managing a correspondent account in the United States for, or on behalf of, a foreign shell bank. A foreign shell bank is defined as a foreign bank without a physical presence in any country.[3] An exception, however, permits a bank to maintain a correspondent account for a foreign shell bank that is a regulated affiliate.[4] Section 313 also requires that a bank take reasonable steps to ensure that a correspondent account for a foreign bank is not being used to provide banking services indirectly to foreign shell banks.

Certifications

A bank that maintains a correspondent account in the United States for a foreign bank must maintain records in the United States identifying the owners of each foreign bank.[5] A bank must also record the name and street address of a person who resides in the United States and who is authorized, and has agreed, to be an agent to accept service of legal process.[6] Under 31 CFR 103.185, a bank must produce these records within seven days upon receipt of a written request from a federal law enforcement officer. The U.S. Treasury, working with the industry and federal banking and law enforcement agencies, developed a "certification process" to assist banks in complying with the record keeping provisions. This process includes certification and re-certification forms. While banks are not required to use these forms, a bank will be "deemed to be in compliance" with the regulation if it obtains a completed certification form from the foreign financial institution and receives a re-certification once every three years.

Account Closure

The regulation also contains specific provisions as to when banks must obtain the required information or close correspondent accounts. Banks must obtain certifications (or re-certifications) or otherwise obtain the required information within 30 calendar days after the date an account is established and at least once every three years thereafter. If the bank is unable to obtain the required information, it must close all correspondent accounts with the foreign bank within a commercially reasonable time.

Verification

A bank should review certifications for reasonableness and accuracy. If a bank at any time knows, suspects, or has reason to suspect that any information contained in a certification (or re-certification), or that any other information it relied on is no longer correct, the bank must request that the foreign bank verify or correct such information, or take other appropriate measures to ascertain its accuracy. Therefore, banks should review certifications for potential problems that may warrant further review, such as use of post office boxes or forwarding addresses. If the bank has not obtained the necessary or corrected information within 90 days, it must close the account within a commercially reasonable time. During this time, the bank may not permit the foreign bank to establish any new financial positions or execute any transactions through the account, other than those transactions necessary to close the account. Also, a bank may not establish any other correspondent account for the foreign bank until it obtains the required information. A bank must also retain the original of any document provided by a foreign bank, and retain the original or a copy of any document otherwise relied on for the purposes of the regulation, for at least five years after the date that the bank no longer maintains any correspondent account for the foreign bank.

Subpoenas

Under section 319(b) of the Patriot Act, the Secretary of the Treasury or the U.S. Attorney General may issue a subpoena or summons to any foreign bank that maintains a correspondent account in the United States to obtain records relating to that account, including records maintained abroad, or to obtain records relating to the deposit of funds into the foreign bank. If the foreign bank fails to comply with the subpoena or fails to initiate proceedings to contest that subpoena, the Secretary of the Treasury or the U.S. Attorney General (after consultations with each other) may, by written notice, direct a bank to terminate its relationship with a foreign correspondent bank. If a bank fails to terminate the correspondent relationship within ten days of receipt of notice, it could be subject to a civil money penalty of up to $10,000 per day until the correspondent relationship is terminated.

Requests for AML Records by Federal Regulator
Also, upon request by its federal regulator, a bank must provide or make available records related to AML compliance of the bank or one of its customers, within 120 hours from the time of the request.

DUE DILIGENCE PROGRAM FOR CORRESPONDENT ACCOUNTS FOR FOREIGN FINANCIAL INSTITUTIONS:
Section 312 of the Patriot Act added new subsection (i) to 31 USC 5318 of the BSA. This section requires each U.S. bank that establishes, maintains, administers, or manages a correspondent account in the United States for a non-U.S. person to take certain AML measures for such accounts. In particular, banks must establish appropriate, specific, and, where necessary, enhanced due diligence policies, procedures, and processes that are reasonably designed to enable the bank to detect and report instances of money laundering through those accounts. This requirement applies to a correspondent relationship with any foreign financial institution, even if it is not a traditional banking institution. In addition to this general requirement, which applies to all correspondent accounts for non-U.S. persons, section 312 of the Patriot Act specifies additional standards for correspondent accounts maintained for certain foreign banks. For a correspondent account maintained for a foreign bank operating under an offshore license or a license granted by a jurisdiction designated as being of concern for money laundering, a bank must take reasonable steps to identify the owners of the foreign financial institution, conduct enhanced scrutiny of the correspondent account to guard against money laundering, and ascertain whether the foreign bank provides correspondent accounts to other foreign banks and, if so, conduct appropriate related due diligence.

USAPA Section 312 FINAL RULE
On August 10, 2007, the U.S. Treasury issued the final rule for the correspondent banking section for USAPA Section 312. The final rule did not dramatically change what had been in place in the interim final rule.

General Due Diligence
31 CFR 103.176(a) requires banks to establish a due diligence program that includes appropriate, specific, risk-based, and, where necessary, enhanced policies, procedures, and controls that are reasonably designed to enable the bank to detect and report, on an ongoing basis, any known or suspected money laundering activity conducted through or involving any correspondent account established, maintained, administered, or managed by the bank in the United States for a foreign financial institution ("foreign correspondent account").

The term "foreign financial institution" as defined in 31 CFR 103.175(h) includes:

- A foreign bank.
- A foreign branch, or office of a U.S. bank, broker/dealer in securities, futures commission merchant, introducing broker, or mutual fund.
- Any other person organized under foreign law that, if located in the United States, would be a broker/dealer in securities, futures commission merchant, introducing broker, or mutual fund.
- Any person organized under foreign law that is engaged in the business of, and is readily identifiable as, a currency dealer or exchanger or a money transmitter.

Due diligence policies, procedures, and controls must include an assessment of each of the following five factors:

- The nature of the foreign financial institution's business and the markets it serves;
- The type, purpose, and anticipated activity of the correspondent account;
- The nature and duration of the covered institution's relationship with the foreign institution;
- The anti-money laundering supervisory regime of the jurisdiction that issued the charter or license to the foreign financial institution and its owners, if applicable, to the extent that such information is reasonably available; and,

- Information known or reasonably available to the covered institution about the foreign institution's AML record.

The Final Rule makes consideration of the foreign institution's AML program an optional requirement driven by whether it would be appropriate given the risk based approach to managing/mitigating the risk for a particular customer. **Note:** It is important for a bank to be able to reasonably demonstrate to regulators that it is effectively exercising this discretion.

The guidance to the Final rule also suggests that the use of a questionnaire "may" be effective to gather information related to a respondent's AML program. For cases where a bank has a history with a respondent bank, a review of the transaction history may also serve to assess the money laundering risk associated with it.

It is not expected that covered institutions request lists of foreign bank customers that use the services of the respondent's account. However, based upon the risk assessment of the foreign bank, as part of the EDD process, appropriate inquiries should be made about such customers as the nature of the foreign bank customers the respondent bank serves (if any), and the extent to which transactions for any foreign bank customer may be conducted through the respondent bank's correspondent account. There may, in the highest risk circumstances, be appropriate to obtain information regarding the identity of these banks directly form the respondent bank. If obtaining such information is not possible, - including by monitoring transaction activity - policies and procedures should be in place to dictate how to proceed in light of the circumstances (pursuant to section 103.176(d)).

Enhanced Due Diligence
The final rule applies a risk based approach to the amount of and need to conduct enhanced scrutiny. Section 103.176(b) requires covered institutions to establish enhanced due diligence procedures to conduct risk based enhanced scrutiny of correspondent accounts, determine whether three is any nesting of correspondent accounts (and take reasonable risk mitigation due diligence steps), and for non publicly traded respondent banks, determine identity of the owners and the extent and nature of the ownership interest.

The enhanced scrutiny must reflect the assessment of the account and include, as appropriate:

- obtaining information related to the foreign bank's AML program;
- monitoring transactions to, from, or through the foreign account;
- obtaining identity information regarding those with access to direct transactions through any correspondent account that is a payable through account, as well as the sources and beneficial owners of funds or assets in the PTA;

Transaction monitoring must also be conducted as part of the enhanced due diligence steps. This may be conducted electronically or manually and may be done on an individual account basis or by product activity, and should reflect the risk assessment conducted on each respondent bank subject to the enhanced due diligence provisions.

Statutory Triggers for Conducting Enhanced Due Diligence
Section 103.176(c) requires that enhanced due diligence ***must*** be conducted if the respondent bank falls into any of these three categories:

1. A bank operating under an offshore banking license;[7]
2. A banking license issued by a foreign country that has been designated as non-cooperative with international AML principles or procedures by an inter-governmental group or organization of which the United States is a member, and with whose designation the United States representative to the group or organization concurs;
3. A banking license issued by a foreign country that has been designated by the Secretary of the Treasury as warranting special measures due to money laundering concerns.

The comments for the final rule suggest that, even for these respondents for whom EDD is required, a risk based approach to the level of EDD is still appropriate. For example, when dealing with an offshore booking location of a bank located in a country with a strong AML regime, a covered institution will not ordinarily be required to conduct EDD to the same degree as it would with a stand-alone offshore bank.

While not cited in the Final Rule, examples of existing sound practices and standards include the following (cited previously in the Interim Final Rule):

- The New York Clearing House Association, L.L.C., "The New York Clearing House Issues Anti-Money Laundering Guidelines for Correspondent Banking," (March 2002) at www.nych.org.
- Basel Committee on Banking Supervision, "Customer Due Diligence for Banks," (October 2001) at www.bis.org.
- Wolfsberg Principles on Correspondent Banking

A due diligence program that does not adopt all of the sound practices and standards described in industry and other available guidance could be considered reasonable if the bank has a justifiable reason for not adopting a particular sound practice or standard, based on the particular type of accounts held by the bank.

Risk Assessment of Foreign Financial Institutions

A bank's general due diligence program should include policies, procedures, and processes to assess the risks posed by the bank's foreign financial institution customers. A bank's resources are most appropriately directed at those accounts that pose a more significant money laundering risk. The following factors may be used to help identify potential risk characteristics of a foreign correspondent customer. Nevertheless, management should weigh and evaluate each risk factor to arrive at a risk determination for each customer and then prioritize oversight resources. Relevant risk factors include the following:

- The foreign financial institution's jurisdiction of organization, chartering, and licensing;
- Products and services offered by the foreign financial institution;
- Markets (including customer base) and locations served by the foreign financial institution.
- Purpose of the account (e.g., a proprietary operating account or a customer-directed account);
- Anticipated activity (e.g., dollar amount, number, and types of transactions) of the account.
- The nature and duration of the bank's relationship with the foreign financial institution (and, if relevant, with any affiliate of the foreign financial institution);
- Any information known or reasonably available to the bank about the foreign financial institution's AML record, including public information in standard industry guides, periodicals, and major publications.
- The AML regime of the jurisdiction issuing an offshore charter or license may be particularly relevant in assessing money laundering risks and may be a mitigating factor for the purposes of complying with the EDD provisions, as also may be the regime of the home jurisdiction of the foreign bank or is parent to the extent relevant information is readily available.

Under subsections 5318(i)(2)(B)(i) through (iii), a bank must establish policies, procedures, and controls to ensure that for each such foreign bank subject to enhanced due diligence, the bank takes reasonable steps to:

- Ascertain, for any such foreign bank whose shares are not publicly traded, the identity of each of the owners of the foreign bank, and the nature and extent of the ownership interest of each such owner;[8]
- Conduct enhanced scrutiny of any accounts held by such banks to guard against money laundering and report any suspicious transactions in accordance with SAR regulations;
- Ascertain whether such foreign bank provides correspondent accounts to other foreign banks and, if so, to ascertain the identity of those foreign banks and conduct due diligence as appropriate under the requirements of subsection 5318(i)(1) (i.e., the bank's general due diligence program). Considering

risk factors such as the location and size of the foreign correspondent bank and number of its foreign financial institution customers, the bank should determine the extent to which enhanced due diligence of a foreign correspondent bank's foreign financial institution customers is necessary.

Banks should focus enhanced due diligence measures on those correspondent accounts that are maintained by a foreign bank deemed by 31 USC 5318(i)(2)(A) to pose a particularly high risk of money laundering on the basis of the bank's overall assessment of the risk posed by the foreign bank. In addition, banks should apply any or all of the steps listed above, as appropriate, to a foreign financial institution identified by the bank's general due diligence program as representing an increased risk of money laundering.

Examiners will seek to determine whether a bank has established a due diligence program that includes appropriate, specific, risk-based, and, where necessary, enhanced policies, procedures, and controls for correspondent accounts established, maintained, administered, or managed in the United States for foreign financial institutions ("foreign correspondent account").

The bank will need to verify for examiners that due diligence policies, procedures, and controls include:

- Determining whether any foreign correspondent account is subject to enhanced due diligence (31 CFR 103.176(a)(1)).
- Assessing the money laundering risks presented by the foreign correspondent account (31 CFR 103.176(a)(2)).
- Applying risk-based procedures and controls to each foreign correspondent account reasonably designed to detect and report known or suspected money laundering activity, including a periodic review of the correspondent account activity sufficient to determine consistency with information obtained about the type, purpose, and anticipated activity of the account (31 CFR 103.176(a)(3)).

The bank will need to verify for examiners that its due diligence program considers the following factors, as appropriate, as criteria in the risk assessment:

- The nature of the foreign financial institution's business and the markets it serves.
- The type, purpose, and anticipated activity of the foreign correspondent account.
- The nature and duration of the bank's relationship with the foreign financial institution and any of its affiliates.
- The AML and supervisory regime of the jurisdiction that issued the charter or license to the foreign financial institution, and, to the extent that information regarding such jurisdiction is reasonably available, of the jurisdiction in which any company that is an owner of the foreign financial institution is incorporated or chartered.
- Information known or reasonably available to the bank about the foreign financial institution's AML record.

---

[1] "Correspondent Banking: A Gateway for Money Laundering," See Senate Hearing 107-84. The report appears on p. 273 of volume 1 of the hearing records entitled "Role of U.S. Correspondent Banking in International Money Laundering" held on March 1, 2, and 6, 2001.

[2] For purposes of 31 CFR 103.177 and 103.185, a "correspondent account" is an account established by a bank for a foreign bank to receive deposits from, to make payments or other disbursements on behalf of a foreign bank, or to handle other financial transactions related to the foreign bank. An "account" means any formal banking or business relationship established to provide regular services, dealings, and other financial transactions. It includes a demand deposit, savings deposit, or other transaction or asset account and a credit account or other extension of credit (31 CFR 103.175(d)).

[3] "Physical presence" means a place of business that:

- Is maintained by a foreign bank.

• Is located at a fixed address (other than solely an electronic address or a post office box) in a country in which the foreign financial institution is authorized to conduct banking activities, at which location the foreign financial institution:

- Employs one or more persons on a full-time basis.
- Maintains operating records related to its banking activities.

• Is subject to inspection by the banking authority that licensed the foreign financial institution to conduct banking activities.

[4] A "regulated affiliate" is a shell bank that is affiliated with a depository institution, credit union, or foreign bank that maintains a physical presence in the United States or in another jurisdiction. The regulated affiliate shell bank must also be subject to supervision by the banking authority that regulates the affiliated entity.

[5] To minimize the record keeping burdens, ownership information is not required for foreign financial institutions that file a form FR Y-7 ("Annual Report of Foreign Banking Organizations") with the Federal Reserve or for those foreign financial institutions that are publicly traded. "Publicly traded" refers to shares that are traded on an exchange or an organized over-the-counter market that is regulated by a foreign securities authority as defined in section 3(a)(50) of the Securities Exchange Act of 1934.

[6] "Service of legal process" means that the agent is willing to accept legal documents, such as subpoenas, on behalf of the foreign bank.

[7] The Patriot Act defines an offshore banking license as a license to conduct banking activities that, as a condition of the license, prohibits the licensed entity from conducting banking activities with the citizens of, or with the local currency of, the country that issued the license. Refer to 31 USC 5318(i)(4)(A).

[8] The preamble to the *Federal Register* notice that accompanied the interim final rule (67 *Federal Register* 48348) stated that for purposes of subsection 5318(i)(2)(B)(i), an owner is deemed to be any person who directly or indirectly owns, controls, or has voting power over 5 percent or more of any class of securities of a foreign bank, the shares of which are not publicly traded. "Publicly traded" means shares that are traded on an exchange or an organized over-the-counter market that is regulated by a foreign securities authority.

1. Has your bank established a due diligence program that includes appropriate, specific, risk-based, and, where necessary, enhanced policies, procedures, and controls that are reasonably designed to enable it to detect and report, on an ongoing basis, any known or suspected money laundering activity conducted through or involving any correspondent account established, maintained, administered, or managed by the bank in the United States for a foreign financial institution?

☐ *Yes*

☐ *No*

Comments:

Follow-up:

2. Are risk-based procedures and controls applied to each correspondent account reasonably designed to detect and report known or suspected money laundering activity, including a periodic review of the correspondent account activity sufficient to determine consistency with information obtained about the type, purpose, and anticipated activity of the account?

☐ *Yes*

☐ *No*

Comments:

Follow-up:

3. Has your bank recorded and maintained records of the names and street addresses of persons who reside in the United States and who are authorized and have agreed to be an agent to accept service of legal process?

☐ *Yes*

☐ *No*

Comments:

Follow-up:

4. Has your bank obtained certifications (or re-certifications) or otherwise obtained the required information within 30 calendar days after the date an account has been established and at least once every three years thereafter?

☐ *Yes*

☐ *No*

Comments:

Follow-up:

5. Does your bank maintain adequate systems for aging and maintaining certifications and re-certifications?

☐ *Yes*

☐ *No*

Comments:

Follow-up:

6. Are procedures and controls in place to request that foreign banks verify or correct information when any information contained in a certification (or recertification) or any other information relied upon is no longer correct?

☐ *Yes*

☐ *No*

Comments:

Follow-up:

7. Are procedures in place and properly followed for reviewing certifications for potential problems that may warrant further review, such as use of post office boxes or forwarding addresses?

☐ ***Yes***

☐ ***No***

Comments:

Follow-up:

8. If your bank cannot obtain the necessary or corrected information for a certification within 90 days, are procedures in place and properly followed to close the account within a commercially reasonable time?

☐ ***Yes***

☐ ***No***

Comments:

Follow-up:

9. During the period referred to in Question #8, does your bank have procedures to prevent the foreign bank from establishing any new financial positions or execute any transactions through the account, other than those transactions necessary to close the account for the foreign bank until it obtains the required information?

☐ *Yes*

☐ *No*

Comments:

Follow-up:

10. During the period referred to in Question #8, does your bank have procedures in place to prevent establishment of any other correspondent account?

☐ *Yes*

☐ *No*

Comments:

Follow-up:

11. Does your bank maintain the original of any document provided by a foreign bank and the original or a copy of any document otherwise relied upon, for at least five years after the date that the institution no longer maintains any correspondent account for the foreign bank?

☐ ***Yes***

☐ ***No***

Comments:

Follow-up:

12. Are your bank's policies and procedures, including the policies for any of its foreign branches, current regarding foreign correspondent accounts?

☐ ***Yes***

☐ ***No***

Comments:

Follow-up:

13. Can your bank provide a list of foreign branches and the steps taken to determine that its accounts with its branches are not used to indirectly provide services to foreign shell banks?

☐ *Yes*

☐ *No*

Comments:

Follow-up:

14. Does your bank maintain a list of all foreign correspondent accounts and relationships with foreign banks that have been closed or terminated due to nonconformance with 31 CFR 103.177 (i.e., service foreign shell banks; records of owners and agents)?

☐ *Yes*

☐ *No*

Comments:

Follow-up:

15. Does your bank maintain a file of requests from federal law enforcement agencies for information regarding foreign correspondent accounts and evidence of compliance?

☐ *Yes*

☐ *No*

Comments:

Follow-up:

16. Does your bank maintain a log of any notices to close foreign correspondent accounts from the Secretary of the Treasury or the U.S. Attorney General and can it present evidence of compliance?

☐ *Yes*

☐ *No*

Comments:

Follow-up:

17. Are copies maintained of any Suspicious Activity Reports (SARs) filed relating to the requirements of 31 CFR 103.177 (i.e., service to foreign shell banks; records of owners and agents)?

☐ *Yes*

☐ *No*

Comments:

Follow-up:

18. Are records of analysis or documentation where a SAR was considered, but where the decision was made not to file a SAR, maintained?

☐ *Yes*

☐ *No*

Comments:

Follow-up:

19. Has a responsible party been designated by your institution for managing the certification and re-certification process?

☐ *Yes*

☐ *No*

Comments:

Follow-up:

20. Are all the following documented, and is the designated responsible person sufficiently trained to handle the process for:

a. Identifying foreign correspondent accounts?
b. Sending, tracking, receiving, and reviewing certification requests/requests for information?
c. Evaluating the quality of the responses/information?
d. Closing accounts?
e. Maintaining and keeping records current?
f. Procedures for determining if and when SARs should be filed?

☐ *Yes*

☐ *No*

Comments:

Follow-up:

21. Is an independent test conducted by your bank to ensure compliance with the regulations regarding correspondent banking activities?

☐ *Yes*

☐ *No*

Comments:

Follow-up:

22. Regarding the collection of required account information, does your bank have procedures to prevent a foreign bank or other customer from establishing any new financial positions or executing any transactions through the new account, other than those transactions necessary to close the account, until your bank receives the required information?

☐ *Yes*

☐ *No*

Comments:

Follow-up:

23. Does your bank's policy provide evidence of its good faith efforts to incorporate due diligence procedures for those correspondent accounts it maintains for foreign financial institutions that pose an increased risk of money laundering?

☐ *Yes*

☐ *No*

Comments:

Follow-up:

24. Does your bank focus enhanced due diligence measures on those correspondent accounts that are maintained by a foreign bank deemed by 31 USC 5318(i)(2)(A) to pose a particularly high risk of money laundering on the basis of the bank's overall assessment of the risk posed by the foreign bank?

☐ *Yes*

☐ *No*

Comments:

Follow-up:

25. Does your IT department adequately support the requirements that, upon request by its federal regulator, the bank must provide or make available records related to AML compliance of the bank or one of its customers within 120 hours from the time of the request?

☐ *Yes*

☐ *No*

Comments:

Follow-up:

26. Each relationship that a U.S. bank has with a foreign correspondent financial institution should be governed by an agreement or a contract describing each party's responsibilities and other relationship details (e.g., products and services provided, acceptance of deposits, clearing of items, forms of payment, and acceptable forms of endorsement). Does your bank's policies and procedures address this guidance and are the contracts periodically reviewed?

☐ *Yes*

☐ *No*

Comments:

Follow-up:

27. Regarding question 26, above, do the agreements or contracts consider the foreign correspondent's AML responsibilities, customer base, due diligence procedures, and customer referrals from the correspondent to the U.S. bank, clearly defining all referral terms (e.g., customer type and business profile, customer's geographic location, and any special terms)?

☐ *Yes*

☐ *No*

Comments:

Follow-up:

28. Does your bank have policies, procedures, and processes to manage the BSA/AML risks inherent with correspondent relationships, and do you closely monitor transactions related to these accounts to detect and report suspicious activities and identify risks associated with "nesting" of correspondent accounts?

☐ *Yes*

☐ *No*

Comments:

Follow-up:

29. As part of your bank's Foreign Correspondent Account Recordkeeping and Due Diligence program, do policies, procedures, and processes address:

a. Intended use of the accounts and expected account activity (e.g., determine whether the relationship will serve as a payable through account)?
b. The foreign correspondent financial institution's other correspondent relationships (e.g., determine whether nested accounts will be utilized)?
c. Assessment of the risks posed by the foreign correspondent financial institution relationships?
d. Conducting adequate and ongoing due diligence on the foreign correspondent financial institution relationships, which may include periodic visits?
e. Ensuring that foreign correspondent financial institution relationships are appropriately included within the U.S. bank's suspicious activity monitoring and reporting systems?
f. Establishment of criteria for closing the foreign correspondent financial institution account?

☐ *Yes*

☐ *No*

Comments:

Follow-up:

30. Has your bank communicated its AML related expectations to its foreign correspondent financial institution customers?

☐ *Yes*

☐ *No*

Comments:

Follow-up:

31. Is your bank aware of and does it understand the AML controls in place at the foreign correspondent financial institutions, including customer due diligence practices and recordkeeping documentation.

☐ *Yes*

☐ *No*

Comments:

Follow-up:

32. In determining whether a correspondent banking account is covered under 31 CFR 103.176, has the bank considered whether the money laundering risk presented by such correspondent account, takes into consideration all relevant factors, including:

a. The nature of the foreign financial institution's business and the markets it serves?
b. The type, purpose, and anticipated activity of such correspondent account?
c. The nature and duration of the covered financial institution's relationship with the foreign financial institution (and any of its affiliates)?
d. The anti-money laundering and supervisory regime of the jurisdiction that issued the charter or license to the foreign financial institution, and, to the extent that information regarding such jurisdiction is reasonably available, of the jurisdiction in which any company that is an owner of the foreign financial institution is incorporated or chartered?
e. Information known or reasonably available to the covered financial institution about the foreign financial institution's anti-money laundering record?

☐ *Yes*

☐ *No*

Comments:

Follow-up:

33. If your bank maintains a correspondent account in the United States for a foreign bank, are records maintained in the United States identifying the owners of each foreign bank?

☐ *Yes*

☐ *No*

Comments:

Follow-up:

34. Where ownership information is not maintained, is documentation kept showing that that either the foreign banks have filed a form FR-7 with the Federal Reserve or are publicly traded?

☐ *Yes*

☐ *No*

Comments:

Follow-up:

35. Does the bank's due diligence include procedures to be followed in circumstances when it cannot perform appropriate due diligence with respect to a correspondent account, including when it should refuse to open the account, suspend transaction activity, file a suspicious activity report, or close the account?

☐ *Yes*

☐ *No*

Comments:

Follow-up:

36. Do your bank's procedures incorporate the best practices of the New York Clearing House and Wolfsberg group, as suggested in the final rule comments for USA PATRIOT Act Section 312?

☐ *Yes*

☐ *No*

Comments:

Follow-up:

37. Do your bank's FCB policies and procedures address the three statutory requirements for performing Enhanced Due Diligence for specific correspondent accounts/customers as required by Section 312 of the PATRIOT Act?

☐ *Yes*

☐ *No*

Comments:

Follow-up:

38. Do your bank's FCB policies and procedures address the requirement that, in cases where any of the three statutory triggers for enhanced due diligence are not applicable, "increased due diligence" should be performed on correspondent banking customers on the basis of a risk based assessment, and are the levels of risk and their appropriate increased due diligence steps specifically documented in the bank's policies and/or procedures?

☐ *Yes*

☐ *No*

Comments:

Follow-up:

Currency Flows & Reporting – Large Cash

Shipment activity regarding currency shipped to and received from the Federal Reserve Bank or correspondent banks, or reflecting currency shipped between branches and their banks' central currency vaults will be examined by regulators. The period of time to examine will be chosen relative to the size and complexity of a bank.

1. Have cash totals shipped to and received from the Federal Reserve Bank, correspondent banks, or between branch offices reviewed within a reasonable period of time (typically three months)?

☐ *Yes*

☐ *No*

Comments:

Follow-up:

2. Have material variances (i.e. variances in totals of currency shipped or received, or large denominations of currency exchanged) been logged and/or investigated?

☐ *Yes*

☐ *No*

Comments:

Follow-up:

3. Is your bank's volume of CTR filings during the current period consistent with changes in the patterns of cash activity?

☐ *Yes*

☐ *No*

Comments:

Follow-up:

Currency Transactions Capturing

A bank's information systems must be able to track and aggregate cash transactions for reporting purposes as well as to adequately aid in detection and investigation of unusual activity. A system need not be an automated one, but must be adequately robust to allow the institution to maintain compliance. Size and complexity of an institution with regard to the volume of cash transactions processed are factors that determine what management information systems should look like.

1, Do your firm's automated systems adequately capture cash transactions (individual and/or multiple transactions) in excess of $10,000 on the same business day by or on behalf of the same individual, or by account?

☐ ***Yes***

☐ ***No***

Comments:

Follow-up:

2, Has the accuracy and validity of the bank's automated large transaction identification system been tested with regard to all points of cash entry and exit?

☐ ***Yes***

☐ ***No***

Comments:

Follow-up:

3. Are CTRs (FinCEN Form 104) properly completed and filed for each transaction in currency deposit, withdrawal, exchange or other payment or transfer) of more than $10,000 by, through, or to the bank?

☐ *Yes*

☐ *No*

Comments:

Follow-up:

4. Are transaction amounts reviewed for consistency with the type and nature of business or occupation of the customer?

☐ *Yes*

☐ *No*

Comments:

Follow-up:

5. Does your bank properly treat, and are systems in place to aggregate multiple currency transactions totaling more than $10,000 during any one business day as a single transaction if the bank has knowledge that they are by or on behalf of the same person?

☐ *Yes*

☐ *No*

Comments:

Follow-up:

6. Are CTRs filed and mailed (or otherwise transmitted) within 15 calendar days after the date of the transaction (25 days if magnetically filed) and does your bank retain copies of CTRs for five years from the date of the report? (31 CFR 103.27(a)(3)).

☐ *Yes*

☐ *No*

Comments:

Follow-up:

7. Do the bank's systems adequately cover discount brokerage, private banking, trust, or any other departments within the bank that engage in currency transactions subject to the regulations?

☐ *Yes*

☐ *No*

Comments:

Follow-up:

8. If your bank does not make use of an automated large transaction identification or aggregation system, does the internal audit program or other independent review include a sample test check of tellers' cash proof sheets or tapes to determine if large cash transactions are being reported?

☐ *Yes*

☐ *No*

Comments:

Follow-up:

Currency Transactions Reporting

A Currency Transaction Report (CTR) must be filed for each deposit, withdrawal, exchange of currency, or other payment or transfer, by, through or to a financial institution, which involves a transaction in currency of *more than* $10,000. Multiple currency transactions must be treated as a single transaction if the financial institution *has knowledge* that: (a) they are conducted by or on behalf of the same person; and, (b) they result in cash received or disbursed by the financial institution of more than $10,000. (31 CFR 103.22).

As of April 30, 1996, banks were not required to file CTRs on large currency transactions conducted by certain "exempt persons" defined as:

- Domestic depository institutions;
- Departments and agencies of the United States, the states, and their political subdivisions;
- Any entity established under the laws of the United States, of any state, or the political subdivision of any state, or under an interstate compact between two or more states, that exercises authority on behalf of the United States or any such state or political subdivision;
- Any entity, other than a bank, whose common stock or analogous equity interests are listed on the New York Stock Exchange, the American Stock Exchange, or whose common stock, or analogous equity interests have been designated as a Nasdaq National Market Security listed on the Nasdaq Stock Market (except stock or interests listed under the separate "Nasdaq Small-Cap Issues" heading);
- Any subsidiary, other than a bank, of any entity described in number four (a "listed entity") that is organized under the laws of the United States or of any state and at least 51 percent of whose common stock is owned by the listed entity. Franchises of listed entities may not be treated as exempt persons, unless they qualify as subsidiaries.

Phase II rules [103.22(d)(2)(vi)-(vii)] allow banks to exempt:

- Any other commercial enterprise (also known under the new exemption procedures as non-listed businesses), to the extent of its domestic operations, other than those ineligible businesses covered by 103.22(d)(6)(viii);
- A customer that holds a payroll account that regularly withdraws more than $10,000 to pay its U.S. employees in currency solely for withdrawals for payroll purposes from existing transaction accounts.

The "Designation of Exempt Person" form, TDF 90-22.53, must be filed to exempt customers under phase I and II rules. Under the phase II rule:

- Twelve months of account history must exist before the customer can be exempted. (The months do not have to be consecutive, but should be recent.)
- The customer must engage frequently in large currency transactions (eight or more a year).
- The customer must be incorporated or organized under the laws of the United States or a state, or registered or eligible to do business in the United States.

Annually, banks must verify whether each exemption continues to meet the exemption eligibility requirements. Banks may develop their own methods and procedures for this annual review. Biennially, banks must file the "Designation of Exempt Person" form for each non-listed business and payroll customer. As part of the biennial filing of the "Designation of Exempt Person" form, a bank must certify that, as part of its BSA compliance program, it has policies and procedures in place for identifying, reviewing, and reporting suspicious activity in accordance with the SAR filing requirements. (31 CFR 103.18 and 12 CFR 21.11) No exemptions under the old rules were permitted after October 20, 1998. However, banks were allowed to treat exemptions granted prior to October 20, 1998 as exempt until June 30, 2000. All exemptions granted by a bank had to be converted to the new exemption procedures by June 30, 2000. For more information about granting, maintaining, and documenting exemptions under the BSA, see 31 CFR 103.22 (d)(2)-(11).

1. Does the compliance office conduct periodic testing/sampling to ensure the efficacy of the bank's policies and procedures for exemptions? (Note: As of July 1, 2000, new Treasury exemption procedures allowing financial institutions to exempt transactions of certain businesses from the requirement to report transactions in currency in excess of $10,000. If a customer's cash deposits or withdrawal amounts do not exceed $10,000 on a "regular and frequent" basis, the customer does not qualify for an exemption.)

☐ *Yes*

☐ *No*

Comments:

Follow-up:

2. Department of the Treasury Administrative Ruling 88-3 states that banks may not exempt "cash back" transactions (transactions involving the deposit of checks where a portion of the deposit is remitted in cash) from the CTR reporting requirements. Therefore, cash received by the customer on "cash-back" transactions should not be included in the exemption limit review. Does your bank's policy and procedure ensure compliance with this ruling?

☐ *Yes*

☐ *No*

Comments:

Follow-up:

3. Has the institution designated any *exempt persons* as defined in the regulations?

☐ ***Yes***

☐ ***No***

Comments:

Follow-up:

4. If your institution has designated any *exempt persons* as defined in the regulations, does the bank have sufficient procedures related to exemptions?

☐ ***Yes***

☐ ***No***

Comments:

Follow-up:

5. If your institution has designated any *exempt persons* as defined in the regulations, does the bank have adequate and knowledgeable personnel sufficient to maintain the exemption process?

☐ *Yes*

☐ *No*

Comments:

Follow-up:

6. Does the bank maintain appropriate and sufficient documentation to support each exemption?

☐ *Yes*

☐ *No*

Comments:

Follow-up:

7. Are controls in place to determine and verify the eligibility of exemptions?

☐ *Yes*

☐ *No*

Comments:

Follow-up:

8. Do all Phase I exemptions meet the established criteria?

a. Bank
b. Government Agency
c. Exchange Listed Business
d. Subsidiary of a Listed Business

☐ *Yes*

☐ *No*

Comments:

Follow-up:

9. Do all Phase II *non-listed business* exemptions meet the established criteria?

a. Maintained a transaction account with the bank for at least 12 months?
b. Frequently engaged in currency transactions in excess of $10,000?
c. Is incorporated or organized under US or State law or is registered and is eligible to do business within the US or a State?

☐ *Yes*

☐ *No*

Comments:

Follow-up:

10. Do all Phase II *payroll customer* exemptions meet the established criteria?

a. Maintained a transaction account with the bank for at least 12 months?
b. Operates a firm that regularly withdraws more than $10,000 in order to pay its US employees in currency?
c. Is incorporated or organized under US or State law or is registered and is eligible to do business within the US or a State?

☐ *Yes*

☐ *No*

Comments:

Follow-up:

11. For each exempt person, has the bank filed a Designation of Exempt Person Form completely and within 30 days of the first reportable transaction that was exempted, and does your firm record that Designation of Exempt Person Forms are filled out within 30 days of the first reportable

☐ *Yes*

☐ *No*

Comments:

Follow-up:

12. For Phase II exemptions, has the bank filed a Designation of Exempt Person biennially by March 15 beginning the second calendar year following the original designation?

☐ *Yes*

☐ *No*

Comments:

Follow-up:

13. Does your bank, at least once per year, review and verify the information supporting each designation of a Phase II exempt person, and, consistent with this annual review, does your bank review and verify at least once each year that management monitors these Phase II accounts for suspicious transactions?

☐ *Yes*

☐ *No*

Comments:

Follow-up:

14. Does documentation exist to evidence your bank's efforts to monitor the volumes, amounts and frequency of large currency transactions for each exempt person such that they are consistent with what is normal and expected and commensurate with lawful activity?

☐ *Yes*

☐ *No*

Comments:

Follow-up:

15. Does the bank have a system to monitor the currency transactions of exempt persons for suspicious activity?

☐ ***Yes***

☐ ***No***

Comments:

Follow-up:

16. Is your firm's monitoring system adequate to identify suspicious activity and is there sufficient documentation evidencing consideration and resolution of all alerts or indications of possible suspicious activity reported by your transaction monitoring system?

☐ ***Yes***

☐ ***No***

Comments:

Follow-up:

17. Has the bank's internal audit department reviewed the exemption process?

☐ *Yes*

☐ *No*

Comments:

Follow-up:

18. Have there been any outstanding issues involving exemptions and if so, have they been documented and resolved?

☐ *Yes*

☐ *No*

Comments:

Follow-up:

19. Have the methods used by exempt customers to withdraw currency in excess of $10,000 been reviewed by the compliance staff?

☐ *Yes*

☐ *No*

Comments:

Follow-up:

20. If either checks payable to *cash*, *counter currency withdrawal tickets*, or *counter checks* are used by exempt customers to withdraw currency in excess of $10,000, has the compliance office reviewed whether the cash portion of the withdrawals are sufficient to qualify the customer for an exemption based upon Treasury's "regular and frequent" requirement for a withdrawal exemption?

☐ *Yes*

☐ *No*

Comments:

Follow-up:

21. Are established dollar limits reasonable as evidenced by reviewing and documenting the customer's cash withdrawal activity?

☐ *Yes*

☐ *No*

Comments:

Follow-up:

22. Are Designation of Exempt Persons Form (TDF 90-22.53) filed in accordance with regulations (within 30 days after the first customer transaction the bank wishes to exempt)?

☐ *Yes*

☐ *No*

Comments:

Follow-up:

23. Does your bank's exemption policy take into consideration FinCEN guidance which states that: a customer being considered for exemption as a non-listed business should be conducting at least eight large currency transactions throughout the year? (**Note:** In essence, this means the customer conducts a large currency transaction approximately every six weeks. The fact a customer conducts fewer than eight large currency transactions annually would generally indicate that any large currency transactions conducted do not relate to a recurring or routine need)

☐ *Yes*

☐ *No*

Comments:

Follow-up:

24. Under the biennial renewal process applicable to Phase II customers, does your bank include the following required information on the biennial renewal:

a. Ay change in control of the exempt person known to the bank (or for which the bank has reason to know); and,
b. A certification that the bank has applied its suspicious activity monitoring system to transactions in currency of the exempt person as necessary, but at least annually?

(Phase II exemptions must be re-filed every two years, on or before March 15, as part of the biennial renewal process.)

☐ *Yes*

☐ *No*

Comments:

Follow-up:

Deposit and Non-Deposit Account Types

Non-deposit investment products (ND IP) include a wide array of investment products (e.g., securities, bonds, and fixed or variable annuities). Sales programs may also include cash management sweep accounts to retail and commercial clients; these programs are offered by the bank directly. Banks offer these investments to increase fee income and provide customers with additional products and services. The manner in which the NDIP relationship is structured and the methods in which the products are offered substantially affect the bank's BSA/AML risks and responsibilities.

Networking Arrangements

Banks typically enter into networking arrangements with securities broker/dealers to offer NDIP on bank premises. For BSA/AML purposes, under a networking arrangement, the customer is a customer of the broker/dealer, although the customer may also be a bank customer for other financial services. Bank examiners recognize that the U.S. Securities and Exchange Commission (SEC) is the primary regulator for NDIP offerings through broker/dealers, and the agencies will observe functional supervision requirements of the Gramm-Leach-Bliley Act.[1] Federal banking agencies are responsible for supervising NDIP activity conducted directly by the bank.

Different types of networking arrangements may include the following:

- Co-branded Products – Co-branded products are offered by another company or financial services corporation[2] in co-sponsorship with the bank. For example, a financial services corporation tailors a mutual fund product for sale at a specific bank. The product is sold exclusively at that bank and bears the name of both the bank and the financial services corporation.

  Because of this co-branded relationship, responsibility for BSA/AML compliance becomes complex. As these accounts are not under the sole control of the bank or financial entity, responsibilities for completing Customer Identification Program (CIP), customer due diligence (CDD), and suspicious activity monitoring and reporting can vary. The bank should fully understand each party's contractual responsibilities and ensure adequate control by all parties.

- Dual-Employee Arrangements – In a dual-employee arrangement, the bank and the financial services corporation such as an insurance agency or a registered broker/dealer have a common (shared) employee. The shared employee may conduct banking business as well as sell NDIP, or sell NDIP full-time. Because of this dual-employee arrangement, the bank retains responsibility over NDIP activities. Even if contractual agreements establish the financial services corporation as being responsible for BSA/AML, the bank remains responsible and needs to ensure proper oversight and compliance with all regulatory requirements.[3]

Under some networking arrangements, registered securities sales representatives are dual employees of the bank and the broker/dealer. When the dual employee is providing investment products and services, the broker/dealer is responsible for monitoring the registered representative's compliance with applicable securities laws and regulations. When the dual employee is providing bank products or services, the bank has the responsibility for monitoring the employee's performance and compliance with BSA/AML.

- Third-Party Arrangements – Third-party arrangements may involve leasing the bank's lobby space to a financial services corporation to sell NDIPs. In this case, the third-party must clearly differentiate itself from the bank. If the arrangement is appropriately implemented, third-party arrangements do not affect the BSA/AML compliance requirements of the bank. As a sound practice, the bank is encouraged to ascertain if the financial services provider has an adequate BSA/AML compliance program as part of its due diligence.

In-House Sales and Proprietary Products

Unlike networking arrangements, the bank is fully responsible for in-house NDIP transactions completed on behalf of its customers, either with or without the benefit of an internal broker/dealer employee.[4] In addition, the bank may also offer its own proprietary NDIPs, which can be created and offered by the bank, its subsidiary, or an affiliate.

With in-house sales and proprietary products, the entire customer relationship and all BSA/AML risks may need to be managed by the bank, depending on how the products are sold. Unlike a networking arrangement, in which all or some of the responsibilities may be assumed by the third party broker/dealer with in-house sales and proprietary products, the bank should manage all of its in-house and proprietary NDIP sales not only on a department-wide basis, but on an enterprise-wide basis.

RISK FACTORS

BSA/AML risks arise because NDIP can involve complex legal arrangements, large dollar amounts, and the rapid movement of funds. NDIP portfolios managed and controlled directly by clients pose a greater money laundering risk than those managed by the bank or by the financial services provider. Sophisticated clients may create ownership structures to obscure the ultimate control and ownership of these investments. For example, customers can retain a certain level of anonymity by creating Private Investment Companies (PICs), offshore trusts, or other investment entities that hide the customer's ownership or beneficial interest.

RISK MITIGATION

Management should develop risk-based policies, procedures, and processes that enable the bank to identify unusual account relationships and circumstances, questionable assets and sources of funds, and other potential areas of risk (e.g., offshore accounts, agency accounts, and unidentified beneficiaries). Management should be alert to situations that need additional review or research.

Networking Arrangements

Before entering into a networking arrangement, banks should conduct an appropriate review of the broker/dealer. The review should include an assessment of the broker/dealer's financial status, management experience, National Association of Securities Dealers (NASD) status, reputation, and ability to fulfill its BSA/AML compliance responsibilities in regards to the bank's retail customers. Appropriate due diligence would include a determination that the broker/dealer has adequate policies, procedures, and processes in place to enable the broker/dealer to meet its legal obligations.

The bank should maintain documentation on its due diligence of the broker/dealer. Furthermore, detailed written contracts should address all facets of the networking arrangement, including the responsibilities of the broker/dealer and its registered representatives. The contract should specifically cover each party's responsibilities for compliance with BSA/AML regulations and laws and for suspicious activity monitoring and reporting.

A bank may also want to mitigate risk exposure by limiting certain investment products offered to its retail customers. Investment products such as PICs, offshore trusts, or offshore hedge funds may involve international funds transfers or offer customers ways to obscure ownership interests.

Bank management should make reasonable efforts to update due diligence information on the broker/dealer. Such efforts may include a periodic review of information on the broker/dealer's compliance with its BSA/AML responsibilities, verification of the broker/dealer's record in meeting testing requirements, and a review of consumer complaints. Bank management is also encouraged, when possible, to review BSA/AML reports generated by the broker/dealer. This review could include information on account openings, transactions, investment products sold, and suspicious activity monitoring and reporting.

In-House Sales and Proprietary Products

Bank management should assess risk on the basis of a variety of factors such as:

- The type of NDIP purchased and the size of the transactions;
- The types and frequency of transactions;
- The country of residence of the principals or beneficiaries, or the country of incorporation, or the source of funds;
- Accounts and transactions that are not usual and customary for the customer or for the bank.

For customers that management considers high risk for money laundering and terrorist financing, more stringent documentation, verification, and transaction monitoring procedures should be established. Enhanced due diligence may be appropriate in the following situations:

- The bank is entering into a relationship with a new customer;
- Non-discretionary accounts have a large asset size or frequent transactions;
- The customer resides in a foreign jurisdiction;
- The customer is a PIC or other corporate structure established in a higher risk jurisdiction;
- Assets or transactions are atypical for the customer;
- Investment type, size, assets, or transactions are atypical for the bank;
- International funds transfers are conducted, particularly from offshore funding sources;
- The identities of the principals or beneficiaries in investments or relationships are unknown or cannot be easily determined;
- Politically exposed persons are parties to any investments or transactions.

---

[1] Functional regulation limits the circumstances in which the federal banking agencies can directly examine or require reports from a bank affiliate or subsidiary whose primary regulator is the SEC, the Commodity Futures Trading Commission, or state issuance authorities. Federal banking agencies are generally limited from examining such an entity unless further information is needed to determine whether the banking affiliate or subsidiary poses a material risk to the bank, to determine compliance with a legal requirement under the federal banking agencies' jurisdiction, or to assess the bank's risk management system covering the functionally regulated activities. These standards require greater reliance on the functional regulator and better cooperation among regulators.

[2] A financial services corporation includes those entities offering NDIP, which may include investment firms, financial institutions, securities brokers/dealers, and insurance companies.

[3] If the bank uses the reliance provision under the CIP, responsibility for CIP shifts to the third-party provider. Refer to core overview section "Customer Identification Program" on page 30 for additional information.

[4] A bank shall not be considered to be a broker, nor need an employee registered as a broker/dealer, because the bank engages in any one or more of the activities under the conditions described:

- The bank effects customer transactions in municipal securities.
- The bank effects not more than 500 transactions in securities for its customers in any calendar year, and such transactions are not effected by an employee of the bank who is also an employee of a broker or dealer.
- The bank deals in commercial paper, banker's acceptances, commercial bills, or exempted securities.
- The bank effects customer transactions in identified banking products as defined in section 206 of the Gramm-Leach-Bliley Act.
- The bank effects customer transactions in certain stock purchase plans such as employee benefit plans, dividend reinvestment plans, and issuer plans.

1. Has the legitimacy of deposit brokers and representatives (corporate documentation, references, background checks, verification of prior employment, database searches, etc.) been verified?

☐ *Yes*

☐ *No*

Comments:

Follow-up:

2. Does your bank's compliance program require or provide training or information to brokers/representatives on money laundering risks and bank procedures?

☐ *Yes*

☐ *No*

Comments:

Follow-up:

3. Do your bank's policies and procedures require review and verification of customer information provided by the deposit broker/representative using call back procedures or conducting meetings with customers?

☐ *Yes*

☐ *No*

Comments:

Follow-up:

4. Does your bank segregate and monitor brokered accounts for unusual activity?

☐ *Yes*

☐ *No*

Comments:

Follow-up:

5. If your bank accepts deposit broker accounts or funds, has it developed appropriate policies, procedures, and processes that establish minimum CDD procedures for all deposit brokers providing deposits to the bank?

☐ *Yes*

☐ *No*

Comments:

Follow-up:

6. In an effort to address the risk inherent in deposit broker relationships, does your bank have require a signed contract with brokers that sets out the roles and responsibilities of each party and restrictions on types of customers (e.g., nonresident or offshore customers, SFPFs, or foreign shell banks).

☐ *Yes*

☐ *No*

Comments:

Follow-up:

7. To manage the BSA/AML risks associated with brokered deposits, do your bank's policies and procedures require it to:

a. Determine whether a deposit broker is a legitimate business, in all operating locations where the business is conducted?
b. Review deposit brokers' business strategies, including targeted customer markets (e.g., foreign or domestic customers) and whether a deposit broker is subject to regulatory oversight?
c. Evaluate whether deposit brokers' BSA/AML/OFAC policies, procedures, and processes are adequate (e.g., ascertain whether the deposit broker performs sufficient CDD and CIP procedures)?
d. Determine whether deposit brokers screen clients for OFAC matches?
e. Evaluate the adequacy of deposit brokers' BSA/AML/OFAC audits and ensure that they address compliance with applicable regulations and requirements?

☐ *Yes*

☐ *No*

Comments:

Follow-up:

8. Do your bank's procedures require monitoring existing deposit broker relationships for any significant changes in business strategies that may influence the broker's risk profile?

☐ *Yes*

☐ *No*

Comments:

Follow-up:

9. Do your bank's procedures require periodically re-verifying and updating each deposit broker's profile to ensure an appropriate risk assessment?

☐ *Yes*

☐ *No*

Comments:

Follow-up:

10. Banks should implement appropriate polices, procedures, and processes to address risks with Independent Sales Organization (ISO) relationships? At a minimum, does your bank's policies include:

a. Verification of an ISO's legitimacy through a review of corporate documentation, licenses, permits, contracts, or references?
b. Review of public databases to determine the existence of issues with the ISO or principal owners?
c. Understanding of the currency servicing arrangements for privately-owned ATMs and whether legitimate currency generation is sufficient to service machines?
d. Documentation of the locations of privately-owned ATMs and determination of the ISO's target geographic market?
e. Expected account activity, including currency withdrawals?

☐ *Yes*

☐ *No*

Comments:

Follow-up:

11. Due diligence on customers that are ISOs, must extend beyond the minimum customer identification program (CIP) requirements. Banks should also perform due diligence on ATM owners. Does your bank's compliance program due diligence steps require the bank to:

a. Verify the ATM owner's legitimacy through a review of corporate documentation, licenses, permits, contracts, or references, including the ATM transaction provider contract?
b. Review public databases for information on the ATM owners?
c. Obtain the addresses of all ATM locations, ascertain the types of businesses where they are located, and identify targeted demographics?
d. Determine expected ATM activity levels, including currency withdrawals?
e. Ascertain the sources of currency for the ATMs by reviewing copies of armored car contracts, lending arrangements, or any other documentation, as appropriate?

☐ *Yes*

☐ *No*

Comments:

Follow-up:

12. Regarding *networking arrangements* for Non-Deposit Investment Products (NDIP) that are co-branded, does your bank's management fully understand each party's contractual responsibilities and ensure adequate control by all parties?

☐ *Yes*

☐ *No*

Comments:

Follow-up:

13. Regarding networking arrangements for Non-Deposit Investment Products (NDIP) and Dual Employee Arrangements, if the bank does not use the *reliance provision* under CIP, does it ensure proper oversight and compliance with all regulatory requirements concerning the arrangement?

☐ *Yes*

☐ *No*

Comments:

Follow-up:

14. When a dual employee is providing bank products or services, does your bank's policies and procedures cover its responsibility for monitoring the employee's performance and compliance with BSA/AML?

☐ *Yes*

☐ *No*

Comments:

Follow-up:

15. Has management developed risk-based policies, procedures, and processes that enable the bank to identify unusual account relationships and circumstances, questionable assets and sources of funds, and other potential areas of risk (e.g., offshore accounts, agency accounts, and unidentified beneficiaries)?

☐ *Yes*

☐ *No*

Comments:

Follow-up:

16. If your bank has entered into a networking arrangement with a broker dealer, has it conducted appropriate due diligence to include a determination that the broker/dealer has adequate policies, procedures, and processes in place to enable the broker/dealer to meet its legal obligations, and has the bank maintained documentation on its due diligence of the broker/dealer?

☐ *Yes*

☐ *No*

Comments:

Follow-up:

17. Does your bank maintain detailed written contracts that address all facets of networking arrangements with broker/dealers, including the responsibilities of broker/dealer and its registered representatives? (**Note:** The contract should specifically cover each party's responsibilities for compliance with BSA/AML regulations and laws and for suspicious activity monitoring and reporting.)

☐ *Yes*

☐ *No*

Comments:

Follow-up:

18. Does your bank conduct periodic reviews of information on the broker/dealer's compliance with its BSA/AML responsibilities, verification of the broker/dealer's record in meeting testing requirements, and a review of consumer complaints?

☐ *Yes*

☐ *No*

Comments:

Follow-up:

19. For insurance product sales, does your bank monitor or review transactions for early policy terminations as well as other unusual and suspicious activity (e.g., a single, large premium payment, a customer's purchase of a product that appears to fall outside the customer's normal range of financial transactions, early redemptions, multiple transactions, payments to apparently unrelated third parties, and collateralized loans)?

☐ *Yes*

☐ *No*

Comments:

Follow-up:

Education/Training/Awareness

Banks must ensure that appropriate personnel are trained in applicable aspects of the BSA. Training should include regulatory requirements and the bank's internal BSA/AML policies, procedures, and processes. At a minimum, the bank's training program must provide training for all personnel whose duties require knowledge of the BSA. The training should be tailored to the person's specific responsibilities. In addition, an overview of the BSA/AML requirements should be given to new staff. Training should encompass information related to applicable operational lines, such as trust services, international, and private banking.

The board of directors and senior management should be informed of changes and new developments in the BSA, its implementing regulations and directives, and the federal banking agencies' regulations. While the board of directors may not require the same degree of training as banking operations personnel, they need to understand the importance of BSA/AML regulatory requirements, the ramifications of noncompliance, and the risks posed to the bank. Without a general understanding of the BSA, the board of directors cannot adequately provide BSA/AML oversight; approve BSA/AML policies, procedures, and processes; or provide sufficient BSA/AML resources.

Training should be ongoing and incorporate current developments and changes to the BSA and any related regulations. Changes to internal policies, procedures, processes, and monitoring systems should also be covered during training. The program should reinforce the importance that the board and senior management place on the bank's compliance with the BSA and ensure that all employees understand their role in maintaining an effective BSA/AML compliance program.

Examples of money laundering activity and suspicious activity monitoring and reporting can and should be tailored to each individual audience. For example, training for tellers should focus on examples involving large currency transactions or other suspicious activities; training for the loan department should provide examples involving money laundering through lending arrangements.

Banks should document their training programs. Training and testing materials, the dates of training sessions, and attendance records should be maintained by the bank and be available for examiner review.

1. Regulations require that financial institutions provide BSA training for appropriate personnel, including, but not limited to, tellers, customer service representatives, lending officers, private and personal banking officers and all other customer contact personnel. Are these requirements properly documented in your firm's operations manuals?

☐ *Yes*

☐ *No*

Comments:

Follow-up:

2. Does your institution's program for educating appropriate employees regarding the BSA establish a program to include reporting of large currency transactions?

☐ *Yes*

☐ *No*

Comments:

Follow-up:

3. Does your institution's program for educating appropriate employees regarding the BSA cover exemptions from large currency transaction reporting?

☐ *Yes*

☐ *No*

Comments:

Follow-up:

4. Does your institution's program for educating appropriate employees regarding the BSA cover identification and reporting of suspicious activities or alleged criminal conduct?

☐ *Yes*

☐ *No*

Comments:

Follow-up:

5. Does your institution's program for educating appropriate employees regarding the BSA cover record retention requirements?

☐ *Yes*

☐ *No*

Comments:

Follow-up:

6. Does your institution's program for educating appropriate employees regarding the BSA cover the sale/purchase of monetary instruments?

☐ *Yes*

☐ *No*

Comments:

Follow-up:

7. Does your institution's program for educating appropriate employees regarding the BSA cover the periodic review of internal policies/procedures?

☐ *Yes*

☐ *No*

Comments:

Follow-up:

8. Does your institution's program for educating appropriate employees regarding the BSA cover examples of money laundering cases and the methods in which activities can be detected/resolved/reported?

☐ *Yes*

☐ *No*

Comments:

Follow-up:

9. Does your institution's program for educating appropriate employees regarding the BSA cover an overview of the different forms that money laundering can take (deposit accounts, wire transfer loans, etc)?

☐ *Yes*

☐ *No*

Comments:

Follow-up:

10. Does your institution's program for educating appropriate employees regarding the BSA cover wire (fund) transfer activity?

☐ *Yes*

☐ *No*

Comments:

Follow-up:

11. Does your institution's program for educating appropriate employees regarding the BSA cover *Know Your Customer* procedures?

☐ *Yes*

☐ *No*

Comments:

Follow-up:

12. Are your firm's training policies sufficient in scope and frequency of training meetings to demonstrate the importance management places in ongoing education and training?

☐ *Yes*

☐ *No*

Comments:

Follow-up:

13. If you were to question operations and/or business personnel right now, would they be able to demonstrate sufficient knowledge concerning the BSA with respect to their specific operating areas?

☐ *Yes*

☐ *No*

Comments:

Follow-up:

14. Can your firm (the Compliance Office, etc.) demonstrate that the firm's training addresses money laundering schemes?

☐ *Yes*

☐ *No*

Comments:

Follow-up:

15. Is *on-going* continuing education provided for all personnel conducting training?

☐ *Yes*

☐ *No*

Comments:

Follow-up:

16. Does your bank's training and education program include information on Mexican bank draft and factored third party check schemes?

☐ *Yes*

☐ *No*

Comments:

Follow-up:

17. Do your business units' procedures provide for detection of red flags for which the bank should investigate further, including high volume of cash activity?

☐ *Yes*

☐ *No*

Comments:

Follow-up:

18. Do your business units' procedures provide for detection of red flags for which the bank should investigate further, including deposit activity followed by lump sum wire transfers?

☐ *Yes*

☐ *No*

Comments:

Follow-up:

19. Do your business units' procedures provide for detection of red flags for which the bank should investigate further, including unusual monetary instrument or check activity?

☐ *Yes*

☐ *No*

Comments:

Follow-up:

20. Do your business units' procedures provide for detection of red flags for which the bank should investigate further, including international wire transfers to known money laundering havens?

☐ *Yes*

☐ *No*

Comments:

Follow-up:

Electronic Cash

E-cash is a digital representation of money. E-cash (or e-money) comes in two basic forms:

- Stored value card e-cash; and,
- Computer e-cash.

Stored value card e-cash is most often downloaded through special terminals (e.g., specially equipped automated teller machines (ATMs), computers, or cellular phones) onto electronic cards. Computer e-cash is downloaded to personal computer hard disks via a modem or stored in an online repository.

Stored value cards can operate in either an open or closed system. Typically, open system cards may be reloaded, allowing the cardholder to add value. Closed system cards are usually limited to the initial value posted to the card, but some may allow the cardholder to add value. Additionally, funds can be prepaid on an open system card by one person, with someone else accessing the currency elsewhere through an ATM. Prepayment involves a transfer of funds to the card (e.g., telephone calling cards). Some domestic and offshore banks offer cards with currency access through ATMs internationally. Since stored value cards are easy to fund and transport without creating a paper trail, they are attractive for abuse by various illegal enterprises and money launderers. For example, drug dealers have been known to load currency onto prepaid cards and send the cards to their drug suppliers outside the country. Phone cards and other closed system prepaid cards can be purchased for currency and transferred from one person to another and resold. Often, a firm independent of a bank processes all card transactions through a "pooled" bank account held in the name of the firm managing the card program.[1]

Consumers use e-cash to access, store, and redeem funds that are maintained electronically. The transfer of funds to the card is a form of prepayment (e.g., telephone calling cards). In addition, e-cash, in the form of payroll cards, is now offered by employers to their employees in place of a check to distribute wages. The value of the funds stored on these cards can be transferred between vendors and individuals using compatible electronic systems, often without using banks. Using special readers, stored monetary value is subtracted from the card. When the monetary value is depleted, the card is either discarded or, in some instances, value is replenished. In the case of computer e-e-cash, monetary value is electronically deducted from the bank account when a purchase is made. Additional information on types of e-cash products is available in the FFIEC Information Technology Examination Handbook.

RISK FACTORS

Transactions using e-cash may pose the following unique risks to the bank:

- Funds may be transferred to or from an unknown third party;
- Customers may be able to avoid border restrictions as the transactions can become mobile and may not be subject to jurisdictional restrictions;
- Transactions may be instantaneous;
- Specific cardholder activity may be difficult to determine by reviewing activity through a pooled account;
- The customer may perceive the transactions as less transparent.

RISK MITIGATION

Banks should establish BSA/AML monitoring, identification, and reporting for unusual and suspicious activities occurring through e-cash. Useful management information systems for detecting unusual activity on high-risk accounts include ATM activity reports (focusing on foreign transactions), funds transfer reports, new account activity reports, change of Internet address reports, Internet Protocol (IP) address reports, and reports to identify related or linked accounts (e.g., common addresses, phone numbers, e-mail addresses, and tax identification numbers). Other controls, such as establishing transaction and account dollar limits that require manual intervention to exceed the preset limit, may also be instituted by the bank.

[1] "Open" system cards can be used to connect to global debit and ATM networks; the cards can be used for purchases at any merchant or to access currency at any ATM that connects to global payment networks. "Closed" system cards are limited in that they can only be used to buy goods or services from the merchant issuing the card or a select group of merchants or service providers that participate in a network.

1. Has your bank's management and risk policy recognized e-banking as a potentially high-risk area and developed adequate policies, procedures, and processes for customer identification and monitoring for specific areas of banking?

☐ *Yes*

☐ *No*

Comments:

Follow-up:

2. Do your bank's transaction monitoring systems adequately capture transactions conducted electronically?

☐ *Yes*

☐ *No*

Comments:

Follow-up:

3. Does your bank have an adequate program for BSA/AML monitoring, identification, and reporting for unusual and suspicious activities occurring through e-banking systems? (**Note:** Useful management information systems for detecting unusual activity in high-risk accounts include ATM activity reports, funds transfer reports, new account activity reports, change of Internet address reports, Internet Protocol (IP) address reports, and reports to identify related or linked accounts (e.g., common addresses, phone numbers, e-mail addresses, and tax identification numbers.))

☐ *Yes*

☐ *No*

Comments:

Follow-up:

4. In determining the level of monitoring required for an account, does your bank's risk program include how the account was opened, as a factor?

☐ *Yes*

☐ *No*

Comments:

Follow-up:

5. Are other controls, such as establishing transaction dollar limits for large items that require manual intervention to exceed the preset limit, also instituted as part of the bank's e-banking risk mitigation program?

☐ *Yes*

☐ *No*

Comments:

Follow-up:

6. Does your bank have policies and procedures for BSA/AML monitoring, identification, and reporting for unusual and suspicious activities occurring through e-cash facilities?

☐ *Yes*

☐ *No*

Comments:

Follow-up:

7. Are controls, such as establishing transaction and account dollar limits that require manual intervention to exceed the preset limit, instituted by the bank in its e-cash monitoring efforts?
(Note: Useful management information systems for detecting unusual activity on high-risk accounts include, ATM activity reports focusing on foreign transactions), funds transfer reports, new account activity reports, change of Internet address reports, Internet Protocol (IP) address reports, and reports to identify related or linked accounts (e.g., common addresses, phone numbers, e-mail addresses, and tax identification numbers.)

☐ *Yes*

☐ *No*

Comments:

Follow-up:

Electronic (3rd Party) Payment Processor Services

Non-bank, or third-party, payment processors (processors) are bank customers that provide payment-processing services to merchants and other business entities. Traditionally, processors contracted primarily with retailers that had physical locations in order to process the retailers' transactions. These merchant transactions primarily included credit card payments but also covered automated clearing house demand drafts[1] (also known as e-checks), and debit and stored value cards transactions. With the expansion of the Internet, retail borders have been eliminated. Processors may now service a variety of merchant accounts, including conventional retail and Internet-based establishments, prepaid travel, and Internet gaming enterprises.

RISK FACTORS

Processors generally are not subject to BSA/AML regulatory requirements. As a result, some processors may be vulnerable to money laundering, identity theft, and fraud schemes.

The bank's BSA/AML risks when dealing with a processor account are similar to risks from other activities in which the bank's customer conducts transactions through the bank on behalf of the customer's clients. When the bank is unable to identify and understand the nature and source of the transactions processed through an account, the risks to the bank and the likelihood of suspicious activity can increase. If a bank has not implemented an adequate processor-approval program that goes beyond credit risk management, it could be vulnerable to processing illicit or sanctioned transactions.

RISK MITIGATION

Banks offering account services to processors should develop and maintain adequate policies, procedures, and processes to address risks related to these relationships. At a minimum, these policies should authenticate the processor's business operations and assess their risk level. Verification and assessment of a processor can be completed by performing the following procedures:

- Reviewing the processor's promotional materials, including its web site, to determine the target clientele. (Businesses with elevated risk may include: offshore companies, online gambling-related operations, and online payday lenders). For example, a processor whose customers are primarily offshore would be inherently riskier than a processor whose customers are primarily restaurants;
- Determining whether the processor re-sells its services to a third party who may be referred to as an "agent or provider of Independent Sales Organization (ISO) opportunities" or "gateway" arrangements;[2]
- Reviewing the processor's policies, procedures, and processes to determine the adequacy of its due diligence standards for new merchants;
- Identifying the processor's major customers;
- Reviewing corporate documentation including independent reporting services and, if applicable, documentation on principal owners;
- Visiting the processor's business operations center. Banks that provide account services should monitor their processor relationships for any significant changes in the processors' business strategies that may affect their risk profile.

Banks should periodically re-verify and update the businesses' profiles to ensure the risk assessment is appropriate. In addition to adequate and effective account opening and due diligence procedures for processor accounts, management should monitor these relationships for unusual and suspicious activities. To effectively monitor these accounts, the bank should have an understanding of the following processor information:

- Merchant base;
- Merchant activities;
- Average number of dollar volume and number of transactions;
- "Swiping" versus "keying" volume for credit card transactions;
- Charge-back history.

---

[1] A demand draft is a substitute for a pre-printed paper check. The draft is produced without a consumer signature but presumably with the consumer's authorization.

[2] Gateway arrangements are similar to an Internet service provider with excess computer storage capacity who sells its capacity to a third party, who would then distribute computer service to various other individuals unknown to the provider. The third party would be making decisions about who would be receiving the service, although the provider would be providing the ultimate storage capacity. Thus, the provider bears all of the risks while receiving a smaller profit.

1. If your bank offers account services to processors (i.e., third party payment processors) has it developed and maintained adequate policies, procedures, and controls to address risks related to these relationships? (Note: At a minimum, these policies should authenticate the processor's business operations and assess their risk level. See the FFIEC examination manual for assessment procedures).

☐ *Yes*

☐ *No*

Comments:

Follow-up:

2. If your Bank provides account services to payment processors, does it monitor the processor relationship for any significant changes in the processors' business strategies that may affect their risk profile?

☐ *Yes*

☐ *No*

Comments:

Follow-up:

3. In addition to adequate and effective account opening and due diligence procedures for processor accounts, does your bank's management monitor these relationships for unusual and suspicious activities and include consideration of all of the following applicable factors:

a. The Merchant's base?
b. The Merchant's activities?
c. The average dollar volume and number of transactions?
d. Swiping versus keying volume for credit card transactions?
e. Charge-back history?

☐ *Yes*

☐ *No*

Comments:

Follow-up:

Embassy & Foreign Government Accounts

Embassies contain the offices of the foreign ambassador, the diplomatic representative, and their staff. The embassy, led by the ambassador, is a foreign government's official representation in the United States (or other country). Foreign consulate offices act as branches of the embassy and perform various administrative and governmental functions (e.g., issuing visas and handling immigration matters). Foreign consulate offices are typically located in major metropolitan areas. In addition, foreign ambassadors' diplomatic representatives, their families, and their associates may be considered politically exposed persons (aka, SFPFs) in certain circumstances.

Embassies and foreign consulates in the United States require access to the banking system to meet many of their day-to-day financial responsibilities. Such services can range from account relationships for operational expenses (e.g., payroll, rent, and utilities) to inter-and intra-governmental transactions (e.g., commercial and military purchases). In addition to official embassy accounts, some banks provide ancillary services or accounts to embassy staff, families, and current or prior foreign government officials. Each of these relationships poses different levels of risk to the bank. Embassy accounts, including those accounts for a specific embassy office such as a cultural or education ministry, a defense attaché or ministry, or any other account, should have a specific operating purpose stating the official function of the foreign government office. Consistent with established practices for business relationships, these embassy accounts should have written authorization by the foreign government.

RISK FACTORS

To provide embassy and foreign consulate services, a U.S. bank may need to maintain a foreign correspondent relationship with the embassy's or foreign consulate's bank. Banks conducting business with foreign embassies or consulates should assess and understand the potential risks of these accounts and should develop appropriate policies, procedures, and processes. Embassy or foreign consulate accounts may pose a higher risk in the following circumstances:

- Accounts are from countries that have been designated as high risk.
- Substantial currency transactions take place in the accounts.
- Account activity is not consistent with the purpose of the account (e.g., pouch activity or payable upon proper identification transactions).
- Accounts directly fund personal expenses of foreign nationals, including but not limited to expenses for college students.
- Official embassy business is conducted through personal accounts.

RISK MITIGATION

Banks should obtain comprehensive due diligence information on embassy and foreign consulate account relationships. For private banking accounts for non-U.S. persons specifically, banks must obtain due diligence information as required by 31 CFR 103.181. The bank's due diligence related to embassy and foreign consulate account relationships should be commensurate with the risk levels presented. In addition, banks are expected to establish policies, procedures, and processes that provide for greater scrutiny and monitoring of all embassy and foreign consulate account relationships. Management should fully understand the purpose of the account and the expected volume and nature of account activity. Ongoing monitoring of embassy and foreign consulate account relationships is critical to ensuring that the account relationships are being used as anticipated.

1. Do account acceptance processes for embassy accounts include written authorization by the foreign government as well as the gathering of comprehensive due diligence information on embassy and foreign consulate account relationships?

☐ *Yes*

☐ *No*

Comments:

Follow-up:

2. Do your bank's policies, procedures, and processes specifically provide for greater scrutiny and monitoring of all embassy and foreign consulate account relationships?

☐ *Yes*

☐ *No*

Comments:

Follow-up:

3. Does management fully understand the purpose of each embassy and/or foreign government account and the expected volume and nature of account activity?

☐ ***Yes***

☐ ***No***

Comments:

Follow-up:

4. Is ongoing monitoring of embassy and foreign consulate account relationships being conducted to ensure that account relationships are being used as anticipated?

☐ ***Yes***

☐ ***No***

Comments:

Follow-up:

Foreign Bank & Financial Account Record

Each person[1] (including a bank) subject to U.S. jurisdiction with a financial interest in or signature authority over, a bank, a securities, or any other financial account in a foreign country must file a Report of Foreign Bank and Financial Accounts (FBAR) with the Internal Revenue Service (IRS) (TD F 90-22.1) if the aggregate value of these financial accounts exceeds $10,000 at any time during the calendar year. A bank must file this form on its own accounts that meet this definition; the bank may be obligated to file these forms for customer accounts in which the bank has a financial interest or over which it has signature authority.

A FBAR must be filed with the commissioner of the IRS on or before June 30 of each calendar year for foreign financial accounts exceeding $10,000 maintained at any time during the previous calendar year.

---

[1] As defined in 31 CFR 103.11(z), the term "person" means an individual, a corporation, a partnership, a trust or estate, a joint stock company, an association, a syndicate, joint venture or other unincorporated organization or group, an Indian Tribe (as that term is defined in the Indian Gaming Regulatory Act), and all entities cognizable as legal personalities.

1. Does your bank's compliance program address the requirement that each person (including a bank) subject to U.S. jurisdiction with a financial interest in, or signature authority over, a bank, a securities, or any other financial account in a foreign country file a Report of Foreign Bank and Financial Accounts (FBAR) with the Internal Revenue Service (IRS) (TD F 90-22.1) if the aggregate value of these financial accounts exceeds $10,000 at any time during the calendar year?
(**Note:** A bank must file this form on its own accounts that meet this definition; the bank may be obligated to file these forms for customer accounts in which the bank has a financial interest or over which it has signature authority.)

☐ *Yes*

☐ *No*

Comments:

Follow-up:

2. Does your bank file FBARs with the commissioner of the IRS on or before June 30 of each calendar year for foreign financial accounts exceeding $10,000 maintained at any time during the previous calendar year?

☐ *Yes*

☐ *No*

Comments:

Follow-up:

Foreign Branches and Offices of US Banks

U.S. banks open foreign branches and offices to meet specific customer demands, to help the bank grow, or to expand products or services offered. Foreign branches and offices vary significantly in size, complexity of operations, and scope of products and services offered. Examiners must take these factors into consideration when reviewing whether the foreign branches and offices adhere to the bank's BSA/AML compliance program. AML policies, procedures, and processes at the foreign office or branch should comply with local requirements and be consistent with the U.S. bank's standards; however, they may need to be tailored for local or business practices.[1]

RISK FACTORS

BSA compliance officers should understand the type of products and services offered at foreign branches and offices, as well as the customers and geographic locations served at the foreign branches and offices. Any service offered by the U.S. bank may be offered by the foreign branches and offices if not prohibited by the host country. Such products and services offered at the foreign branches and offices may have a different risk profile from that of the same product or service offered in the U.S. bank (e.g., money services businesses are regulated in the United States; however, similar entities in another country may not be regulated). Therefore, the compliance officers should be aware that risks associated with foreign branches and offices may differ (e.g., wholesale versus retail operations). A BSA officer should understand the foreign jurisdictions' various AML requirements. Secrecy laws or their equivalent may affect the ability of the foreign branch or office to share information with the U.S. parent bank, or the ability of the bank auditor (or compliance department) to examine onsite. Although specific BSA requirements are not applicable at foreign branches and offices, banks are expected to have policies, procedures, and processes in place at all their branches, including affiliates and subsidiaries. Considerations should include

- The risk profile of the foreign branch or office and whether the profile is stable or hanging as a result of a reorganization, the introduction of new products or services, or other factors, including the risk profile of the jurisdiction itself;
- The effectiveness and quality of bank supervision in the host country;
- Existence of information sharing agreement between the host country and the U.S. supervisor;
- The history of examination or audit concerns at the foreign branch or office;
- The size and complexity of the foreign branch's or office's operations;
- Effectiveness of internal controls, including systems for managing AML risks on a consolidated basis and internal audit;
- The capability of management at the foreign branch or office to protect the entity from money laundering or terrorist financing;
- The availability of the foreign branch or office records in the United States.

U.S.-Based Examinations

U.S.-based, or off-site examinations, generally require greater confidence in the AML program at the foreign branch or office, as well as the ability to access sufficient records. Such off-site examinations should include discussions with senior bank management at the head and foreign offices which are crucial to the understanding of the foreign branches or offices' operations, AML risks, and AML programs. Also, the examination of the foreign branch or office should include a review of the U.S. bank's involvement in managing or monitoring the foreign branch's operations, internal control systems (e.g., policies, procedures, and monitoring reports), and, where available, the host country supervisors' examination findings, audit findings, and work-papers. As with all BSA/AML examinations, the extent of transaction testing and activities where it is performed is based on various factors including the examiner's judgment of risks, controls, and the adequacy of the independent testing.

Host Jurisdiction-Based Examinations

AML reporting requirements are likely to be different, as they will be adjusted to local regulatory requirements. In addition, on-site work in the host jurisdiction will enable examiners to better understand the role of the U.S. bank in relation to its foreign branch or office.

For both U.S.-based and host-based examinations of foreign branches and offices, the procedures used for specific products, services, and customers are those found in the FFIEC Examination manual. For example, if an examiner is looking at pouch activities at foreign branches and offices, he or she should would the applicable expanded examination procedures.

---

[1] For additional information refer to "Consolidated Know Your Customer (KYC) Risk Management," Basel Committee on Banking Supervision, 2004, at www.bis.org/publ.

1. Does your bank have policies, procedures, and processes in place at all its foreign branches and offices?

☐ *Yes*

☐ *No*

Comments:

Follow-up:

2. Does your bank have a program in place to review involvement in managing or monitoring foreign branches' operations, internal control systems (e.g., policies, procedures, and monitoring reports), and, where available, the host country supervisors' examination findings, audit findings, and work papers?

☐ *Yes*

☐ *No*

Comments:

Follow-up:

3. Does your bank's monitoring program for its foreign branches and offices consider transaction testing and activities based on various factors including judgment of risks, controls, and the adequacy of the independent testing?

☐ *Yes*

☐ *No*

Comments:

Follow-up:

Funds/Wire Transfer

Funds transfer systems enable the instantaneous transfer of funds, including both domestic and cross-border transfers. Consequently these systems can present an attractive method to disguise the source of funds derived from illegal activity. The BSA was amended by the Annunzio-Wylie Anti-Money Laundering Act of 1992 to authorize the U.S. Treasury and the Federal Reserve Board to prescribe regulations for domestic and international funds transfers.

Banks need to have sound policies, procedures, and processes to manage the BSA/AML risks of its funds transfer activities. Such policies may encompass more than regulatory record-keeping minimums and be expanded to cover OFAC.

Obtaining customer due diligence (CDD) information is an important mitigant of risk in providing funds transfer services. Because of the nature of funds transfers, adequate and effective CDD policies, procedures, and processes are critical in detecting unusual and suspicious activities. Equally important is an effective risk-based suspicious activity monitoring and reporting system.

Originating and beneficiary banks should establish effective and appropriate policies, procedures, and processes for PUPID activity including:

- Specifying the type of identification that is acceptable;
- Maintaining documentation of individuals consistent with the bank's record-keeping policies;
- Defining which bank employees may conduct PUPID transactions;
- Establishing limits on the amount of funds that may be transferred to or from the bank for non-customers (including type of funds accepted (i.e., currency or official check) by originating bank);
- Monitoring and reporting suspicious activities.
- Providing enhanced scrutiny for transfers to or from certain jurisdictions.
- Identifying disbursement method (i.e., by currency or official check) for proceeds from beneficiary bank.

Banks should consider all three stages of money laundering when evaluating or assessing funds transfer risks.

In 1995, the U.S. Treasury and the Board of Governors of the Federal Reserve System issued a final rule on record-keeping requirements concerning payment orders by banks (31 CFR 103.33).[1] The rule requires each bank involved in funds transfers[2] to collect and retain certain information in connection with funds transfers of $3,000 or more.[3] The information required to be collected and retained depends on the bank's role in the particular funds transfer (originator's bank, intermediary bank, or beneficiary's bank).[4]
The requirements may also vary depending on whether an originator or beneficiary is an established customer of a bank and whether a payment order is made in person or otherwise.

Also in 1995, the U.S. Treasury issued a final rule that requires all financial institutions to include certain information in transmittal orders for funds transfers of $3,000 or more (31 CFR 103.33).[5] This requirement is commonly referred to as the "Travel Rule."

[1] 31 CFR 103.33(e) is the record-keeping rule for banks, and 31 CFR 103.33(f) imposes similar requirements for non-bank financial institutions that engage in funds transfers. The procedures in this core overview address only the rules for banks in 31 CFR 103.33(e).

[2] Funds transfer is defined under 31 CFR 103.11. Funds transfers governed by the Electronic Fund Transfer Act of 1978, as well as any other funds transfers that are made through an automated clearing house, an automated teller machine, or a point-of-sale system, are excluded from this definition and exempt from the requirements of 103.33(e), (f) and (g).

[3] 31 CFR 103.33(e)(6) provides exceptions to the funds transfer requirements. Funds transfers where both the originator and the beneficiary are the same person and the originator's bank and the beneficiary's bank are the same bank are not subject to the record-keeping requirements for funds transfers. Additionally, exceptions are provided from the record-keeping requirements for funds transfers where the originator and beneficiary are: a bank; a wholly owned domestic subsidiary of a bank chartered in the United States; a broker or dealer in securities; a wholly-owned domestic subsidiary of a broker or dealer in securities; the United States; a state or local government; or a federal, state or local government agency or instrumentality.

[4] These terms are defined under 31 CFR 103.11.

[5] The rule applies to both banks and non-banks (31 CFR 103.33(g)). Because it is broader in scope, the Travel Rule uses more expansive terms, such as "transmittal order" instead of "payment order" and "transmittor's financial institution" instead of "originating bank." The broader terms include the bank specific terms.

1. Is there adequate separation of duties or compensating controls to ensure proper authorization for sending and receipt of transfers, correct posting to accounts and an audit trail of activities?

☐ *Yes*

☐ *No*

Comments:

Follow-up:

2. Does the institution accept cash for funds transfers and, if so, does the institution require identification, maintain documentation, and file CTRs, if applicable?

☐ *Yes*

☐ *No*

Comments:

Follow-up:

3. Does your institution send or receive fund transfers to/from financial institutions in other countries, especially countries with strict privacy and secrecy laws, and, if so, are amounts, frequency, and countries of origin/destination consistent with the nature of the business or occupation of the customer? Are internal audits conducted periodically, or are systems in place to monitor these on an ongoing basis?

☐ *Yes*

☐ *No*

Comments:

Follow-up:

4. Does your institution have procedures to monitor accounts conducting frequent cash deposits and subsequent wire transfers of funds to a larger institution or out of the country?

☐ *Yes*

☐ *No*

Comments:

Follow-up:

5. Does your bank use a customer's true name and address to comply with the Travel Rule? (**Note:** From 1998 to 2004, a conditional exception to the Travel Rule generally permitted banks to include a customer's coded name or pseudonym in a transmittal order, provided that the bank maintained the customer's full information in an automated customer information file (CIF). FinCEN revoked this exception, known as the "CIF exception," as of July 1, 2004.)

☐ *Yes*

☐ *No*

Comments:

Follow-up:

6. For funds transfer activities, if your bank acts as an originator or beneficiary bank, are effective and appropriate policies, procedures, and processes for PUPID activity in place, including:

a. Specifying the type of identification that is acceptable?
b. Maintaining documentation of individuals consistent with the bank's recordkeeping policies?
c. Defining which bank employees may conduct PUPID transactions?
d. Establishing limits on the amount of funds that may be transferred to or from the bank for non-customers (including type of funds accepted (i.e., currency or official check) by originating bank)?
e. Monitoring and reporting suspicious activities?
f. Providing enhanced scrutiny for transfers to or from certain jurisdictions?
g. Identifying disbursement method (i.e., by currency or official check) for proceeds from beneficiary bank?

☐ *Yes*

☐ *No*

Comments:

Follow-up:

Funds/Wire Transfer - Beneficiary Banks

Record-keeping Requirements

For each payment order of $3,000 or more that a bank accepts as a beneficiary's bank, the bank must retain a record of the payment order. If the beneficiary is not an established customer of the bank, the beneficiary's institution must retain the following information for each payment order of $3,000 or more.

Proceeds Delivered in Person

If proceeds are delivered in person to the beneficiary or its representative or agent, the institution must verify the identity of the person receiving the proceeds and retain a record of the following:

- Name and address;
- The type of document reviewed;
- The number of the identification document;
- The person's TIN, or, if none, the alien identification number or passport number and country of issuance, or a notation in the record of the lack thereof;
- If the institution has knowledge that the person receiving the proceeds is not the beneficiary, the institution must obtain and retain a record of the beneficiary's name and address, as well as the beneficiary's identification.

Proceeds Not Delivered in Person

If proceeds are not delivered in person, the institution must retain a copy of the check or other instrument used to effect the payment, or the institution must record the information on the instrument. The institution must also record the name and address of the person to which it was sent.

Retrievability

Information retained must be retrievable by reference to the name of the beneficiary. When the beneficiary is an established customer of the institution and has an account used for funds transfers, information retained must also be retrievable by account number (31 CFR 103.33(e)(4)).

There are no Travel Rule requirements for beneficiary banks.

EXPIRATION OF THE CONDITIONAL CUSTOMER INFORMATION FILE EXCEPTION - TRAVEL RULE

From 1998 to 2004, a conditional exception to the Travel Rule generally permitted banks to include a customer's coded name or pseudonym in a transmittal order, provided that the bank maintained the customer's full information in an automated customer information file (CIF). FinCEN revoked this exception, known as the "CIF exception," as of July 1, 2004. After that date institutions must use a customer's true name and address to comply with the Travel Rule. At this time, banks may still be examined where transactions subject to the CIF exception may be included in the examiner's sample for transaction testing.

ABBREVIATIONS AND ADDRESSES

Although the Travel Rule does not permit the use of coded names or pseudonyms, the rule does allow the use of abbreviated names, names reflecting different accounts of a corporation (e.g., XYZ Payroll Account), and trade and assumed names of a business (doing business as) or the names of unincorporated divisions or departments of the business.

Customer Address

The term "address," as used in 31 CFR 103.33(g), is not defined. Previously issued guidance from FinCEN had been interpreted as not allowing the use of mailing addresses in a transmittal order when a street address is known to the transmittor's financial institution. However, in the November 28, 2003, *Federal Register* notice FinCEN issued a regulatory interpretation that states the Travel Rule should allow the use of mailing addresses, including post office boxes, in the transmittor address field of transmittal orders in certain circumstances.

The regulatory interpretation states that, for purposes of 31 CFR 103.33(g), the term "address" means either the transmittor's street address or the transmittor's address maintained in the financial institution's automated CIF (such as a mailing address including a post office box) as long as the institution maintains the transmittor's address[1] on file and the address information is retrievable upon request by law enforcement.

---

[1] Consistent with the final rules issued under section 326 of the Patriot Act an "address" for purposes of the Travel Rule is as follows: for a person, is a residential or business street address, an Army Post Office ox or a Fleet Post Office Box, or the residential or business street address of next of kin or another contact person for persons who do not have a residential or business address. For a person other than an individual (such as a corporation, partnership, or trust), "address" is a principal place of business, local office, or other physical location. However, while the section 326 rules apply only to new customers opening accounts on or after October 1, 2003, and while the rule exempt funds transfers from the definition of "account," for banks, the Travel Rule applies to all transmittals of funds of $3,000 or more, whether or not the transmitter is a customer for purposes of the section 326 rules.

1. For each payment order of $3,000 or more that your institution accepts as a beneficiary's bank, does the institution retain either the original or a microfilm, other copy, or electronic record of the payment order? (31 CFR 103.33(e)(1)(iii))

☐ *Yes*

☐ *No*

Comments:

Follow-up:

2. For transmittals of funds of $3,000 or more, does your institution include in the transmittal order to the next receiving financial institution the following, if received from the sender (31 CFR 103.33(g)(2)):

a. The name and account number of the transmittor?
b. The address of the transmittor, except for transmittal orders through Fedwire until such time as the bank that sends the order to the Federal Reserve Bank completes its conversion to the expanded Fedwire format;
c. The amount of the transmittal order?
d. The date of the transmittal order?
e. The identity of the recipient's financial institution?
f. As many of the following items as are received with the transmittal order:
   - The name and address of the recipient?
   - The account number of the recipient?
   - Any other specific identifier of the recipient; and either the name and address or numeric identifier of the transmittor's financial institution?

☐ *Yes*

☐ *No*

Comments:

Follow-up:

3. For transmittals of funds of $3,000 or more, does your institution include in the transmittal order to the next receiving financial institution the following, if received from the sender (31 CFR 103.33(g)(2)):

a. The name and account number of the transmittor?

b. The address of the transmittor, except for transmittal orders through Fedwire until such time as the bank that sends the order to the Federal Reserve Bank completes its conversion to the expanded Fedwire format?

☐ *Yes*

☐ *No*

Comments:

Follow-up:

4. Is information retained retrievable by reference to the name of the beneficiary?

☐ *Yes*

☐ *No*

Comments:

Follow-up:

5. If the beneficiary is an established customer of the institution and has an account used for funds transfers, is information retained also retrievable by account number, as required? (31 CFR 103.33(e)(4))?

☐ *Yes*

☐ *No*

Comments:

Follow-up:

Funds/Wire Transfer - Intermediary Banks

Record-keeping Requirements

For each payment order of $3,000 or more that a bank accepts as an intermediary bank, the bank must retain a record of the payment order.

Travel Rule Requirements

For transmittals of $3,000 or more, the intermediary financial institution must include the following information if received from the sender in a transmittal order at the time that order is sent to a receiving financial institution (31 CFR 103.33(g)(2)):

- Name and account number of the transmittor.
- Address of the transmittor.
- Amount of the transmittal order.
- Date of the transmittal order.
- Identity of the recipient's financial institution.
- As many of the following items as are received with the transmittal order:
    – Name and address of the recipient.
    – Account number of the recipient.
    – Any other specific identifier of the recipient.
- Either the name and address or the numerical identifier of the transmittor's financial institution.

Intermediary financial institutions must pass on all of the information received from a transmittor's financial institution or the preceding financial institution, but they have no duty to obtain information not provided by the transmittor's financial institution or the preceding financial institution.

1. For each payment order of $3,000 or more that your firm accepts as an intermediary bank, does your bank retain a record of the payment order?

☐ *Yes*

☐ *No*

Comments:

Follow-up:

2. When acting as an Intermediary financial institutions, does your bank pass on all of the information received from a transmittor's financial institution or the preceding financial institution in accordance with the travel rule requirements?

☐ *Yes*

☐ *No*

Comments:

Follow-up:

Funds/Wire Transfer - Originating Banks

Record-keeping Requirements

For each payment order in the amount of $3,000 or more that a bank accepts as an originator's bank, the bank must obtain and retain the following records (31 CFR 103.33(e)(1)(i)):

- Name and address of the originator
- Amount of the payment order
- Date of the payment order
- Any payment instructions
- Identity of the beneficiary's institution
- As many of the following items as are received with the payment order:
  - Name and address of the beneficiary;
  - Account number of the beneficiary;
  - Any other specific identifier of the beneficiary.

Additional Records for Non-Established Customers

If the originator is not an established customer of the bank, collect and retain the information listed above. In addition, the originator's bank must collect and retain other information, depending on whether the payment order is made in person.

Payment Orders Made in Person

If the payment order is made in person, the originator's bank must verify the identity of the person placing the payment order before it accepts the order. If it accepts the payment order, the originator's financial institution must obtain and retain the following records:

- Name and address of the person placing the order.
- Type of identification reviewed.
- The person's taxpayer identification number (TIN) (e.g., Social Security number (SSN) or employer identification number (EIN)) or, if none, the alien identification number or passport number and country of issuance, or a notation in the record of the lack thereof. If the originator's bank has knowledge that the person placing the payment order is not the originator, the originator's bank must obtain and record the originator's TIN (e.g., SSN or EIN) or, if none, the alien identification number or passport number and country of issuance, or a notation of the lack thereof.

Payment Orders Not Made in Person

If a payment order is not made in person, the originator's bank must obtain and retain the following records:

- Name and address of the person placing the payment order.
- The person's TIN (e.g., SSN or EIN) or, if none, the alien identification number or passport number and country of issuance , or a notation in the record of the lack thereof, and a copy or record of the method of payment (e.g., check or credit card transaction) for the funds transfer. If the originator's bank has knowledge that the person placing the payment order is not the originator, the originator's bank must obtain and record the originator's TIN (e.g., SSN or EIN) or, if none, the alien identification number or passport number and country of issuance, or a notation of the lack thereof.

Retrievability

Information retained must be retrievable by reference to the name of the originator. When the originator is an established customer of the bank and has an account used for funds transfers, information retained must also be retrievable by account number (31 CFR 103.33(e)(4)). Records must be maintained for five years.

Travel Rule Requirement

For funds transmittals of $3,000 or more, the transmittor's financial institution must include the following information in the transmittal order at the time that a transmittal order is sent to a receiving financial institution (31 CFR 103.33(g)(1)):

- Name of the transmittor, and, if the payment is ordered from an account, the account number of the transmittor.
- Address of the transmittor.
- Amount of the transmittal order.
- Date of the transmittal order.
- Identity of the recipient's financial institution
- As many of the following items as are received with the transmittal order:
  - Name and address of the recipient.
  - Account number of the recipient.
  - Any other specific identifier of the recipient.
- Either the name and address or the numerical identifier of the transmittor's financial institution.

There are no record-keeping requirements in the Travel Rule.

1. For funds transfer originations of $3,000 or more, does your institution retain all of the following records (this information may be with the payment order or in the institution's files if the originator has an established relationship with the institution) (31 CFR 103.33(e)(1)(i)):

a. The name and address of the originator?
b. The amount of the funds transfer?
c. The date of the funds transfer?
d. The identity of the beneficiary's bank?
e. As many of the following items as are received with the payment order:
- The name and address of the beneficiary?
- The account number of the beneficiary?
- Any other specific identifier of the beneficiary?

☐ *Yes*

☐ *No*

Comments:

Follow-up:

2. For funds transfers of $3,000 or more, where payments are made in person and for originators that do not have an established relationship with the institution, in addition to the requirements above, does your bank obtain and retain the following information:

a. Name and address of the person placing the order?
b. Type of identification reviewed?
c. Number of the identification document (e.g., driver's license)?
d. The person's taxpayer identification number (TIN) (e.g., Social Security number (SSN) or employer identification number (EIN)) or, if none, the alien identification number or passport number and country of issuance, or a notation in the record of the lack thereof?

☐ *Yes*

☐ *No*

Comments:

Follow-up:

3. For funds transfers of $3,000 or more for originators that do not have an established relationship with the institution and payment is not made in person, does the bank obtain and retain the following information:

a. Name and address of the person placing the payment order?
b. The person's TIN (e.g., SSN or EIN) or, if none, the alien identification number or passport number and country of issuance , or a notation in the record of the lack thereof, and a copy or record of the method of payment (e.g., check or credit card transaction) for the funds transfer?

☐ *Yes*

☐ *No*

Comments:

Follow-up:

4. Does your institution verify the identity of persons placing orders on behalf of a third party?

☐ *Yes*

☐ *No*

Comments:

Follow-up:

5. For funds transfers of $3,000 or more for originators that do not have an established relationship with the institution, in addition to the requirements in Question #1 above:

–If the payment order is not made in person, does the institution obtain and retain a record of name and address of the person placing the payment order, as well as the person's taxpayer identification number (e.g., social security or employer identification number) or, if none, alien identification number or passport number and country of issuance, or a notation in the record of the lack thereof, and a copy or record of the method of payment (e.g., check or credit card transaction) for the funds transfer? (31CFR 03.33(e)(2)(ii))?

☐ *Yes*

☐ *No*

Comments:

Follow-up:

6. Is the information that the institution must retain for originators retrievable by reference to the name of the originator and retained for five years?

☐ *Yes*

☐ *No*

Comments:

Follow-up:

7. If the originator is an established customer of the institution and has an account used for funds transfers, is the information also retrievable by account number and retained for five years? (31 CFR 103.33(e)(4))?

☐ *Yes*

☐ *No*

Comments:

Follow-up:

8. For transmittals of funds of $3,000 or more, does the institution include all of the following information in the transmittal order (31 CFR 103.33(g)(1)) (the "Travel Rule")

a. The name and, if the payment is ordered from an account, the account number of the transmittor?
b. The address of the transmittor, except for transmittal orders through Fedwire (until such time as the bank that sends the order to the Federal Reserve Bank completes its conversion to the expanded Fedwire format?)
c. The amount of the transmittal order?
d. The date of the transmittal order?
e. The identity of the recipient's financial institution?
f. As many of the following items as are received with the transmittal order?
   - The name and address of the recipient?
   - The account number of the recipient?
   - Any other specific identifier of the recipient; and either the name and address or numeric identifier of the transmittor's financial institution?

☐ *Yes*

☐ *No*

Comments:

Follow-up:

Information Sharing

On September 26, 2002, final regulations (31 CFR 103.100 and 31 CFR 103.110) implementing section 314 of the Patriot Act became effective. The regulations established procedures for information sharing to deter money laundering and terrorist activity.

INFORMATION SHARING BETWEEN LAW ENFORCEMENT AND FINANCIAL INSTITUTIONS - SECTION 314(a) OF THE PATRIOT ACT (31 CFR 103.100)

A federal law enforcement agency investigating terrorist activity or money laundering may request that FinCEN solicit, on its behalf, certain information from a financial institution or a group of financial institutions. The law enforcement agency must provide a written certification to FinCEN attesting that there is credible evidence of engagement or reasonably suspected engagement in terrorist activity or money laundering for each individual, entity, or organization about which the law enforcement agency is seeking information. The law enforcement agency also must provide specific identifiers, such as a date of birth and address, which would permit a financial institution to differentiate among common or similar names. Upon receiving a completed written certification from a law enforcement agency, FinCEN may require a financial institution to search its records to determine whether it maintains or has maintained accounts for, or has engaged in transactions with, any specified individual, entity, or organization.

Upon receiving an information request, a financial institution must conduct a one-time search of its records to identify accounts or transactions of a named suspect. Unless otherwise instructed by an information request, financial institutions must search their records for current accounts, accounts maintained during the preceding 12 months, and transactions conducted outside of an account by or on behalf of a named suspect during the preceding six months. The financial institution must search its records and report any positive matches to FinCEN within 14 days, unless otherwise specified in the information request.

In March 2005, FinCEN began posting section 314(a) subject lists through the 314(a) Secure Information Sharing System. Every two weeks, or more frequently if an emergency request is transmitted, the financial institution's designated point(s) of contact will receive notification from FinCEN that there are new postings to FinCEN's secure web site. The point of contact will be able to access the current section 314(a) subject list (and one prior) and download the files in various formats for searching. Financial institutions should report all positive matches via the Secure Information Sharing System. Those financial institutions choosing to receive the section 314(a) subject lists by facsimile will continue to receive the lists in that manner. For those financial institutions, positive matches should be indicated on the respective subject information form and faxed to FinCEN

FinCEN has provided financial institutions with General Instructions and Frequently Asked Questions (FAQs) relating to the section 314(a) process. Unless otherwise instructed by an information request, financial institutions must search the records specified in the General Instructions. A financial institution may obtain additional or replacement copies of the General Instructions or FAQs by contacting FinCEN. If a financial institution identifies any account or transaction, it must report to FinCEN that it has a match. No details should be provided to FinCEN other than the fact that the financial institution has a match. A negative response is not required. A financial institution may provide a list of named suspects to a third-party service provider or vendor to perform or facilitate record searches as long as the institution takes the necessary steps, through the use of an agreement or procedures, to ensure that the third party safeguards and maintains the confidentiality of the information. Financial institutions should develop and implement comprehensive policies, procedures, and processes for responding to section 314(a) requests. The regulation restricts the use of the information provided in a section 314(a) request (31 CFR 103.100(b)(2)(iv)). A financial institution may only use the information to report the required information to FinCEN, to determine whether to establish or maintain an account or engage in a transaction, or to assist in BSA/AML compliance. While the section 314(a) list could be used to determine whether to establish or maintain an account, FinCEN strongly discourages financial institutions from using this as the sole factor in reaching a decision to do so unless the request specifically states otherwise. Unlike the OFAC lists, section 314(a) lists are not permanent "watch lists." In fact, section 314(a) lists generally relate to one-time inquiries and are not updated or corrected if an investigation is dropped, a prosecution is declined, or a subject is exonerated. Further, the names do not correspond to convicted or indicted persons; rather a 314(a) subject need only be "reasonably suspected" based on credible evidence of engaging in terrorist acts or money laundering. Moreover, FinCEN advises that inclusion on a section 314(a) list should not be the sole factor used to determine whether to file a Suspicious Activity Report (SAR). Financial institutions should establish a process for determining when and if a SAR should be filed. Actions taken pursuant to information provided in a request from FinCEN do not affect a financial institution's obligations to comply with all of the rules and regulations of OFAC nor do they affect a financial institution's obligations to respond to any legal process. Additionally, actions taken in response to a request do not relieve a financial institution of its obligation to file a SAR and immediately notify law enforcement, if necessary, in accordance with applicable laws and regulations.

A financial institution cannot disclose to any person, other than to FinCEN, the institution's primary bank regulator, or the federal law enforcement agency on whose behalf FinCEN is requesting information, the fact that FinCEN has requested or obtained information. A financial institution should designate one or more point-of-contacts for receiving information requests. FinCEN has stated that an affiliated group of financial institutions may establish one point-of-contact to distribute the section 314(a) list to respond to requests. However, the section 314(a) lists cannot be shared with any foreign office, branch or affiliate (unless the request specifically states otherwise), and the lists cannot be shared with affiliates, or subsidiaries of bank holding companies, if the affiliates or subsidiaries are not financial institutions as described in 31 USC 5312(a)(2). Each financial institution must maintain adequate procedures to protect the security and confidentiality of requests from FinCEN. The procedures to ensure confidentiality will be considered adequate if the financial institution applies procedures similar to those it has established to comply with section 501 of the Gramm-Leach-Bliley Act (15 USC 6801) for the protection of its customers' nonpublic personal information. Financial institutions may keep a log of all section 314(a) requests received and of any positive matches identified and reported to FinCEN.

Documentation

Additionally, documentation that all required searches were performed is essential. This may be accomplished by maintaining copies of the cover page of the request with a bank sign-off that the records were checked, the date of the search, and search results (e.g., positive or negative). For positive matches, copies of the form returned to FinCEN and the supporting documentation should be retained. If the financial institution elects to maintain copies of the section 314(a) requests, it should not be criticized for doing so, as long as it appropriately secures them and protects their confidentiality. Audits should include an evaluation of compliance with these guidelines within their scope. In March 2005, FinCEN began distributing section 314(a) subject lists through a secure web site. Every two weeks, or if an emergency request is transmitted, the bank's designated point of contact will receive notification from FinCEN that there are new postings to FinCEN's secure site. The point of contact will be able to access the current, and one prior, section 314(a) subject lists and download the files in various formats for searching. In addition, the banks can use FinCEN's web site to notify FinCEN of positive matches. Those banks receiving the section 314(a) subject lists by facsimile transmission will continue to receive the lists in that manner.
Each bank should contact its primary federal regulator for guidance to ensure it obtains the section 314(a) list and for updating contact information.

VOLUNTARY INFORMATION SHARING - SECTION 314(b) OF THE PATRIOT ACT (31 CFR 103.110)

Section 314(b) encourages financial institutions and associations of financial institutions located in the United States to share information in order to identify and report activities that may involve terrorist activity or money laundering. Section 314(b) also provides specific protection from civil liability. To avail itself of this statutory safe harbor from liability, a financial institution or an association must notify FinCEN of its intent to engage in information sharing and that it has established and will maintain adequate comply with the requirements of 31 CFR

103.110 will result in loss of safe harbor protection for information sharing and may result in a violation of privacy laws or other laws and regulations.

If a financial institution chooses to voluntarily participate in section 314(b), policies procedures, and processes should be developed and implemented for sharing and receiving of information.

A notice to share information is effective for one year The financial institution should designate a point-of-contact for receiving and providing information. A financial institution should establish a process for sending and receiving information sharing requests. Additionally, a financial institution must take reasonable steps to verify that the other financial institution or association of financial institutions with which it intends to share information has also submitted the required notice to FinCEN. FinCEN provides participating financial institutions with access to a list of other participating financial institutions and their related contact information.

If a financial institution receives such information from another financial institution, it must also limit use of the information and maintain its security and confidentiality (see 31 CFR 103.110(b)(4)). Such information may be used only to identify and, where appropriate, report on money laundering and terrorist activities; to determine whether to establish or maintain an account; to engage in a transaction; or to assist in BSA compliance. The procedures to ensure confidentiality will be considered adequate if the financial institution applies procedures similar to the ones it has established to comply with section 501 of the Gramm-Leach-Bliley Act (15 USC 6801) for the protection of its customers' nonpublic personal information. The safe harbor does not extend to sharing of information across international borders. In addition, section 314(b) does not authorize a financial institution to share a SAR, nor does it permit the financial institution to disclose the existence or nonexistence of a SAR. If a financial institution shares information under section 314(b) about the subject of a prepared or filed SAR, the information shared should be limited to underlying transactional and customer information. A financial institution may use information obtained under section 314(b) to determine whether to file a SAR, but the intention to prepare or file a SAR cannot be shared with another financial institution. Financial institutions should establish a process for determining when and if a SAR should be filed.

Actions taken pursuant to information obtained through the voluntary information sharing process do not affect a financial institution's obligations to respond to any legal process. Additionally, actions taken in response to information obtained through the voluntary information sharing process do not relieve a financial institution of its obligation to file a SAR and to immediately notify law enforcement, if necessary, in accordance with all applicable laws and regulations.

1. Are procedures in place to protect the security and confidentiality of requests from FinCEN (The procedures to ensure confidentiality will be considered adequate if the financial institution applies procedures similar to those it has established to comply with section 501 of the Gramm-Leach-Bliley Act (15 USC 6801) for the protection of its customers' nonpublic personal information).

☐ *Yes*

☐ *No*

Comments:

Follow-up:

2. Does your financial institution's policy and procedures address receiving and responding to FinCEN section 314(a) requests for information regarding terrorist activities or money laundering and for sharing suspected terrorist activity or money laundering information pursuant to section 314(b) and receiving such information and protecting its confidentiality?

☐ *Yes*

☐ *No*

Comments:

Follow-up:

3. Is documentation of any positive match with a section 314(a) request maintained and properly reported?

☐ *Yes*

☐ *No*

Comments:

Follow-up:

4. Are copies of any vendor confidentiality agreements regarding section 314(a) services maintained, if applicable?

☐ *Yes*

☐ *No*

Comments:

Follow-up:

5. Do your bank's policies and procedures designate a contact person and a responsible party for handling section 314(a) requests and procedures and managing 314b processes?

☐ *Yes*

☐ *No*

Comments:

Follow-up:

6. Is ongoing training for section 314 processes documented and in place as part of your bank's training program?

☐ *Yes*

☐ *No*

Comments:

Follow-up:

7. Is your bank's 314 program independently tested?

☐ *Yes*

☐ *No*

Comments:

Follow-up:

8. Are all of the required types of records and appropriate categories of accounts and transactions searched? (31 CFR 103.100(b)(2)(i))

☐ *Yes*

☐ *No*

Comments:

Follow-up:

9. Is documentation available to verify that a response was provided to FinCEN within the designated time period? (31 CFR 103.100(b)(2)(ii))

☐ *Yes*

☐ *No*

Comments:

Follow-up:

10. If your financial institution uses a third-party vendor to perform or facilitate searches, are written agreements and/or procedures maintained to ensure confidentiality?

☐ *Yes*

☐ *No*

Comments:

Follow-up:

11. Are internal control processes documented sufficiently to evidence that there is adequate compliance? (Such documentation could include, for example, copies of the 314(a) requests; a log that records the tracking numbers with a sign-off column; or copies of the request cover page with a sign-off, indicating that the records were checked, along with the date of the search and search results (e.g., positive/negative). For positive matches, copies of the form returned to FinCEN along with supporting documentation should be retained).

☐ *Yes*

☐ *No*

Comments:

Follow-up:

12. If your bank has chosen to voluntarily share information under the provisions of Section 314b, has notification been communicated to FinCEN of the bank's intent to engage in information sharing and that it has established and will maintain adequate procedures to protect the security and confidentiality of the information?

☐ *Yes*

☐ *No*

Comments:

Follow-up:

13. If your financial institution has chosen to voluntarily participate in section 314(b), have policies, procedures, and processes been developed and implemented for sharing and receiving of information?

☐ *Yes*

☐ *No*

Comments:

Follow-up:

14. If your financial institution receives 314b information from another financial institution, does it limit use of the information and maintain its security and confidentiality in accordance with 31CFR 103.110(b)(4)) and Gramm-Leach-Bliley Act (15 USC 6801)?

☐ *Yes*

☐ *No*

Comments:

Follow-up:

Internal Audit/Independent Review

Those persons responsible for conducting an objective independent evaluation of the written BSA/AML compliance program should perform testing for specific compliance with the BSA, and evaluate pertinent management information systems (MIS). The audit should be risk based and evaluate the quality of risk management for all banking operations, departments, and subsidiaries. Risk-based audit programs will vary depending on the bank's size, complexity, scope of activities, risk profile, quality of control functions, geographic diversity, and use of technology. An effective risk-based auditing program will cover all of the bank's activities. The frequency and depth of each activity's audit will vary according to the activity's risk assessment. Risk-based auditing enables the board of directors and auditors to use the bank's risk assessment to focus the audit scope on the areas of greatest concern. The testing should assist the board of directors and management in identifying areas of weakness or areas where there is a need for enhancements or stronger controls.

Independent testing should, at a minimum, include:

- An evaluation of the overall integrity and effectiveness of the BSA/AML compliance program, including policies, procedures, and processes;
- A review of the bank's risk assessment for reasonableness given the bank's risk profile (products, services, customers, and geographic locations);
- Appropriate transaction testing to verify the bank's adherence to the BSA record-keeping and reporting requirements (e.g., CIP, SARs, CTRs, and CTR exemptions, information sharing requests);
- An evaluation of management's efforts to resolve violations and deficiencies noted in previous audits and regulatory examinations, including progress in addressing outstanding supervisory actions, if applicable;
- A review of staff training for adequacy, accuracy, and completeness;
- A review of the effectiveness of the suspicious activity monitoring systems (manual, automated, or a combination) used for BSA/AML compliance. Related reports may include, but are not limited to:
    - Suspicious activity monitoring reports.
    - Large currency aggregation reports.
    - Monetary instrument records.
    - Funds transfer records.
    - Non-sufficient funds (NSF) reports.
    - Large balance fluctuation reports.
    - Account relationship reports.

- An assessment of the overall process for identifying and reporting suspicious activity, including a review of filed or prepared SARs to determine their accuracy, timeliness, completeness, and effectiveness of the bank's policy. Auditors should document the audit scope, procedures performed, transaction testing completed, and findings of the review. All audit documentation and work papers should be available for examiner review. Any violations, policy or procedures exceptions, or other deficiencies noted during the audit should be included in an audit report and reported to the board of directors or a designated committee in a timely manner. The board or designated committee and the audit staff should track audit deficiencies and document corrective actions.

1. Does your institution have an independent review process for its BSA program?

☐ *Yes*

☐ *No*

Comments:

Follow-up:

2. If your institution does not have an internal audit function, has a program of management reviews or self audits been established which include all the requirements of the BSA?

☐ *Yes*

☐ *No*

Comments:

Follow-up:

3. Does your compliance testing program include confirmation of the integrity and accuracy of the systems for the reporting of large currency transactions?

☐ *Yes*

☐ *No*

Comments:

Follow-up:

4. Does your compliance testing program include a review of tellers' work and Forms 4789/104 and 4790?

☐ *Yes*

☐ *No*

Comments:

Follow-up:

5. Does your compliance testing program include confirmation of the integrity and accuracy of the institution's recordkeeping activities?

☐ *Yes*

☐ *No*

Comments:

Follow-up:

6. Does your compliance testing program include a test of adherence to your bank's record retention schedule?

☐ *Yes*

☐ *No*

Comments:

Follow-up:

7. Does your compliance testing program include steps necessary to ascertain that your bank is maintaining documentation of exempt customers as required by the regulations?

☐ *Yes*

☐ *No*

Comments:

Follow-up:

8. Does your compliance testing program include a test of the reasonableness of the CTR exemptions granted?

☐ *Yes*

☐ *No*

Comments:

Follow-up:

9. Are those performing the independent testing function sufficiently qualified to ensure that the bank can rely upon the findings and conclusions?

☐ *Yes*

☐ *No*

Comments:

Follow-up:

10. Does your compliance testing program include steps requiring an auditor to ascertain that your institution has filed a Report of Foreign Bank Financial Accounts, (Treasury Form 90-22.1) declaring interests in foreign financial accounts?

☐ *Yes*

☐ *No*

Comments:

Follow-up:

11. Does your compliance testing program include steps necessary to ascertain that your institution has procedures in place for obtaining and maintaining required information for the sale/purchase of monetary instruments for cash in amounts between $3,000 and $10,000 inclusive, and that appropriate customer identification measures are in place?

☐ *Yes*

☐ *No*

Comments:

Follow-up:

12. Does your bank's audit program review the integrity and accuracy of management information systems (MIS) used in the BSA/AML compliance (e.g., MIS includes reports used to identify large currency transactions, aggregate daily currency transactions, funds transfer transactions, and monetary instrument sales transactions).

☐ *Yes*

☐ *No*

Comments:

Follow-up:

13. Has your bank's audit staff determined that management's supervision of BSA compliance is sufficient?

☐ *Yes*

☐ *No*

Comments:

Follow-up:

14. Is your bank's independent testing program sufficiently comprehensive and are the results reported to the Board and/or senior management on a periodic and timely basis?

☐ *Yes*

☐ *No*

Comments:

Follow-up:

15. If an automated system is not used to identify or aggregate large transactions, does the audit or independent review include a sample test check of tellers' cash proof sheets, tapes, or other documentation to determine whether large currency transactions are accurately identified and reported?

☐ *Yes*

☐ *No*

Comments:

Follow-up:

16. Does the bank's independent audit review of suspicious activity monitoring systems include an evaluation of the system's ability to identify unusual activity, and includes:

a. Evaluation of the system's methodology for establishing and applying expected activity or filtering criteria?
b. Evaluation of the system's ability to generate monitoring reports?
c. Determination whether the system filtering criteria are reasonable?

☐ *Yes*

☐ *No*

Comments:

Follow-up:

17. Does the bank's independent testing include a review of policies, procedures, and processes for referring unusual activity from all business lines (e.g., legal, private banking, foreign correspondent banking) to the personnel or departments responsible for evaluating unusual activity?

☐ *Yes*

☐ *No*

Comments:

Follow-up:

18. Does the bank's internal auditor track previously identified deficiencies and ensure that management corrects them?

☐ *Yes*

☐ *No*

Comments:

Follow-up:

Internal Controls

Internal controls are the means by which a financial institution's resources are directed, monitored and measured. They are directly related to the reliability of the core functions of an anti-money laundering program, such as monitoring transactions, suspicious activity reporting, aggregation of transactions, etc. There are more items related to internal controls in the FFIEC Examination manual than any other single topic. This should not be too surprising, as the regulators assign importance of control functions for every element of a BSA program. So, while it may appear that the questions below appear elsewhere, keep in mind that the answers to these questions relate less to the specifics of individual topics of examination and more to how those topics are implemented and their activities accounted for in practice.

1. Do controls exist to maintain an up-to-date written compliance program?

☐ *Yes*

☐ *No*

Comments:

Follow-up:

2. Does your written BSA compliance program provide for a system of internal controls to ensure ongoing compliance?

☐ *Yes*

☐ *No*

Comments:

Follow-up:

3. Does your written BSA program provide for independent testing to be conducted by either bank personnel or an outside party? Is a list of person(s) designated to conduct independent testing available for inspection?

☐ *Yes*

☐ *No*

Comments:

Follow-up:

4. Does your written BSA compliance program provide for designation of a qualified individual(s) responsible for coordinating and monitoring day-to-day compliance? Is a list of the individual(s) responsible for compliance along with the appropriateness of qualifications (i.e. training, experience) available for inspection?

☐ *Yes*

☐ *No*

Comments:

Follow-up:

5. Does your written BSA compliance program provide for training for appropriate personnel and controls to ensure that appropriate training is administered to those who should receive it?

☐ *Yes*

☐ *No*

Comments:

Follow-up:

6. Is your compliance program approved in writing (and noted in the minutes) by the institution's board of directors, and do the board of directors and senior management receive adequate reports on BSA/AML compliance and SAR filings?

☐ *Yes*

☐ *No*

Comments:

Follow-up:

7. If required per USA PATRIOT Act Section 326, has your Customer Identification Program been approved by the institution's board of directors and approval noted in the minutes?

☐ *Yes*

☐ *No*

Comments:

Follow-up:

8. If your firm is a foreign institution, was the compliance program approved at the highest level of United States management as well as by the home office board of directors?

☐ *Yes*

☐ *No*

Comments:

Follow-up:

10. Does your institution's written compliance program include procedural guidelines for the detection, prevention and reporting of suspicious transactions related to money laundering activities?

☐ *Yes*

☐ *No*

Comments:

Follow-up:

11. Does your institution's compliance program include written procedural guidelines for meeting the reporting and recordkeeping requirements of the BSA regulations and provide for the filing of a report of each deposit, withdrawal, exchange of currency or other payment or transfer, by, through or to the financial institution, which involves a transaction in currency of more than $10,000? (FinCEN Form 104) (31 CFR 103.22(a)(1))

☐ *Yes*

☐ *No*

Comments:

Follow-up:

12. Does your institution's compliance program include written procedural guidelines for meeting the reporting and recordkeeping requirements of the BSA regulations and provide for the maintenance of a centralized list containing each exemption granted, with the supporting information prescribed in 31 CFR 103.22(f)? (Each exemption granted after October 27, 1986, shall be accompanied by the required statement and attendant language in 31 CFR 103.22(d) (31 CFR 103.22(b)(2))

☐ *Yes*

☐ *No*

Comments:

Follow-up:

13. Does your institution's compliance program include written procedural guidelines for meeting the reporting and recordkeeping requirements of the BSA regulations and provide for the filing of a report (U.S. Customs Form 4790) of each shipment of currency or other monetary instrument(s) in excess of $10,000 out of the United States or into the United States on behalf of the institution (not its customers), except via common carrier by, or to the institution (31 CFR 103.23(a))? (In most cases, this refers to the institution's cash shipments.)

☐ *Yes*

☐ *No*

Comments:

Follow-up:

14. Does your institution's compliance program include written procedural guidelines for meeting the reporting and record keeping requirements of the BSA regulations and provide for the maintenance of required records for each monetary instrument purchase/sale for currency in amounts between $3,000 and $10,000 inclusive, with the supporting information prescribed in 31 CFR 103.29? (31 CFR 103.29(a))

☐ *Yes*

☐ *No*

Comments:

Follow-up:

15. Do procedural guidelines include provisions for the retention of either the original, microfilm, copy or other reproduction of the each Currency Transaction Report (CTR, IRS Form 4789 or FinCEN Form 104), and is each item retained for a period of at least five years?

☐ *Yes*

☐ *No*

Comments:

Follow-up:

16. Do procedural guidelines include provisions for the retention of either the original, microfilm, copy or other reproduction of documentation to support each exemption and a requirement to retain such documentation for a period of five years from the date it was discontinued? (31 CFR 103.22(d))

☐ *Yes*

☐ *No*

Comments:

Follow-up:

17. Do the procedural guidelines include provisions for the retention of either the original, microfilm, copy or other reproduction of each extension of credit in an amount over $10,000, except when the extension is secured by an interest in real property? (31 CFR 103.33(a))

☐ *Yes*

☐ *No*

Comments:

Follow-up:

18. Do procedural guidelines include provisions for the retention of either the original, microfilm, copy or other reproduction of each advice, request, or instruction received regarding a transaction which results in the transfer of funds, currency, checks, investment securities, other monetary instruments or credit, of more than $10,000, to a person, account or place outside the United States? (31 CFR 103.33(b))

☐ *Yes*

☐ *No*

Comments:

Follow-up:

19. Do procedural guidelines include provisions for the retention of either the original, microfilm, copy or other reproduction of each advice, request, or instruction given to another financial institution or other person located within or outside the United States, regarding a transaction intended to result in a transfer of funds, currency, checks, investment securities, other monetary instruments or credit of more than $10,000 to a person, account or place outside the United States? (31 CFR 103.33(c))

☐ *Yes*

☐ *No*

Comments:

Follow-up:

20. Do procedural guidelines include provisions for the retention of either the original, microfilm, copy or other reproduction of each payment order that a financial institution accepts as an originator's, intermediary, or beneficiary's bank with respect to a funds transfer in the amount of $3,000 or more? (31 CFR 103.33(e))

☐ *Yes*

☐ *No*

Comments:

Follow-up:

21. Do procedural guidelines include provisions for the retention of either the original, microfilm, copy or other reproduction of a list of each individual, including the name, address and account number, who holds a deposit account for which the bank has been unable to secure a taxpayer identification number from that person after making a reasonable effort to obtain the number? (31 CFR 103.34(a)(1)(ii))

☐ *Yes*

☐ *No*

Comments:

Follow-up:

22. Do procedural guidelines include provisions for the retention of either the original, microfilm, copy or other reproduction of each item relating to any transaction of more than $10,000 received on any one occasion directly and not through a domestic financial institution, from a bank, broker or dealer n foreign exchange outside the United States? (31 CFR 103.34(b)(8)and(9))

☐ *Yes*

☐ *No*

Comments:

Follow-up:

23. Do procedural guidelines include provisions for the retention of either the original, microfilm, copy or other reproduction of each document granting signature authority over each deposit account? (31 CFR 03.34(b)(1))

☐ *Yes*

☐ *No*

Comments:

Follow-up:

24. Do procedural guidelines include provisions for the retention of either the original, microfilm, copy or other reproduction of each statement, ledger card or other record of each deposit account showing each transaction involving the account, excepting those items listed in 31 CFR 103.34(b)(3) (31 CFR 103.34(b)(2),(3)and(4))?

☐ *Yes*

☐ *No*

Comments:

Follow-up:

25. Do procedural guidelines include provisions for the retention of either the original, microfilm, copy or other reproduction of each document relating to a transaction of more than $10,000 remitted or transferred to a person, account or place outside the United States? (31 CFR 103.34(b)(5) and (6))

☐ *Yes*

☐ *No*

Comments:

Follow-up:

26. Do procedural guidelines include provisions for the retention of either the original, microfilm, copy or other reproduction of each check or draft in an amount in excess of $10,000 drawn on or issued by a foreign bank which the domestic bank has paid or presented to a non-bank drawee for payment? (31 CFR 103.34 (b)(7))

☐ *Yes*

☐ *No*

Comments:

Follow-up:

27. Do procedural guidelines include provisions for the retention of either the original, microfilm, copy or other reproduction of records prepared or received by a bank in the ordinary course of business which would be needed to reconstruct a demand deposit account and to trace a check in excess of $100 deposited in such demand deposit account? (31 CFR 103.34(b)(10))

☐ *Yes*

☐ *No*

Comments:

Follow-up:

28. Do procedural guidelines include provisions for the retention of either the original, microfilm, copy or other reproduction of records containing the name, address and taxpayer identification number, if available, of any person presenting a certificate of deposit for payment, as well as a description of the instrument and the date of the transaction? (31 CFR 103.34(b)(12)

☐ *Yes*

☐ *No*

Comments:

Follow-up:

29. Do procedural guidelines include provisions for the retention of either the original, microfilm, copy or other reproduction of each deposit slip or credit ticket reflecting a transaction in excess of $100 or the equivalent record for direct deposit or other wire transfer deposit transactions? Does the slip or ticket record the amount of any currency involved? (31 CFR 103.34(b)(13))

☐ *Yes*

☐ *No*

Comments:

Follow-up:

30. Are your bank's system of internal controls sufficient to ensure ongoing compliance?

☐ *Yes*

☐ *No*

Comments:

Follow-up:

31. Are procedures in place to control changes in processes, including forms, contracts, software programs, etc?

☐ *Yes*

☐ *No*

Comments:

Follow-up:

32. Are all policies and procedures updated to account for all types of products or services offered, including those offered to persons or businesses that do not hold accounts?

- ☐ *Yes*
- ☐ *No*

Comments:

Follow-up:

33. Do your bank's procedures and controls take into full account the locations and markets which it operates in?

- ☐ *Yes*
- ☐ *No*

Comments:

Follow-up:

34. Does the compliance office consider internal or external factors that could affect BSA, AML, or OFAC compliance?

☐ *Yes*

☐ *No*

Comments:

Follow-up:

35. Is it evident that management is sufficiently aware of the provisions of the applicable laws and regulations?

☐ *Yes*

☐ *No*

Comments:

Follow-up:

36. Do the bank's policies specifically describe the reporting lines of the BSA Compliance officer?

☐ *Yes*

☐ *No*

Comments:

Follow-up:

37. Are responsibilities of BSA, AML, and OFAC compliance distributed throughout all areas of the bank?

☐ *Yes*

☐ *No*

Comments:

Follow-up:

38. Are the bank's employees encouraged to report suspicious activity directly to the BSA Compliance Office, and do escalation procedures cover contingencies, such as what to do when key compliance or other executives are not available or should not be notified of a particular event because of possible conflicts of interest?

☐ *Yes*

☐ *No*

Comments:

Follow-up:

39. Are procedures in place to account for the reporting of significant changes in policies, personnel, or controls?

☐ *Yes*

☐ *No*

Comments:

Follow-up:

40. Do procedures provide for dual controls and the segregation of duties? (For example, employees that complete the reporting forms (e.g., SARs, CTRs, and CTR exemptions) should not also be responsible for filing the reports or granting the exemptions.)

☐ *Yes*

☐ *No*

Comments:

Follow-up:

41. Do your bank's policies and procedures provide that high-risk areas, products, and services are targeted specifically?

☐ *Yes*

☐ *No*

Comments:

Follow-up:

42. Are corrective actions timely, appropriate, and reported to management and the board?

☐ *Yes*

☐ *No*

Comments:

Follow-up:

43. Are regular periodic audits or reviews prescribed by the BSA program, and are they actually performed at regular and appropriate intervals?

☐ *Yes*

☐ *No*

Comments:

Follow-up:

44. Do controls provide for adequate supervision of employees that handle currency transactions, complete reports, grant exemptions, monitor for suspicious activity, or engage in any other activity covered by the BSA and its implementing regulations?

☐ *Yes*

☐ *No*

Comments:

Follow-up:

45. Do your policies and procedures identify banking operations (products, services, customers, and geographic locations) more vulnerable to abuse by money launderers and criminals; provide for periodic updates to the bank's risk profile; and provide for a BSA/AML compliance program tailored to manage risks?

☐ *Yes*

☐ *No*

Comments:

Follow-up:

46. Do your bank's policies, procedures and controls consider the specific risks arising from the type(s) of market its products are catering to and the locations where it is conducting business?

☐ *Yes*

☐ *No*

Comments:

Follow-up:

47. Are policies and procedures effective to ensure that when business offerings change (including those to non-account holders), ongoing compliance is maintained?

☐ *Yes*

☐ *No*

Comments:

Follow-up:

48. Are policies and procedures in place to test for and prevent potential abuses by insiders?

☐ *Yes*

☐ *No*

Comments:

Follow-up:

International Transportation of Currency

Each person (including a bank) who physically transports, mails, or ships currency or monetary instruments in excess of $10,000 at one time out of or into the United States (and each person who causes such transportation, mailing, or shipment), must file a Report of International Transportation of Currency or Monetary Instruments (CMIR) (FinCEN Form 105). A CMIR must be filed with the appropriate Bureau of Customs and Border Protection officer or with the commissioner of Customs at the time of entry into or departure from the United States. When a person receives currency or monetary instruments in an amount exceeding $10,000 at one time that have been shipped from any place outside the United States, a CMIR must be filed with the appropriate Bureau of Customs and Border Protection officer or with the commissioner of Customs within 15 days of receipt of the instruments (unless a report has already been filed). The report is to be completed by or on behalf of the person requesting transfer of the currency or monetary instruments. However, banks are not required to report these items if they are mailed or shipped through the postal service or by common carrier.[1] In addition, a commercial bank or trust company organized under the laws of any state or of the United States is not required to report overland shipments of currency or monetary instruments if they are shipped to or received from an established customer maintaining a deposit relationship with the bank and if the bank reasonably concludes the amounts do not exceed what is commensurate with the customary conduct of the business, industry, or profession of the customer concerned.

Management should implement applicable policies, procedures, and processes for CMIR filing. Management should review the international transportation of currency and monetary instruments and determine whether a customer's activity is usual and customary for the type of business. If not, a Suspicious Activity Report should be considered.

---

[1] In contrast, a bank is required to file a CMIR to report shipments of currency or monetary instruments to foreign offices when those shipments are performed directly by bank personnel, such as currency shipments handled by bank employees using bank-owned vehicles.

1. Has your bank documented and implemented applicable policies, procedures, and processes for CMIR (Report of International Transportation of Currency or Monetary Instruments FinCEN Form 105) filing?

☐ *Yes*

☐ *No*

Comments:

Follow-up:

2. As part of its ongoing suspicious activity efforts, does management review the international transportation of currency and monetary instruments and determine whether customers' activity is usual and customary for the type of business?

☐ *Yes*

☐ *No*

Comments:

Follow-up:

3. Regarding question #2, above, does your bank's SAR filing policy include CMIR reviews?

☐ ***Yes***

☐ ***No***

Comments:

Follow-up:

KYC & CIP

As of October 1, 2003, all banks and their operating subsidiaries must have a written Customer Information Program (CIP).[1] The CIP rule implements section 326 of the Patriot Act and requires each bank to implement a written CIP that is appropriate for its size and type of business and that includes certain minimum requirements. The CIP must be incorporated into the bank's BSA/AML compliance program, which is subject to approval by the bank's board of directors.[2]

The CIP is intended to enable the bank to form a reasonable belief that it knows the true identity of each customer. The CIP must include account opening procedures that specify the identifying information that will be obtained from each customer. It must also include reasonable and practical risk-based procedures for verifying the identity of each customer. Banks should conduct a risk assessment of their customer base and product offerings, and in determining the risks, consider:

- The types of accounts offered by the bank;
- The bank's methods of opening accounts;
- The types of identifying information available; and,
- The bank's size, location, and customer base.

Pursuant to the CIP rule, an "account" is a formal banking relationship to provide or engage in services, dealings, or other financial transactions, and includes a deposit account, a transaction or asset account, a credit account, or another extension of credit. An account also includes a relationship established to provide a safe deposit box or other safekeeping services or to provide cash management, custodian, or trust services. An account does not include:

- Products or services for which a formal banking relationship is not established with a person, such as check cashing, funds transfer, or the sale of a check or money order;
- Any account that the bank acquires. This may include single or multiple accounts as a result of a purchase of assets, acquisition, merger, or assumption of liabilities;
- Accounts opened to participate in an employee benefit plan established under the Employee Retirement Income Security Act of 1974.

The CIP rule applies to a "customer." A customer is a person (an individual, a corporation, partnership, a trust, an estate, or any other entity recognized as a legal person) who opens a new account, an individual who opens a new account for another individual who lacks legal capacity, and an individual who opens a new account for an entity that is not a legal person (e.g., a civic club). A customer does not include a person who does not receive banking services, such as a person whose loan application is denied.[3] The definition of *customer* also does not include an existing customer as long as the bank has a reasonable belief that it knows the customer's true identity.[4] Excluded from the definition of customer are federally regulated banks, banks regulated by a state bank regulator, governmental entities, and publicly traded companies (as described in 31 CFR 103.22(d)(2)(ii) through (iv)).

CUSTOMER INFORMATION REQUIRED

The CIP must contain account opening procedures detailing the identifying information that must be obtained from each customer.[5] At a minimum, the bank must obtain the following basic information from each customer before opening the account:[6]

- Name
- Date of birth, for individuals Address[7]
- Identification number[8]

Based on its risk assessments, a bank may require identifying information in addition to the items above for certain customers or product lines.

CUSTOMER VERIFICATION

The CIP must contain risk-based procedures for verifying the identity of the customer within a reasonable period of time after the account is opened. The verification procedures must use "the information obtained in accordance with [31 CFR 103.121] paragraph (b)(2)(i)," namely the identifying information obtained by the bank. A bank need not establish the accuracy of every element of identifying information obtained, but it must verify enough information to form a reasonable belief that it knows the true identity of the customer. The bank's procedures must describe when it will use documents, non-documentary methods, or a combination of both.

Verification Through Documents

A bank using documentary methods to verify a customer's identity must have procedures that set forth the minimum acceptable documentation. The CIP rule gives examples of types of documents that have long been considered primary sources of identification. The rule reflects the federal banking agencies' expectations that banks will review an unexpired government-issued form of identification from most customers. This identification must provide evidence of a customer's nationality or residence and bear a photograph or similar safeguard; examples include a driver's license or passport. However, other forms of identification may be used if they enable the bank to form a reasonable belief that it knows the true identity of the customer. Nonetheless, given the availability of counterfeit and fraudulently obtained documents, a bank is encouraged to review more than a single document to ensure that it has a reasonable belief that it knows the customer's true identity.

For a person other than an individual (such as a corporation, partnership, or trust), the bank should obtain documents showing the legal existence of the entity, such as certified articles of incorporation, an unexpired government-issued business license, a partnership agreement, or a trust instrument.

Verification Through Non-documentary Methods

Banks are not required to use non-documentary methods to verify a customer's identity. However, a bank using non-documentary methods to verify a customer's identity must have procedures that set forth the methods the bank will use. Non-documentary methods may include contacting a customer; independently verifying the customer's identity through the comparison of information provided by the customer with information obtained from a consumer reporting agency, public database, or other source; checking references with other financial institutions; and obtaining a financial statement.

The bank's non-documentary procedures must also address the following situations:

- An individual is unable to present an unexpired government-issued identification document that bears a photograph or similar safeguard;
- The bank is not familiar with the documents presented; the account is opened without obtaining documents (e.g., the bank obtains the required information from the customer with the intent to verify it); the customer opens the account without appearing in person; or,
- The bank is otherwise presented with circumstances that increase the risk that it will be unable to verify the true identity of a customer through documents.

Additional Verification for Certain Customers

The CIP must address situations where, based on its risk assessment of a new account opened by a customer that is not an individual, the bank will obtain information about individuals with authority or control over such accounts, including signatories, in order to verify the customer's identity. This verification method applies only when the bank cannot verify the customer's true identity using documentary or non-documentary methods. For example, a bank may need to obtain information about and verify the identity of a sole proprietor or the principals in a partnership when the bank cannot otherwise satisfactorily identify the sole proprietorship or the partnership.

Lack of Verification

The CIP must also have procedures for circumstances in which the bank cannot form a reasonable belief that it knows the true identity of the customer. These procedures should describe:

- Circumstances in which the bank should not open an account;
- The terms under which a customer may use an account while the bank attempts to verify the customer's identity;
- When the bank should close an account, after attempts to verify a customer's identity have failed;
- When the bank should file a SAR in accordance with applicable law and regulation.

RECORDKEEPING REQUIREMENTS AND RETENTION

A bank's CIP must include record-keeping procedures. At a minimum, the bank must retain the identifying information (name, address, date of birth for an individual, TIN, and any other information required by the CIP) obtained at account opening for a period of five years after the account is closed.[9] For credit cards, the retention period is five years after the account closes or becomes dormant.

The bank must also keep a description of the following for five years after the record was made:

- Any document that was relied on to verify identity, noting the type of document, the identification number, the place of issuance and, if any, the date of issuance and expiration date;
- The method and the results of any measures undertaken to verify identity;
- The results of any substantive discrepancy discovered when verifying identity.

COMPARISON WITH GOVERNMENT LISTS

The CIP must include procedures for determining whether the customer appears on any federal government list of known or suspected terrorists or terrorist organizations.[10] Banks will be contacted by the U.S. Treasury in consultation with their federal banking agency when a list is issued. At such time, banks must compare customer names against the list within a reasonable time of account opening or earlier, if required by the government, and they must follow any directives that accompany the list.

---

[1] See 12 CFR 208.63(b), 211.5(m), 211.24(j) (Board of Governors of the Federal Reserve System); 12 CFR 326.8(b) (Federal Deposit Insurance Corporation); 12 CFR 748.2(b) (National Credit Union Administration); 12 CFR 21.21 (Office of the Comptroller of the Currency); 12 CFR 563.177(b) (Office of Thrift Supervision); and 31 CFR 103.121 (FinCEN).

[3] When the account is a loan, the account is considered to be "opened" when the bank enters into an enforceable agreement to provide a loan to the customer.

[4] The bank may demonstrate that it knows an existing customer's true identity showing that before the issuance of the final CIP rule, it had comparable procedures in place to verify the identity of persons who had accounts with the bank as of October 1, 2003, though the bank may not have gathered the very same information about such persons as required by the final CIP rule. Alternative means include showing that the bank has had an active and longstanding relationship with a particular person, as evidenced by such things as a history of account statements sent to the person, information sent to the Internal Revenue Service (IRS) about the person's accounts without issue, loans made and repaid, or other services performed for the person over a period of time. Alternative means, however, may not suffice for persons
that the bank has deemed to be high risk.

[5] When an individual opens a new account for an entity that is not a legal person or for another individual who lacks legal capacity, the identifying information for the individual opening the account must be obtained. By contrast, when an account is opened by an agent on behalf of another person, the bank must obtain the identifying information of the person on whose behalf the account is being opened.

[6] For credit card customers, the bank may obtain identifying information from a third-party source before extending credit.

[7] For an individual: a residential or business street address, or if the individual does not have such an address, an Army Post Office (APO) or Fleet Post Office (FPO) box number, the residential or business street address of next of kin or of another contact individual, or a description of the customer's physical location. For a "person" other

than an individual (such as a corporation, partnership, or trust): a principal place of business, local office, or other physical location.

[8] An identification number for a U.S. person is a taxpayer identification number (TIN) (or evidence of an application for one), and for a non-U.S. person is one or more of the following: a TIN; a passport number and country of issuance; an alien identification card number; or a number and country of issuance of any other unexpired government-issued document evidencing nationality or residence and bearing a photograph or similar safeguard. TIN is defined by section 6109 of the Internal Revenue Code of 1986 (26 USC 6109) and the IRS regulations implementing that section (e.g., Social Security number or employer identification number).

[9] Banks are not required to make and retain photocopies of any documents used in the verification process. However, if a bank does choose to do so, it should ensure that these photocopies are physically secured to adequately protect against possible identity theft. In addition, such photocopies should not be maintained with files and documentation relating to credit decisions to avoid any potential problems with consumer compliance regulations.

[10] As of the publication date of this manual, there are no designated government lists to verify specifically for CIP purposes. Customer comparisons to lists required by OFAC and the Patriot Act section 314(a) (31 CFR 103.100) requests remain separate and distinct requirements.

1. If your institution uses fictitious names for customers on the general ledger or other institution documents, does the institution maintain files containing the customers' real names and other identifying information and does the institution have knowledge of these customers' activities? (The use of fictitious names is customarily found in private or foreign banking)

☐ ***Yes***

☐ ***No***

Comments:

Follow-up:

2. Does your bank have adequate ongoing monitoring systems in place to identify suspicious transactions, i.e., structuring, transactions inconsistent with the nature of a customer's stated business purpose, unusual wire transfer activities, etc.?

☐ *Yes*

☐ *No*

Comments:

Follow-up:

3. Does your firm's CIP include account opening procedures that specify the identifying information that will be obtained from each customer?

☐ *Yes*

☐ *No*

Comments:

Follow-up:

4. Does your CIP include reasonable and practical risk-based procedures for verifying the identity of each customer?

☐ *Yes*

☐ *No*

Comments:

Follow-up:

5. Has your bank conducted a risk assessment of its customer base and product offerings, and in determining the risks, considered the following factors:

a. The various types of accounts maintained by the bank?
b. The bank's various methods of opening accounts?
c. The various types of identifying information available?
d. The bank's size, location, and customer base?

☐ *Yes*

☐ *No*

Comments:

Follow-up:

6. Does your CIP contain account-opening procedures detailing the identifying information it must obtain from each customer?

☐ *Yes*

☐ *No*

Comments:

Follow-up:

7. If an individual opens a new account for an entity that is not a legal person or for another individual who lacks legal capacity, is the identifying information for the individual opening the account obtained?

☐ *Yes*

☐ *No*

Comments:

Follow-up:

8. When an account is opened by an agent on behalf of another person, does the bank obtain the identifying information of the person on behalf of whom the account is being opened?

☐ *Yes*

☐ *No*

Comments:

Follow-up:

9. Does your CIP capture the following basic information from the customer prior to opening the account:

a. Name?
b. Date of birth, for individuals?
c. Address?
d. Identification number?

☐ *Yes*

☐ *No*

Comments:

Follow-up:

10. Does your bank, based on its assessment of risk, require identifying information in addition to the items in question #9 for certain customers or product lines?

☐ *Yes*

☐ *No*

Comments:

Follow-up:

11. Do your bank's procedures describe when it will use documents, non-documentary methods or a combination of both, and also describe the documents it will use?

☐ *Yes*

☐ *No*

Comments:

Follow-up:

12. For existing customers (i.e. prior to implementation of the final rule's (Sec. 312) provisions), has your bank verified the identity of its high risk customers as well as all those for whom the bank cannot form a reasonable belief as to the accounts' identity?

☐ *Yes*

☐ *No*

Comments:

Follow-up:

13. If using documentary methods to verify a customer's identity, does your bank have procedures that set forth the documents that the bank will use?

☐ *Yes*

☐ *No*

Comments:

Follow-up:

14. For a person other than an individual (such as a corporation, partnership, or trust), does your bank obtain documents showing the legal existence of the entity, such as certified articles of incorporation, an unexpired government-issued business license, a partnership agreement, or a trust instrument?

☐ *Yes*

☐ *No*

Comments:

Follow-up:

15. If your bank uses non-documentary methods to verify a customer's identity does it have procedures that set forth the methods that the bank will use?

☐ *Yes*

☐ *No*

Comments:

Follow-up:

16. Do your bank's non-documentary procedures address situations where:

a. An individual s unable to present an unexpired government-issued identification document that bears a photograph or similar safeguard;
b. The bank is not familiar with the documents presented; the account is opened without obtaining documents (e.g., the bank obtains the required information from the customer with the intent to subsequently verify it);
c. The customer opens the account without appearing in person at the bank; and,
d. The bank is otherwise presented with circumstances that increase the risk that the bank will be unable to verify the true identity of a customer through documents?

☐ *Yes*

☐ *No*

Comments:

Follow-up:

17. Does your CIP address situations where, based on its risk assessment of a new account opened by a customer that is not an individual, the bank will obtain information about the individuals with authority or control over such accounts, including signatories, in order to verify the customer's identity? (Note: This verification method applies only when the bank cannot verify the customer's true identity using documentary or non-documentary methods.)

☐ *Yes*

☐ *No*

Comments:

Follow-up:

18. Does the CIP have procedures that respond to circumstances in which the bank cannot form a reasonable belief that it knows the true identity of the customer?

☐ *Yes*

☐ *No*

Comments:

Follow-up:

19. Do the procedures described in Question #18 describe:

a. Circumstances in which the bank should not open an account?
b. The terms under which a customer may use an account while the bank attempts to verify the customer's identity?
c. When the bank should close an account, after attempts to verify a customer's identity have failed?

☐ *Yes*

☐ *No*

Comments:

Follow-up:

20. Does the bank retain the identifying information (name, address, date of birth for an individual, tax identification number (TIN), and any other information required by the CIP) obtained at account opening for a period of five years after the account is closed?

☐ *Yes*

☐ *No*

Comments:

Follow-up:

21. Does your bank retain identifying information for credit card accounts, for five years after the account closes or becomes dormant?

☐ *Yes*

☐ *No*

Comments:

Follow-up:

22. Does your bank keep a description of the following for five years after the record was made:

a. Any document that was relied upon to verify identity, noting the type of document, the identification number, the place of issuance and, if any, the date of issuance and expiration date?
b. The method and the results of any measures undertaken to verify identity?
c. The results of any substantive discrepancy discovered when verifying identity?

☐ *Yes*

☐ *No*

Comments:

Follow-up:

23. Does your CIP include procedures for determining whether the customer appears on any federal government list of known or suspected terrorist or terrorist organizations should this requirement be initiated?

☐ *Yes*

☐ *No*

Comments:

Follow-up:

24. Does your bank's CIP detail procedures for providing customers with adequate notice that the bank is requesting information to verify their identities and are those procedures in effect?

☐ *Yes*

☐ *No*

Comments:

Follow-up:

25. If your bank relies on other parties for fulfillment of CIP obligations, are all the following criteria met:

a. The relied-upon financial institution is subject to an anti-money laundering program rule (31 U.S.C. 5318(h)) and is regulated by a federal functional regulator;
b. The customer has an account at the bank and the other functionally regulated financial Institution;
c. Reliance is reasonable, under the circumstances;
d. The other financial institution enters into a contract requiring it to certify annually to the bank that it has implemented its anti-money laundering program, and that it will perform (or its agent will perform) the specified requirements of the bank's CIP?

☐ *Yes*

☐ *No*

Comments:

Follow-up:

26. Does the bank's CIP contain written rationale for exempting existing customer from its CIP and does the bank's policy specifically prohibit staff from making or approving CIP exceptions?

☐ *Yes*

☐ *No*

Comments:

Follow-up:

27. Does the bank have a written CIP training program in effect?

☐ *Yes*

☐ *No*

Comments:

Follow-up:

28. Can your bank produce a list of any accounts opened with an application for a tax identification number (TIN)?

☐ ***Yes***

☐ ***No***

Comments:

Follow-up:

29. If such accounts exist (those referred to in Question #28 above), can your bank produce a list of any accounts opened where verification has not been completed or opened with exceptions to the CIP?

☐ ***Yes***

☐ ***No***

Comments:

Follow-up:

30. Can your bank produce a list of accounts identified as high-risk for CIP by the bank?

☐ *Yes*

☐ *No*

Comments:

Follow-up:

31. If your bank is using the *reliance provision* to rely on another financial institution to perform some or all of its CIP on any new accounts, can the bank provide the following:

a. Copies of any contracts signed between the parties?
b. A copy of the CIP or procedures used by the other party?
c. Any certifications made by the other party?

☐ *Yes*

☐ *No*

Comments:

Follow-up:

32. Does your bank's CIP contain procedures specifying a reasonable period of time by which verification of enough of the customer's identity information allows it to form a reasonable belief as to the customer's true identity?

☐ *Yes*

☐ *No*

Comments:

Follow-up:

33. Does your bank's CIP contain procedures to resolve situations where customer identity could not be reasonably established?

☐ *Yes*

☐ *No*

Comments:

Follow-up:

34. Does your CIP provide for review of unexpired government-issued form of identification from customers and does this identification provide required evidence of a customer's nationality or residence, and bear a photograph or similar safeguard (examples include a driver's license or passport)?

☐ *Yes*

☐ *No*

Comments:

Follow-up:

35. If your bank retains photocopies of any documents used in the verification process, are policies and procedures in place to ensure that these photocopies are physically secured to adequately protect against possible identity theft?

☐ *Yes*

☐ *No*

Comments:

Follow-up:

36. In addition to question 35, above, are such photocopies maintained separately from files and documentation relating to credit decisions (in order to avoid any potential problems with consumer compliance regulations)?

☐ *Yes*

☐ *No*

Comments:

Follow-up:

37. Regarding reliance on a third party for verification, do your bank's policies reflect that your bank is ultimately responsible for that third party's compliance with the requirements of the bank's CIP? (Note: This requirement contrasts with the *reliance provision* of the rule that permits the relied-upon

☐ *Yes*

☐ *No*

Comments:

Follow-up:

Know Your Employee

The principal of knowing your employees (KYE) is designed to avoid conflict of interests that may give rise to BSA risk (such as, for example, when commissioned private bankers' compensation depends on volume or dollar amount of business conducted,) or potential for insider complicity/fraud.

Complicity is defined as "the state of being an accomplice, partnership or involvement in wrong doing." When an insider is involved in wrong doing, the detection of the suspicious or unusual activity is difficult. Tests for insider complicity must be incorporated into a bank's internal control systems. The cornerstone of such a process is a stringent employee screening process that alerts management to any potential issues prior to hiring. Many banks use external search firms to aid in this process.

In addition to an effective employment screening process, management should ensure that internal controls address insider complicity on an *ongoing* basis. Employees assigned to higher risk areas of the bank and higher risk accounts (both discussed elsewhere in this handbook) should be subject to heightened scrutiny. Their accounts should be reviewed routinely for any unusual or suspicious activity. Lifestyle vs. salary should be emphasized. Tests for insider complicity should also be part of a bank's audit program.

1 Do policies and procedures exist, and are proper controls and special due diligence exercised for accounts from the highest compensated employees, recent high performers, and/or new employees?

☐ *Yes*

☐ *No*

Comments:

Follow-up:

2. Has Management (or the Compliance Office) assessed the knowledge and technical skills of bank management and personnel with respect to BSA, AML, and OFAC laws and regulations? (To include those who work in BSA compliance, branches, audit, safekeeping and safe deposit, lending, trust, correspondent banking, private banking, international, and the wire transfer room)

☐ *Yes*

☐ *No*

Comments:

Follow-up:

3. Has management's employment screening process been examined for reasonableness and to identify safeguards (e.g., background checks and references) implemented to protect the bank from hiring individuals with questionable or possibly suspicious backgrounds?

☐ *Yes*

☐ *No*

Comments:

Follow-up:

4. Have personnel files been recently reviewed to determine adherence to established policies and procedures?

☐ *Yes*

☐ *No*

Comments:

Follow-up:

5. Have descriptions of account officer and manager positions, the compensation program, and recruitment program been reviewed and commented upon from a BSA perspective?

☐ *Yes*

☐ *No*

Comments:

Follow-up:

6. Does a code of ethics policy exist for signature by staff involved in private banking activities?

☐ *Yes*

☐ *No*

Comments:

Follow-up:

7. Has the bank's private banking and trust employees' compensation program been reviewed to determine whether it includes qualitative measures that provide incentives to comply with account opening and suspicious activity monitoring requirements?

☐ *Yes*

☐ *No*

Comments:

Follow-up:

8. Do written job descriptions include compliance with anti-money laundering laws, regulations, policies, and procedures?

☐ *Yes*

☐ *No*

Comments:

Follow-up:

9. Are procedures in place to detect and report unusual behavior by employees (for example, an employee leads a lavish lifestyle that cannot be supported by his salary, is reluctant to take a vacation, or will not conform to policies or internal controls)

☐ *Yes*

☐ *No*

Comments:

Follow-up:

Lending Activities

Lending to high net worth individuals and their business concerns often takes on unique banking characteristics. The majority of private banking lending is fully secured—often by cash, securities and other assets held by the private banking function. Thus, the extensions of credit to high net worth individuals on a secured basis should not result in compromising sound underwriting standards. If credit is extended based on collateral, even if the collateral is cash, repayment is not assured. For example, collateral derived from illicit activities may be subject to government forfeiture. Accordingly, when extending secured private banking loans, institutions should be satisfied as to the source and legitimacy of the client's collateral, the borrower's intended use of the proceeds and the source of repayment. Some institutions have appropriately recognized that, when lending to high net worth individuals, whether on a secured or unsecured basis, the creditworthiness determination is bolstered by a thorough and well-structured KYC process.

Lending activities include, but are not limited to, real estate, trade finance, cash secured, credit card, consumer, commercial, and agricultural. Lending activities can include multiple parties (e.g., guarantors, signatories, principals, or loan participants).

RISK FACTORS

The involvement of multiple parties may increase the risk of money laundering or terrorist financing when the source and use of the funds are not transparent. This lack of transparency can create opportunities in any of the three stages of money laundering or terrorist financing schemes. These schemes could include the following:

- To secure a loan, an individual purchases a certificate of deposit with illicit funds;
- Loans are made for an ambiguous or illegitimate purpose;
- Loans are made for, or are paid for, a third party;
- The bank or the customer attempts to sever the paper trail between the borrower and the illicit funds;
- Loans are extended to persons located outside the United States, particularly to those in high-risk jurisdictions and geographic locations. Loans may also involve collateral located outside the United States.

RISK MITIGATION

All loans are considered to be accounts for purposes of the Customer Identification Program (CIP) regulations. For loans that may pose a higher risk for money laundering and terrorist financing, including the loans listed above, the bank should complete due diligence on related account parties (i.e., guarantors, signatories, or principals). Due diligence beyond what is required for a particular lending activity will vary according to the BSA/AML risks present but could include performing reference checks, obtaining credit references, verifying the source of collateral, and obtaining tax or financial statements on the borrower and any or all of the various parties involved in the loan.

1. For loans that may pose a higher risk for money laundering and terrorist financing –including real estate, trade finance, cash secured, credit card, consumer, commercial, and agricultural– does your bank complete due diligence on related account parties (i.e., guarantors, signatories, or principals)?

☐ *Yes*

☐ *No*

Comments:

Follow-up:

2. Does the sophistication of the bank's systems used to monitor lending account activity conform to the size and complexity of the bank's lending business?

☐ *Yes*

☐ *No*

Comments:

Follow-up:

Management Awareness

While there are certain requirements that management be kept in the information loop for certain things, in general, it is management's responsibility to foster a culture of compliance. This means that it should be aware of both the specific requirements and general provisions for running an enterprise-wide anti-money laundering compliance program. Evidence that senior management and board of directors have received training regarding the institution's AML program requirements, as well as procedures that reflect ongoing notifications to management by AML compliance staff are examples that might evidence awareness.

1 Is evidence available to demonstrate to examiners that management is aware of the provisions of the applicable laws and regulations?

☐ *Yes*

☐ *No*

Comments:

Follow-up:

NBFIs

NBFIs are broadly defined as institutions that offer financial services. The Patriot Act has defined a variety of entities as financial institutions. Common examples of NBFIs include, but are not limited to:

- Casinos and card clubs.
- Securities and commodities firms (e.g., brokers/dealers, investment advisers, mutual funds, hedge funds, or commodity traders).
- Money services businesses (e.g., certain check cashers; currency dealers or exchangers; issuers, sellers, or redeemers of traveler's checks, money orders, or stored value cards; money transmitters).
- Insurance companies
- Other financial institutions (e.g., dealers in precious metals, stones, or jewels; pawnbrokers; loan or finance companies).

Some NBFIs are currently required to develop an AML program, comply with the reporting and record-keeping requirements of the BSA, and report suspicious activity, as are required by banks. NBFIs typically require a bank account in order to operate. Although NBFIs maintain operating accounts at banks, the BSA does not require, and neither FinCEN nor the federal banking agencies expect, banks to serve as the *de facto* regulator of any NBFI industry or individual NBFI customer. Furthermore, while banks are expected to manage risk associated with all accounts, including NBFI accounts, banks will not be held responsible for their customers' compliance with the BSA and other applicable federal and state laws and regulations.

RISK FACTORS

NBFI industries are extremely diverse, ranging from large multi-national corporations to small, independent businesses that offer financial services only as an ancillary component to its primary business (e.g., grocery store that offers check cashing). The range of products and services offered, and the customer bases served by NBFIs, are equally diverse.

Banks that maintain account relationships with NBFIs may be exposed to a higher risk for potential money laundering activities because many NBFIs:

- Lack ongoing customer relationships and require minimal or no identification by customers;
- Maintain limited or inconsistent record-keeping on customers and transactions
- Engage in frequent currency transactions;
- Are subject to varying levels of regulatory requirements and oversight;
- Can quickly change their product mix or location and quickly enter or exit an operation;
- Sometimes operate without proper registration or licensing.

RISK MITIGATION

Banks that maintain account relationships with NBFIs should develop policies, procedures, and processes to:

- Identify NBFIs relationships;
- Assess the potential risks posed by the NBFI relationships;
- Conduct adequate and ongoing due diligence on the NBFI relationships when necessary;
- Ensure NBFI relationships are appropriately considered within the bank's suspicious activity monitoring and reporting systems.

Risk Assessment Factors

Banks should assess the risks posed by their NBFI customers and direct their resources most appropriately to those accounts that pose a more significant money laundering risk. The following factors may be used to help identify the relative risks within the NBFI portfolio. Nevertheless, management should weigh and evaluate each risk assessment factor to arrive at a risk determination for each customer and to prioritize oversight resources. Relevant risk factors include:

- Types of products and services offered by the NBFI;
- Locations and markets served by the NBFI;
- Anticipated account activity;
- Purpose of the account.

A bank's due diligence should be commensurate with the level of risk of the NBFI customer identified through its risk assessment. If a bank's risk assessment indicates potential for a heightened risk of money laundering or terrorist financing, it will be expected to conduct further due diligence in a manner commensurate with the heightened risk.

Providing Banking Services to Money Services Businesses

FinCEN and the federal banking agencies issued interpretive guidance[1] on April 26, 2005, to clarify the BSA requirements and supervisory expectations as applied to accounts opened or maintained for MSBs.[2] With limited exceptions, many MSBs are subject to the full range of BSA regulatory requirements, including the anti-money laundering program rule, suspicious activity and currency transaction reporting rules, and various other identification and recordkeeping rules.[3] Existing FinCEN regulations require certain MSBs to register with FinCEN.[4] Finally, many states have established supervisory requirements, often including the requirement that an MSB be licensed with the state(s) in which it is incorporated or does business.

The following regulatory expectations apply to banks with MSB customers:

- The BSA does not require, and neither FinCEN nor the federal banking agencies expect, banks to serve as the de facto regulator of any type of NBFI industry or individual NBFI customer, including MSBs.
- While banks are expected to manage risk associated with all accounts, including MSB accounts, banks will not be held responsible for the MSB's BSA/AML program.
- Not all MSBs pose the same level of risk, and not all MSBs will require the same level of due diligence. Accordingly, if a bank's assessment of the risks of a particular MSB relationship indicates a low risk of money laundering or other illicit activity, a bank is not routinely expected to perform further due diligence (such as reviewing information about an MSB's BSA/AML program) beyond the minimum due diligence expectations. Unless indicated by the risk assessment of the MSB, banks are not expected to routinely review an MSB's BSA/AML program.

MSB Risk Assessment

An effective risk assessment should be a composite of multiple factors, and depending upon the circumstances, certain factors may be given more weight than others. The following factors may be used to help identify the level of risk presented by each MSB customer:

- Purpose of the account.
- Anticipated account activity (type and volume).
- Types of products and services offered by the MSB.
- Locations and markets served by the MSB.

Bank management may tailor these factors based on their customer base or the geographic locations in which the bank operates. Management should weigh and evaluate each risk assessment factor to arrive at a risk determination for each customer. A bank's due diligence should be commensurate with the level of risk assigned to the MSB customer, after consideration of these factors. If a bank's risk assessment indicates potential for a heightened risk of money laundering or terrorist financing, the bank will be expected to conduct further due diligence in a manner commensurate with the heightened risk.

MSB Risk Mitigation

A bank's policies, procedures, and processes should provide for sound due diligence and verification practices, adequate risk assessment of MSB accounts, and ongoing monitoring and reporting of unusual or suspicious activities. A bank that establishes and maintains accounts for MSBs should apply appropriate, specific, risk-based, and where necessary, enhanced due diligence (EDD) policies, procedures, and controls. The factors below, while not all inclusive, may reduce or mitigate the risk in some MSB accounts:

- The MSB is registered with FinCEN and licensed with the appropriate state(s), if required.
- The MSB confirms it is subject to examination for AML compliance by the Internal Revenue Service (IRS) or the state(s), if applicable.
- The MSB affirms the existence of a written BSA/AML program and provides the BSA officer's name and contact information.
- The MSB has an established banking relationship and/or account activity consistent with expectations.
- The MSB is an established business with an operating history.
- The MSB is a principal with one or a few agents, or is acting as an agent for one principal.
- The MSB provides services only to local residents.
- Most of the MSB's customers conduct routine transactions in low dollar amounts.
- The expected (low-risk) transaction activity for the MSB's business operations is consistent with information obtained by bank at account opening. Examples include the following:
- Check cashing activity is limited to payroll or government checks (any dollar amount).
- Check cashing service is not offered for third-party or out-of-state checks.
- Money-transmitting activities are limited to domestic entities (e.g., domestic bill payments) or limited to lower dollar amounts (domestic or international).

MSB Due Diligence Expectations

Registration with FinCEN, if required, and compliance with any state-based licensing requirements represent the most basic of compliance obligations for MSBs. As a result, it is reasonable and appropriate for a bank to require an MSB to provide evidence of compliance with such requirements, or to demonstrate that it is not subject to such requirements due to the nature of its financial services or status exclusively as an agent of another MSB(s).

Given the importance of licensing and registration requirements, a bank should file a SAR if it becomes aware that a customer is operating in violation of the registration or state licensing requirement. There is no requirement in the BSA regulations for a bank to close an account that is the subject of a SAR. The decision to maintain or close an account should be made by bank management under standards and guidelines approved by its board of directors.

The extent to which the bank should perform further due diligence beyond the minimum due diligence obligations set forth below will be dictated by the level of risk posed by the individual MSB customer. Because not all MSBs present the same level of risk, not all MSBs will require further due diligence. For example, a local grocer that also cashes payroll checks for customers purchasing groceries may not present the same level of risk as a money transmitter specializing in cross-border funds transfers. Therefore, the customer due diligence requirements will differ based on the risk posed by each MSB customer. Based on existing BSA requirements applicable to banks, the minimum due diligence expectations associated with opening and maintaining accounts for any MSB[230] are:

- Apply the bank's Customer Identification Program;
- Confirm FinCEN registration, if required. (Note: registration must be renewed every two years.);
- Confirm compliance with state or local licensing requirements, if applicable;
- Confirm agent status, if applicable;

- Conduct a basic BSA/AML risk assessment to determine the level of risk associated with the account and whether further due diligence is necessary.

If the bank determines that the MSB customer presents a higher level of money laundering or terrorist financing risk, increased due measures should be conducted in addition to the minimum due diligence procedures. Depending on the level of perceived risk, and the size and sophistication of the particular MSB, banking organizations may pursue some or all of the following actions as part of an appropriate enhanced due diligence review:

- Review the MSB's BSA/AML program;
- Review results of the MSB's independent testing of its AML program;
- Review written procedures for the operation of the MSB;
- Conduct onsite visits;
- Review list of agents, including locations, within or outside the United States, that will be receiving services directly or indirectly through the MSB account;
- Review written agent management and termination practices for the MSB;
- Review written employee screening practices for the MSB.

FinCEN and the federal banking agencies do not expect banks to uniformly require any or all of the actions identified above for all MSBs

---

[1] Refer to "Interagency Interpretive Guidance on Providing Banking Services to Money Services Businesses Operating in the United States," available at www.fincen.gov.

[2] Refer to Interagency Interpretive Guidance on Providing Banking Services to Money Services Businesses Operating in the United States, April 26, 2005, available at www.fincen.gov.

[3] See 31 CFR 103.125 (requirement for money services businesses (MSBs) to establish and maintain an anti-money laundering program); 31 CFR 103.22 (requirement for MSBs to file Currency Transaction Reports); 31 CFR 103.20 (requirement for MSBs to file Suspicious Activity Reports, other than for check cashing and stored value transactions); 31 CFR 103.29 (requirement for MSBs that sell money orders, traveler's checks, or other monetary instruments for currency to verify the identity of the customer and create and maintain a record of each currency purchase between $3,000 and $10,000, inclusive); 31 CFR 103.33(f) and (g) (rules applicable to certain transmittals of funds); and 31 CFR 103.37 (additional recordkeeping requirement for currency exchangers including the requirement to create and maintain a record of each exchange of currency in excess of $1,000).

[4] See 31 CFR 103.41. All MSBs must register with FinCEN (whether or not licensed as an MSB by any state) except: a business that is an MSB solely because it serves as an agent of another MSB; a business that is an MSB solely as an issuer, seller, or redeemer of stored value; the U.S. Postal Service; and agencies of the United States, of any state, or of any political subdivision of any state. A business that acts as an agent for a principal or principals engaged in MSB activities, and that does not on its own behalf perform any other services of a nature or value that would cause it to qualify as an MSB, is not required to register with FinCEN. FinCEN has issued guidance on MSB registration and de-registration. See FIN-2006-G006, Registration and De-Registration of Money Services Businesses, February 3, 2006, at www.fincen.gov.

1. According to interpretive guidance issued on April 26, 2005 to clarify the BSA requirements and supervisory expectations as applied to accounts opened or maintained for money services businesses, does your bank follow these minimum due diligence expectations when opening or maintaining accounts for money services businesses:

a. Confirm FinCEN registration, if required;
b. Confirm state licensing, if applicable;
c. Confirm agent status, if applicable;
d. Conduct a risk assessment to determine the level of risk associated with each account and whether further due diligence is required?

☐ *Yes*

☐ *No*

Comments:

Follow-up:

2. Does your bank have policies, procedures, and processes to:

a. Identify NBFIs relationships;
b. Assess the potential risks posed by the NBFI relationships;
c. Conduct adequate and ongoing due diligence on the NBFI relationships when necessary;
d. Ensure NBFI relationships are appropriately considered within the bank's suspicious activity monitoring and reporting systems?

☐ *Yes*

☐ *No*

Comments:

Follow-up:

3. Are the following risk assessment factors considered in your bank's risk scoring and subsequent treatment of NBFIs:

a. Types of products and services offered by the NBFI;
b. Locations and markets served by the NBFI;
c. Anticipated account activity;
d. Purpose of the account?

☐ *Yes*

☐ *No*

Comments:

Follow-up:

4. Is your bank's due diligence effort commensurate with the level of risk of its NBFI customers, are the risks routinely identified through the bank's risk assessment process, and, is further due diligence conducted as required in a manner commensurate with the heightened risk?

☐ *Yes*

☐ *No*

Comments:

Follow-up:

NGOs and Charities

NGOs are private nonprofit organizations that pursue activities intended to serve the public good. NGOs may provide basic social services, work to relieve suffering, promote the interests of the poor, bring citizen concerns to governments, encourage political participation, protect the environment, or undertake community development to serve the needs of citizens, organizations, or groups in one or more of the communities that the NGO operates. An NGO can be any nonprofit organization that is independent from government.

NGOs can range from large regional, national, or international charities to community based self-help groups. NGOs also include research institutes, churches, professional associations, and lobby groups. NGOs typically depend, in whole or in part, on charitable donations and voluntary service for support.

RISK FACTORS

Since NGOs can be used to obtain funds for charitable organizations, the flow of funds both into and out of the NGO can be complex, making them susceptible to abuse by money launderers and terrorists. Consequently, law enforcement has increased their scrutiny of NGOs.

RISK MITIGATION

To assess the risk of NGO customers, a bank should conduct adequate due diligence on the organization. In addition to required Customer Identification Program (CIP) information, due diligence for NGOs should focus on other aspects of the organization, such as the following:

- Purpose or ideology;
- The geographic areas served (including headquarters and operational areas);
- The organizational structure;
- The donor and volunteer base;
- Funding and disbursement criteria (including basic beneficiary information);
- Record-keeping requirements;
- Its affiliation with other NGOs, governments, or groups;
- Internal controls and audits.

For accounts that bank management considers to be high risk, stringent documentation, verification, and transaction monitoring procedures should be established. NGO accounts that are at higher risk for BSA/AML concerns include those operating or providing services internationally, conducting unusual or suspicious activities, or lacking proper documentation. Enhanced due diligence for these accounts should include:

- Evaluating the principals;
- Obtaining and reviewing the financial statements and audits;
- Verifying the source and use of funds;
- Evaluating large contributors or grantors of the NGO;
- Conducting reference checks.

1. Does your bank's due diligence for NGOs focus on aspects of the organization, such as the following:

a. Purpose or ideology;
b. The geographic areas served (including headquarters and operational areas);
c. The organizational structure;
d. The donor and volunteer base;
e. Funding and disbursement criteria (including basic beneficiary information);
f. Recordkeeping requirements;
g. Its affiliation with other NGOs, governments, or groups?

☐ ***Yes***

☐ ***No***

Comments:

Follow-up:

2. For accounts that bank management considers to be high risk, stringent documentation, verification, and transaction monitoring procedures should be established. Are all the following part of due diligence requirements for NGOs:

a. Evaluating the principals;
b. Obtaining and reviewing the financial statements and audits;
c. Verifying the source and use of funds;
d. Evaluating large contributors or grantors of the NGO;
e. Conducting reference checks?

☐ ***Yes***

☐ ***No***

Comments:

Follow-up:

NRAs and Foreign Individuals

Foreign individuals maintaining relationships with U.S. banks can be divided into two categories: resident aliens and nonresident aliens. For definitional purposes, an NRA is a non-U.S. citizen who: (i) is not a lawful permanent resident of the United States during the calendar year and who does not meet the substantial presence test,[1] or (ii) has not been issued an alien registration receipt card, also known as a green card. The Internal Revenue Service determines the tax liabilities of a foreign person and officially defines the person as a "resident" or "nonresident."

Although NRAs are not permanent residents, they may have a legitimate need to establish an account relationship with a U.S. bank. NRAs use bank products and services for asset preservation (e.g., mitigating losses due to exchange rates), business expansion, and investments. The amount of NRA deposits in the U.S. banking system has been estimated to range from hundreds of billions of dollars to about $1 trillion. Even at the low end of the range, the magnitude is substantial, both in terms of the U.S. banking system and the economy.

RISK FACTORS

Banks may find it more difficult to verify and authenticate an NRA account-holder's identification, source of funds, and source of wealth, which may result in BSA/AML risks. The NRA's home country may also heighten the account risk, depending on the secrecy laws of that country. Since the NRA is expected to reside outside of the United States, funds transfers or the use of foreign automated teller machines (ATMs) may be more frequent. The BSA/AML risk may be further heightened if the NRA is a politically exposed person (SFPF). Refer to the expanded procedures section "Politically Exposed Persons," on page 259 for further information.

RISK MITIGATION

Banks should establish policies, procedures, and processes that provide for sound due diligence and verification practices, adequate risk assessment of NRA accounts, and ongoing monitoring and reporting of unusual or suspicious activities. The following factors are to be considered when determining the risk level of an NRA account:

- The account-holder's home country
- The types of products and services used
- Forms of identification
- The source of wealth and funds
- Unusual account activity

NRA customers may request W-8 status for U.S. tax withholding. In such cases, the NRA customer completes a W-8 form, which attests to the customer's foreign and U.S. tax-exempt status. While it is an Internal Revenue Service (IRS) form, a W-8 is not sent to the IRS, but is maintained on file at the bank to support the lack of any tax withholding from earnings.[2]

The bank's Customer Identification Program (CIP) should detail the identification requirements for opening an account for an NRA. The program should include the use of documentary and non-documentary methods to verify a customer. In addition, the Patriot Act amended the BSA to require special due diligence for private banking accounts for non-U.S. persons, including those held for SFPFs or senior foreign political figures.

---

[1] A foreign national is a resident alien if the individual is physically present in the United States for at least 31 days in the current calendar year and present 183 days or more based on counting: all days present during the current year, plus 1/3 of the days present in the preceding year, plus 1/6 of the days present in the second preceding year. Certain days of presence are disregarded, such as (i) days spent in the United States for a medical condition that developed while the foreign national was present in the United States and unable to leave, (ii) days regular commuters spend traveling to or from Canada or Mexico, (iii) a day of less than 24 hours spent while in transit between two locations outside the United States., and (iv) days when the foreign national was an exempt individual. The individual is considered a resident alien for federal income and employment tax purposes from the

first day of physical presence in the United States in the year that the test is satisfied. Refer to the Internal Revenue Service web site: www.irs.gov.

[2] Additional information can be found at www.irs.gov/formspubs.

1 Has your bank established policies, procedures, and processes that provide for sound due diligence and verification practices and adequate risk assessment of NRA accounts, including ongoing monitoring and reporting of unusual or suspicious activities?

☐ *Yes*

☐ *No*

Comments:

Follow-up:

2. Does your bank's calculation of risks for NRA accounts consider all of the following:

a. The accountholder's home country.
b. The types of products and services used.
c. Forms of identification.
d. The source of wealth and funds.
e. Unusual account activity.

☐ *Yes*

☐ *No*

Comments:

Follow-up:

3. Does your bank's Customer Identification Program (CIP) specifically detail the identification requirements for opening an account for an NRA?

☐ *Yes*

☐ *No*

Comments:

Follow-up:

4. Does your bank's EDD program require special due diligence for private banking accounts for non-U.S. persons, including those held for SFPFs?

☐ *Yes*

☐ *No*

Comments:

Follow-up:

OFAC

OFAC requirements are separate and distinct from the BSA, but both OFAC and the BSA share a common national security goal. For this reason, many financial institutions view compliance with OFAC sanctions as related to BSA compliance obligations; supervisory examination for BSA compliance is logically connected to the examination of a financial institution's compliance with OFAC sanctions.

Evaluation of OFAC compliance is frequently included in BSA/AML examinations. It is not the federal banking agencies' primary role to identify OFAC violations, but rather to evaluate the sufficiency of a bank's implementation of policies, procedures, and processes to ensure compliance with OFAC laws and regulations. To facilitate the examiner's understanding of the bank's risk profile and to adequately establish the scope of the OFAC examination, the regulatory examiners will complete the following steps as part of their examinations:

- Review the bank's OFAC risk assessment. The risk assessment should consider the various types of products, services, customers, transactions, and geographic locations in which the bank is engaged, including those that are processed by, through, or to the bank to identify potential OFAC exposure.
- Review the bank's independent testing of its OFAC program.
- Review correspondence received from OFAC and, as needed, the civil penalties area on OFAC's web site to determine whether the bank had any warning letters, fines, or penalties imposed by OFAC since the most recent examination.
- Review correspondence between the bank and OFAC (e.g., periodic reporting of prohibited transactions and, if applicable, annual OFAC reports on blocked property).

All U.S. banks, federal branches and agencies, international banking facilities, and overseas branches, offices and subsidiaries of U.S. banks must comply with the laws and OFAC-issued regulations. In general, these regulations:

- Require the blocking of accounts and other assets of specified countries, entities, and individuals.
- Prohibit unlicensed trade and financial transactions with specified countries, entities, and individuals.

Banks should establish and maintain effective OFAC compliance programs. This program should include written policies and procedures for filtering transactions for possible OFAC violations, designating an individual responsible for day-to-day compliance, establishing and maintaining strong lines of communication between departments of the bank, and an annual in-depth audit of OFAC compliance.

The compliance program should also include procedures for maintaining current lists of blocked countries, entities, and individuals and disseminating such information throughout the bank's domestic operations and its offshore branches and offices. New deposit, loan, trust, and discount brokerage accounts should be compared with the OFAC lists prior to being opened, and established accounts should be compared regularly with the current and updated OFAC lists. Wire transfer, letters of credit, and non-customer transactions, such as security or funds transfers should be compared with the OFAC lists before being conducted.

1. Has your institution established and maintained an effective, written OFAC program commensurate with its OFAC risk profile (based on products, services, customers, and geographic locations), and does the program:

a. Identify high-risk areas;
b. Provide for appropriate internal controls for screening and reporting;
c. Establish independent testing for compliance;
d. Designate a bank employee or employees as responsible for OFAC compliance;
e. Create training programs for appropriate personnel in all relevant areas of the bank?

☐ *Yes*

☐ *No*

Comments:

Follow-up:

2. Does the U.S. bank maintain a current listing of prohibited countries, entities and individuals?

☐ *Yes*

☐ *No*

Comments:

Follow-up:

3. Is the OFAC information disseminated to foreign country offices?

☐ *Yes*

☐ *No*

Comments:

Follow-up:

4. If your bank uses a third party, such as an agent or service provider, to perform OFAC checks on its behalf, has your bank established adequate controls and review procedures for such relationships?

☐ *Yes*

☐ *No*

Comments:

Follow-up:

5. Are established accounts regularly compared to current OFAC listings? (**Note:** banks should have policies, procedures and processes in place to check existing customers when there are additions or changes to the OFAC list. The frequency of the review should be based on the bank's OFAC risk.)

☐ *Yes*

☐ *No*

Comments:

Follow-up:

6. Are procedures documented in your Customer Identification Program for comparing account names to the OFAC lists?

☐ *Yes*

☐ *No*

Comments:

Follow-up:

7. For any blocked transaction, does documentation exist (and does written policy address) that your bank reported such blocking to OFAC within ten days of the occurrence and annually by September 30 concerning those assets blocked (as of June 30)?

☐ ***Yes***

☐ ***No***

Comments:

Follow-up:

8. Have all prohibited transactions identified and rejected by your bank been reported to OFAC within ten days of the occurrence?

☐ ***Yes***

☐ ***No***

Comments:

Follow-up:

9. Has your bank kept a full and accurate record of each blocked or rejected transaction for at least five years after the date of the transaction?

☐ *Yes*

☐ *No*

Comments:

Follow-up:

10. For blocked property, have records been maintained for the period the property is blocked and for five years after the date the property is unblocked?

☐ *Yes*

☐ *No*

Comments:

Follow-up:

11. Does your bank periodically reassess its OFAC risks, as suggested by Federal guidance?

☐ ***Yes***

☐ ***No***

Comments:

Follow-up:

12. Do your bank's policies, procedures, and processes address how the bank will flag and review transactions and accounts for possible OFAC violations, whether conducted manually, through interdiction software, or a combination of both?

☐ ***Yes***

☐ ***No***

Comments:

Follow-up:

13. For screening purposes, does your bank clearly define its criteria for comparing names provided on the OFAC list with the names in the bank's files (or on transactions) and for flagging transactions or accounts involving sanctioned countries?

☐ *Yes*

☐ *No*

Comments:

Follow-up:

14. Do your bank's policies, procedures, and processes address how it will determine whether an initial OFAC hit is a valid match or a false hit?

☐ *Yes*

☐ *No*

Comments:

Follow-up:

15. New accounts should be compared with the OFAC lists prior to being opened or shortly thereafter (e.g., during nightly processing). If your bank performs OFAC checks after account opening, are controls in place to prevent transactions, other than initial deposits, from occurring until the OFAC check is completed?

☐ *Yes*

☐ *No*

Comments:

Follow-up:

16. Does your bank's OFAC program include policies, procedures, and processes for timely updating of the lists of blocked countries, entities, and individuals and disseminating such information throughout the bank's domestic operations and its offshore offices, branches and, in the case of Cuba and North Korea, foreign subsidiaries?

☐ *Yes*

☐ *No*

Comments:

Follow-up:

17. In the cases of interdictions related to narcotics trafficking or terrorism, do your bank's policies and procedures address notification of OFAC as soon as possible by phone or e-hotline about potential hits with a follow-up in writing within ten days?

☐ *Yes*

☐ *No*

Comments:

Follow-up:

18. Are total amounts blocked, *including interest*, reported to OFAC by September 30 of each year (information as of June 30)?

☐ *Yes*

☐ *No*

Comments:

Follow-up:

19. Does your bank maintain copies of customers' OFAC licenses on file for five years, following the most recent transaction conducted in accordance with the license?

☐ *Yes*

☐ *No*

Comments:

Follow-up:

20. Have independent tests of your OFAC program been performed at least once per year or more, in accordance with the perceived risk of given business areas?

☐ *Yes*

☐ *No*

Comments:

Follow-up:

21. Has your bank designated a qualified individual(s) to be responsible for the day-to day compliance of the OFAC program, including the reporting of blocked or rejected transactions to OFAC and the oversight of blocked funds?

☐ *Yes*

☐ *No*

Comments:

Follow-up:

22. Has your bank provide adequate training for all appropriate employees, the scope and frequency of which is consistent with the bank's OFAC risk profile and appropriate to employee responsibilities?

☐ *Yes*

☐ *No*

Comments:

Follow-up:

Parallel Banking

A parallel banking organization exists when at least one U.S. bank and one foreign financial institution are controlled either directly or indirectly by the same person or group of persons who are closely associated in their business dealings or otherwise acting together, but are not subject to consolidated supervision by a single home country supervisor. The foreign financial institution will be subject to different money laundering rules and regulations and a different supervisory oversight structure, both of which may be less stringent than in the United States. The regulatory and supervisory differences heighten the BSA/AML risk associated with parallel banking organizations.

RISK FACTORS

Parallel banking organizations may have common management, share policies and procedures, cross-sell products, or generally be linked to a foreign parallel financial institution in a number of ways. The key money laundering concern regarding parallel banking organizations is that the U.S. bank may be exposed to greater risk through transactions with the foreign parallel financial institution. Transactions may be facilitated and risks heightened because of the lack of arm's-length dealing or reduced controls on transactions between banks that are linked or closely associated. For example, officers or directors may be common to both entities or may be different but nonetheless work together.

RISK MITIGATION

The U.S. bank's policies, procedures, and processes for parallel banking relationships should be consistent with those for other foreign correspondent bank relationships. In addition, parallel banks should:

- Provide for independent lines of decision-making authority;
- Guard against conflicts of interest;
- Ensure independent and arm's-length dealings between the related entities.

1. Are your bank's policies, procedures, and processes for parallel banking relationships consistent with those for other foreign correspondent bank relationships?

☐ *Yes*

☐ *No*

Comments:

Follow-up:

2. For parallel banking relationships, does your bank provide for independent lines of decision-making authority?

☐ *Yes*

☐ *No*

Comments:

Follow-up:

3. Do bank policies and procedures adequately guard against conflicts of interest with respect to parallel banking relationships that may exist ?

☐ *Yes*

☐ *No*

Comments:

Follow-up:

4. Do your bank's policies, procedures and processes ensure independent and arm's-length dealings between the related parallel banking entities?

☐ *Yes*

☐ *No*

Comments:

Follow-up:

Payable-Through Accounts

Foreign financial institutions use payable-through accounts (PTAs), also known as "pass-through" or "pass-by" accounts, to provide their customers with access to the U.S. banking system. Some U.S. banks offer these accounts as a service to foreign financial institutions. Generally, a foreign financial institution requests a PTA for its customers that want to conduct banking transactions in the United States through the foreign financial institution's account at a U.S. bank. The foreign financial institution provides its customers, commonly referred to as "sub-accountholders," with checks that allow them to draw funds from the foreign financial institution's account at the U.S. bank.[1] The sub-accountholders, who may number several hundred or in the thousands for one PTA, all become signatories on the foreign financial institution's account at the U.S. bank. While payable through customers are able to write checks and make deposits at a bank in the United States like any other account-holder, they might not be directly subject to the bank's account opening requirements in the United States.

PTA activities should not be confused with traditional international correspondent banking relationships, in which a foreign financial institution enters into an agreement with a U.S. bank to process and complete transactions on behalf of the foreign financial institution and its customers. Under the latter correspondent arrangement, the foreign financial institution's customers do not have direct access to the correspondent account at the U.S. bank, but they do transact business through the U.S. bank. This arrangement differs significantly from a PTA with sub-accountholders who have direct access to the U.S. bank by virtue of their independent ability to conduct transactions with the U.S. bank through the PTA.

RISK FACTORS

PTAs may be prone to higher risk because U.S. banks do not typically implement the same due diligence requirements for PTAs that they require of domestic customers who want to open checking and other accounts. For example, some U.S. banks merely request a copy of signature cards completed by the payable through customers (the customer of the foreign financial institution). These U.S. banks then process thousands of sub-account-holder checks and other transactions, including currency deposits, through the foreign financial institution's PTA. In most cases, little or no independent effort is expended to obtain or confirm information about the individual and business sub-accountholders that use the PTAs Foreign financial institutions' use of PTAs, coupled with inadequate oversight by U.S. banks, may facilitate unsound banking practices, including money laundering and related criminal activities. The potential for facilitating money laundering or terrorist financing, OFAC violations, and other serious crimes increases when a U.S. bank is unable to identify and adequately understand the transactions of the ultimate users (all or most of whom are outside of the United States) of its account with a foreign correspondent. PTAs used for illegal purposes can cause banks serious financial losses in criminal and civil fines and penalties, seizure or forfeiture of collateral, and reputation damage.

RISK MITIGATION

U.S. banks offering PTA services should develop and maintain adequate policies, procedures, and processes to guard against possible illicit use of these accounts. At a minimum, policies, procedures, and processes should enable each U.S. bank to identify the ultimate users of its foreign financial institution PTA and should include the bank's obtaining (or having the ability to obtain through a trusted third-party arrangement) substantially the same information on the ultimate PTA users as it obtains on its direct customers.

Policies, procedures, and processes should include a review of the foreign financial institution's processes for identifying and monitoring the transactions of sub-accountholders and for complying with any AML statutory and regulatory requirements existing in the host country and the foreign financial institution's master agreement with the U.S. bank. In addition, U.S. banks should have procedures for monitoring transactions conducted in foreign financial institutions' PTAs. In an effort to address the risk inherent in PTAs, U.S. banks should have a signed contract (i.e., master agreement) that includes:

- Roles and responsibilities of each party;

- Limits or restrictions on transaction types and amounts (e.g., currency deposits, funds transfers, check cashing);
- Restrictions on types of sub-accountholders (e.g., casas de cambio, finance companies, funds remitters, or other non-bank financial institutions);
- Prohibitions or restrictions on multi-tier sub-accountholders;
- Access to the foreign financial institution's internal documents and audits that pertain to its PTA activity. U.S. banks should consider closing the PTA in the following circumstances:
- Insufficient information on the ultimate PTA users;
- Evidence of substantive or ongoing suspicious activity;
- Inability to ensure that the PTAs are not being used for money laundering or other illicit purposes.

---

[1] In this type of relationship, the foreign financial institution is commonly referred to as the "master account-holder."

1. Do existing payable-through account contracts/arrangements with foreign banks address procedures for opening sub-accounts?

☐ *Yes*

☐ *No*

Comments:

Follow-up:

2. Do existing payable through account contracts/arrangements with foreign banks require the master account holder to provide the U.S.-based bank with the true identity of sub-account holders?

☐ *Yes*

☐ *No*

Comments:

Follow-up:

3. Do existing payable through account contracts/arrangements with foreign banks allow cash transactions by sub-account holders within the U.S. borders?

☐ *Yes*

☐ *No*

Comments:

Follow-up:

4. Do existing payable through account contracts/arrangements with foreign banks require the foreign bank to investigate suspicious transactions and report findings to the U.S. based bank?

☐ *Yes*

☐ *No*

Comments:

Follow-up:

5. Do existing payable through account contracts/arrangements with foreign banks clearly state the liability of both the U.S.-based bank and the foreign bank to which the payable through service is being offered?

☐ *Yes*

☐ *No*

Comments:

Follow-up:

6. Do existing payable through account contracts/arrangements with foreign banks have approval of personnel with appropriate authority?

☐ *Yes*

☐ *No*

Comments:

Follow-up:

7. Do internal controls for opening and monitoring payable through accounts include written procedures for procedures for opening accounts?

☐ *Yes*

☐ *No*

Comments:

Follow-up:

8. Does your U.S. based bank apply its know-your-customer policy to both payable through accounts and sub-account holders?

☐ *Yes*

☐ *No*

Comments:

Follow-up:

9. Does the U.S.-based bank prohibit foreign banks from opening sub-accounts (second tier) for other foreign banks, casas de cambios, finance companies or other financial intermediaries?

☐ *Yes*

☐ *No*

Comments:

Follow-up:

10. If question #9 is no, are adequate procedures in place for the U.S. bank to understand the identity of these second-tier sub-accounts holders and the nature of the business transactions?

☐ *Yes*

☐ *No*

Comments:

Follow-up:

11. Does the U.S. based bank review the listing of account and sub-account holders to ensure that no accounts have been opened for individuals or businesses located in countries that are prohibited from doing business with the U.S. including Specially Designated Nationals or Specially Designated Narcotics Traffickers as determined by the Treasury's Office of Foreign Assets Control?

☐ *Yes*

☐ *No*

Comments:

Follow-up:

12. Do the foreign banks that maintain the payable-through relationship properly review and explain

☐ *Yes*

☐ *No*

Comments:

Follow-up:

13. Does the U.S.-based bank allow cash transactions by sub-account holders? If so, does the U.S. bank properly report CTRs for large cash transactions?

☐ *Yes*

☐ *No*

Comments:

Follow-up:

14. Does the U.S.-based bank conduct audits of payable-through accounts to ensure compliance with the contract and appropriate laws and regulations?

☐ *Yes*

☐ *No*

Comments:

Follow-up:

15. Does the U.S. based bank conduct audits of the foreign bank, or review in some other way that:

a. There are available for inspection, written procedures of the foreign bank for opening accounts, to determine if they are consistent with U.S. requirements, and,

b. There are available for inspection, written procedures for the foreign bank's monitoring of sub-account holder activities to detect and report suspicious or unusual transactions?

☐ *Yes*

☐ *No*

Comments:

Follow-up:

16. Does the U.S. based bank maintain adequate documentary information (i.e. financial statements, licensing confirmation, etc.) regarding the foreign bank?

☐ ***Yes***

☐ ***No***

Comments:

Follow-up:

17. Does home country supervisor of the foreign bank require banks in that jurisdiction to identify and monitor the transactions of its own customers consistent with U.S. requirements?

☐ ***Yes***

☐ ***No***

Comments:

Follow-up:

18. Has the U.S.-based bank determined whether the home country supervisor of the foreign bank requires banks in that jurisdiction to identify and monitor the transactions of its own customers consistent with U.S. requirements?

☐ *Yes*

☐ *No*

Comments:

Follow-up:

19. Does the U.S.-based bank obtain adequate information about the ultimate users of the payable-through accounts?

☐ *Yes*

☐ *No*

Comments:

Follow-up:

20. Is the U.S. based bank able to rely on the home country supervisor to require the foreign bank to identify and monitor the transactions of its own customers?

☐ *Yes*

☐ *No*

Comments:

Follow-up:

Senior Foreign Political Figures

Section 312 USA PATRIOT Act (final rule) defines a Senior Foreign Political Figure as[1]:
(i) A current or former senior official in the executive, legislative, administrative or judicial branches of a foreign government (whether elected or not); a senior official of a major foreign political party; or a senior executive of a foreign government-owned commercial enterprise; (ii) a corporation, business or other entity that has been formed by, or for the benefit of, any such individual; (iii) an immediate family member of any such individual; and (iv) a person who is widely and publicly known (or is actually known by the relevant covered financial institution) to maintain a close personal or professional relationship with any such individual. (It is important to note that while government-owned corporations may present risks of their own, the government-owned corporations themselves are not within the definition of a senior foreign political figure.). In addition, a senior foreign political figure includes any corporation, business, or other entity that has been formed by, or for the benefit of, a senior foreign political figure.

- The "immediate family" of a senior foreign political figure typically includes the figure's parents, siblings, spouse, children, and in-laws.
- A "close associate" of a senior foreign political figure is a person who is widely and publicly known to maintain an unusually close relationship with the senior foreign political figure, and includes a person who is in a position to conduct substantial domestic and international financial transactions on behalf of the senior foreign political figure. While close associates are more difficult for banks to identify, they include individuals who due to the nature of their relationship with the SFPF, are in a position to conduct significant domestic and international financial transactions on behalf of the PEP.

The definition of senior official or executive must remain sufficiently flexible to capture the range of individuals who, by virtue of their office or position, potentially pose a risk that their funds may be the proceeds of foreign corruption.[2] Titles alone may not provide sufficient information to determine if an individual is a SFPF, since governments are organized differently from jurisdiction to jurisdiction.

Banks should establish risk-based controls and procedures that include reasonable steps to ascertain the status of an individual as a SFPF and to conduct risk-based scrutiny of accounts held by these individuals. Banks should consider various factors when determining if an individual is a SFPF, including:

- Official responsibilities of the individual's office.
- The nature of the title (e.g., honorary or salaried).
- Level of authority over government activities or other officials.
- Access to significant government assets or funds.

In determining the acceptability of high-dollar or high-risk accounts, a bank should be able to obtain sufficient information to determine whether an individual is or is not a SFPF. For example, when conducting due diligence on a high-dollar or high-risk account, it would be usual for a bank to review a customer's income sources, financial information, and professional background. These factors would likely require some review of past and present employment as well as general references that may identify a customer's status as a SFPF. Moreover, a bank should always keep in mind that identification of a customer's status as a SFPF should not automatically result in a high-risk determination; it is only one factor the bank should consider in assessing the risk of a relationship.

Ascertaining whether a customer has a close association with a senior foreign political figure can be difficult, although focusing on those relationships that are "widely and publicly known" provides a reasonable limitation on expectations to identify close associates as SFPFs. However, banks that have actual knowledge of a close association should consider their customer a SFPF, even if such association is not otherwise widely or publicly known. Banks are expected to follow reasonable steps to ascertain the status of an individual, and the federal banking agencies and FinCEN recognize that these steps may not uncover all close associations.

RISK FACTORS
In high-profile cases over the past few years, SFPFs have used banks as conduits for their illegal activities, including corruption, bribery, and money laundering. However, not all SFPFs present the same level of risk. This risk will vary depending on numerous factors, including the geographic locations involved and the individual's position or authority. Risk will also vary depending on other factors including products and services used, or size or complexity of the account relationship. As a result of these factors, some SFPFs may be lower risk and some may be higher risk for foreign corruption or money laundering. Banks that conduct business with dishonest SFPFs face substantial reputation risk, additional regulatory scrutiny, and possible supervisory action. Red flags regarding transactions that may be related to the proceeds of foreign corruption are listed in the January 2001 inter-agency guidance. Banks also should be alert to a SFPF's control or influence over state-owned government or corporate accounts.

RISK MITIGATION
Banks should exercise reasonable judgment in designing and implementing policies, procedures, and processes regarding SFPFs. Banks should obtain risk-based due diligence information on SFPFs and establish policies, procedures, and processes that provide for appropriate scrutiny and monitoring. Having appropriate risk-based account opening procedures for large-dollar or high-risk products and services are critical, as this is the prime opportunity for the bank to gather information for all customers, including SFPFs. Commensurate with the identified level of risk, due diligence procedures should include, but are not necessarily limited to, the following:

- Identify the accountholder and beneficial owner;
- Seek information directly from the individual regarding possible PEP status;
- Identify the accountholder's country of residence;
- Obtain information regarding employment or other sources of funds;
- Check references, as appropriate, to determine whether the individual is or has been a SFPF;
- Identify the source of wealth;
- Obtain information on immediate family members or close associates having transaction authority over the account;
- Determine the purpose of the account and the expected volume and nature of account activity;
- Make reasonable efforts to review public sources of information. These sources will vary depending upon each situation; however, banks should check the accountholder against reasonably accessible public databases.

SFPF accounts are not limited to large or internationally focused banks. A SFPF can open an account at any bank, regardless of its size or location. Banks should have risk-based procedures for identifying SFPF accounts and assessing the degree of risks involved, which will vary. Management should be involved in the decision to accept a SFPF account. If management determines after-the-fact that an account is a SFPF account, it should evaluate the risks and take appropriate steps. The bank should exercise additional, reasonable due diligence with regard to such accounts. For example, the bank may increase reference inquiries, obtain additional background information on the SFPF from branches or correspondents operating in the client's home country, and make reasonable efforts to consult publicly available information sources. Ongoing risk-based monitoring of PEP accounts is critical to ensuring that the accounts are being used as anticipated.

---

[1] "Guidance on Enhanced Scrutiny for Transactions that may Involve the Proceeds for Foreign Official Corruption" issued by the U.S. Treasury, Board of Governors of the Federal Reserve System, Federal Deposit Insurance Corporation, Office of the Comptroller of the Currency, Office of Thrift Supervision, and the Department of State, January 2001.
[2] 71 Federal Register 495-515

1. Does your bank obtain comprehensive due diligence information on SFPFs and has it established policies, procedures, and processes that provide for greater scrutiny and monitoring of all SFPF customers?

☐ *Yes*

☐ *No*

Comments:

Follow-up:

2. Federal guidance states that account opening procedures are critical, as this is the prime opportunity for the bank to gather the following information on a SFPF. Are all the following obtained upon account opening?

a. The identity of the accountholder and beneficial owner?
b. The source of funds?
c. The source of wealth?
d. Information on immediate family members or close associates having transaction authority over the account?
e. The purpose of the account and the expected volume and nature of account activity?

☐ *Yes*

☐ *No*

Comments:

Follow-up:

3. Does your bank specifically identify SFPF accounts and assess the degree of risks involved?

☐ *Yes*

☐ *No*

Comments:

Follow-up:

4. Is your bank's senior management involved in the decision to accept a SFPF account?

☐ *Yes*

☐ *No*

Comments:

Follow-up:

Pouch Activity

Pouch activity entails the use of a carrier, courier (either independent or common), or a referral agent employed by the courier,[1] to transport currency, monetary instruments, and other documents from outside the United States to a bank in the United States. Pouches can be sent by another bank or individuals. Pouch services are commonly offered in conjunction with foreign correspondent banking services. Pouches can contain loan payments, transactions for demand deposit accounts, or other types of transactions.

RISK FACTORS

Banks should be aware that bulk amounts of monetary instruments purchased in the United States that appear to have been structured to avoid the BSA-reporting requirements often have been found in pouches or cash letters received from foreign financial institutions. This is especially true in the case of pouches and cash letters received from jurisdictions with lax or deficient AML structures. The monetary instruments involved are frequently money orders, traveler's checks, and bank checks that usually have one or more of the following characteristics in common:

- The instruments were purchased on the same or consecutive days at different locations;
- They are numbered consecutively in amounts just under $3,000 or $10,000;
- The payee lines are left blank or made out to the same person (or to only a few people);
- They contain little or no purchaser information;
- They bear the same stamp, symbol, or initials;
- They are purchased in round denominations or repetitive amounts;
- The depositing of the instruments is followed soon after by a funds transfer out in the same dollar amount.

RISK MITIGATION

Banks should have policies, procedures, and processes related to pouch activity that should:

- Outline criteria for opening a pouch relationship with an individual or a foreign financial institution (e.g., customer due diligence requirements, type of institution or person, acceptable purpose of the relationship);
- Detail acceptable and unacceptable transactions (e.g., monetary instruments with blank payees, unsigned monetary instruments, and a large number of consecutively numbered monetary instruments);
- Detail procedures for processing the pouch, including employee responsibilities, dual control, reconciliation and documentation requirements, and employee sign off;
- Detail procedures for reviewing for unusual or suspicious activity, including elevating concerns to management. (Contents of pouches may be subject to Currency Transaction Report (CTR), Report of International Transportation of Currency or Monetary Instruments (CMIR), and Suspicious Activity Report (SAR) reporting requirements.);
- Discuss criteria for closing pouch relationships.

The above factors should be included within an agreement or contract between the bank and the courier that details the services to be provided and the responsibilities of both parties.

---

[1] Referral agents are foreign individuals or corporations, contractually obligated to the U.S. bank. They provide representative-type services to the bank's clients abroad for a fee. Services can range from referring new customers to the bank, to special mail handling, obtaining and pouching documents, distributing the bank's brochures and applications or forms, notarizing documents for customers, and mailing customers' funds to the bank in the United States for deposit.

1. Are logs or other documents adequately maintained by your bank with regard to pouch activity?

☐ ***Yes***

☐ ***No***

Comments:

Follow-up:

2. Are procedures in place to identify any suspicious patterns (for example, sequentially numbered items), and determine whether CTRs, CMIRs and/or SARs should be filed?

☐ ***Yes***

☐ ***No***

Comments:

Follow-up:

3. Are logs maintained for pouch contents containing currency or monetary instruments?

☐ *Yes*

☐ *No*

Comments:

Follow-up:

4. Do your bank's policies and procedures outline criteria for opening a pouch relationship with an individual or a foreign financial institution (e.g., customer due diligence requirements, type of institution or person, acceptable purpose of the relationship)?

☐ *Yes*

☐ *No*

Comments:

Follow-up:

5. Does your bank's Pouch Activity policy detail acceptable and unacceptable transactions (e.g., monetary instruments with blank payees, unsigned monetary instruments, and a large number of consecutively numbered monetary instruments)?

☐ *Yes*

☐ *No*

Comments:

Follow-up:

6. Are procedures detailed for processing a pouch, including employee responsibilities, dual control, reconciliation and documentation requirements, and employee sign off?

☐ *Yes*

☐ *No*

Comments:

Follow-up:

7. Do procedures discuss criteria for closing pouch relationships?

☐ *Yes*

☐ *No*

Comments:

Follow-up:

8. Are all factors relating to risk mitigation of pouch activity included within the agreements or contracts between the bank and the couriers that detail the services to be provided and the responsibilities of both parties?

☐ *Yes*

☐ *No*

Comments:

Follow-up:

Private Banking

Private banking can be broadly defined as providing personalized financial services to wealthy clients. Section 312 of the Patriot Act added new subsection (i) to 31 USC 5318 of the BSA. This subsection requires each U.S. financial institution that establishes, maintains, administers, or manages a private banking account in the United States for a non-U.S. person to take certain AML measures with respect to these accounts. In particular, a bank must establish appropriate, specific, and, where necessary, enhanced due diligence policies, procedures, and controls that are reasonably designed to enable the bank to detect and report instances of money laundering through such accounts. In addition, section 312 mandates enhanced scrutiny to detect and, if appropriate, report transactions that may involve proceeds of foreign corruption for private banking accounts that are requested or maintained by or on behalf of a senior foreign political figure or the individual's immediate family and close associates. On January 4, 2006, FinCEN issued a final regulation (31 CFR 103.178) to implement the private banking requirements of 31 USC 5318(i).

Private banking can be broadly defined as personalized financial services to wealthy clients. The PATRIOT Act amended the BSA to define a "private banking account" as an account, or combination of accounts, that meets the following criteria:

- Requires a minimum aggregate deposit of funds or other assets of not less than $1 million.
- Is established on behalf of one or more individuals who have a direct or beneficial ownership interest in the account.
- Is assigned to, or administered or managed by, in whole or in part, an officer, employee, or agent of a financial institution acting as a liaison between the financial institution and the direct and beneficial owner of the account.[1]

Note: With regard to the minimum deposit requirement, a "private banking account" is an account (or combination of accounts) that *requires* a minimum deposit of not less than $1,000,000. A bank may offer a wide range of services that are generically termed private banking, and even if certain (or any combination, or all) of the bank's private banking services do not require a minimum deposit of not less than $1,000,000, these relationships may be subject to a greater level of due diligence under the bank's risk-based BSA/AML compliance program but are not subject to 31 CFR 103.178.

In particular, banks must establish appropriate, specific, and, where necessary, enhanced due diligence policies, procedures, and controls that are reasonably designed to enable the bank to detect and report instances of money laundering through private banking accounts established, administered, or maintained in the United States for non-U.S. persons. In addition to this general requirement, section 312 described minimum standards for private banking accounts requested or maintained by, or on behalf of, non-U.S. persons, to ensure that, at a minimum, the bank takes reasonable steps to:

- Ascertain the identity of the nominal and beneficial owners of, and the source of funds deposited into, private banking accounts, as needed to guard against money laundering and report any suspicious transactions.
- Conduct enhanced scrutiny of any private banking account that is requested or maintained by, or on behalf of, a senior foreign political figure, or any immediate family member or close associate of a senior foreign political figure. This enhanced scrutiny is reasonably designed to detect and report transactions that may involve the proceeds of foreign corruption.

DUE DILIGENCE

A private banking due diligence program must be reasonably designed to detect and report money laundering and the existence of the proceeds of foreign corruption. In the interim, a reasonable due diligence policy is one that (i) comports with existing sound practices and standards for banks that maintain private banking accounts for non-U.S. persons, (ii) evidences good faith efforts to incorporate the minimum due diligence standards described previously, and (iii) focuses on those private banking accounts that present a high risk of money laundering. Examples of existing sound practices and standards include the following:

- The Board of Governors of the Federal Reserve System, "Private Banking Activities" (SR letter 97-19 (SUP), June 30, 1997) at www.federalreserve.gov.
- U.S. Treasury, the federal bank regulators, and the U.S. Department of the State, "Guidance on Enhanced Scrutiny for Transactions that May Involve the Proceeds of Foreign Corruption," (January 2001) at www.treas.gov/press/releases/docs/guidance.htm.
- The Wolfsberg Group, "Wolfsberg AML Principles on Private Banking" (1st revision May 2002) at www.wolfsberg-principles.com.
- Bank for International Settlements (BIS) Basel Committee on Banking Supervision, "Customer Due Diligence for Banks" (October 2001) at www.treas.gov/press/releases/docs/guidance.htm.

A due diligence program that does not adopt all of the sound practices and standards described in the government and industry guidance listed previously could be considered reasonable. An institution should have a justifiable reason for not adopting a particular sound practice or standard, based on the particular type of accounts held by the bank.

Risk Assessment of Private Banking Accounts for Non-U.S. Persons

A bank must establish and maintain a due diligence program that includes policies, procedures, and controls that are reasonably designed to detect and report any known or suspected money laundering or suspicious activity conducted through or involving any private banking account for a non-U.S. person that is established, maintained, administered, or managed in the United States by the bank. The due diligence program must ensure that, at a minimum, the bank takes reasonable steps to do each of the following:

- Ascertain the identity of all nominal and beneficial owners of a private banking account;
- Ascertain whether the nominal or beneficial owner of any private banking account is a senior foreign political figure;
- Ascertain the source(s) of funds deposited into a private banking account and the purpose and expected use of the account;
- Review the activity of the account to ensure that it is consistent with the information obtained about the client's source of funds, and with the stated purpose and expected use of the account, and to file a Suspicious Activity Report (SAR), as appropriate, to report any known or suspected money laundering or suspicious activity conducted to, from, or through a private banking account.

Banks should develop policies, procedures, and processes to assess the risks posed by private banking accounts for non-U.S. persons and direct their resources most appropriately at those accounts that pose a more significant money laundering risk. The following factors may be used to help identify potential risk characteristics of a private banking customer. Nevertheless, management should weigh and evaluate each risk factor to arrive at a risk determination for each customer. Relevant risk factors may include the following:

- Nature of customer's business (i.e., source of wealth). The nature of the private banking customer's business, the source of the customer's wealth, and the extent to which the customer's business history presents an increased risk for money laundering. This factor should be considered for private banking accounts opened for senior foreign political figures, to the extent needed to reasonably detect and report transactions that may involve the proceeds of foreign corruption.
- Purpose of an account and anticipated activity. The size, purpose, type of accounts involved in the relationship, and anticipated activity of the account (e.g., dollar amount, number, and types of transactions).
- Customer history. The nature and duration of the bank's relationship with the private banking customer.
- Jurisdiction. The private banking customer's location of domicile and business. This review would include considering the extent to which the relevant jurisdiction is internationally recognized as

presenting a greater risk for money laundering or, conversely, if it is considered to have more robust AML standards.

- Available information. Any information known or reasonably available to the institution about the private banking customer. The scope and depth of such a review will depend on the nature of the information uncovered.

The nature and extent of due diligence conducted on private banking accounts for non-U.S. persons will likely vary for each client depending on the presence of potential risk factors. More extensive due diligence, for example, may be appropriate for new clients; clients who operate in, or whose funds are transmitted from or through, jurisdictions with weak AML controls; and clients whose lines of business are primarily currency-based (e.g., casinos or currency exchangers). Due diligence should also be commensurate with the size of the account. Accounts with relatively more deposits and assets should be subject to greater due diligence. In addition, if the bank at any time learns of information that casts doubt on previous information, further due diligence would be appropriate.

Ascertaining Source of Funds and Monitoring Account Activity

Banks that provide private banking services generally obtain considerable information about their clients, including the purpose for which the customer establishes the private banking account. This information can establish a baseline for account activity that will enable a bank to better detect suspicious activity and to assess situations where additional verification regarding the source of funds may be necessary. Banks are not expected, in the ordinary course of business, to verify the source of every deposit placed into every private banking account. However, banks should monitor deposits and transactions as necessary to ensure that activity is consistent with information that the bank has received about the client's source of funds and with the stated purpose and expected use of the account. Such monitoring will facilitate the identification of accounts that warrant additional scrutiny.

For private banking accounts for which a senior foreign political figure is a nominal or beneficial owner, the bank's due diligence program must include enhanced scrutiny that is reasonably designed to detect and report transactions that may involve the proceeds of foreign corruption. The term "proceeds of foreign corruption" means any asset or property that is acquired by, through, or on behalf of a senior foreign political figure through misappropriation, theft, or embezzlement of public funds, the unlawful conversion of property of a foreign government, or through acts of bribery or extortion, and includes any other property into which any such assets have been transformed or converted.

Enhanced scrutiny of private banking accounts for senior foreign political figures should be risk-based. Reasonable steps to perform enhanced scrutiny may include consulting publicly available information regarding the home country of the client, contacting branches of the U.S. bank operating in the home country of the client to obtain additional information about the client and the political environment, and conducting greater scrutiny of the client's employment history and sources of income. For example, funds transfers from a government account to the personal account of a government official with signature authority over the government account may raise a bank's suspicions of possible political corruption. In addition, if a bank's review of major news sources indicates that a client may be or is involved in political corruption, the bank should review the client's account for unusual activity.

---

[1] *Beneficial owner* of an account means an individual who has a level of control over, or entitlement to, the funds or assets in the account that, as a practical matter, enables the individual, directly or indirectly, to control, manage or direct the account. The ability to fund the account or the entitlement to the funds of the account alone, however, without any corresponding authority to control, manage or direct the account (such as in the case of a minor child beneficiary), does not cause the individual to be a beneficial owner.

1. Is your private banking due diligence program reasonably designed to detect and report money laundering and the existence of or suspicious activity conducted through or involving any private banking account that is established, maintained, administered, or managed in the United States?

☐ *Yes*

☐ *No*

Comments:

Follow-up:

2. Has your bank developed policies, procedures, and processes to assess the risks posed by private banking accounts for non-U.S. persons and are resources directed appropriately at those accounts that pose a more significant money laundering risk?

☐ *Yes*

☐ *No*

Comments:

Follow-up:

3. Are your bank's systems adequate to manage the risks associated with private banking activities and support management's ability to implement effective due diligence, monitoring, and reporting?

☐ *Yes*

☐ *No*

Comments:

Follow-up:

4. Does your bank assess the risks that its private banking activities pose on the basis of the scope of operations and the complexity of the bank's customer relationships?

☐ *Yes*

☐ *No*

Comments:

Follow-up:

5. Regarding private banking accounts, does your bank's management establish a risk profile for each customer to be used in prioritizing oversight resources and for ongoing monitoring of relationship activities?

☐ *Yes*

☐ *No*

Comments:

Follow-up:

6. Are the following factors considered when identifying risk characteristics of private banking customers:

a. Nature of the customer and the customer's business?
b. The source of the customer's wealth, the nature of the customer's business, and the extent to which the customer's business history presents an increased risk for money laundering and terrorist financing? (**Note**: This factor should be considered for private banking accounts opened for SFPFs.)
c. The size, purpose, types of accounts, products, and services involved in the relationship?
d. The nature and duration of the bank's relationship (including relationships with affiliates) with the private banking customer?
e. Type of corporate structure (e.g., IBCs, shell corporations (domestic or foreign), or PICs)?
f. The location and jurisdiction of the private banking customer's domicile and business (domestic or foreign)? (**Note:** The review should consider the extent to which the relevant jurisdiction is internationally recognized as presenting a greater risk for money laundering or, conversely, is considered to have robust AML standards.) Information known or reasonably available to the bank about the private banking customer?

☐ *Yes*

☐ *No*

Comments:

Follow-up:

7. Do policies, procedures, and processes for private banking accounts define acceptable CDD for different types of products (e.g., PICs), services, and accountholders?

☐ *Yes*

☐ *No*

Comments:

Follow-up:

8. Has your bank taken reasonable steps to establish the identity of its private banking clients and, as appropriate, the beneficial owners of accounts?

☐ *Yes*

☐ *No*

Comments:

Follow-up:

9. Does your compliance policy detail additional steps to verify the identity of a customer that is not an individual (e.g., a PIC) by obtaining information about individuals with ownership or control over the account in order to verify a customer's identity and to determine whether the account is maintained for non-U.S. persons?

☐ *Yes*

☐ *No*

Comments:

Follow-up:

10. Before opening private banking accounts, does your bank collect the following information from the Private banking clients:

a. The purpose of the account?
b. The type of products and services to be used?
c. Anticipated account activity?
d. A description and history of the source of the client's wealth?
e. The client's estimated net worth, including financial statement?
f. The current source of funds for the account?
g. The references or other information to confirm the reputation of the client?

☐ *Yes*

☐ *No*

Comments:

Follow-up:

11. The board of director's and senior management's active oversight of private banking activities and the creation of an appropriate corporate oversight culture are crucial elements of a sound risk management and control environment. Are the purpose and objectives of your organization's private banking activities clearly identified and communicated by the board and senior management?

☐ *Yes*

☐ *No*

Comments:

Follow-up:

12. Do your bank's goals and objectives describe the target client base in terms of minimum net worth, investable assets, and types of products and services sought?

☐ *Yes*

☐ *No*

Comments:

Follow-up:

13. Do goals and objectives also specifically describe the types of clients your bank will and will not accept and establish appropriate levels of authorization for new-client acceptance?

☐ *Yes*

☐ *No*

Comments:

Follow-up:

14. Are Board and senior management actively involved in establishing control and risk management goals for private banking activities, including effective audit and compliance reviews?

☐ *Yes*

☐ *No*

Comments:

Follow-up:

15. Has your bank ensured that its policies, procedures, and processes for conducting private banking activities are evaluated and updated regularly and ensure that roles, responsibilities, and accountability are clearly delineated?

☐ *Yes*

☐ *No*

Comments:

Follow-up:

16. Has your bank's Board and senior management ensured that compensation plans do not create incentives for employees to ignore appropriate due diligence and account opening procedures or possible suspicious activity relating to the account?

☐ *Yes*

☐ *No*

Comments:

Follow-up:

17. Does your bank thoroughly investigate the background of newly hired private banking relationship managers and established ongoing monitoring of their personal financial condition to detect any indications of inappropriate activities?

☐ *Yes*

☐ *No*

Comments:

Follow-up:

18. When private banking relationship managers change employers, their customers often move with them. Are these accounts promptly reviewed using the bank's procedures for establishing new account relationships?

☐ *Yes*

☐ *No*

Comments:

Follow-up:

19. Do the bank's policies and procedures require Board and senior management review of relationship manager compensation reports, budget or target comparison reports, and applicable risk management reports?

☐ *Yes*

☐ *No*

Comments:

Follow-up:

20. Do Private banker Management Information System (MIS) reports enable the relationship manager to view and manage the whole client and any related client relationships?

☐ *Yes*

☐ *No*

Comments:

Follow-up:

21. Does your bank's compliance policy for private banking define Beneficial Owner of an account as an individual who has a level of control over, or entitlement to, the funds or assets in the account that, as a practical matter, enables the individual, directly or indirectly, to control, manage or direct the account?

☐ *Yes*

☐ *No*

Comments:

Follow-up:

22. Has the identity of all nominal and beneficial owners of each private banking account been established?

☐ *Yes*

☐ *No*

Comments:

Follow-up:

23. Has your bank ascertained whether any person receiving private banking account services is a senior foreign political figure?

☐ *Yes*

☐ *No*

Comments:

Follow-up:

24. Do your bank's account opening and ongoing monitoring policies and procedures include reviews of the activity of each private banking account to ensure that it is consistent with the information obtained about the client's source of funds, and with the stated purpose and expected use of the account?

☐ *Yes*

☐ *No*

Comments:

Follow-up:

25. Do your bank's policies and procedures call for enhanced scrutiny when a private banking account involves a senior foreign political figure?

☐ *Yes*

☐ *No*

Comments:

Follow-up:

26. Does your bank's due diligence program include procedures to be followed in circumstances in which a covered financial institution cannot perform appropriate due diligence with respect to a private banking account, including when the covered financial institution should refuse to open the account, suspend transaction activity, file a suspicious activity report, or close the account?

☐ *Yes*

☐ *No*

Comments:

Follow-up:

Professional Service Providers

A professional service provider acts as an intermediary between its client and the bank. Professional service providers include lawyers, accountants, investment brokers, and other third parties that act as financial liaisons for their clients. These providers may conduct financial dealings for their clients. For example, an attorney may perform services for a client, or arrange for services to be performed on the client's behalf, such as: settlement of real estate transactions, asset transfers, management of client monies, investment services, and trust arrangements.

A typical example is interest on lawyers' trust accounts (IOLTA). These accounts contain funds for a lawyer's various clients, but act as a standard bank account with one unique feature: The interest earned on the account is ceded to the state bar association or another entity for public interest and pro bono purposes.

RISK FACTORS

In contrast to escrow accounts that are set up to serve individual clients, professional service provider accounts allow for ongoing business transactions with multiple clients. Generally, a bank has no direct relationship with or knowledge of the beneficial owners of these accounts, who may be a constantly changing group of individuals and legal entities.

As with any account that presents third-party risk, the bank could be more vulnerable to potential money laundering abuse. Some potential examples of abuse could include:

- Laundering illicit currency.
- Structuring currency deposits and withdrawals.
- Opening any third-party account for the primary purpose of masking the underlying client's identity.

As such, the bank should establish an effective due diligence program for the professional service provider as summarized below.

RISK MITIGATION

When establishing and maintaining relationships with professional service providers, banks should adequately assess account risk and monitor the relationship for suspicious or unusual activity. At account opening, the bank should have an understanding of the intended use of the account, including anticipated transaction volume, products and services used, and geographic locations involved in the relationship. Professional service providers cannot be exempted from currency transaction reporting requirements.

1. When establishing and maintaining relationships with professional service providers, does your bank adequately assess account risk and monitor the relationship for suspicious or unusual activity?

☐ *Yes*

☐ *No*

Comments:

Follow-up:

2. At account opening, does your bank have an understanding of the intended use of the account, including anticipated transaction volume, products and services used, and geographic locations involved in the relationship?

☐ *Yes*

☐ *No*

Comments:

Follow-up:

3. Does your bank's Currency Transaction Reporting Exemptions policy specifically prohibit, as required, granting exemptions to professional service providers, and are proper training, controls and oversight in place to enforce this restriction?

☐ ***Yes***

☐ ***No***

Comments:

Follow-up:

Purchases/Sales of Monetary Instruments

Banks sell a variety of monetary instruments (e.g., bank checks or drafts, including foreign drafts, money orders, cashier's checks, and traveler's checks) in exchange for currency. Purchasing these instruments in amounts of less than $10,000 is a common method used by money launderers to evade large currency transaction reporting requirements. Once converted from currency, criminals typically deposit these instruments in accounts with other banks to facilitate the movement of funds through the payment system. In many cases, the persons involved do not have an account with the bank from which the instruments are purchased.

PURCHASER VERIFICATION

Under 31 CFR 103.29 banks are required to verify the identity of persons purchasing monetary instruments for currency in amounts between $3,000 and $10,000, inclusive, and to maintain records of all such sales.

Banks may either verify that the purchaser of monetary instruments is a deposit account-holder with identifying information on record with the bank or a bank may verify the identity of the purchaser by viewing a form of identification that contains the customer's name and address and that the financial community accepts as a means of identification when cashing checks for non-customers. The bank must obtain additional information for purchasers who do not have deposit accounts. The method used to verify the identity of the purchaser must be recorded.

ACCEPTABLE IDENTIFICATION

The U.S. Treasury's Administrative Ruling 92-1 provides guidance on how a bank can verify the identity of an elderly or disabled customer who does not possess the normally acceptable forms of identification. A bank may accept a Social Security card or a Medicare/Medicaid card along with another form of documentation bearing the customer's name and address. Additional forms of documentation include a utility bill, a tax bill, or a voter registration card. The forms of alternate identification a bank decides to accept should be included in its formal policies, procedures, and processes.

CONTEMPORANEOUS PURCHASES

Contemporaneous purchases of the same or different types of instruments totaling $3,000 or more must be treated as one purchase. Multiple purchases during one business day totaling $3,000 or more must be aggregated and treated as one purchase if the bank has knowledge that the purchases have occurred.

INDIRECT CURRENCY PURCHASES OF MONETARY INSTRUMENTS

Banks may implement a policy requiring customers who are deposit accountholders and who want to purchase monetary instruments in amounts between $3,000 and $10,000 with currency to first deposit the currency into their deposit accounts. Nothing within the BSA, or its implementing regulations prohibits a bank from instituting such a policy. However, FinCEN takes the position that when a customer purchases a monetary instrument in amounts between $3,000 and $10,000 using currency that the customer first deposits into the customer's account, the transaction is still subject to the record-keeping requirements of 31 CFR 103.29. This requirement applies whether the transaction is conducted in accordance with a bank's established policy or at the request of the customer. Generally, when a bank sells monetary instruments to deposit accountholders, the bank will already maintain most of the information required by 31 CFR 103.29 in the normal course of its business.

RECORDKEEPING AND RETENTION REQUIREMENTS

Under 31 CFR 103.29, a bank's records of sales must contain, at a minimum, the following information:

- If the purchaser **has a deposit account** with the bank:
  - Name of the purchaser.
  - Date of purchase.
  - Types of instruments purchased.
  - Serial numbers of each of the instruments purchased.

- Dollar amounts of each of the instruments purchased in currency.
- Specific identifying information, if applicable.[1]

• If the purchaser **does not have a deposit account** with the bank:
- Name and address of the purchaser.
- Social Security or alien identification number of the purchaser.
- Date of birth of the purchaser.
- Date of purchase.
- Types of instruments purchased.
- Serial numbers of each of the instruments purchased.
- Dollar amounts of each of the instruments purchased.
- Specific identifying information for verifying the purchaser's identity (e.g., state of issuance and number on driver's license).

If the purchaser cannot provide the required information at the time of the transaction or through the bank's own previously verified records, the transaction should be refused. The records of monetary instrument sales must be retained for five years and be available to the appropriate agencies upon request.

RISK FACTORS

The purchase or exchange of monetary instruments at the placement and layering stages f money laundering can conceal the source of illicit proceeds. As a result, banks have been major targets in laundering operations because they provide and process monetary instruments through deposits. For example, customers or non-customers have been known to purchase monetary instruments in amounts below the $3,000 threshold to avoid having to provide adequate identification. Subsequently, monetary instruments are then placed into deposit accounts to circumvent the Currency Transaction Report (CTR) filing threshold.

RISK MITIGATION

Banks selling monetary instruments should have appropriate policies, procedures, and processes in place to mitigate risk. Policies should define:

- Acceptable and unacceptable monetary instrument transactions (e.g., non-customer transactions, monetary instruments with blank payees, unsigned monetary instruments, identification requirements for structured transactions or the purchase of multiple sequentially numbered monetary instruments for the same payee).
- Procedures for reviewing for unusual or suspicious activity, including elevating concerns to management.
- Criteria for closing relationships or refusing to do business with non-customers who have consistently or egregiously been involved in suspicious activity.

---

[1] The bank must verify that the person is a deposit account-holder or must verify the person's identity. Verification may be either through a signature card or other file or record at the bank, provided the deposit account-holder's name and address were verified previously and that information was recorded on the signature card or other file or record, or by examination of a document that is normally acceptable within the banking community and that contains the name and address of the purchaser. If the deposit account-holder's identity has not been verified previously, the bank shall record the specific identifying information (e.g., state of issuance and number of driver's license) of the document examined.

1. For purchasers of monetary instruments for currency in amounts between $3,000 and $10,000, inclusive, who have deposit accounts with the bank, do your bank's records include ALL the following required information (31 CFR 103.29(a)(1)):

a. The name of the purchaser?
b. Date of purchase?
c. The type(s) of instrument(s) purchased?
d. The serial number(s) of each of the instrument(s) purchased?
e. The dollar amount(s) of each of the instrument(s) purchased in currency?
f. Method of verification of identity (either at the time of purchase or when the deposit account was opened)?

☐ *Yes*

☐ *No*

Comments:

Follow-up:

2. For purchasers of monetary instruments for currency in amounts between $3,000 and $10,000, inclusive, who do not have deposit accounts with your bank, do the bank's records include the following required information (31 CFR 103.29(a)(2)):

a. The name and address of the purchaser?
b. The social security or alien identification number of the purchaser?
c. The date of birth of the purchaser?
d. The date of purchase?
e. The type(s) of instrument(s) purchased?
f. The serial number(s) of each of the instrument(s) purchased?
g. The dollar amount(s) of each of the instrument(s) purchased?
h. Method of verifying the purchaser's specific identifying information (e.g., state of issuance and number of driver's license)?

☐ *Yes*

☐ *No*

Comments:

Follow-up:

3. Contemporaneous purchases of the same or different types of instruments totaling $3,000 or more must be treated as one purchase. Does your bank have an effective automated or manual system to detect multiple sales of monetary instruments in one day, in amounts totaling $3,000 or more? (**Note:** Multiple purchases during one business day totaling $3,000 or more must be aggregated and treated as one purchase if the bank has knowledge that the purchases have occurred.)

☐ *Yes*

☐ *No*

Comments:

Follow-up:

4. Does your bank have appropriate procedures in place for conducting appropriate follow up, including filing SARs, when structuring is apparent? Is the required documentation maintained? 31 CFR 103.29(b)

☐ *Yes*

☐ *No*

Comments:

Follow-up:

5. Are your bank's transaction monitoring systems (either automated or manual) adequately monitoring

☐ *Yes*

☐ *No*

Comments:

Follow-up:

6. Are records of monetary instrument sales retained for five years and readily available to the appropriate agencies upon request?

☐ *Yes*

☐ *No*

Comments:

Follow-up:

7. Do your bank's procedures state (and does training for relevant employees address) that if a purchaser of monetary instruments cannot provide required information at the time of the transaction or through the bank's own previously verified records, the transaction must be refused?

☐ *Yes*

☐ *No*

Comments:

Follow-up:

8. Do your bank's policies for purchases and sales of monetary instruments define:

a. Acceptable and unacceptable monetary instrument transactions (e.g., non-customer transactions, monetary instruments with blank payees, unsigned monetary instruments, identification requirements for structured transactions or the purchase of multiple sequentially numbered monetary?
b. Instruments for the same payee)?
c. Procedures for reviewing for unusual or suspicious activity, including elevating concerns to management?
d. Criteria for closing relationships or refusing to do business with non-customers who have consistently or egregiously been involved in suspicious activity?

☐ *Yes*

☐ *No*

Comments:

Follow-up:

Quality of Risk Management

Quality refers to how effective the policies and procedures already in place are at accomplishing the objectives of the BSA. While the questions below may be covered in greater detail in other specific sections of the BSA Exam Manual, regulators use these to take a high level look at the overall quality of your bank's attempt at risk management. Often, in the interest of time, they will do this first, rather than use the more detailed, topic specific questions. Problems noted by examiners in this section will lead them to drill down, as appropriate.

1. Has the Board of Directors formally adopted, and has management implemented adequate policies and procedures to maintain compliance with the BSA, AML, and OFAC laws and regulations?

☐ *Yes*

☐ *No*

Comments:

Follow-up:

2. Do policies and procedures address identifying and reporting money laundering in its different forms (e.g., placement, layering, and integration)?

☐ *Yes*

☐ *No*

Comments:

Follow-up:

3. Do policies and procedures address potential high-risk activities, businesses, and countries?

☐ *Yes*

☐ *No*

Comments:

Follow-up:

4. Is coverage for BSA and other regulations sufficiently documented and in effect for teller and currency operations?

☐ *Yes*

☐ *No*

Comments:

Follow-up:

5. Is coverage for BSA and other regulations sufficiently documented and in effect for sales of monetary instruments?

☐ *Yes*

☐ *No*

Comments:

Follow-up:

6. Is coverage for BSA and other regulations sufficiently documented and in effect for all lending activities?

☐ *Yes*

☐ *No*

Comments:

Follow-up:

7. Are processes and responsibilities for responding to changes in laws and regulations documented and in effect?

☐ *Yes*

☐ *No*

Comments:

Follow-up:

8. Are employee consequences for noncompliance well documented and communicated to employees at hiring and as part of your bank's ongoing education programs?

☐ *Yes*

☐ *No*

Comments:

Follow-up:

9. Do policies and procedures address the specific requirements of 31 CFR 103 (Financial Record Keeping and Reporting of Currency and Foreign Transactions)?

☐ *Yes*

☐ *No*

Comments:

Follow-up:

10. Do bank compliance policies address the specific requirements of 12 CFR 21.21 (BSA Compliance)?

☐ *Yes*

☐ *No*

Comments:

Follow-up:

11. Do policies and procedures address the specific requirements of 12 CFR 21.11 (Reports of Suspicious Activities)?

☐ *Yes*

☐ *No*

Comments:

Follow-up:

12. Do policies and procedures address the specific requirements of 18 USC 1956 and 1957 (Money Laundering Statutes)?

☐ *Yes*

☐ *No*

Comments:

Follow-up:

13. Do policies and procedures address the specific requirements of 18 USC 981 and 982 (Civil and Criminal Forfeiture Statutes)?

☐ *Yes*

☐ *No*

Comments:

Follow-up:

14. Do policies and procedures address the specific requirements of 31 CFR 500 et seq. (Office of Foreign Assets Control)?

☐ *Yes*

☐ *No*

Comments:

Follow-up:

15. Is coverage for BSA and other regulations sufficiently documented and in effect for all credit card transactions/operations?

☐ *Yes*

☐ *No*

Comments:

Follow-up:

16. Is coverage for BSA and other regulations sufficiently documented and in effect for all funds transfer activities/operations?

☐ *Yes*

☐ *No*

Comments:

Follow-up:

17. Is coverage for BSA and other regulations sufficiently documented and in effect for all private banking activities/operations?

☐ *Yes*

☐ *No*

Comments:

Follow-up:

18. Is coverage for BSA and other regulations sufficiently documented and in effect for all correspondent banking activities/operations?

☐ *Yes*

☐ *No*

Comments:

Follow-up:

19. Is coverage for BSA and other regulations sufficiently documented and in effect for all payable through account(s) operations?

☐ *Yes*

☐ *No*

Comments:

Follow-up:

20. Is coverage for BSA and other regulations sufficiently documented and in effect for all trust activities/operations?

☐ *Yes*

☐ *No*

Comments:

Follow-up:

21. Is coverage for BSA and other regulations sufficiently documented and in effect for all international activities/operations?

☐ *Yes*

☐ *No*

Comments:

Follow-up:

22. Is coverage for BSA and other regulations sufficiently documented and in effect for all special use account activities/operations?

☐ *Yes*

☐ *No*

Comments:

Follow-up:

23. Is coverage for BSA and other regulations sufficiently documented and in effect for all brokerage account activities/operations?

☐ *Yes*

☐ *No*

Comments:

Follow-up:

24. Do policies and procedures address the specific requirements of USA PATRIOT Act Sec. 313 regarding certification and re-certification of banks?

☐ *Yes*

☐ *No*

Comments:

Follow-up:

25. Do policies and procedures address the specific requirements of USA PATRIOT Act Sec. 311 and 312?

☐ *Yes*

☐ *No*

Comments:

Follow-up:

26. Do policies and procedures address the specific requirements of USA PATRIOT Act Sec. 326 regarding all Know-your-customer requirements to include record retention requirements?

☐ *Yes*

☐ *No*

Comments:

Follow-up:

27. Do policies and procedures address the specific requirements of USA PATRIOT Act Sec. 314a regarding FinCEN requests, including security of the information contained in the requests?

☐ *Yes*

☐ *No*

Comments:

Follow-up:

28. Do policies and procedures address the specific requirements of USA PATRIOT Act Sec. 314b regarding information sharing, and are the required documents needed to share information under this provision available for review?

☐ *Yes*

☐ *No*

Comments:

Follow-up:

Report Filing

Accounting for the various reports required by the BSA should be a simple task, yet there have been instances where financial institutions filled out forms and never sent them in (for example, MGM failing to send in 15,000 CTRs which had been dutifully filled out!), or didn't fill out forms when required, or filled them out so sloppily that they may as well have not done so at all.

1. Are CMIR (Customs Form 4790) and/or logs evidencing submission readily available for inspection?

☐ *Yes*

☐ *No*

Comments:

Follow-up:

2. Are FBAR (TDF 90-22.1) and/or logs evidencing submission readily available for inspection?

☐ *Yes*

☐ *No*

Comments:

Follow-up:

3. Are SARs (TDF 90-22.47) and/or logs evidencing submission readily available for inspection?

☐ *Yes*

☐ *No*

Comments:

Follow-up:

4. Are CTR's (IRS Form 4789 and/or FinCEN Form 104) and/or logs evidencing submission readily available for inspection?

☐ *Yes*

☐ *No*

Comments:

Follow-up:

5. Are Designation of Exempt Persons Form (TDF 90-22.53) and/or logs evidencing submission readily available for inspection?

☐ *Yes*

☐ *No*

Comments:

Follow-up:

6. For international accounts, was a CMIR (U.S. Customs Form 4790) filed for each shipment of cash, except by common carrier, of currency or other monetary instrument(s) in excess of $10,000 from the United States or into the United States, by, or to the bank? 31 CFR 103.23(a) and (b) (In most cases, this refers to the bank's cash shipments.)

☐ *Yes*

☐ *No*

Comments:

Follow-up:

7. Does your bank have a financial interest in, or signature authority over, a bank, securities, or other financial account in a foreign country and if so, has the bank filed within the required time frame the Report of Foreign Bank and Financial Accounts (FBAR: Treasury Form 90-22.1)? Reference: (31CFR 103.24)

☐ *Yes*

☐ *No*

Comments:

Follow-up:

8. Has your bank retained for at least five years either the original, microfilm, or other copy, or reproduction of the records required by the BSA? Reference: 31 CFR 103.22(d), 103.27(a)(3), 103.29(c), 103.33(a)-(c), 103.34(a)(1)(ii), and 103.34(b)(1)-(13)?

☐ *Yes*

☐ *No*

Comments:

Follow-up:

Significant Changes

The BSA compliance environment is dynamic. Rules are promulgated, re-noticed, and changed, watch-lists are constantly updated, and even your own financial institution on occasion offers new products and services or banks different customer types. BSA regulators want to be sure that your policies, procedures and controls address all the necessary elements of change with respect to BSA concern.

1. Does your bank have procedures or systems in place for communicating the requirements of, and any subsequent changes to, BSA, AML, and OFAC laws and regulations in a manner adequate to ensure ongoing compliance?

☐ *Yes*

☐ *No*

Comments:

Follow-up:

2. Does your bank have a system or procedure for updating policies and procedures to ensure compliance with current laws and regulations?

☐ *Yes*

☐ *No*

Comments:

Follow-up:

3. Does your bank have documented procedures in use to ensure compliance when new products are implemented or operational changes occur (e.g., changes in software programs)?

☐ *Yes*

☐ *No*

Comments:

Follow-up:

4. Are version controls or other audit trail controls provided for critical documents for all operations and business areas?

☐ *Yes*

☐ *No*

Comments:

Follow-up:

5. Are methods in place to communicate changes in laws or regulations and are controls in place to assure that required changes to operations manuals and/or procedures have taken place accordingly?

☐ ***Yes***

☐ ***No***

Comments:

Follow-up:

Miscellaneous Due Diligence

Various degrees of due diligence that guidance and regulations prescribe for different customer types can be confusing. For example, there are statutory triggers for *Special* (aka enhanced) Due Diligence (which is described and narrowly defined in the final rule implementing Section 312 of the PATRIOT Act), and increased due diligence (also prescribed by Section 312) for when special due diligence does not apply statutorily. Section 311 may describe *specific special measures*. The BSA Exam Manual and most literature dispose with the formality and use the term enhanced due diligence (EDD) generically to describe any steps beyond the usual CDD practices that are applied to accounts posing higher BSA risks. The questions in this section are meant to ensure that the latter definition is appropriately applied where regulatory examiners expect it should be. Additionally, regulators look to see if due diligence is applied by BSA staff with respect to implementation and control within their own financial institutions. Amazingly, financial institutions have been cited in enforcement actions for not executing basic KYC principals and being unaware of customers that engage in certain high risk activities or unable to produce lists by customer activity or category. Questions in this section address these issues as well.

1. Do policies and procedures exist, and are proper controls and special due diligence exercised for customers who deal in large cash transactions?

☐ *Yes*

☐ *No*

Comments:

Follow-up:

2. Do policies and procedures exist, and are proper controls and increased due diligence exercised for customers from high-risk countries?

☐ *Yes*

☐ *No*

Comments:

Follow-up:

3. Do policies and procedures exist, and are proper controls and increased due diligence exercised for customers who are foreign clients and government officials from high-risk countries?

☐ *Yes*

☐ *No*

Comments:

Follow-up:

4. Have business or strategic plans for private banking and trust activities been reviewed by the compliance department to assess how compliance policies and procedures are implemented in the business units?

☐ *Yes*

☐ *No*

Comments:

Follow-up:

5. Are methods in place to aggregate customer holdings and activities across business units throughout the organization?

☐ *Yes*

☐ *No*

Comments:

Follow-up:

6. Are reports received regularly by management on private banking and trust activities?

☐ *Yes*

☐ *No*

Comments:

Follow-up:

7. Does a list of accounts exist for the bank's private banking and trust customers who are foreign government officials, export/import business owners, money transmitters, private investment companies (PICs), financial advisors, offshore entities, or money managers (when an intermediary is acting on behalf of customers)?

☐ *Yes*

☐ *No*

Comments:

Follow-up:

8. Do lists exist of private banking and trust customer accounts brought to the bank by account officers who were previously employed by other financial institutions?

☐ *Yes*

☐ *No*

Comments:

Follow-up:

9. Is a list maintained for accounts where a third-party investment advisor referred the accounts to the bank?

☐ *Yes*

☐ *No*

Comments:

Follow-up:

10. Is a list maintained of accounts for whom nominee names are used?

☐ *Yes*

☐ *No*

Comments:

Follow-up:

11. Do written policies, procedures, and systems of internal controls for opening and monitoring private banking and trust accounts provide for:

a. Procedures for opening accounts?
b. Operational procedures?
c. Periodic reviews?
d. Staff responsibility and accountability?
e. Training?
f. Monitoring for unusual or suspicious transactions?
g. Reporting of unusual or suspicious transactions?

☐ *Yes*

☐ *No*

Comments:

Follow-up:

12. Have management information systems supporting private banking and trust activities been reviewed as to whether the reports they generate are adequate, useful, timely, aggregated across departments and products, as needed, and provided to senior management and the board of directors, as needed?

☐ *Yes*

☐ *No*

Comments:

Follow-up:

13. Regarding Question #12, Do MIS reports encompass all of the following?

a. Customer aggregation reports (all holdings throughout the institution, including overseas and nominee name holdings)?
b. Profitability reports?
c. Policy exception and missing document reports?
d. Customer risk classification reports?
e. Unusual account activity (including cash and non-cash, funds transfer, asset management, loan payments, offshore activities, etc.)?
f. Suspicious activity reports?

☐ *Yes*

☐ *No*

Comments:

Follow-up:

14. Are account transactions regularly reviewed to determine if they are consistent with *expectations* (i.e., not just thresholds for the group of customers)?

☐ *Yes*

☐ *No*

Comments:

Follow-up:

15. Does your bank have a well documented system to identify suspicious activity associated with private banking and trust customers?

☐ *Yes*

☐ *No*

Comments:

Follow-up:

16. Does your bank have documented systems and procedures in place to detect, investigate, and report suspicious loan transactions?

☐ *Yes*

☐ *No*

Comments:

Follow-up:

17. Are loan activities periodically reviewed and/or are procedures effectively in place address/monitor:

a. Cash-secured loans?
b. Loans that do not fit the customer's general business profile?
c. Premature cancellation of debt, particularly with cash?

☐ *Yes*

☐ *No*

Comments:

Follow-up:

18. Has your bank's management considered money laundering implications and prevention measures associated with safe deposit activity, and are ample policies, procedures and controls documented to address these?

☐ *Yes*

☐ *No*

Comments:

Follow-up:

19. Could investigators identify the ultimate owner and address of the owner of the items held in safe custody?

☐ *Yes*

☐ *No*

Comments:

Follow-up:

20. Do policies and procedures exist, and are proper controls and increased due diligence exercised for customers who have accounts offshore or with offshore entities, including PICs?

☐ *Yes*

☐ *No*

Comments:

Follow-up:

21. Do policies and procedures exist, and are proper controls and increased due diligence exercised for customers who have large and frequent funds transfer activity?

☐ *Yes*

☐ *No*

Comments:

Follow-up:

22. Do policies and procedures exist, and are proper controls and increased due diligence exercised for the grantors of private banking and trust accounts that direct loans from their accounts to other parties or business interests of account principals or beneficiaries?

☐ *Yes*

☐ *No*

Comments:

Follow-up:

23. Do policies and procedures exist, and are proper controls and special due diligence exercised for accounts that appear to act as pass-through accounts with high volumes of credits and debits and low average monthly balances?

☐ *Yes*

☐ *No*

Comments:

Follow-up:

24. Do policies and procedures exist, and are proper controls and increased due diligence exercised for customers listed on unusual or suspicious activity monitoring reports as well as customers on whom SARs have been filed?

☐ *Yes*

☐ *No*

Comments:

Follow-up:

25. Do policies and procedures exist, and are proper controls and special due diligence exercised for clients with nondiscretionary accounts (e.g., custodial accounts, investment advisory accounts, and revocable trusts)?

☐ *Yes*

☐ *No*

Comments:

Follow-up:

Special Measures

Section 311 of the PATRIOT Act added 31 USC 5318A to the BSA, which authorizes the Secretary of the Treasury to require domestic financial institutions and domestic financial agencies to take certain special measures against foreign jurisdictions, foreign financial institutions, classes of international transactions, or types of accounts of primary money laundering concern. Section 311 provides the Secretary of the Treasury with a range of options that can be adapted to target specific money laundering and terrorist financing concerns. Section 311 is implemented through various orders and regulations that are incorporated into 31 CFR Part 103. As set forth in section 311, certain special measures may be imposed by an order without prior public notice and comment, but such orders must be of limited duration and must be issued together with a Notice of Proposed Rulemaking.

Section 311 establishes a process for the Secretary of the Treasury to follow, and identifies federal agencies to consult before the Secretary of the Treasury may conclude that a jurisdiction, financial institution, class of transactions, or type of account is of primary money laundering concern. The statute also provides similar procedures, including factors and consultation requirements, for selecting the specific special measures to be imposed against a jurisdiction, financial institution, class of transactions, or type of account that is of primary money laundering concern. It is important to note that, while a jurisdiction, financial institution, class of transactions, or type of account may be designated of primary money laundering concern in an order issued together with a Notice of Proposed Rulemaking, special measures of unlimited duration can only be imposed by a final rule issued after notice and an opportunity for comment.

TYPES OF SPECIAL MEASURES

The following five special measures can be imposed, either individually, jointly, or in any combination:

Record-keeping and Reporting of Certain Financial Transactions

Under the first special measure, banks may be required to maintain or to file reports concerning the aggregate amount of transactions or the specifics of each transaction with respect to a jurisdiction, financial institution, class of transactions, or type of account that is of primary money laundering concern. The statute contains minimum information requirements for these records and reports and permits the Secretary of the Treasury to impose additional information requirements.

Information Relating to Beneficial Ownership

Under the second special measure, banks may be required to take reasonable and practicable steps, as determined by the Secretary of the Treasury, to obtain and retain information concerning the beneficial ownership of any account opened or maintained in the United States by a foreign person (other than a foreign entity whose shares are subject to public reporting requirements or are listed and traded on a regulated exchange or trading market), or a representative of such foreign person, that involves a jurisdiction, financial institution, class of transactions, or type of account that is of primary money laundering concern.

Information Relating to Certain Payable Through Accounts

Under the third special measure, banks that open or maintain a payable through account involving a jurisdiction, financial institution, class of transactions, or type of account that is of primary money laundering concern, may be required to: (i) identify each customer (and representative) who is permitted to use the account or whose transactions are routed through the account; and (ii) obtain information about each such customer (and representative) that is substantially comparable to that which a United States depository institution obtains in the ordinary course of business with respect to its customers residing in the United States.

Information Relating to Certain Correspondent Accounts

Under the fourth special measure, banks that open or maintain a correspondent account in the United States involving a jurisdiction, financial institution, class of transactions, or type of account that is of primary money laundering concern may be required to: (i) identify each customer (and representative) who is permitted to use the account or whose transactions are routed through the account; and (ii) obtain information about each such customer (and representative) that is substantially comparable to that which a United States depository institution obtains in the ordinary course of business with respect to its customers residing in the United States.

Prohibitions or Conditions on Opening or Maintaining Certain Correspondent or Payable Through Accounts

Under the fifth, and strongest, special measure, banks may be prohibited from opening or maintaining any correspondent account or payable through account for, or on behalf of, a foreign financial institution if the account involves a jurisdiction, financial institution, class of transactions, or type of account that is of primary money laundering concern. The imposition of this measure can prohibit U.S. banks from establishing, maintaining, administering or managing a correspondent or payable through account for, or on behalf of, any financial institution from a specific foreign jurisdiction. This measure may also be applied to specific foreign financial institutions and their subsidiaries.

The regulations that implement these prohibitions may require banks to review their account records to determine that they maintain no accounts directly for, or on behalf of, such entities. In addition to the direct prohibition, banks may also be:

- Prohibited from knowingly providing indirect access to the specific entities through its other banking relationships.
- Required to notify correspondent accountholders that they must not provide the specific entity with access to the account maintained at the U.S. bank.
- Required to take reasonable steps to identify any indirect use of its accounts by the specific entity.

SPECIAL MEASURES GUIDANCE

Orders and regulations implementing specific special measures taken under section 311 of the PATRIOT Act are not static; they can be issued or rescinded over time as the Secretary of the Treasury determines that a subject jurisdiction, institution, class of transactions, or type of account is no longer of primary money laundering concern. In addition, special measures imposed against one jurisdiction, institution, class of transactions, or type of account may vary from those imposed in other situations. Examiners and BSA Officers should also note that compliance with special measures is not necessarily absolute; an order or rule imposing a special measure may establish a standard of due diligence that banks must apply to comply with the particular special measure.

BSA Officers reviewing compliance with this section should visit FinCEN's web site www.fincen.gov for current information on final special measures. Examiners should only examine for those special measures that are final, and should not review banks against those that are proposed.

1. For final special measures implementing Section 311 of the PATRIOT Act, does your bank have written policies, procedures and controls addressing such compliance?

☐ *Yes*

☐ *No*

Comments:

Follow-up:

Special Use Accounts

Special use accounts (SUAs) are in-house accounts established to facilitate the processing and settlement of multiple or individual customer transactions within the bank, usually on the same day. These accounts have several different names, including concentration, omnibus, suspense, settlement, intra-day, sweep, and collection accounts. SUAs are used widely in private banking, wire transfer, and other bank departments.

Money laundering risk can arise in these accounts because customer-identifying information, such as address and account number ,can be separated from financial transactions. If that happens, an effective audit trail is lost, and accounts can be misused or administered improperly.

Banks that use SUAs should implement adequate procedures and controls covering access to and operation of those accounts, including being able to identify, measure, monitor, and control the associated risks. The bank must be aware of and understand fully the activities of its customers and report transactions that have no apparent lawful purpose or are not the sort in which a particular customer would normally be expected to engage. This includes those customers whom, for whatever reason, are users of these types of special use accounts.

1. Are policies, procedures and controls documented and in place describing who within your bank can access (debit or credit) special use account(s) and whether two signatures are required for access?

☐ *Yes*

☐ *No*

Comments:

Follow-up:

2. Are policies, procedures and controls documented and in place describing whether customers have the ability to access special use accounts?

- ☐ *Yes*
- ☐ *No*

Comments:

Follow-up:

3. Are customer transactions also captured in the customer's account statements?

- ☐ *Yes*
- ☐ *No*

Comments:

Follow-up:

4. Are proper controls in place to ensure frequency of reconcilements according to your bank's policies and procedures?

☐ ***Yes***

☐ ***No***

Comments:

Follow-up:

5. Is your bank's process to resolve discrepancies well documented and followed?

☐ ***Yes***

☐ ***No***

Comments:

Follow-up:

Suspicious Activity Detection & Reporting

Banks, bank holding companies, and their subsidiaries are required by federal regulations[1] to file a SAR with respect to:

- Criminal violations involving insider abuse in any amount.
- Criminal violations aggregating $5,000 or more when a suspect can be identified.
- Criminal violations aggregating $25,000 or more regardless of a potential suspect.
- Transactions conducted or attempted by, at, or through the bank (or an affiliate) and aggregating $5,000 or more, if the bank or affiliate knows, suspects, or has reason to suspect that the transaction:
  - May involve potential money laundering or other illegal activity (e.g., terrorism financing).
  - Is designed to evade the BSA or its implementing regulations
  - Has no business or apparent lawful purpose or is not the type of transaction that the particular customer would normally be expected to engage in, and the bank knows of no reasonable explanation for the transaction after examining the available facts, including the background and possible purpose of the transaction.

A transaction includes a deposit; a withdrawal; a transfer between accounts; an exchange of currency; an extension of credit; a purchase or sale of any stock, bond, certificate of deposit, or other monetary instrument or investment security; or any other payment, transfer, or delivery by, through, or to a bank.

SYSTEMS TO IDENTIFY, RESEARCH, AND REPORT SUSPICIOUS ACTIVITY

Policies, procedures, and processes should indicate the persons responsible for the identification, research, and reporting of suspicious activities. Appropriate policies, procedures, and processes should be in place to monitor and identify unusual activity. The level of monitoring should be dictated by the bank's assessment of risk, with particular emphasis on high-risk products, services, customers, and geographic locations. Monitoring systems typically include employee identification or referrals, manual systems, automated systems, or any combination. The bank should ensure adequate staff is assigned to the identification, research, and reporting of suspicious activities taking into account the bank's overall risk profile and the volume of transactions. Upon identification of unusual activity, additional research is typically conducted. Customer due diligence (CDD) information will assist banks in evaluating if the unusual activity is considered suspicious. After thorough research and analysis, decisions to file or not to file a SAR should be documented. If applicable, reviewing and understanding suspicious activity monitoring across the organization's affiliates, business lines, and risk types (e.g., reputation, compliance, or transaction) may enhance a banking organizations' ability to detect suspicious activity and thus minimize the potential for financial losses, increased expenses, and reputational risk to the organization.

Manual Transaction Monitoring

A manual transaction monitoring system consists of a review of various reports generated by the bank's management information systems (MIS) or vendor systems. Some bank's MIS are supplemented by vendor systems designed to identify reportable currency transactions and to maintain required funds transfer records. Many of these vendor systems include filtering models for identification of unusual activity. Examples of MIS reports include currency activity reports, funds transfer reports, monetary instrument sales reports, large item reports, significant balance change reports, and non-sufficient funds (NSF) reports. The process may involve review of daily reports, reports that cover a period of time (e.g., rolling 30-day reports, monthly reports), or a combination of both types of reports. The type and frequency of reviews and resulting reports used should be commensurate with the bank's BSA/AML risk profile and appropriately cover its high risk products, services, customers, and geographic locations.

MIS or vendor system-generated reports typically use a discretionary dollar threshold. Thresholds selected by management for the production of transaction reports should enable management to detect unusual activity. Upon identification of unusual activity, assigned personnel should review CDD and other pertinent information to determine whether the activity is suspicious. Management should periodically evaluate the appropriateness of filtering criteria and thresholds used in the monitoring process. Each bank should evaluate and identify filtering criteria most appropriate for their bank. Typical manual transaction monitoring reports are as follows. In addition, the programming of the bank's monitoring systems should be independently reviewed for reasonable filtering criteria.

Currency Activity Reports: Most vendors offer reports that identify all currency activity or currency activity greater than $10,000. These reports assist bankers with filing Currency Transaction Reports (CTRs) and identifying suspicious currency activity. Most bank information service providers offer currency activity reports that can filter transactions using various parameters, for example:

- Currency activity including multiple transactions greater than $10,000.
- Currency activity (single and multiple transactions) below the $10,000 reporting requirement (e.g., between $7,000 and $10,000).
- Currency transactions involving multiple lower dollar transactions (e.g., $3,000) that over a period of time (e.g., 15 days) aggregate to a substantial sum of money (e.g., $30,000).

Such filtering reports, whether implemented through a purchased vendor software system or through requests from information service providers, will significantly enhance a bank's ability to identify and evaluate unusual currency transactions.

Funds Transfer Records

The BSA requires banks to maintain records of funds transfer in amounts of $3,000 and above. Periodic review of this information can assist banks in identifying patterns of unusual activity. A periodic review of the funds transfer records in banks with low funds transfer activity is usually sufficient to identify unusual activity. For banks with more significant funds transfer activity, use of spreadsheet or vendor software is an efficient way to review funds transfer activity for unusual patterns. Most vendor software systems include standard suspicious activity filter reports. These reports typically focus on identifying certain high-risk geographic locations and larger dollar funds transfer transactions for individuals and businesses. Each bank should establish its own filtering criteria for both individuals and businesses. Non-customer funds transfer transactions and payable upon proper identification (PUPID) transactions should also be reviewed for unusual activity.

Monetary Instrument Records: Records for monetary instrument sales are required by the BSA. Such records can assist the bank in identifying possible currency structuring through the purchase of cashier's checks, official bank checks, money orders, or traveler's checks in amounts of $3,000 to $10,000. A periodic review of these records can also help identify frequent purchasers of monetary instruments and common payees.

Automated Account Monitoring

Automated account-monitoring systems typically use computer programs, developed in-house or purchased from vendors, to identify individual transactions, patterns of unusual activity, or deviations from expected activity. These systems can capture a wide range of account activity, such as deposits, withdrawals, funds transfers, automated clearing house (ACH) transactions, and automated teller machine (ATM) transactions, directly from the bank's core data processing system. Banks that are large, operate in many locations, or have a large volume of high-risk customers typically use automated account-monitoring systems.

Current types of automated systems include rule-based and intelligent systems. Rule based systems detect unusual transactions that are outside of system-developed or management-established "rules." Such systems can consist of few or many rules, depending on the complexity of the in-house or vendor product. These rules are applied using a series of transaction filters or a rules engine. Rule-based automated systems are more sophisticated than the basic manual system, which only filters on one rule (e.g., transaction greater than $10,000). Rule-based automated monitoring systems can apply complex or multiple filters. For example, rules-based automated monitoring systems can apply first to all accounts, then to a subset or risk category of accounts (such as all customers with direct deposit or all restaurants). Rule-based monitoring systems can also filter individual customer-account profiles.

Intelligent systems are adaptive systems that can change their analysis over time on the basis of activity patterns, recent trends, changes in the customer base, and other relevant data. Intelligent systems review transactions in context with other transactions and the customer profile. In doing so, these systems increase their information database on the customer, account type, category, or business, as more transactions and data are stored in the system.

Understanding the filtering criteria of a software-based monitoring system is critical to assessing the effectiveness of automated account monitoring systems. System filtering criteria should be developed through a review of specific high-risk customers, products, and services. System filtering criteria, including specific profiles and rules, should be based on what is reasonable and expected for each type of customer. Monitoring customers purely on the basis of historical activity can be misleading if their activity is not actually consistent with similar types of customers. For example, a customer may have a historical transaction activity that is substantially different from what would normally be expected from that type of customer (e.g., a check-cashing business that deposits large sums of currency versus withdrawing currency to fund the cashing of checks).

The authority to establish or change expected activity profiles should be clearly defined and should generally require the approval of the BSA compliance officer or senior management. Controls should ensure limited access to the monitoring system. Management should document or be able to explain filtering criteria, thresholds used, and how both are appropriate for the bank's risks. Management should also periodically review the filtering criteria and thresholds established to ensure that they are still effective. In addition, the bank's programming methodology should be independently validated.

Identifying Underlying Crime

Banks are required to report suspicious activity that may involve money laundering, BSA violations, terrorist financing,[2] and certain other crimes above prescribed dollar thresholds. However, banks are not obligated to investigate or confirm the underlying predicate crime (e.g., terrorist financing, money laundering,, identity theft, and various types of fraud). Investigation is the responsibility of law enforcement. When evaluating suspicious activity and completing the SAR, banks should, to the best of their ability, identify the characteristics of the suspicious activity. Part III, section 35, of the SAR provides 20 different characteristics of suspicious activity. Although an "Other" category is available, the use of this category should be limited to situations that cannot be broadly identified within the 20 characteristics provided.

Law Enforcement Inquiries and Requests

Banks should establish policies, procedures, and processes for identifying subjects of law enforcement requests, monitoring the transaction activity of those subjects, identifying unusual or suspicious activity related to those subjects, and filing, as applicable, SARs related to those subjects. Law enforcement inquiries and requests can include criminal subpoenas, national security letters (NSLs), and section 314(a) requests. ere receipt of any law enforcement inquiry, does not, by itself, require the filing of a SAR by the bank. Nonetheless, a law enforcement inquiry may be relevant to a bank's overall risk assessment of its customers and accounts. It is incumbent upon a bank to assess all of the information it knows about its customer, including the receipt of a law enforcement inquiry, in accordance with its risk-based BSA/AML compliance program. The bank should determine whether a SAR should be filed based on all customer information available.

National Security Letters

NSLs are written investigative demands that may be issued by the local Federal Bureau of Investigation (FBI) and other federal governmental authorities in counter-intelligence and counter-terrorism investigations to obtain the following:

- Telephone and electronic communications records from telephone companies and Internet service providers.[3]
- Information from credit bureaus.[4]
- Financial records from financial institutions.[5]

NSLs are highly confidential.[6] Pursuant to 12 USC 3414(a)(3) and (5)(D), no bank, or officer, employee or agent of the institution, can disclose to any person that a government authority or the FBI has sought or obtained access to records through a Right to Financial Privacy Act NSL. Banks that receive NSLs must take appropriate measures to ensure the confidentiality of the letters and should have procedures in place for processing and maintaining the confidentiality of NSLs.

If a bank files a SAR after receiving a NSL, the SAR should not contain any reference to the receipt or existence of the NSL. The SAR should reference only those facts and activities that support a finding of unusual or suspicious transactions identified by the bank.

Questions regarding NSLs should be directed to the bank's local FBI field office.
Contact information for the FBI field offices can be found at www.fbi.gov.

SAR DECISION-MAKING PROCESS

The bank should have policies, procedures, and processes for referring unusual activity from all business lines to the personnel or department responsible for evaluating unusual activity. The process should ensure that all applicable information (e.g., criminal subpoenas, NSLs, or section 314(a) requests) is effectively evaluated.

Banks are encouraged to document SAR decisions. Thorough documentation provides a record of the SAR decision-making process, including final decisions not to file a SAR. he decision to file a SAR is an inherently subjective judgment. Examiners should focus on whether the bank has an effective SAR decision-making process, not individual SAR decisions. Examiners may review individual SAR decisions as a means to test the effectiveness of the SAR monitoring, reporting, and decision-making process. In those instances where the bank has an established SAR decision-making process, has followed existing policies, procedures, and processes and has determined not to file a SAR, the bank should not be criticized for the failure to file a SAR unless the failure is significant or accompanied by evidence of bad faith.

TIMING OF A SAR FILING

The SAR rules require that a SAR be filed no later than 30 calendar days from the date of the initial detection of the suspicious activity, unless no suspect can be identified. In that case, the time period for filing a SAR is extended to 60 days. Organizations may need to review transaction or account activity for a customer to determine whether to file a SAR.

The need for a review of customer activity or transactions does not necessarily indicate a need to file a SAR. The time period for filing a SAR starts when the organization, during its review or because of other factors, knows or has reason to suspect that the activity or transactions under review meet one or more of the definitions of suspicious activity.[7] Whenever possible, an expeditious review of the transaction or the account is recommended and can be of significant assistance to law enforcement. In any event, the review should be completed in a reasonable period of time. For violations requiring immediate attention, such as when a reportable violation is ongoing, a bank is required to immediately notify, by telephone, an "appropriate law enforcement authority" and as necessary the bank's primary regulator, in addition to filing a timely SAR. An "appropriate law enforcement authority" would generally be the local office of the Internal Revenue Service Criminal Investigation Division or the FBI. Notifying law enforcement of a suspicious activity does not relieve a bank of its obligation to file a SAR.

BOARD OF DIRECTORS' NOTIFICATION

Banks are required by the SAR regulations of their federal banking agency to notify the board of directors or an appropriate board committee that SARs have been filed.[8] However, the regulations do not mandate a particular notification format and banks should have flexibility in structuring their format. Therefore, banks may, but are not required to, provide actual copies of SARs to the board of directors or a board committee. Alternatively, banks may opt to provide summaries, tables of SARs filed for specific violation types, or other forms of notification. Regardless of the notification format used by the bank, management should provide sufficient information on its SAR filings to the board of directors or an appropriate committee in order to fulfill its fiduciary duties.[9]

SAR FILING ON CONTINUING ACTIVITY

One purpose of filing SARs is to identify violations or potential violations of law to the appropriate law enforcement authorities for criminal investigation. This objective is accomplished by the filing of a SAR that identifies the activity of concern. If this activity continues over a period of time, such information should be made known to law enforcement (and the federal banking agencies). FinCEN's guidelines suggest that banks should report continuing suspicious activity by filing a report at least every 90 days. This practice will notify law enforcement of the continuing nature of the activity, as well as remind the bank that it should continue to review the suspicious activity to determine whether other actions may be appropriate, such as bank management determining that it is necessary to terminate a relationship with the customer or employee that is the subject of the filing.

The bank should develop policies, procedures, and processes indicating when to escalate issues or problems identified as result of repeat SAR filings on accounts. The procedures should include:

- Review by senior management and legal staff (e.g., BSA compliance officer or SAR committee).
- Criteria for when analysis of the overall customer relationship is necessary.
- Criteria for when to close the account.
- Criteria for when to notify law enforcement, if applicable.

SAR QUALITY

Banks are required to file SAR forms that are complete, thorough, and timely. Banks should include all known suspect information on the SAR form, and the importance of the accuracy of this information cannot be overstated. Inaccurate information on the SAR form, or an incomplete or disorganized narrative, may make further analysis difficult, if not impossible. However, there may be legitimate reasons why certain information may not be provided in a SAR, such as when the filer does not have the information. A thorough and complete narrative may make the difference in whether the described conduct and its possible criminal nature are clearly understood by law enforcement. Because the SAR narrative section is the only area summarizing suspicious activity, the narrative section, as stated on the SAR form, is "critical." Thus, a failure to adequately describe the factors making a transaction or activity suspicious undermine the purpose of the SAR.

By their nature, SAR narratives are subjective, and examiners generally should not criticize the bank's interpretation of the facts. Nevertheless, banks should ensure that SAR narratives are complete, thoroughly describe the extent and nature of the suspicious activity, and is included within the SAR form (e.g., no attachments to the narrative section will be included within the BSA-reporting database). More specific guidance is available in Appendix L ("SAR Quality Guidance") to assist banks in writing and assist examiners in evaluating, SAR narratives. In addition, comprehensive guidance is available from FinCEN ("Guidance on Preparing a Complete & Sufficient Suspicious Activity Report Narrative") at www.fincen.gov.

PROHIBITION OF SAR DISCLOSURE

No bank, and no director, officer, employee, or agent of a bank, that reports a suspicious transaction may notify any person involved in the transaction that the transaction has been reported. Thus, any person subpoenaed or otherwise requested to disclose a SAR or the information contained in a SAR, except when such disclosure is requested by FinCEN or an appropriate law enforcement or federal banking agency, shall decline to produce the SAR or to provide any information that would disclose that a SAR has been prepared or filed, citing 31 CFR 103.18(e) and 31 USC 5318(g)(2). FinCEN and the bank's federal banking agency should be notified of any such request and of the bank's response. Furthermore, FinCEN and the federal banking agencies take the position that banks' internal controls for the filing of SARs should minimize the risks of disclosure.

RECORD RETENTION
Banks must retain copies of SARs and supporting documentation for five years from the date of the report.

---

[1] See 12 CFR 208.62, 211.5(k), 211.24(f), and 225.4(f) (Board of Governors of the Federal Reserve System); 12 CFR 353 (Federal Deposit Insurance Corporation); 12 CFR 748 (National Credit Union Administration); 12 CFR 21.11 (Office of the Comptroller of the Currency); 12 CFR 563.180 (Office of Thrift Supervision) (does not apply to Savings and Loan Holding Companies); and 31 CFR 103.18 (FinCEN). FFIEC BSA/AML Examination Manual 40 6/23/2005

[2] If a bank knows, suspects, or has reason to suspect that a customer may be linked to terrorist activity against the United States, the bank should immediately call FinCEN's Financial Institutions Terrorist Hotline at the toll-free number: 1-866-556-3974. Similarly, if any other suspected violation - such as an ongoing money laundering scheme - requires immediate attention, the bank should notify the appropriate federal banking and law enforcement agencies. In either case, the bank must also file a SAR.

[3] Electronic Communications Privacy Act, 18 USC 2709.

[4] Fair Credit Reporting Act, 15 USC 1681u.

[5] Right to Financial Privacy Act of 1978, 12 USC 3401 *et seq.*

[6] Refer to the *SAR Activity Review*, Issue 8, April 2005 for further information on NSLs which is available at www.fincen.gov

[7] Bank Secrecy Act Advisory Group, "Section 5 – Issues and Guidance" *The SAR Activity Review – Trends, Tips & Issues*, October 2000, page 27.

[8] Credit unions do not have a regulatory requirement to notify the board of directors of SAR filings, although many take this action as a matter of a sound practice.

[9] As noted in the *SAR Activity Review*, Issue 2, June 2001, "In the rare instance when suspicious activity is related to an individual in the organization, such as the president or one of the members of the board of directors, the established policy that would require notification of a SAR filing to such an individual should not be followed. Deviations to established policies and procedures so as to avoid notification of a SAR filing to a subject of the SAR should be documented and appropriate uninvolved senior organizational personnel should be so advised."

1. Does your bank have an ongoing program to monitor for and detect suspicious activity in all its business lines and is an audit/testing program in place to ensure the quality of the system(s), either manual or automatic, employed to detect and report suspicious activity?

☐ *Yes*

☐ *No*

Comments:

Follow-up:

2. Do your bank's policies and procedures reflect the requirement for banks, bank holding companies, and their subsidiaries, by federal regulations, to file a SAR with respect to:

a. Criminal violations involving insider abuse in any amount?
b. Criminal violations aggregating $5,000 or more when a suspect can be identified?
c. Criminal violations aggregating $25,000 or more regardless of a potential suspect?
d. Transactions conducted or attempted by, at, or through the bank (or an affiliate) and aggregating $5,000 or more, if the bank or affiliate knows, suspects, or has reason to suspect that the transaction
   - May involve potential money laundering or other illegal activity (e.g., terrorism financing)?
   - Is designed to evade the BSA or its implementing regulations?
   - Has no business or apparent lawful purpose or is not the type of transaction that the particular customer would normally be expected to engage in, and the bank knows of no reasonable explanation for the transaction after examining the available facts, including the background and possible purpose of the transaction?

☐ *Yes*

☐ *No*

Comments:

Follow-up:

3. Do your bank's policies, procedures, and processes indicate the persons responsible for the identification, research, and reporting of suspicious activities?

☐ *Yes*

☐ *No*

Comments:

Follow-up:

4. Are appropriate policies, procedures, and processes should be in place to monitor and identify unusual activity?

☐ *Yes*

☐ *No*

Comments:

Follow-up:

5. Do your bank's policies and procedures address the level of monitoring dictated by the bank's assessment of risk, with particular emphasis on high-risk products, services, customers, and geographic locations? (**Note:** Monitoring systems typically include employee identification or referrals, manual systems, automated systems, or any combination.)

☐ *Yes*

☐ *No*

Comments:

Follow-up:

6. Does your bank's AML policy describe the thorough research and analysis surrounding the decision process to file or not to file a SAR, and is each case documented?

☐ *Yes*

☐ *No*

Comments:

Follow-up:

7. If your bank uses a manual transaction monitoring process, does the process include review of daily reports, reports that cover a period of time (e.g., rolling 30-day reports, monthly reports), or a combination of both types of reports?

☐ *Yes*

☐ *No*

Comments:

Follow-up:

8. Regarding Question #7, above, are the type and frequency of reviews conducted and the resulting reports commensurate with the bank's BSA/AML risk profile and appropriately cover its high risk products, services, customers, and geographic locations?

☐ *Yes*

☐ *No*

Comments:

Follow-up:

9. For either manual or automated transaction monitoring, does your bank's management periodically evaluate the appropriateness of filtering criteria and thresholds used in the monitoring process, and is evidence of such monitoring documented?

☐ *Yes*

☐ *No*

Comments:

Follow-up:

10. Are non-customer funds transfer transactions and payable upon proper identification (PUPID) transactions reviewed for unusual activity as part of your bank's transaction monitoring procedures?

☐ *Yes*

☐ *No*

Comments:

Follow-up:

11. Does your bank's compliance department and management understand the filtering criteria of its software based monitoring system (if applicable) and conduct reviews to assess the effectiveness of its automated account monitoring systems?

☐ *Yes*

☐ *No*

Comments:

Follow-up:

12. Does documentation exist to substantiate that your bank's system filtering criteria was developed through a review of specific high-risk customers, products, and services? (Note: System filtering criteria, including specific profiles and rules, should be based on what is reasonable and expected for each type of customer.)

☐ *Yes*

☐ *No*

Comments:

Follow-up:

13. Do policies, procedures and controls exist documenting the authority to establish or change expected activity profiles and do they require the approval of the BSA compliance officer or senior management? (Note: Controls should ensure limited access to the monitoring system. Management should document or be able to explain filtering criteria, thresholds used, and how both are appropriate for the bank's risks.)

☐ *Yes*

☐ *No*

Comments:

Follow-up:

14. Do system level controls provide for limited access to your bank's transaction monitoring system?

☐ *Yes*

☐ *No*

Comments:

Follow-up:

15. Has management documented filtering criteria, thresholds used, and how both are appropriate for the bank's risks?

☐ *Yes*

☐ *No*

Comments:

Follow-up:

16. Has your bank established policies, procedures, and processes for identifying subjects of law enforcement requests, monitoring the transaction activity of those subjects, identifying unusual or suspicious activity related to those subjects, and filing, as applicable, SARs related to those subjects?

☐ *Yes*

☐ *No*

Comments:

Follow-up:

17. Do your bank's policies and procedures document who within the bank determines whether a SAR should be filed? (Note: It is incumbent upon a bank to assess all of the information it knows about its customer, including the receipt of a law enforcement inquiry based on all customer information it has available.)

☐ *Yes*

☐ *No*

Comments:

Follow-up:

18. Do your bank's policies and procedures address controls regarding receipt of National Security Letters and the appropriate measures to ensure the confidentiality of the letters as well as procedures for processing and maintaining the confidentiality of NSLs?

☐ *Yes*

☐ *No*

Comments:

Follow-up:

19. Does your bank have written policies, procedures, and processes for referring unusual activity from all business lines to the personnel or department responsible for evaluating unusual activity?

☐ *Yes*

☐ *No*

Comments:

Follow-up:

20. Do your bank's compliance procedures specifically describe the SAR filing decision process, and does the process provide for documenting why, for each specific case, a SAR was not filed?

☐ *Yes*

☐ *No*

Comments:

Follow-up:

21. Does your bank's SAR policy address the 30 and 60 day provisions for SAR filing?

☐ *Yes*

☐ *No*

Comments:

Follow-up:

22. Does your compliance policy, as required by the SAR regulations of its federal banking agency, address the requirement for notifying your board of directors or an appropriate board committee that a SAR(s) have been filed?

☐ *Yes*

☐ *No*

Comments:

Follow-up:

23. For suspicious activity identified and noted as continuing over a period of time, do your bank's policies address FinCEN's guidelines suggesting that banks report continuing suspicious activity by filing a report at least every 90 days?

☐ *Yes*

☐ *No*

Comments:

Follow-up:

24. Do your bank's policies, procedures, and processes indicate when to escalate issues or problems identified as result of repeat SAR filings on accounts, and do these procedures include:

a. Review by senior management and legal staff (e.g., BSA compliance officer or SAR committee)?
b. Criteria for when analysis of the overall customer relationship is necessary?
c. Criteria for when to close the account?
d. Criteria for when to notify law enforcement, if applicable?

☐ *Yes*

☐ *No*

Comments:

Follow-up:

25. In the rare instance when suspicious activity is related to an individual in the organization, such as the president or one of the members of the board of directors, the established policy that would require notification of a SAR filing to such an individual should not be followed. Are deviations to established policies and procedures (so as to avoid notification of a SAR filing to a subject of the SAR) documented in the compliance program, and are provisions in place such that an appropriate uninvolved senior organizational person be so advised?

☐ *Yes*

☐ *No*

Comments:

Follow-up:

26. Are SARs filled out and reviewed such that the narrative section adequately describes the factors making a transaction or activity suspicious? (**Note:** banks should ensure that SAR narratives are complete, thoroughly describe the extent and nature of the suspicious activity, and is included within the SAR form. No attachments to the narrative section should be included.)

☐ *Yes*

☐ *No*

Comments:

Follow-up:

27. Do your bank's internal controls for the filing of SARs minimize the risks of disclosure and do your policies and procedures address FinCEN's and the bank's federal banking agencies' requirement for notification of any request to disclose information pertaining to a SAR?

☐ *Yes*

☐ *No*

Comments:

Follow-up:

28. Does your bank retain copies of SARs and supporting documentation for five years from the date of each report?

☐ *Yes*

☐ *No*

Comments:

Follow-up:

29. Does your bank have either manual or automated systems and procedures in place to look for cash transactions and deposits (usually of monetary instruments with individual face values of less than $3,000) that appear to have been structured before reaching the bank)?

☐ *Yes*

☐ *No*

Comments:

Follow-up:

30. Does your bank have either manual or automated systems and procedures in place to look for possible suspicious activity in the accounts of nonresident aliens from countries and jurisdictions considered to be at high risk for money laundering? (**Note:** These accounts are characterized by small cash deposits and checks written to purchase large ticket items, sometimes located in the Florida and Panama free trade zones. These accounts also lack typical payments for housing, utilities, and credit cards, etc.)

☐ *Yes*

☐ *No*

Comments:

Follow-up:

31. Does your bank have either manual or automated systems and procedures in place to screen wire transfers, especially those that involve any type of import/export business and are to or from Colombia, Panama, Aruba or Mexico, for suspicious activity?

☐ *Yes*

☐ *No*

Comments:

Follow-up:

32. Does your bank have either manual or automated systems and procedures in place to monitor unusual check activity (e.g., structuring, followed by lump sum payments to U.S. appliance manufacturers or import/export companies in Florida and Panama).

☐ *Yes*

☐ *No*

Comments:

Follow-up:

Systems and IT Support

BSA compliance has become complicated, and it is rare that at least part of the process, such as transaction monitoring or watch list scanning is not automated. For transaction monitoring, as noted in a question in the previous section, it is important that compliance management have a full understanding of the monitor's capabilities and features. This awareness requirement is meant to ensure that your bank is not overly reliant on technology or has not placed unfounded confidence in its systems' capabilities. This section deals not only with issues related to installed compliance systems themselves, but also how these systems are integrated into your bank's system architecture and how changes to system parameters are made.

1. Does your bank's system architecture schematic diagram properly reflect that all front office systems are interfaced to the bank's transaction monitoring software?

☐ ***Yes***

☐ ***No***

Comments:

Follow-up:

2. Can the bank's IT department produce a list of accounts as well as all account activity for each account?

☐ ***Yes***

☐ ***No***

Comments:

Follow-up:

3. Are any systems in use at your bank for which transactions are booked offshore? Do these transactions pass through your transaction monitoring system?

☐ *Yes*

☐ *No*

Comments:

Follow-up:

4. Does your bank's IT department have a formally documented software development lifecycle methodology and have all Compliance Office requests to IT for support regarding systems implementations, changes, data management issues, etc., been documented according to the bank's adopted development/change methodology?

☐ *Yes*

☐ *No*

Comments:

Follow-up:

5. Have all modifications to software or systems been properly documented?

☐ *Yes*

☐ *No*

Comments:

Follow-up:

6. Have operations manuals for each business unit affected been updated to reflect software system changes? Are revision histories present in those documents?

☐ *Yes*

☐ *No*

Comments:

Follow-up:

7. Have IT projects sponsored by the compliance department (e.g., implementation of software, data accuracy, etc.) been properly documented to include sign-off procedures and user testing and acceptance plans/tests?

☐ *Yes*

☐ *No*

Comments:

Follow-up:

8. Has your bank's internal audit program examined IT support of BSA compliance issues?

☐ *Yes*

☐ *No*

Comments:

Follow-up:

9. Have customer information files been reconciled periodically to ensure integrity and accuracy of the bank's data from system to system?

☐ *Yes*

☐ *No*

Comments:

Follow-up:

10. Does your bank's disaster recovery plan address critical systems and database backups of KYC systems and other critical systems supporting BSA compliance?

☐ *Yes*

☐ *No*

Comments:

Follow-up:

11. Have reports developed for BSA compliance purposes by your bank's IT department been adequately tested prior to implementation? Does documentation exist to support the tests and were results noted by senior management?

☐ *Yes*

☐ *No*

Comments:

Follow-up:

12. Has your bank's data security department been involved with your BSA compliance program to ensure data security, password integrity, and privacy requirements per the regulations?

☐ *Yes*

☐ *No*

Comments:

Follow-up:

13. Do your operations manuals contain detailed operational mapping of products and activities feeding accounting and counterparty databases/systems?

☐ *Yes*

☐ *No*

Comments:

Follow-up:

14. Do Human Resource Department systems adequately support the requirements of Know-Your-Employee best practices as required by your compliance program?

Yes

☐ *Yes*

☐ *No*

Comments:

Follow-up:

15. Is your internal audit department routinely and formally notified of all new IT projects and software modifications?

☐ *Yes*

☐ *No*

Comments:

Follow-up:

16. Is OFAC monitoring conducted for transactions booked offshore?

☐ *Yes*

☐ *No*

Comments:

Follow-up:

17. Are tolerance levels programmed into transaction monitoring systems realistic and adequate?

☐ *Yes*

☐ *No*

Comments:

Follow-up:

18. Does your bank have a segregation of duties policy for BSA purposes?

☐ *Yes*

☐ *No*

Comments:

Follow-up:

19. Does your bank's KYC database provide for issue tracking or aging to ensure that required documentation, account termination, etc., is being performed timely and in accordance with internal policy or regulation?

☐ *Yes*

☐ *No*

Comments:

Follow-up:

20. Does the appropriate bank system track initial account screening information (e.g., expected activity) versus actual business transactions conducted by an account?

☐ *Yes*

☐ *No*

Comments:

Follow-up:

Trade Finance Activities

Trade finance typically involves short-term financing to facilitate the import and export of goods. These operations can involve the transmission of funds to enable the transaction (e.g., letter of credit), or may instead only involve the payment of funds if the commercial terms of the transactions are not met (e.g., guarantees or standby letters of credit). In both cases, a bank's involvement in trade finance minimizes payment risk to importers and exporters. The nature of trade finance activities requires the active involvement of multiple parties on both sides of the transaction. In addition to the basic exporter/importer relationship at the center of any particular trade activity, relationships may exist between the exporter and the suppliers and between the importer and the customers.

Both the exporter and importer may also have other banking relationships. Furthermore, many other intermediary financial and non-financial institutions may provide conduits and services to expedite the underlying documents and payment flows associated with trade transactions. As an example, in a letter of credit arrangement, a bank can serve as the issuing bank, allowing its customer (the buyer) to purchase goods locally or internationally, or the bank can act as an advising bank, enabling their customer (the exporter) to sell their goods locally or internationally. The relationship between the two banks will vary, and in some cases it may be similar to a correspondent relationship.

Financial institutions can participate in trade financing by providing pre-export financing, helping in the collection process, confirming or issuing letters of credit, discounting drafts and acceptances, or offering fee-based services such as providing credit and country information on buyers. Although most trade financing is short-term and self-liquidating in nature, medium-term loans (one to five years) or long-term loans (more than five years) may be used to finance the import and export of capital goods such as machinery and equipment.

In transactions that are covered by letters of credit, participants can take the following roles:

- **Applicant** - The buyer or party who requests the issuance of a letter of credit.

- **Issuing Bank** - Issues the letter of credit on behalf of the Applicant and forwards it to the Advising Bank for notification to the Beneficiary. The Applicant is the Issuing Bank's customer.

- **Confirming Bank** - Typically in the country of the Beneficiary, at the request of the Issuing Bank, joins the Issuing Bank in honoring draws made by the Beneficiary, provided the terms and conditions of the letter of credit are met.

- **Advising Bank** - Branch or correspondent bank near the Beneficiary's domicile, to which the Issuing Bank sends the letter of credit or notification of its issuance, with instructions to notify the Beneficiary. The Advising Bank advises the Beneficiary without taking other active engagement in the letter of credit.

- **Beneficiary (Drawer)** - The seller or party to whom the letter of credit is addressed.

- **Negotiating Bank** - Usually the Beneficiary's bank. Agrees to purchase the draft and pay the Beneficiary after satisfying itself that documentary requirements have been met.

- **Accepting Bank** - Incurs a legal obligation to pay the draft at maturity. Drafts are drawn on the Accepting Bank that dates and signs the instrument.

- **Discounting Bank** - Discounts a draft for the Beneficiary after it has been accepted by an Accepting Bank.

- **Reimbursing Bank** - Authorized by the Issuing Bank to reimburse the Drawee Bank submitting claims under the letter credit.

- **Paying (Drawee) Bank** - As named in the letter of credit, the bank where drafts are to be paid. The Paying Bank is typically the Issuing Bank, but is often a branch or correspondent of the Issuing Bank. Once paid or accepted by the Paying or Drawee Bank, there is no recourse to the drawers.

In a letter of credit arrangement, a bank can serve as the Issuing Bank, allowing its customer (the buyer) to purchase goods locally or internationally, or the bank can act as an Advising Bank, enabling its customer (the exporter) to sell its goods locally or internationally. The relationship between any two banks may vary and could include any of the roles listed above.

RISK FACTORS

The involvement of multiple parties can make the process of due diligence more difficult. As such, the bank should conduct a thorough review and fully understand all trade finance documentation and related values. Since the trade finance business can be more document-based than other areas of banking, it can be susceptible to documentary fraud, which can be linked to money laundering, terrorist financing, or the circumvention of OFAC sanctions or other prohibitions. Banks should be alert to transactions involving higher risk goods (e.g., trade in weapons or nuclear equipment).

While banks should be alert to transactions involving higher risk goods (e.g., trade in weapons or nuclear equipment), they need to be aware that goods may be over- or under-valued in an effort to evade AML or customs regulations. For example, an importer may pay a large sum of money from the proceeds of an illegal activity for goods that are essentially worthless and are subsequently discarded. Alternatively, trade documents, such as invoices, may be fraudulently altered to hide the scheme. Variations on this theme include double invoicing, partial shipment of goods, and the use of fictitious goods. Illegal proceeds transferred in such transactions thereby appear sanitized and enter the realm of legitimate commerce.

The Applicant may substitute third-party nominees, such as shell companies, to disguise the Applicant's role in a trade finance agreement. This substitution results in a lack of transparency, effectively hiding the identity of the purchasing party, thus increasing the risk of money laundering activity.

RISK MITIGATION

Sound customer due diligence (CDD) procedures are needed to gain a thorough understanding of the customer's underlying business and locations served. The banks in the letter of credit process need to undertake varying degrees of due diligence depending upon their role in the transaction. For example, issuing banks should conduct sufficient due diligence on prospective import or export customers before establishing the letter of credit. The due diligence should include gathering sufficient information on Applicants and Beneficiaries, including their identities, nature of business, and sources of funding. This may require the use of background checks or investigations, particularly in higher-risk jurisdictions. As such, banks should conduct a thorough review and reasonably know their customers prior to facilitating trade-related activity and should have a thorough understanding of trade finance documentation. Refer to the core overview section, "Customer Due Diligence," page 56, for additional guidance. Likewise, guidance provided by the Financial Action Task Force on Money Laundering (FATF) has helped set important industry standards and is a resource for banks that provide trade finance services.[1]

Banks taking other roles in the letter of credit process should complete due diligence that is commensurate with their roles in each transaction. Banks need to be aware that because of the frequency of transactions in which multiple banks are involved, Issuing Banks may not always have correspondent relationships with the Advising or Confirming Bank.

To the extent feasible, banks should review documentation, not only for compliance with the terms of the letter of credit, but also for anomalies or red flags that could indicate unusual or suspicious activity. Reliable documentation is critical in identifying potentially suspicious activity. When analyzing applicable trade transactions, banks should consider obtaining copies of official U.S. or foreign government import and export forms to assess the reliability of documentation provided.[2] These anomalies could appear in shipping documentation, obvious under- or over-invoicing, government licenses (when required), or discrepancies in the description of goods on various documents. Identification of these elements may not, in itself, require the filing of a Suspicious Activity Report (SAR), but may suggest the need for further research and verification. In circumstances where a SAR is warranted, the bank is not expected to stop trade or discontinue processing the transaction. However, stopping the trade may be required to avoid a potential violation of an OFAC sanction.

---

[1] Refer to Trade Based Money Laundering, June 23, 2006, at www.fatf-gafi.org/dataoecd/60/25/37038272.pdf.

[2] For instance, U.S. Customs and Border Protection Form 7501 (Entry Summary) (www.cbp.gov/linkhandler/cgov/toolbox/forms/7501.ctt/7501.pdf) and U.S. Department of Commerce Form 7525-V (Shipper's Export Declaration) (www.census.gov/foreign-trade/regulations/forms/new7525v.pdf) classify all U.S. imports and exports by 10-digit harmonized codes. (Refer to www.census.gov/foreign-trade/faq/sb/sb0008.html for additional guidance.)

1. Has your bank conducted a thorough review and fully understand all trade finance documentation and related values?

☐ *Yes*

☐ *No*

Comments:

Follow-up:

2. Does your bank perform sufficient customer due diligence on prospective import/export customers, including gathering information on principals and beneficiaries including their identities, nature of the customer's business, and source of wealth and funds before establishing a credit relationship?

☐ *Yes*

☐ *No*

Comments:

Follow-up:

3. Do policies, procedures, and processes require a thorough review of all applicable trade finance documentation to enable your bank to monitor and report unusual and suspicious activity?

☐ *Yes*

☐ *No*

Comments:

Follow-up:

4. Is the sophistication of your bank's reporting systems and management information systems commensurate with the size and complexity of the bank's trade finance activities?

☐ *Yes*

☐ *No*

Comments:

Follow-up:

5. In addition to financial transaction monitoring and OFAC filtering, does your bank's review of trade finance activities detect:

a. Shipping items that are inconsistent with the nature of the customer's business?
b. Customers conducting business with jurisdictions designated as high risk?
c. Customers conducting transactions with businesses involved in higher-risk activities (i.e., weapons dealers, nuclear materials, or chemical)?
d. Goods entering or exiting ports of non-cooperative countries?
e. Irregular pricing of goods?
f. Excessively amended letters of credit?
g. Transactions designed to evade home country legal restrictions?

☐ *Yes*

☐ *No*

Comments:

Follow-up:

6. With regard to monitoring for irregular pricing of goods, does your bank conduct reviews of documentation related to trade finance transactions to determine whether the prices are generally consistent with market prices?

☐ *Yes*

☐ *No*

Comments:

Follow-up:

Trust and Asset Management Services

Trust[1] accounts are generally defined as a legal arrangement in which one party (the truster or grantor) transfers ownership of assets to a person or bank (the trustee) to be held or used for the benefit of others. These arrangements include the broad categories of court-supervised accounts (i.e., executorships and guardianships), personal trusts (i.e., living trusts, trusts established under a will, and charitable trusts), and corporate trusts (i.e., bond trusteeships).

Unlike trust arrangements, agency accounts are established by contract and governed by contract law. Assets are held under the terms of the contract, and legal title or ownership does not transfer to the bank as agent. Agency accounts include custody, escrow, investment management,[2] and safekeeping relationships. Agency products and services may be offered in a traditional trust department or through other bank departments.

CUSTOMER IDENTIFICATION PROGRAM

Customer Identification Program (CIP) rules, which became effective October 1, 2003, apply to substantially all bank accounts opened after that date. The CIP rule defines an "account" to include cash management, safekeeping, custodian, and trust relationships. However, the CIP rule excludes employee benefit accounts established pursuant to the Employee Retirement Income Security Act of 1974 (ERISA).

For purposes of the CIP, a bank is not required to search the trust, escrow, or similar accounts to verify the identities of beneficiaries but instead is only required to verify the identity of the named account-holder (the trust). In the case of a trust account, the customer is the trust whether or not the bank is the trustee for the trust. However, the CIP rule also provides that, based on the bank's risk assessment of a new account opened by a customer that is not an individual, the bank may need "to obtain information about" individuals with authority or control over such an account, including signatories, in order to verify the customer's identity.[3] For example, in certain circumstances involving revocable trusts, the bank may need to gather information about the settlor, grantor, trustee, or other persons with the authority to direct the trustee, and who thus have authority or control over the account, in order to establish the true identity of the customer.

In the case of an escrow account, if a bank establishes an account in the name of a third party, such as a real estate agent, who is acting as escrow agent, then the bank's customer is the escrow agent. If the bank is the escrow agent, then the person who establishes the account is the bank's customer. For example, if the purchaser of real estate directly opens an escrow account and deposits funds to be paid to the seller upon satisfaction of specified conditions, the bank's customer will be the purchaser. Further, if a company in formation establishes an escrow account for investors to deposit their subscriptions pending receipt of a required minimum amount, the bank's customer will be the company in formation (or if not yet a legal entity, the person opening the account on its behalf). However, the CIP rule also provides that, based on the bank's risk assessment of a new account opened by a customer that is not an individual, the bank may need "to obtain information about" individuals with authority or control over such an account, including signatories, in order to verify the customer's identity.[4]

RISK FACTORS

Trust and asset management accounts, including agency relationships, present BSA/AML concerns similar to those of deposit taking, lending, and other traditional banking activities. Concerns are primarily due to the unique relationship structures involved when the bank handles trust and agency activities such as:

- Personal and court-supervised accounts;
- Trust accounts formed in the private banking department;
- Asset management and investment advisory accounts;
- Global and domestic custody accounts;
- Securities lending;
- Employee benefit and retirement accounts;

- Corporate trust accounts;
- Other related business lines.[5]

As in any account relationship, money laundering risk may arise from trust and asset management activities. When misused, trust and asset management accounts can conceal the sources and uses of funds, as well as the identity of beneficial and legal owners. Customers and account beneficiaries may try to remain anonymous in order to move illicit funds or avoid scrutiny. For example, customers may seek a certain level of anonymity by creating Private Investment Companies (PICs), offshore trusts, or other investment entities that hide the true ownership or beneficial interest of the trust.

RISK MITIGATION

Management should develop policies, procedures, and processes that enable the bank to identify unusual account relationships and circumstances, questionable assets and sources of assets, and other potential areas of risk (e.g., offshore accounts, PICs, asset protection trusts (APTs),142 agency accounts, and unidentified beneficiaries). While the majority of traditional trust and asset management accounts will not need enhanced due diligence, management should be alert to those situations that need additional review or research.

Customer Comparison Against Lists

The bank must be capable of maintaining required CIP information and completing the required one-time check of trust account names against section 314(a) search requests. The bank should also be able to identify customers who may be politically exposed persons (PEPs), doing business with or located in jurisdictions designated as "special money laundering concern" under section 311 of the Patriot Act, or match OFAC lists.[6] As a sound practice, the bank should also determine the identity of other parties that may have control over the account, such as grantors or co-trustees.

Circumstances Warranting Increased Due Diligence

Management should assess account risk on the basis of a variety of factors which may include:

- The type of trust or agency account and its size;
- The types and frequency of transactions;
- The country of residence of the principals or beneficiaries, or the country where established, or source of funds;
- Accounts and transactions that are not usual and customary for the customer or for the bank.

Stringent documentation, verification, and transaction monitoring procedures should be established for accounts that management considers as high risk. Typically, employee benefit accounts and court-supervised accounts are among the lowest BSA/AML risks.

The following are examples of situations in which increased due diligence may be appropriate:

- The bank is entering into a relationship with a new customer;
- The account principals or beneficiaries reside in a foreign jurisdiction, or the trust or its funding mechanisms are established offshore;
- Assets or transactions are atypical for the type and character of the customer;
- The account type, size, assets, or transactions are atypical for the bank;
- International funds transfers are conducted, particularly through offshore funding sources;
- Accounts are funded with easily transportable assets such as gemstones, precious metals, coins, artwork, rare stamps, or negotiable instruments;
- Accounts or relationships are maintained in which the identities of the principals, or beneficiaries, or sources of funds are unknown or cannot easily be determined;
- Accounts benefit charitable organizations or other non-governmental organizations (NGOs) that may be used as a conduit for illegal activities;

- Interest on lawyers' trust accounts (IOLTA) holding and processing significant dollar amounts;
- Account assets which include PICs;
- SFPFs are parties to any accounts or transactions.

Note: Asset management accounts can be trust or agency accounts managed by the bank.

[1] The OCC and OTS use the broader term "fiduciary capacity" instead of "trust." Fiduciary capacity includes a trustee, an executor, an administrator, a registrar of stocks and bonds, a transfer agent, a guardian, an assignee, a receiver, or a custodian under a uniform gifts to minors act; an investment adviser, if the bank receives a fee for its investment advice; any capacity in which the bank possesses investment discretion on behalf of another (12 CFR 9.2(e) and 12 CFR 550.30).

[2] For purposes of national banks and OTS-regulated savings associations, certain investment management activities, such as providing investment advice for a fee, are "fiduciary" in nature.

[3] Refer to 31 CFR 103.121(b)(2)(ii)(C).

[4] Refer to the appropriate federal banking agency's manuals for specific definitions of these products.

[5] APTs are a special form of irrevocable trust, usually created (settled) offshore for the principal purposes of preserving and protecting part of one's wealth against creditors. Title to the asset is transferred to a person named as the trustee. APTs are generally tax neutral with the ultimate function of providing for the beneficiaries.

[6] Management and examiners should be aware that OFAC list matching is not a BSA requirement. However, since trust systems are typically separate and distinct from bank systems, verification of these checks on the bank system is not sufficient to ensure that these checks are also completed in the trust and asset management department.

1. Has management developed policies, procedures, and processes that enable the bank to identify unusual account relationships and circumstances, questionable assets and sources of assets, and other potential areas of risk (e.g., offshore accounts, PICs, asset protection trusts (APTs),142 agency accounts, and unidentified beneficiaries)?

☐ *Yes*

☐ *No*

Comments:

Follow-up:

2. Is your bank alert to transactions involving higher risk goods (e.g., trade in weapons or nuclear equipment)?

☐ *Yes*

☐ *No*

Comments:

Follow-up:

3. Does your bank determine the identity of other parties that may have control over an account, such as grantors or co-trustees?

☐ *Yes*

☐ *No*

Comments:

Follow-up:

4 Does bank management assess account risk on the basis of a variety of factors which may include:

a. The type of trust or agency account and its size?
b. The types and frequency of transactions?
c. The country of residence of the principals or beneficiaries, or the country where established, or source of funds?
d. Accounts and transactions that are not usual and customary for the customer or for the bank?

☐ *Yes*

☐ *No*

Comments:

Follow-up:

US Dollar Drafts

A U.S. dollar draft is a bank draft or check denominated in U.S. dollars and made available at foreign financial institutions. These drafts are drawn on a U.S. correspondent account by a foreign financial institution. Drafts are frequently purchased to pay for commercial or personal transactions and to settle overseas obligations.

RISK FACTORS

The majority of U.S dollar drafts are legitimate; however, drafts have proven, to be vulnerable to money laundering abuse. Such schemes involving U.S. dollar drafts could involve the smuggling of U.S. currency to a foreign financial institution for the purchase of a check or draft denominated in U.S. dollars. The foreign financial institution accepts the U.S. currency and issues a U.S. dollar draft drawn against its U.S. correspondent bank account. Once the currency is in bank draft form, the money launderer can more easily conceal the source of funds. The ability to convert illicit proceeds to a bank draft at a foreign financial institution makes it easier for a money launderer to transport the instrument either back into the United States or to endorse it to a third party in a jurisdiction where money laundering laws or compliance are lax. In any case, the individual has laundered illicit proceeds; ultimately, the draft or check will be returned for processing at the U.S. correspondent bank.

RISK MITIGATION

A U.S. bank's policies, procedures, and processes should include the following:

- Outline criteria for opening a U.S. dollar draft relationship with a foreign financial institution or entity (e.g., jurisdiction; products, services, target market; purpose of account and anticipated activity; or customer history);
- Detail acceptable and unacceptable transactions (e.g., structuring transactions or the purchase of multiple sequentially numbered drafts for the same payee);
- Detail the monitoring and reporting of suspicious activity associated with U.S. dollar drafts;
- Discuss criteria for closing U.S. dollar draft relationships.

1 Does your bank's US Dollar Draft policy and procedure include all of the following:

a. Outline criteria for opening a U.S. dollar draft relationship with a foreign financial institution or entity (e.g., jurisdiction; products, services, target market; purpose of account and anticipated activity; or customer history)?

b. Detail acceptable and unacceptable transactions (e.g., structuring transactions or the purchase of multiple sequentially numbered drafts for the same payee)?

c. Detail the monitoring and reporting of suspicious activity associated with U.S. dollar drafts?

d. Discuss criteria for closing U.S. dollar draft relationships?

☐ *Yes*

☐ *No*

Comments:

Follow-up:

www.ingramcontent.com/pod-product-compliance
Ingram Content Group UK Ltd.
Pitfield, Milton Keynes, MK11 3LW, UK
UKHW051450290926
15471UKWH00008B/1123